FIRST AID FOR THE®

Pediatrics Clerkship

Fifth Edition

MARK D. HORMANN, MD
Professor of Pediatrics
Division of Community and General Pediatrics
Department of Pediatrics
Vice Dean for Educational Programs
McGovern Medical School at UTHealth Houston
Houston, Texas

ROBERT J. YETMAN, MD
Professor of Pediatrics
Director, Division of Community and General Pediatrics
Vice-Chair for Clinical Operations
Assistant Chief Medical Officer, Children's Memorial Hermann Hospital
Department of Pediatrics
McGovern Medical School at UTHealth Houston
Houston, Texas

LATHA GANTI, MD, MS, MBA, FACEP
Professor of Emergency Medicine and Neurology
University of Central Florida College of Medicine
Vice Chair for Research and Academic Affairs
HCA UCF Emergency Medicine Residency of Greater Orlando
Orlando, Florida

MATTHEW S. KAUFMAN, MD
Associate Director
Department of Emergency Medicine
Richmond University Medical Center
Staten Island, New York

New York   Chicago   San Francisco   Athens   London   Madrid   Mexico City
Milan   New Delhi   Singapore   Sydney   Toronto

First Aid for the®: Pediatrics Clerkship, Fifth Edition

Copyright © 2023 by McGraw Hill LLC. All rights reserved. Printed in China. Except as permitted under the United States Copyright Act of 1976, no part of this publication may be reproduced or distributed in any form or by any means, or stored in a data base or retrieval system, without the prior written permission of the publisher.

First Aid for the® is a registered trademark of McGraw Hill LLC.

1 2 3 4 5 6 7 8 9   DSS   27 26 25 24 23 22

ISBN 978-1-264-26449-0
MHID 1-264-26449-6

This book was set in Electra LT Std by MPS Limited.
The editors were Bob Boehringer and Kim J. Davis.
The production supervisor was Catherine Saggese.
Project management was provided by Vishal Prakash, MPS Limited.

This book is printed on acid-free paper.

Library of Congress Cataloging-in-Publication Data

Names: Hormann, Mark, editor. | Yetman, Robert, editor. | Ganti, Latha, author. |
  Kaufman, Matthew S., editor.
Title: First aid for the pediatrics clerkship / Robert J. Yetman, Mark D.
  Hormann, Latha Ganti, Matthew Kaufman.
Description: Fifth edition. | New York : McGraw Hill, [2022] | Latha's name
  appears first in the previous edition. | Summary: "The goals of this
  book are to assist students in success on the clerkship exam and also to
  help guide them in the clinical diagnosis and treatment of many of the
  problems seen by pediatricians"—Provided by publisher.
Identifiers: LCCN 2022002749 (print) | LCCN 2022002750 (ebook) |
  ISBN 9781264264490 (paperback; alk. paper) | ISBN 1264264496 (paperback;
  alk. paper) | ISBN 9781264264506 (ebook) | ISBN 126426450X (ebook)
Subjects: MESH: Pediatrics | Clinical Clerkship | Study Guide
Classification: LCC RJ48.3 (print) | LCC RJ48.3 (ebook) | NLM WS 18.2 |
  DDC 618.92/0025—dc23/eng/20220323
LC record available at https://lccn.loc.gov/2022002749
LC ebook record available at https://lccn.loc.gov/2022002750

McGraw Hill books are available at special quantity discounts to use as premiums and sales promotions or for use in corporate training programs. To contact a representative, please visit the Contact Us pages at www.mhprofessional.com.

Contents

Contributing Editors

Mohammad Alnoor, MD
Fellow, Pediatric Cardiology
Doernbecher Children's Hospital
Oregon Health & Sciences University
Portland, Oregon

Michelle S. Barratt, MD, MPH
Professor of Pediatrics
Division of Community and General Pediatrics &
    Division of Adolescent Medicine
Associate Residency Program Director
Department of Pediatrics
McGovern Medical School at UTHealth Houston
Houston, Texas

Elizabeth A. Hillman, MD, MEd
Assistant Professor of Pediatrics
Program Director, Neonatal-Perinatal Fellowship
Division of Neonatal-Perinatal Medicine
Department of Pediatrics
McGovern Medical School at UTHealth Houston
Houston, Texas

Paul R. Hillman, MD, PhD
Assistant Professor of Pediatrics
Assistant Program Director, Combined Pediatrics and
    Medical Genetics Residency
Division of Medical Genetics
Department of Pediatrics
McGovern Medical School at UTHealth Houston
Houston, Texas

LaTanya Love, MD
Associate Professor of Pediatrics
Division of Community and General Pediatrics
Department of Pediatrics
Dean of Education
McGovern Medical School at UTHealth Houston
Executive Vice President for Student Affairs and Diversity
The University of Texas Health Science Center at Houston
Houston, Texas

Neethu M. Menon, MD
Assistant Professor of Pediatrics
Division of Hematology
Department of Pediatrics
McGovern Medical School at UTHealth Houston
Houston, Texas

Peter T. Scully, MD
Assistant Professor of Pediatrics
Division of Critical Care Medicine
Department of Pediatrics
McGovern Medical School at UTHealth Houston
Houston, Texas

How to Succeed in the Pediatrics Clerkship

Introduction

This clinical study aid was designed in the tradition of the First Aid series of books. The goals of this book are to help you succeed on the clerkship exam and to help guide you in the clinical diagnosis and treatment of many of the problems pediatricians see. The book's content is based on the objectives for medical students laid out by the Council on Medical Student Education in Pediatrics (COMSEP). Each of the chapters contains the major topics central to the practice of pediatrics; the chapters have been designed for the third-year medical-student learning level.

The content format is similar to other First Aid series texts. Topics are listed by bold headings, which include essential topic information. Included are mnemonics, diagrams, summaries or warning statements, and tips. Tips are categorized into: Typical Scenario , Exam Tips , and Ward Tips ✋.

Even if you are sure you do not want to be a pediatrician, the rotation can be a fun and rewarding experience. The three key components to the rotation are: (1) what to do on the wards, (2) what to do in outpatient clinics, and (3) how to study for the exam.

On the Wards

Be on time. If you are expected to "pre-round," give yourself at least 15 minutes per patient to see the patient, review tests, and learn about the events that occurred overnight. Like all working professionals, you will face occasional obstacles to punctuality, but make sure these are only occasional. When you begin a rotation, try to arrive at least an extra 15 minutes early until you figure out the routine. "Table rounds" followed by walking rounds may be employed, but typically, the emphasis is patient- and family-centered (a model of communicating and learning between the patient, family, medical professionals, and students).

Find a way to keep your patient information organized and handy. You may have previously identified a successful strategy for tracking your patients, including a focused physical, medications, labs, test results, and daily progress. If not, ask other medical students or the interns what methods work for them, potentially copying their template. Many students use index cards, a notebook, or a page-long template kept on a clipboard for each patient. Treat these documents with care since the information is legally protected; losing your patient notes can result in financial penalties to you and your institution.

Dress in a professional manner. Regardless of what the residents and the attending wear, dress in a professional, conservative manner. Wear a short white coat over your clothes unless otherwise discouraged. Wearing scrubs during overnight call is often permitted, but do not make this attire your uniform.

Act in a pleasant manner. Inpatient rotations can be difficult, stressful, and tiring. Introduce yourself to the team with whom you will be working, including the attendings, residents, nurses, and ancillary staff. Smile and try to learn everyone's name. Be nice! If you do not understand—or disagree with—a treatment plan or diagnosis, do not "challenge." Instead, say, "I'm sorry. I don't quite understand; could you please explain . . . ." Be empathetic toward patients.

Be aware of the hierarchy. In general, address your questions regarding ward functioning to interns or residents. Address your medical questions to residents, your senior, or the attending. Try to be informed on your subject before you ask attendings any medical questions.

Address patients and staff respectfully. Address your pediatric patients by using their first name. Address their parents as sir, ma'am, or Mr., Mrs., or Miss. Do not address parents or patients as "honey," "sweetie," and the like. Although you may feel these names are friendly, parents will think you have forgotten their name, that you are being inappropriately familiar, or both. Address all physicians as "doctor" unless told otherwise. Nurses, technicians, and other staff are indispensable and can teach you a lot. Treat them respectfully.

Take responsibility for your patients. Know everything there is to know about your patients—their history, test results, details about their medical problem, and prognosis. Keep your intern or resident informed of new developments about which they might not be aware; ask for updates from them. Assist the team in developing a plan, including speaking to radiology, consultants, and family. Never give bad news to patients or family members without the assistance of your supervising resident or attending.

Respect patients' rights.

- All patients, *including pediatric patients*, have the right to keep their personal medical information private. Maintaining privacy means not discussing the patient's information with unapproved family members without consent (especially with adolescents) and never discussing patient information in public areas.
- Generally speaking, all patients have the right to refuse treatment. They can refuse treatment by a specific individual (e.g., the medical student) or refuse a specific type of treatment (e.g., no nasogastric tube). Patients can even refuse lifesaving treatment. Exceptions are patients deemed to lack the capacity to make decisions or understand situations (in which case, a healthcare proxy is assigned), patients who are suicidal or homicidal, or patients who are not old enough to consent (in which case, a parent is the decision maker).

Volunteer. Be self-motivated. Volunteer to help with a procedure or a difficult task. Volunteer to give a brief talk on a topic of your choice. Volunteer to take additional patients. Volunteer to stay late. Bring in relevant articles regarding patients and their issues—this shows your enthusiasm, curiosity, outside reading, and interest in evidence-based medicine. However, be sure to "read the room." If your team is busy with several new admissions, for example, choose another time to present your outside reading.

Be a team player. Help other medical students with their tasks; teach them information you have learned. Support your supervising intern or resident. Never steal the spotlight, steal a procedure, or make a fellow medical student or resident look bad. Before leaving for the day, ask your team if you can do anything else to help.

Be prepared. Always have these things readily available: medical tools (stethoscope, reflex hammer, penlight, measuring tape), medical tape, pocket references (often electronic), patient information, a small toy for distraction/gaze tracking, and stickers for rewards. Not only will you have what you need, but also you may have what someone else needs! Aim to have the necessary items with you without looking as if you can barely haul around your heavy white coat!

Be honest. If you do not understand, do not know, or did not do it, make sure you say that. Never say or document false information (e.g., "bowel sounds normal" when you did not listen). Trust is foundational to the practice of medicine; the repercussions for lying or presenting false data are always more severe than the brief embarrassment you experience for not having the requested data.

Present patient information in an organized manner. The presentation of a new patient will be more thorough than the update given on daily rounds. Vital information included in a presentation differs by age group. Begin with a line stating the succinct chief complaint, including identifiers (age, gender) and a symptom, not a diagnosis (e.g., "wheezing," not "asthma")—and its duration. The next line should include important diagnoses carried (e.g., here is where you could state "known asthmatic" or other important information for a wheezer).

Here is a template for the "bullet" presentation for inpatients for the days subsequent to admission:

> This is day of hospitalization number [days] for this [age] year old [gender] with a history of [major/pertinent history such as asthma, prematurity, etc. or otherwise healthy] who presented with [major symptoms, such as cough, fever, and chills], and was found to have [working diagnosis]. [Tests done] showed [results]. Yesterday/overnight the patient [state important changes, new plan, new tests, new medications]. This morning, the patient feels [state the patient's words], and the physical exam is significant for [state major findings]. Plan is [state plan].

Some patients have extensive histories. The entire history should be present in the admission note; but, in a ward presentation, it can be challenging to absorb. In these situations, a good summary that maintains an accurate picture of the patient often is appreciated. This summary usually takes some thought, but it is worth it.

How to Present a Chest Radiograph (CXR)

Always take time to look at each of your patients' radiographs; do not rely only on the report. It is good clinical practice, and your attending will likely ask you if you did. Plus, it will help you look like a star on rounds if you have already seen the film.

- First, confirm that the CXR belongs to your patient and is the most recent one.
- If possible, compare it to a previous film.

Then, present in a systematic manner:

1. *Technique*
   Comment on rotation, anteroposterior (AP) or posteroanterior (PA), penetration, inspiratory effort (number of ribs visible in lung fields).
2. *Bony structures*
   Look for rib, clavicle, scapula, and sternum fractures.
3. *Airway*
   Look at the glottal area (steeple sign, thumbprint, foreign body, etc), as well as for tracheal deviation, pneumothorax, and pneumomediastinum.
4. *Pleural space*
   Look for fluid collections, which can represent hemothorax, chylothorax, or pleural effusion.

5. *Lung parenchyma*
   Look for infiltrates and consolidations. These can represent pneumonia, pulmonary contusions, hematoma, or aspiration. The location of an infiltrate can provide a clue to the location of a pneumonia:
   - Obscured right (R) costophrenic angle = right lower lobe
   - Obscured left (L) costophrenic angle = left lower lobe
   - Obscured R heart border = right middle lobe
   - Obscured L heart border = left upper lobe

6. *Mediastinum*
   - Look at size of mediastinum—a widened one (>8 cm) suggests aortic rupture.
   - Look for enlarged cardiac silhouette (>½ thoracic width at base of heart), which may represent congestive heart failure (CHF), cardiomyopathy, hemopericardium, or pneumopericardium.
   - Identify the thymus ("sail" sign) in smaller children.

7. *Diaphragm*
   - Look for free air under the diaphragm (which suggests intestinal perforation).
   - Look for stomach, bowel, or NG tube (NGT) above diaphragm (which suggests diaphragmatic rupture).

8. *Tubes and lines*
   - Identify all tubes and lines.
   - Ensure an endotracheal tube is 2 cm above the carina. A common misplacement occurs with right-mainstem bronchus intubation.
   - Ensure a chest tube (including the most proximal hole) is in the pleural space (not in the lung parenchyma).
   - Ensure an NGT is in the stomach and uncoiled.

A sample CXR presentation may sound like:

This is the CXR of [child's name]. The film is an AP view with good inspiratory effort. There is an isolated fracture of the 8th rib on the right. There is no tracheal deviation or mediastinal shift. There is no pneumo- or hemothorax. The cardiac silhouette appears to be of normal size. The diaphragm and heart borders on both sides are clear; no infiltrates are noted. A nasogastric tube is present, the tip of which is in the stomach. This CXR shows improvement over the CXR from [number of days ago] as the right lower lobe infiltrate is no longer present.

How to Present an Electrocardiogram (ECG)

See the chapter on cardiovascular disease for specific rhythms.

- First, confirm that the ECG belongs to your patient and is the most recent one.
- If possible, compare this ECG to a previous tracing.
- An electronic reading often is included on the ECG output; do not rely on this reading alone because it may not be age specific!

Then, present in a systematic manner:

1. Rate (see Figure 1-1)
   "The rate is [number of] beats per minute."
   - The ECG paper is scored so that one big box is 0.20 seconds. These big boxes consist of five little boxes, each of which represents 0.04 seconds.
   - A quick way to calculate rate when the rhythm is regular is the mantra: 300, 150, 100, 75, 60, 50 (= 300/# large boxes), which is measured as the number

(continued)

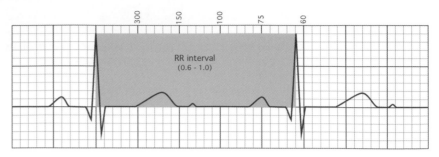

FIGURE 1-1.   **ECG rate.**

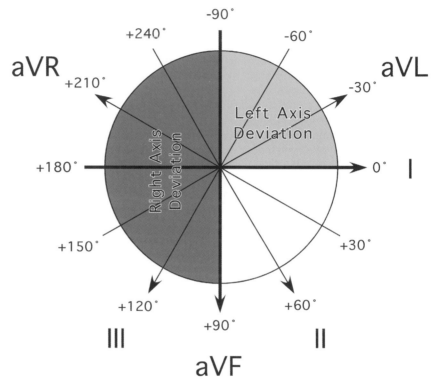

FIGURE 1-2.   **ECG axes.**

of large boxes between two QRS complexes. Therefore, a distance of one large box between two adjacent QRS complexes would be a rate of 300, while a distance of five large boxes between two adjacent QRS complexes would be a rate of 60.

■ For irregular rhythms, count the number of complexes that occur in a 6-second interval (30 large boxes) and multiply by 10 to get a rate in beats per minute (bpm).

2. Rhythm

"The rhythm is [sinus]/[atrial fibrillation]/[atrial flutter]."

■ If *p* waves are present in all leads, and upright in leads I & AVF, then the rhythm is sinus. The lack of *p* waves usually suggests a non-atrial rhythm. A ventricular rhythm (V Fib or V Tach) is an unstable one (and could spell imminent death)—and you should be getting ready for advanced cardiac life support (ACLS, or pediatric advanced life support, or PALS).

3. Axis (see Figure 1-2)

"The axis is [normal]/[deviated to the right]/[deviated to the left]."

■ If I and aVF are both upright or positive, then the axis is normal.

■ If I is upright and aVF is upside down, then there is left-axis deviation (LAD).

- If I is upside down and aVF is upright, then there is right-axis deviation (RAD).
- If I and aVF are both upside down or negative, then there is extreme RAD.

4. Intervals (see Figure 1-3)

"The [PR]/[QRS] intervals are [normal]/[shortened]/[widened]."
- Normal PR interval = 0.12–0.20 seconds.
- Short PR is associated with Wolff-Parkinson-White syndrome (WPW).
- Long PR interval is associated with heart block, of which there are three types:
  - First-degree block: PR interval > 0.20 seconds (one big box).
  - Second-degree (Wenckebach) block: PR interval lengthens progressively until a QRS is dropped.
  - Second-degree (Mobitz) block: PR interval is constant, but one QRS is dropped at a fixed interval.
  - Third-degree block: Complete AV dissociation; prolonged presence is incompatible with life.
- Normal QRS interval ≤ 0.12 seconds.
- Prolonged QRS is seen when the beat is initiated in the ventricle rather than the sinoatrial node, when there is a bundle branch block, and when the heart is artificially paced with longer QRS intervals. Prolonged QRS is also noted in tricyclic overdose and WPW.

5. Wave morphology (see Figure 1-4)
   a. Ventricular hypertrophy
      - "There [is/is no] [left/right] [ventricular/atrial] hypertrophy."
   b. Atrial hypertrophy
      - The clue is the presence of tall *p* waves.
   c. Ischemic changes
      - "There [are/are no] S-T wave [depressions/elevations] or [flattened/inverted] T waves." Presence of Q wave indicates an old infarct.
   d. Bundle branch block (BBB)
      - "There [is/is no] [left/right] bundle branch block."
      - Clues:
        - There is a presence of RSR′ wave in leads V1–V3 with ST depression, and the T wave inversion goes with RBBB.
        - There is a presence of notched R wave in leads I, aVL, and V4–V6 goes with LBBB.

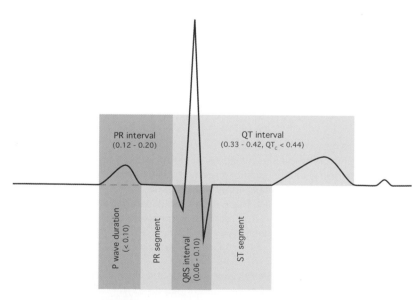

FIGURE 1-3. **ECG segments.**

(continued)

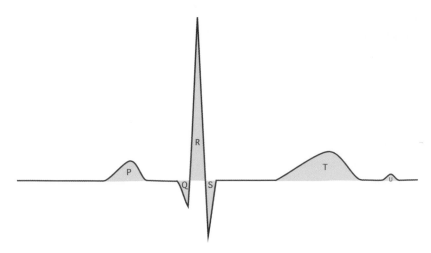

FIGURE 1-4. ECG waves.

On Outpatient

The ambulatory part of the rotation consists of mainly two groups of patients—focused histories and physicals for acute problems, and complete histories and physicals for well-child visits. In the general pediatrics clinic, you will see the common childhood illnesses, but do not overlook the possibility of less common conditions. Usually, you will see the patient first when performing the initial history and physical exam. Strike a balance between obtaining a thorough exam and not upsetting the child so much that the attending will be unable to recheck any pertinent parts. For acute illness visits, present the patient succinctly, including an appropriate differential diagnosis and plan. For presentation of well-child visits, cover all the bases, but focus on the patients' concerns and your findings. Depending on the child's age, specific issues are discussed. Past history and development are important, but so is anticipatory guidance (prevention and expectations for what is to come). The goals for the outpatient rotation are to be both efficient and thorough.

Pediatric History and Physical Exam

HISTORY

ID/CC: Age, sex, symptom, duration

HPI: Present the history of the present illness, or HPI, in an organized and concise way, leading up to the day of admission or the day of presentation. Avoid using actual dates and days of the week. Avoid superfluous details.

A good opening line for your HPI: This is a 4-year-old male with no significant past medical history, who was in his usual state of good health until 3 days prior to [admission or arrival to clinic] when . . .

In the HPI, include:

Symptoms—location, quality, quantity, aggravating and alleviating factors (Make sure to include all pertinent positive and pertinent negative symptoms.)

Time course—onset, duration, frequency, change over time

Rx/Intervention—medications, medical help sought, other actions taken, exposures, ill contacts, travel

Current Health:

Nutrition—breast milk/formula/food, quantity, frequency, supplements, problems (poor suck/swallow, reflux)

Sleep—quantity, quality, disturbances (snoring, apnea, bedwetting, restlessness), intervention, wakes up refreshed

Elimination—bowel movement frequency/quality, urination frequency, problems, toilet training

Behavior—toward family, friends, discipline

Development—gross motor, fine motor, language, cognition, social/emotional

Prior Medical History, or PMH:

Pregnancy, especially for younger children (be sensitive to adoption issues)—gravida/para status, maternal age, duration, exposures (medications, alcohol, tobacco, drugs, infections, radiation); complications (bleeding, gestational diabetes, hypertension, etc); occurred on contraception?, planned?; emotions regarding pregnancy; problems with past pregnancies

Labor and delivery, especially for younger children—length of labor, rupture of membranes, fetal movement, medications, presentation/delivery, mode of delivery, assistance (forceps, vacuum), complications, Apgar scores, immediate breath/cry, oxygen requirement/intubation, and duration

Neonatal—birth height/weight, abnormalities/injuries, length of hospital stay, complications (respiratory distress, cyanosis, anemia, jaundice, seizures, anomalies, infections), behavior, maternal concerns

Infancy—temperament, feeding, family reactions to infant

Illnesses/hospitalizations/surgeries/accidents/injuries—dates, medications/interventions, impact on child/family—don't forget circumcision

Medications—past (antibiotics, especially), present, reactions

Allergies—include reaction

Immunizations—status, reactions; review card if available

Family history—relatives, ages, health problems, deaths (age/cause), miscarriages/stillbirths/deaths of infants or children, health status of parents and siblings, pertinent negative family history

Social history—parents' education and occupation, living arrangements, pets, water (city or well), lead exposure (old house, paint), smoke exposure, religion, finances, family dynamics, risk-taking behaviors, school/daycare, other caregivers, HEEADDSSS exam for adolescents (HEEADDSSS: home, education, eating, activities, drugs and alcohol, depression, safety, sex, and suicide) (see Health Supervision and Adolescent chapters)

Review of Systems, or ROS:

General—fever, activity, growth

Head—trauma, size, shape

Eyes—erythema, drainage, acuity, tearing, trauma

Ears—infection, drainage, hearing

Nose—drainage, congestion, sneezing, bleeding, frequent colds

Mouth—eruption/condition of teeth, lesions, infection, odor

Throat—sore, tonsils

Neck—stiff, lumps, tenderness

Respiratory—cough, wheeze, chest pain, pneumonia, retractions, apnea, stridor

Cardiovascular—murmur, exercise intolerance, diaphoresis, syncope

Gastrointestinal—appetite, constipation, diarrhea, poor suck, swallow, abdominal pain, jaundice, vomiting, change in bowel movements, blood, food intolerances

Genitourinary, or GU—urine output, stream, urgency, frequency, discharge, blood, pain during menstruation, sexually active

Endocrine—polyuria/polydipsia/polyphagia, puberty, thyroid, growth/stature

Musculoskeletal—pain, swelling, redness, warmth, movement, trauma

Neurologic—headache, dizziness, convulsions, visual changes, loss of consciousness, gait, coordination, handedness

Skin—bruises, rash, itching, hair loss, color (cyanosis)

Lymphatics—swelling, redness, tender glands

(continued)

PHYSICAL EXAM

General—smiling, playful, cooperative, irritable, lethargic, tired, hydration status

Vitals—temperature, heart rate, respiratory rate, blood pressure and percentiles, pulse ox

Growth—weight, height, head circumference (include percentiles), BMI if applicable

Skin—inspect, palpate, birthmarks, rash, jaundice, cyanosis

Head—normocephalic, atraumatic, anterior fontanelle, sutures

Eyes—redness, swelling, discharge, red reflex, strabismus, scleral icterus

Ears—external anatomy, tympanic membranes (Ears are often examined last.)

Nose—patent nares, flaring nostrils

Mouth—teeth, palate, thrush

Throat—oropharynx (red, moist, injection, exudate)

Neck—range of motion, meningeal signs

Lymph—cervical, axillary, inguinal

Cardiovascular—heart rate, murmur, rub, pulses (central/peripheral; bilateral upper and lower extremities including femoral), perfusion/color

Respiratory—rate, retractions, grunting, crackles, wheezes

Abdomen—bowel sounds, distention, tenderness, hepatosplenomegaly, masses, umbilicus, rectal

Back—scoliosis, dimples

Musculoskeletal—joints—erythema, warmth, swelling tenderness, range of motion

Neurologic—gait, symmetric extremity movement, strength/tone/bulk, reflexes (age-appropriate and deep tendon reflexes), sensation, mentation, coordination

Genitalia—circumcision, testes, labia, hymen, Sexual Maturity Rating (SMR, aka Tanner staging)

Diversity, Inclusion, and Equity Considerations

Patients will have diverse backgrounds, expectations, beliefs, and values. It is important that each patient encounter is free of potential bias and that all patients are treated equitably.

Cultural competency is the ability to interact effectively with people of different cultures; strive to provide culturally competent care in all patient encounters. Familiarize yourself with religious or cultural beliefs that your patients and families may have that may affect their healthcare-related decisions or perceptions.

Examples of cultural factors that should be considered in patient care include:
- Religious beliefs
- Preferred language
- Distrust of healthcare system and healthcare providers
- Alternative medicine preferences
- Geography
- Healthcare decision maker in the family

Always have a nonjudgmental attitude toward a patient's different beliefs.

COMMUNICATION

Communication between patients and families should be in their preferred language. Familiarize yourself with the options for medical-language interpreters.
- Do not rely on patients, family members, or nontrained interpreters.
- Children should never be used as interpreters for their parents or families.

- Sites may use in-person interpreters, telephone interpreters, or video interpreters.
- Not using a trained medical interpreter can lead to medical errors and miscommunication between the healthcare team and patients.
- Whenever possible, provide patient education materials in the preferred language.

SEXUAL ORIENTATION AND GENDER IDENTITY

- **Sexual orientation** relates to whom an individual is attracted to sexually.
- **Gender identity** is how an individual perceives themselves and can be different from their gender assigned at birth.

Do not make assumptions about your patients' gender identity or sexual orientation. Gender identity can be obtained by asking your youth patients their preferred pronouns; ideally, this conversation would happen in a confidential interview. Questions regarding sexual orientation should be included in the HEEADDSSS portion of the history. Respecting a patient's gender identity and sexual orientation leads to more inclusive healthcare.

UNCONSCIOUS BIAS

An unconscious bias is a positive or negative mental attitude toward a person, thing, or group that a person holds at an unconscious level. This attitude is also called "implicit" bias. Everyone has unconscious biases. Negative associations can be unlearned and replaced with positive associations. Examples of unconscious bias on pediatric clerkships include:

- Making assumptions about the type of insurance the patient may have.
- Assuming that the pediatric patient's mother is the primary caregiver.
- A patient assuming that a female attending is a nurse and not a doctor.
- Making assumptions based on a person's race, gender, or socioeconomic status.

Reflect on your own beliefs to ensure that they do not unintentionally interfere with patient interactions and delivery of care.

- Avoid making assumptions about patients.
- Recognize and acknowledge any biases that you may have.
- Unconscious bias in healthcare can lead to healthcare disparities.

SOCIAL DETERMINANTS OF HEALTH

The World Health Organization defines social determinants of health as the conditions in which people are born, grow, work, live, and age, and the wider set of forces and systems shaping the conditions of daily life. Identify opportunities to evaluate the social determinants of health; the social history may allow better insight of your patients and their social situation.

Examples of social determinants of health include:

- Housing
- Food insecurity
- Early childhood development
- Education
- Income

Familiarize yourself with the Women, Infants, and Children (WIC) nutrition program, transportation options, and low-cost prescription options in your community.

Standardized screening tools may be used to gain more insight. Examples of screening tools include:

- Accountable Health Communities Health-Related Social Needs (HRSN) Screening Tool
- Safe Environment for Every Kid (SEEK) Parent Questionnaire
- The Health Leads Screening Toolkit

Ensure that you know clinic or hospital protocols for patients who may screen positive. If social workers are available, they are typically an excellent resource to help patients obtain needed services.

Your Rotation Grade

Usually, the clerkship grade is broken down into three or four components. (Every medical school divides grades differently; check with your school's grading policy.)

- *Inpatient evaluation:* This component includes evaluation of your ward time by residents and attendings and is based on your performance on the ward.
- *Ambulatory evaluation:* This component includes your performance in clinic, including clinic notes and any procedures performed in the outpatient setting.
- *National Board of Medical Examiners (NBME) examination:* This portion of the grade is anywhere from 20% to 50%, so performance on this multiple-choice test is vital to achieving a high final grade in the clerkship.
- *Objective Structured Clinical Examination (OSCE) or oral exam:* Some schools now include an OSCE or oral exam as part of their clerkship evaluation. This exam involves standardized patients and allows assessment of a student's bedside manner and physical examination skills.

How to Study

Make a list of core material to learn. This list should reflect common symptoms, illnesses, and areas in which you have particular interest or in which you feel particularly weak. Do not try to learn every possible topic.

Symptoms

- Fever
- Failure to thrive
- Sore throat
- Wheezing/cough
- Vomiting
- Diarrhea
- Abdominal pain
- Jaundice
- Fluid and electrolyte imbalance
- Seizures

The knowledge you need on the wards is day-to-day management "know-how." The knowledge you want by the end-of-rotation examination is the epidemiology, risk factors, pathophysiology, diagnosis, and treatment of major pediatric diseases.

As you see patients, note their major symptoms and diagnosis for review. Your reading on the symptom-based topics above should be done with a specific patient in mind. For example, if a patient comes in with diarrhea, check a review book or trusted online source that night for common infectious causes of gastroenteritis—and the differences between and complications of them—and noninfectious causes and dehydration.

Prepare a talk on a topic. You may be asked to give a small talk once or twice during your rotation. If not, you should volunteer! Feel free to choose a topic that is on your list. The ideal topic is slightly uncommon but not rare, for example, Kawasaki disease. To prepare a talk, read about it in a major textbook and a review article not more than 2 years old. Then search online or in the library for recent developments or changes in treatment.

Procedures. You may have the opportunity to perform procedures. Be sure to volunteer to do them whenever you can, and at least actively observe if participation is not allowed. These procedures may include the following:
- Lumbar puncture
- Intravenous line placement
- NGT placement
- Venipuncture (blood draw)
- Foley (urinary) catheter placement
- Transillumination of scrotum
- IM/SQ (intramuscular or subcutaneous) immunization injections
- Rapid strep or throat culture
- Nasopharyngeal swabs or cultures

How to Prepare for the Clinical Clerkship Examination

If you have read about the core illnesses and core symptoms, you will know a great deal about pediatrics. It is difficult but vital to balance reading about your specific patients and covering all the core topics of pediatrics. To study for the clerkship exam, consider these tactics:

2–3 weeks before exam: Read this entire review book, taking notes.
10 days before exam: Read the notes you took during the rotation on your core content list, as well as the corresponding review book sections.
5 days before exam: Read the entire review book, concentrating on lists and mnemonics.
2 days before exam: Exercise, eat well, skim the book, and go to bed early.
1 day before exam: Exercise, eat well, review your notes and the mnemonics, and go to bed on time. Do not have any caffeine after 2 PM.

Throughout all your studying, do practice questions from a reliable source of questions.

Other helpful studying strategies include:

Study with friends. Group studying can be very helpful. Other people may point out areas that you have not studied enough and may help you focus on the goal. If you tend to get distracted by other people, limit this type of studying to less than half of your study time.

Study in a bright room. Find the room that has the best, brightest light. A bright room will help prevent you from falling asleep. If you don't have a bright light, get a halogen desk lamp or a light that simulates sunlight (not a tanning lamp).

Eat light, balanced meals. Make sure your meals are balanced, with lean protein, fruits and vegetables, and fiber. A high-sugar, high-carbohydrate meal will give you an initial burst of energy for 1 to 2 hours, but then your energy levels will drop.

Take practice exams. The point of practice exams is not so much the content that is contained in the questions, but the training of sitting still for 3 hours and trying to pick the best answer for every question.

Tips for answering questions. All questions are intended to have one best answer. Remember—children are not just small adults. They present with a whole new set of medical and social issues. More than ever, you are treating families, not just individual patients.

Pocket Card

The following "card" contains information that is often helpful during the pediatrics rotation (Table 1). We advise that you make a copy of the card, cut it out, and carry it in your coat pocket.

Table 1   Recommended Child and Adolescent Immunization Schedule for ages 18 years or younger, United States, 2022

These recommendations must be read with the notes that follow. For those who fall behind or start late, provide catch-up vaccination at the earliest opportunity as indicated by the green bars. To determine minimum intervals between doses, see the catch-up schedule (Table 2).

Vaccine	Birth	1 mo	2 mos	4 mos	6 mos	9 mos	12 mos	15 mos	18 mos	19–23 mos	2–3 yrs	4–6 yrs	7–10 yrs	11–12 yrs	13–15 yrs	16 yrs	17–18 yrs
Hepatitis B (HepB)	1st dose	←— 2nd dose —→			←——————— 3rd dose ———————→												
Rotavirus (RV): RV1 (2-dose series), RV5 (3-dose series)			1st dose	2nd dose	See Notes												
Diphtheria, tetanus, acellular pertussis (DTaP <7 yrs)			1st dose	2nd dose	3rd dose		←——— 4th dose ———→					5th dose					
Haemophilus influenzae type b (Hib)			1st dose	2nd dose	See Notes		3rd or 4th dose, See Notes										
Pneumococcal conjugate (PCV13)			1st dose	2nd dose	3rd dose		←——— 4th dose ———→										
Inactivated poliovirus (IPV <18 yrs)			1st dose	2nd dose	←——————— 3rd dose ———————→							4th dose					
Influenza (IIV4)						Annual vaccination 1 or 2 doses								Annual vaccination 1 dose only			
or Influenza (LAIV4)											Annual vaccination 1 or 2 doses			**or** Annual vaccination 1 dose only			
Measles, mumps, rubella (MMR)					See Notes	←— 1st dose —→						2nd dose					
Varicella (VAR)						←— 1st dose —→						2nd dose					
Hepatitis A (HepA)					See Notes		2-dose series, See Notes										
Tetanus, diphtheria, acellular pertussis (Tdap ≥7 yrs)														1 dose			
Human papillomavirus (HPV)														See Notes			
Meningococcal (MenACWY-D ≥9 mos, MenACWY-CRM ≥2 mos, MenACWY-TT ≥2years)							See Notes							1st dose		2nd dose	
Meningococcal B (MenB-4C, MenB-FHbp)															See Notes		
Pneumococcal polysaccharide (PPSV23)														See Notes			
Dengue (DEN4CYD; 9-16 yrs)														Seropositive in endemic areas only (See Notes)			

Range of recommended ages for all children   Range of recommended ages for catch-up vaccination   Range of recommended ages for certain high-risk groups   Recommended vaccination can begin in this age group   Recommended vaccination based on shared clinical decision-making   No recommendation/ not applicable

Source: Centers for Disease Control and Prevention. Immunization Schedules. https://www.cdc.gov/vaccines/schedules/index.html.

High-Yield Facts

Gestation and Birth

Placenta

DEVELOPMENT

- Fertilization usually occurs in the fallopian tube ampulla.
- Zygote inner cell mass becomes the embryo.
- Zygote outer cell mass becomes cytotrophoblast and syncytiotrophoblast, which become the placenta.

HORMONES PRODUCED BY THE PLACENTA

- β-human chorionic gonadotropin (β-hCG) is produced by syncytiotrophoblast and can be detected within 9 days following ovulation to test for pregnancy.
- Human placental lactogen (aka human chorionic somatomammotropin) supports fetal nutrition:
    - Increases maternal lipolysis, making free fatty acids available for mother.
    - Anti-insulin maternal effect allows greater fetal glucose availability.

TRANSPORT

- Endometrial arteries bring oxygenated blood into intervillous space. Endometrial veins remove deoxygenated blood and waste.
- Nutrients, electrolytes, water, gases, and many medications and drugs are diffused or transported across the placental villi to the umbilical vein.
    - Most drugs pass through placenta and can be detected in fetal plasma (e.g., warfarin, morphine, propylthiouracil, and drugs of abuse).
    - A few substances cannot pass due to their size or charge (e.g., heparin, insulin).

EXAM TIP

Folic acid supplements during pregnancy reduce the incidence of neural tube defects.

EXAM TIP

The main sources of energy for a growing fetus are maternal glucose and placental lactate.

Embryologic Milestones

TABLE 2-1. Gestational/Embryologic Landmarks

Week 1	Fertilization, usually in fallopian tube ampulla
	Implantation begins
Week 2	Implantation complete
	Endoderm and ectoderm formed (bilaminar embryo)
Week 3	Mesoderm formed (trilaminar embryo)
Week 5	Subdivisions of forebrain, midbrain, and hindbrain are formed
Week 7	Heart formed
Week 8	Primary organogenesis complete
	Placentation occurs
Week 9	Permanent kidneys begin functioning
Week 10	Midgut returns from umbilical cord, where it was developing, to abdominal cavity, while undergoing counterclockwise rotation
Week 24	Primitive alveoli are formed and surfactant production begins
Week 26	Testicles descend

Fetal Circulation

- Oxygenated placental blood flows through the umbilical vein to the ductus venosus and then to the inferior vena cava (IVC). The ductus venosus is a fetal structure found beyond the branching of the left and right portal veins (see Figure 2-1).
- Blood from the IVC and superior vena cava (SVC) returns to the right atrium. The oxygenated blood from the IVC is preferentially shunted through the foramen ovale to the left atrium to provide oxygenated blood to the brain. Blood from the SVC enters the right ventricle.
- The major portion of blood exiting the right ventricle is then shunted to the aorta through the ductus arteriosus; the lungs are collapsed, and pulmonary artery pressures are high.
- Most of the blood in the descending aorta returns to the umbilical arteries for placental reoxygenation; some supplies the inferior part of the body.
- After birth, pulmonary artery pressure drops with lung expansion, reducing ductus arteriosus flow and stimulating its closure, usually within first few days of life. The left atrium pressure becomes higher than the right atrium due to the increased pulmonary return, which stimulates closure of the foramen ovale.

WARD TIP

Closure of the ductus arteriosus can be prevented by prostaglandin E1 and facilitated by indomethacin (via inhibition of prostaglandin synthesis).

WARD TIP

Umbilical vein = oxygenated blood
Umbilical artery = deoxygenated blood

Fetal Fluid

Amniotic fluid comes primarily from fetal urine starting at week 9 of gestation.

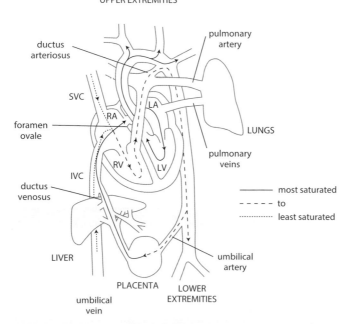

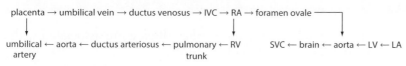

FIGURE 2-1. Fetal circulation.

Bilateral renal agenesis, a failure of both kidneys to develop, leads to oligohydramnios and severe pulmonary hypoplasia. Prenatal ultrasound may show absence of bladder and oligohydramnios.

EXAM TIP

The failure of kidneys to migrate can lead to ectopic kidneys.
A horseshoe kidney gets caught on the inferior mesenteric artery during ascent.

EXAM TIP

Elevation of maternal glucose causes elevated fetal glucose, leading to fetal hyperinsulinism, which can result in hypoglycemia in the newborn after placental supply of glucose is removed.

EXAM TIP

Vascular diseases of the placenta, caused by maternal illness (such as diabetes, lupus, or preeclampsia), can cause an insufficient supply of nutrients to the fetus and result in intrauterine growth restriction.

OLIGOHYDRAMNIOS

- Abnormally small amount of amniotic fluid defined as an amniotic fluid index (AFI) of <5 cm or a single deepest pocket <2 cm.
- Found in 4% of pregnancies and is associated with an increased risk for congenital anomalies.
- Can lead to fetal deformities such as club feet, facial deformities, or pulmonary hypoplasia.
- The most common causes are:
  - Premature rupture of membranes (PROM).
  - Fetal urinary-tract abnormalities.
  - Placental insufficiency or abruption.
  - Twin-Twin transfusion syndrome.
  - Maternal medications.

POLYHYDRAMNIOS

- Abnormally large amount of amniotic fluid is defined as an AFI >24 cm.
- Increases risk for abnormal fetal positioning, placental abruption, and PROM.
- The majority of cases are idiopathic; other common causes are:
  - Gastrointestinal anomalies.
  - Fetal hydrops.
  - Maternal diabetes.

Maternal Conditions and Exposures

MATERNAL DIABETES

- Fetal complications are related to the degree of maternal diabetes control:
  - Poor control early on can lead to caudal regression syndrome.
  - Poor control later on can lead to macrosomia and risk for birth injury.
- Infants of diabetic mothers are at risk for:
  - Hyperinsulinism and hypoglycemia.
  - Metabolic disorders (hypoglycemia, hypocalcemia, and hypomagnesemia).
  - Surfactant deficiency, perinatal asphyxia, respiratory distress syndrome.
  - Polycythemia leading to hyperbilirubinemia and hyperviscosity.
  - Congenital malformations, including cardiac, renal, gastrointestinal, neurologic, and skeletal defects.

MATERNAL LUPUS

- High risk of spontaneous first trimester miscarriage is possible.
  - Nonreversible heart block may occur in affected infants.
  - Neonatal lupus syndrome may result.

OTHER MATERNAL CONDITIONS

- Hypertension, renal disease, and cardiac disease are associated with small-for-gestational-age babies and prematurity.

DRUGS OF ABUSE

- Alcohol is the most common teratogen.
  - Causes neurocognitive impairment, with an unknown dose-response threshold
  - Fetal alcohol spectrum disorder (FASD)—intrauterine growth restriction (IUGR), microcephaly, short palpebral fissures, thin upper lip, and smooth nasal philtrum (See Figure 2-2).
- Cocaine and amphetamines cause increased risk of miscarriage and placental abruption, and ischemic consequences, such as ileal atresia or cutis aplasia.
- Tobacco is associated with IUGR, preterm delivery, and placental abnormalities; dose related.
- Opiates and heroin are associated with:
  - Miscarriage, IUGR, placental abruption and still birth.
  - Neonatal opiate withdrawal syndrome
    - Symptoms include hypertonia, tremors, irritability, sleep disturbance, diarrhea, poor feeding, sneezing, and nasal stuffiness.
    - Treatment includes a quiet dark room, swaddling, pacifier, and frequent feeding. Infants may need morphine or methadone.

> A term, 5-lb, 2-day-old infant has irritability, nasal stuffiness, and coarse tremors. He feeds poorly and has diarrhea. *Think: Opiate or heroin withdrawal.*
> Opiates readily crosses the placental barrier, placing the fetus at risk. Symptoms of opiate withdrawal include tremors, high-pitched cry, irritability, excess suck, apnea, and tachycardia, which can become evident within the first 72 hours of life. Vague autonomic symptoms such as yawning and sneezing are often present. Obtain urine drug screen and meconium screen if opioid use in the mother is suspected.

TERATOGENIC MEDICATIONS

- Phenytoin is associated with IUGR, digit and nail hypoplasia, dysmorphic facies, and cognitive delay.
- Tetracycline causes tooth discoloration and inhibits long bone formation.
- Isotretinoin (retinoic acid) is associated with miscarriage and stillbirth, significant cardiac anomalies, microtia or anotia, hydrocephalus, and limb reduction.
- Warfarin causes nail hypoplasia, stippled bone epiphyses, severe cognitive delay, microcephaly, and seizures. Heparin does not cross the placenta; it is preferred in pregnant women.

Delivery Room

DELIVERY ROOM CARE

- After the head is delivered, the obstetrician may suction the nose and mouth.
- After the whole-body delivery, the newborn is held at table level and the umbilical cord is clamped. Clamping may be delayed for up to 1 minute in vigorous infants to increase hemoglobin and iron stores.
- The newborn is then placed under a radiant warmer and is dried with warm towels. Warming and drying the baby prevents hypothermia.
- The mouth and nose are gently suctioned, if needed.
- Gentle back rubbing or sole flicking can stimulate breathing.
- Any further support is advanced neonatal resuscitation.

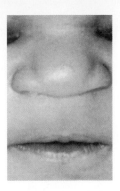

FIGURE 2-2. Fetal alcohol syndrome. Notice the depressed nasal bridge, flat philtrum, long upper lip, and thin vermillion border. (Reproduced with permission from Stoler JM, Holmes LB. Underrecognition of prenatal alcohol effects in infants of known alcohol abusing women, *J Pediatr.* 1999; 135(4): 430–436.)

WARD TIP

Cocaine use is associated with placental abruption.

WARD TIP

Infants of narcotic-abusing mothers should never be given naloxone because it may precipitate seizures.

TABLE 2-2. **Apgar Scoring**

	ACTIVITY (MUSCLE TONE)	PULSE	GRIMACE (REFLEX IRRITABILITY)	APPEARANCE (SKIN COLOR)	RESPIRATION
0	Absent	Absent	No response	Blue-gray, pale all over	Absent
1	Arms and legs flexed	Below 100 bpm	Grimace	Normal, except for extremities	Slow, irregular
2	Active movement	Above 100 bpm	Sneeze, cough, pull away	Normal all over	Good crying

APGAR SCORING

- Traditional method of assessing newborn infants at 1 and 5 minutes of life with a scale of 0–10 (see Table 2-2).
- Apgar scores do not predict the overall infant outcome, nor are they diagnostic.
- Further assessments are recorded at 5-minute intervals until a score of at least 7 is achieved.

Newborn Exam

SMALL FOR GESTATIONAL AGE (SGA)

- Defined as birth weight <10th percentile for gestational age.
- Can be due to constitutionally small infant or intrauterine growth restriction.
- At risk for hypoglycemia.
- IUGR occurring in early gestation:
  - Head circumference and height are proportionally small-sized (symmetric).
  - Seen in infants born to mothers with severe vascular disease with hypertension, renal diseases, congenital anomalies, infections, and chromosomal abnormalities.
- IUGR occurring late in gestation:
  - Head circumference is spared (asymmetric).
  - Can occur with multiple gestation, nutritional deficiency, or placental insufficiency.

LARGE FOR GESTATIONAL AGE (LGA)

- Birth weight is greater than 90th percentile for gestational age.
- Those at risk are infants of diabetic mothers, postmature infants, and those with Beckwith-Wiedemann syndrome.
- Macrosomic infants are generally defined as those with a birth weight of greater than 4.5 kg.
- At risk for hypoglycemia and birth trauma.

SKIN

- Plethora, a ruddy skin appearance, is due to a high hematocrit, which can be secondary to chronic fetal hypoxia.
- Erythema toxicum is a migrating pustular rash over the trunk, face, and extremities; it is benign and resolves within a week. Microscopic examination reveals eosinophils.
- Congenital dermal melanocytosis is the presence of gray-slate or bluish macules over the buttocks and back, seen more often in infants with darker pigmentation; these tend to fade within a year.
- Nevus simplex or salmon patches ("stork bites" on the nape of the neck and "angel kisses" on the eyelids) are pink spots over the eyelids, forehead, and back of the neck that tend to fade with time.
- See Dermatologic Disease chapter.

HEAD

- The anterior fontanelle typically closes between 9 and 24 months; the posterior fontanelle is sometimes closed at birth and should be closed by 4 months.
- A large fontanelle is seen in hypothyroidism, osteogenesis imperfecta, and some chromosomal abnormalities.
- Absent anterior fontanel is associated with craniosynostosis.

WARD TIP

A bulging fontanelle is seen with increased intracranial pressure, such as with hydrocephalus or meningitis.

FACE

- Mouth—look and feel for cleft lip/palate and macroglossia (large tongue is seen with hypothyroidism, Down syndrome, and Beckwith-Wiedemann syndrome).
- Look for dysmorphic features, including micrognathia, forehead bossing, hypertelorism (widely spaced eyes), and low-set ears (associated with many genetic disorders) (see Congenital Malformations and Chromosomal Abnormalities chapter).

EYES

- Check for red reflex with ophthalmoscope. An absent red reflex (leukocoria) in one or both eyes signifies blockage of the passageway between the cornea and retina, such as associated with cataracts or eye tumor (retinoblastoma).
- Look for cataracts, Brushfield spots (salt-and-pepper speckling of the iris seen in Down syndrome), and subconjunctival hemorrhage, which can occur after a traumatic delivery.
- See Special Organs—Eye, Ear, Nose chapter.

EARS

- Check for ear shape, presence of ear canal.
- Identify low set ears, posteriorly rotated ears, ear tags, or ear pits.

NECK

- Inspect for thyroid enlargement and palpate along the sternocleidomastoid for hematoma.
- Check for fistula or tracts (associated with branchial closure malformations).

CHEST

- Check for symmetry/equality of breath sounds.
- Retractions, grunting, tachypnea, nasal flaring, intercostal retractions, and use of accessory muscles may signify respiratory distress.
- Breasts may be enlarged from the effects of maternal estrogens.

HEART

- Check heart rate rhythm, quality of heart sounds, and the presence of a murmur. Murmurs in a newborn infant can be due to patent ductus arteriosus or other pathology.
- Check pulses. Compare brachial with femoral pulse to get an estimate of vascular volume and also to rule out aortic arch obstruction (aortic stenosis, coarctation of aorta), where the femoral pulses will be weak or absent.

ABDOMEN

- Palpate abdomen for masses; evaluate abdominal wall for gastroschisis and muscle tone.
- Examine umbilicus for omphalocele, drainage, erythema.
- Inspect the umbilical cord:
  - The umbilical vein is single open hole; umbilical arteries are two white wormlike structures.
  - If only one artery is present, it may indicate congenital anomalies, especially renal abnormalities.

EXTREMITIES

- Check both clavicles for any step off or crepitus, especially in the midclavicular area where most clavicle fractures occur.
- Check primitive reflexes (see Growth and Development chapter).
- Examine for congenital hip dysplasia with Ortolani and Barlow maneuvers.

BACK

Look for dimples or tufts of hair that may indicate subtle signs of spina bifida.

GENITALIA

- Girls may have a hymenal tag. Vaginal bleeding and swollen labia secondary to maternal estrogen withdrawal can occur.
- In boys, palpate for testicles in scrotum and look for hypo- or epispadias (urethral opening on the ventral or dorsal penile surface).
- Examine anal opening and tone to assess for possibility of imperforate anus.

Birth Trauma

MOLDING

- Molding is a temporary skull asymmetry caused by bone overlapping that occurs following prolonged labor and vaginal deliveries.
- Normal head shape is regained within a week.

CAPUT SUCCEDANEUM

- Area of edema due to pressure of the head from the uterus or cervix (Figure 2-3).
- Can be associated with bruising, petechiae, or abrasions.
- Can cross suture lines.
- Resolves in a few days.

CEPHALOHEMATOMA

- Caused by bleeding that occurs below the periosteum of the underlying bone (Figure 2-3).
- Associated with skull fractures in 5–10%, most often linear.
- Imaging not routine, but obtained in the presence of CNS symptoms or exceedingly large cephalohematoma.
- Contained within the periosteum: does *not* cross suture lines.

SUBGALEAL HEMORRHAGE

- Bleeding due to emissary veins rupturing between the aponeurosis and periosteum layers; large potential space (Figure 2-3).
- Crosses suture lines, feels boggy, localization to dependent areas.
- Infants can lose up to 40% of blood volume and develop hypovolemic shock; the mortality rate can be high.
- Usually associated with delivery trauma, instrumental delivery, or a bleeding disorder.

WARD TIP

Layers of the skull can be remembered by this mnemonic:

SCALP
Skin
Cutaneous tissue
Aponeurosis
Loose areolar tissue
Periosteum

WARD TIP

Caput succedaneum is external to the periosteum. Caput crosses the midline of the skull and suture lines, unlike a cephalohematoma, which is below the periosteum and does not cross suture lines.

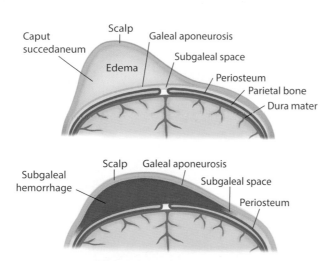

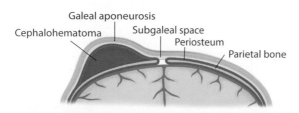

FIGURE 2-3. **Schematic of extracranial lesions in the neonate that include caput succedaneum, subgaleal hemorrhage, and cephalohematoma.** (Reproduced, with permission, from Cunningham F, Leveno KJ, Bloom SL, et al, eds. *Williams Obstetrics*, 25th ed. New York, McGraw Hill, 2018, Figure 33-2.)

WARD TIP

All macrosomic infants should be examined for signs of birth trauma and hypoglycemia.

WARD TIP

Complete clavicular fracture may diminish the ipsilateral Moro reflex.

WARD TIP

The degree of functional return in birth brachial plexus injuries depends on the severity of the nerve injury: stretch, rupture (nerve torn in two pieces), or avulsion (nerves torn away from spinal cord).

WARD TIP

Brachial plexus injuries can occur during birth when traction is used with shoulder dystocia.

CLAVICULAR FRACTURE

- Most common bone fracture during delivery.
- Symptoms can include gross clavicle deformity, tenderness on palpation, localized crepitus, and decreased or absent arm movement and Moro reflex.
- Greenstick (partial) fractures may have no symptoms; the diagnosis is often made at 7–10 days when the callus begins to form.
- Management includes pinning the arm to the chest using the shirt sleeve to decrease movement.

SKULL FRACTURE

- Skull fractures are uncommon.
- If linear, they usually do not require intervention.
- If depressed, they can be associated with instrumented deliveries and may have intracranial bleeding that requires surgical evaluation.

ERB-DUCHENNE PALSY

- Most common brachial plexus injury, caused by lateral traction of the C5 and C6 nerve roots.
- The arm is adducted and internally rotated, but the grasp reflex is intact (see Figure 2-4).
- If C7 is involved, the wrist is held in a flexed position (waiter's tip).

KLUMPKE PALSY

- Least frequent brachial plexus injury, caused by lateral traction of C8–T1 nerve roots.
- The wrist and hand are weak (claw-hand) and lack a grasp reflex.
- If sympathetic nerves are involved, unilateral miosis (Horner syndrome) may result.

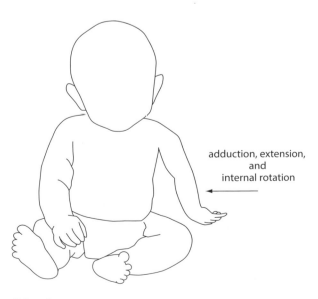

adduction, extension, and internal rotation

FIGURE 2-4. Erb palsy.

Perinatal Infections

Perinatal infections occur in a higher incidence in infants who are small for gestational age or who have hepatosplenomegaly, congenital defects, microcephaly, or intracranial calcifications. Perinatal infections are associated with the rupture of membranes longer than 18 hours, intra-amniotic infection (diagnosed by the OB), intrapartum maternal fever, maternal group B streptococcus (GBS) colonization, or maternal gram negative UTI.

TOXOPLASMOSIS

- Asymptomatic maternal infection due to oocyst ingestion from infected cat feces.
- Fetal features include chorioretinitis, intracranial calcifications, hydrocephalus, microcephaly, hearing loss, and seizures.
- Can lead to vision loss, hearing impairment, and learning disabilities.

PARVOVIRUS

- Maternal infection can present with rash and "slapped cheek" appearance, mild fever, malaise, myalgia and headache, or mild upper respiratory tract infection.
- Fetal effects can include severe anemia, hydrops, intrauterine growth restriction, or death.

HEPATITIS B

- Perinatal transmission occurs from blood exposures during birth, not during gestation.
- If the mother is positive or the status is unknown, the infant should receive hepatitis B vaccine AND hepatitis B immune globulin within 12 hours of birth.

RUBELLA

- Congenital rubella syndrome is rare and usually caused by infection early in pregnancy in an unvaccinated mother.
- Symptoms include cataracts, microphthalmos, glaucoma, meningoencephalitis, microcephaly, sensorineural hearing loss, patent ductus arteriosus, pulmonary artery stenosis, or blueberry muffin rash.

CYTOMEGALOVIRUS (CMV)

- Most infections in adults and infants are asymptomatic.
- Some 10% of infants with congenital CMV have symptoms at birth including: IUGR, jaundice, direct hyperbilirubinemia, petechiae and thrombocytopenia, hepatosplenomegaly, periventricular intracranial calcifications, chorioretinitis, and progressive sensorineural hearing loss.
- Congenital CMV is the most common nongenetic cause of hearing loss, resulting in 20% of all hearing loss at birth and 25% of all hearing loss at 4 years of age.
- CMV may be transmitted through breast milk.

 WARD TIP

Prenatal infections that most commonly cause birth defects:

TORCH
 Toxoplasmosis
 Other: Parvo, hepatitis B, syphilis, varicella-zoster virus, Zika
 Rubella
 Cytomegalovirus
 Herpes simplex virus/human immunodeficiency virus (HSV/HIV)

 WARD TIP

Among women infected with toxoplasmosis, only 50% will give birth to an infected neonate.

 WARD TIP

Pregnant women should not change a cat's litter box due to the risk of toxoplasmosis.

 WARD TIP

Blueberry muffin rash is caused by dermal erythropoiesis.

WARD TIP

Twenty percent of pregnant women are colonized with GBS. It is recommended that all pregnant women be screened (using vaginal, rectal swabs) at 35–37 weeks of gestation and given intrapartum antibiotics if positive. Colonization may recur if treated before labor.

WARD TIP

Intrapartum prophylaxis helps reduce early onset GBS disease, not late onset GBS disease.

GROUP B *STREPTOCOCCUS* (GBS)

- GBS is a major cause of severe systemic neonatal infection, divided into early and late-onset disease.
- Early-onset disease: usually in the first 24–48 hours:
  - Systemic symptoms include respiratory distress, apnea, shock, pneumonia, or meningitis.
  - Transmission occurs shortly before or during delivery.
  - All pregnant women should be screened for GBS at 35–37 weeks. Women should receive intrapartum prophylactic antibiotics if they screen positive for GBS, have GBS bacteriuria during pregnancy, or have a previous child with GBS disease. If the GBS status is unknown, prophylaxis is indicated for women delivering prior to 37 weeks, if rupture of membranes occurs longer than 18 hours prior to delivery, or the woman has an intrapartum fever greater than 100.4°F. Intravenous penicillin G is the preferred agent, with intravenous ampicillin or cefazolin as acceptable options.
- Late-onset disease (7–89 days) usually 3–4 weeks:
  - Late-onset disease most often manifests as bacteremia without a source or meningitis, but it can present as osteomyelitis, septic arthritis, or pneumonia. Half of all infants with GBS meningitis will have neurologic sequelae.

ESCHERICHIA COLI

- Principal cause of gram-negative sepsis and meningitis in newborn.
- Risk factors include maternal urinary tract infection (UTI) during the last month of pregnancy.
- Clinical manifestations include sepsis, meningitis, UTI, and pneumonia.
- Treatment should be based on antibiotic sensitivity data, but a third-generation cephalosporin should be used as an empiric agent.
- *Infants* with galactosemia are at high risk for *E. coli* sepsis and death.

LISTERIA MONOCYTOGENES

- Relatively uncommon but potentially severe infection in neonates.
- Foodborne illness found in soft cheeses, unpasteurized milk, and ready-to-eat meats.
- Can be asymptomatic in mother or present as a mild nonspecific illness.
- Clinical manifestations include fetal death, preterm delivery, sepsis, meningitis, or erythematous rash with granulomas.

HERPES SIMPLEX

- Neonatal infections are associated with high morbidity and mortality despite therapy.
- The risk of neonatal disease is much higher with primary (25–60%) compared to recurrent (2%) maternal infection. More than half of infants with HSV disease are born to women with no HSV symptoms; a negative maternal history does not eliminate HSV as a consideration in a newborn.
- Most infections occur through contact with infected secretions during birth.
- There are three distinct patterns of disease:
  - Skin, eyes, and/or mouth (SEM) disease.
    - About 45% of neonatal disease presentation.

- Typically presents in the first and second weeks of life, with 80% of neonates having vesicular lesions.
- Can progress to disseminated disease if not recognized promptly.
- Disseminated disease
  - About 25% of neonatal disease presentation.
  - Sepsis-like clinical picture: apnea, irritability, hypotonia, hypotension, liver dysfunction, and coagulopathy; must consider in any febrile neonate.
  - Typically presents in the first and second weeks of life; cutaneous lesions may be absent.
- Central nervous system disease
  - About 30% of neonatal disease presentation, typically occurring at second to third week of life.
  - Clinical signs include lethargy, irritability, poor suck, seizures; cutaneous lesions may be absent.

DIAGNOSIS

- Polymerase chain reaction (PCR) from the blood or CSF is the gold standard.
- HSV can be isolated in cell culture from skin lesions or nasopharyngeal swabs.

TREATMENT

- Acyclovir is the treatment.
- The course of treatment is often prolonged (21 days) for encephalitic and disseminated forms.

EXAM TIP

Cesarean section is performed for women with primary genital herpes and vaginal lesions in late gestation.

CHLAMYDIA

A 3-week-old infant presents with staccato cough and tachypnea, but no fever; bilateral diffuse crackles, hyperinflation, and patchy infiltrates on x-ray; he had conjunctivitis at 10 days of age. *Think: Chlamydia trachomatis.*

The incubation period of chlamydial conjunctivitis is usually at least a week and manifests later than gonococcal conjunctivitis (occurs 2–5 days after birth). It is commonly acquired during delivery. It is the most common infectious cause of neonatal conjunctivitis. Generally, gonococcal conjunctivitis has a more rapid, severe, and progressive course than *Chlamydia*.

- Acquired most often during passage through the birth canal of an infected mother.
- Causes conjunctivitis (several days to 2 weeks) and pneumonia (between 2 and 19 weeks) after birth.
- Respiratory symptoms may include congestion, characteristic "staccato" cough and tachypnea.
- Usually presents without fever.

DIAGNOSIS

Culture conjunctival swab or posterior pharynx.

TREATMENT

Administer erythromycin orally for 14 days or azithromycin for 3 days, especially for pneumonia or for patients in whom follow-up is not guaranteed.

EXAM TIP

Oral macrolide (e.g., erythromycin) use in infancy has been associated with development of pyloric stenosis.

SYPHILIS

- Results from transplacental transfer of *Treponema pallidum*.
- Intrauterine infection can manifest as hydrops, stillbirth, or may be asymptomatic. Children with untreated infections may develop symptoms in the first 2 years of life.
- Birth presentation may include hepatosplenomegaly, thrombocytopenia, pneumonia, lymphadenopathy, or a maculopapular rash of the palms and the soles.
- Late manifestations include a saddle nose deformity, saber shins, frontal bossing, Hutchison teeth, 8th cranial nerve deafness, and Clutton's joints (painless joint effusions).

DIAGNOSIS

- Nontreponemal tests include rapid plasma reagin (RPR) titers and the Venereal Disease Research Laboratory (VDRL) slide test. The treponemal test used most frequently is the fluorescent treponemal antibody-absorption test (FTA-ABS).
- Treponemes can also be seen on darkfield microscopy.

TREATMENT

Penicillin G is used, and the treatment length depends on disease stage and clinical presentation.

HUMAN IMMUNODEFICIENCY VIRUS (HIV)

- Mother-to-child transmission is rare in the United States due to screening and treatment. In an untreated mother, the risk of newborn infection is up to 25%. Most transmission occurs in the intrapartum period. For every hour of ruptured membranes, the risk of transmission increases.
- Transmission from infected breast milk can occur.
- Clinical features of infant infection can include persistent thrush, lymphadenopathy and hepatosplenomegaly, severe diarrhea, failure to thrive, and recurrent infections.
- Strategies to reduce transmission:
  - Maternal treatment with zidovudine (AZT) during pregnancy.
  - Cesarean section prior to the onset of labor and rupture of membranes if maternal viral load is unknown or over 1000 copies/mL.
  - Mothers who are HIV positive should avoid breast-feeding.

DIAGNOSIS

- PCR testing for HIV-1 qualitative is used, or, if not available, HIV-1 RNA qualitative.
- Historically, positive antibodies at 18 months indicated infection; however, a small number of children still display maternal antibodies at 2 years of age.

TREATMENT

- Exposed neonates should receive AZT within 6–12 hours of birth and continue for 4–6 weeks.
- High-risk infants (mother without antiretroviral antepartum treatment) should also receive 3 doses of nevirapine beginning as soon as possible.

EXAM TIP

Antiretroviral therapy during pregnancy reduces the rate of perinatal transmission from almost 25% in untreated mothers to about 1% in treated mothers.

Newborn Care

ROUTINE PROPHYLAXIS

- Erythromycin eye ointment is recommended for prophylaxis against ophthalmia neonatorum due to gonococcal (but not chlamydial) infections. Maternal treatment is best prevention of chlamydial infant infections.
- Vitamin K is given intramuscularly (IM) to prevent hemorrhagic disease of the newborn.
- Hepatitis B vaccine is routinely given to all infants within the first 12 hours of life.
  - Hepatitis B immune globulin (HBIG) is also administered to infants of mothers with hepatitis B to minimize transmission risk.

NEWBORN METABOLIC SCREENING

- Newborn screening varies by state, but all have a program designed to detect diseases that can be life threatening or cause significant newborn morbidity before they become symptomatic.
- Typically, blood is collected by heel stick onto filter paper.
- This testing can detect inborn errors of metabolism, endocrine disorders, hemoglobinopathies, immunodeficiency, and cystic fibrosis.

EXAM TIP

Early diagnosis of hypothyroidism and treatment with thyroid hormone prior to 3 months of age can greatly improve intellectual outcome.

AUDITORY SCREENING

- Neonates are screened for hearing loss since early intervention can improve language development.
- Hearing screens include otoacoustic emissions (OAE) or automated auditory brainstem response (AABR). OAE measures sound waves generated by hair cells in the inner ear. It is easier to administer and can detect sensorineural hearing loss, but it does not identify auditory neuropathy. The AABR measures action potentials from the cochlear nerve to the midbrain. It detects neural hearing loss and auditory neuropathy, but it is somewhat more difficult to administer. All NICU infants should be screened with an AABR since they have more risk factors for hearing loss.

CRITICAL CONGENITAL HEART DISEASE (CCHD) SCREENING

- Up to 30% of infants with CCHD may appear normal on a routine exam. Therefore, all infants should be screened for congenital cardiac disease after 24 hours of age.
- Oxygen saturation is measured in the right hand and in one foot to evaluate for low oxygen saturations or a difference in the preductal (right hand) and postductal (foot) saturations.

DEVELOPMENTAL DYSPLASIA OF THE HIP (DDH)

- DDH is a spectrum of abnormal development of the acetabulum and proximal femur that leads to instability of the hip joint.
- Risk factors include: female gender, breech presentation, and family history. DDH is more likely to be unilateral and involve the left hip.

- Signs include asymmetry of the skin folds in the groin, shortening of the affected leg, or asymmetric gait.
- Evaluation maneuvers eliciting a "clunk" in either suggests DDH:
  - Ortolani—hip abduction using gentle inward and upward pressure over the greater trochanter; a "clunk" is the femoral head relocation into the acetabulum.
  - Barlow—hip adduct using the thumb to apply outward and backward pressure; a "clunk" is femoral head dislocation.
- Diagnosis can be made by an abnormal ultrasound at 6 weeks of age. A normal ultrasound does not rule out DDH, and clinical suspicion can necessitate further imaging.
- Can be treated with a brace (Pavlik harness) or casting. (See Musculoskeletal Disease chapter.)

Prematurity and the Critically Ill Neonate

Meconium Aspiration

A full-term male infant was born after a prolonged second stage of labor and had thick meconium at delivery. He was depressed at birth and required positive pressure ventilation. His condition improved quickly, and he was vigorous at 3 minutes of life. The Apgar score was 3 at 1 minute and 7 at 5 minutes. He was doing well until 3 hours of life, when he was noted to have a dusky episode with an oxygen saturation of 82% on room air. Despite supplemental O_2 his saturation remained in the 80s. He was intubated and started on mechanical ventilation. His chest x-ray is shown in Figure 3-1. *Think: meconium aspiration.*

This infant has characteristic meconium-aspiration syndrome, as seen by the nodular appearance of both lung fields on the chest x-ray. He is developing persistent pulmonary hypertension of the newborn (PPHN), management of which includes aggressive ventilation, inhaled nitric oxide, and close monitoring of gas exchange. An echocardiogram is useful to provide details on the elevated pulmonary pressures and to rule out any cardiac defects. Infants are at risk of shunting the pulmonary flow via the ductus arteriosus into the systemic circulation, resulting in different O_2 saturations in the upper and lower extremities.

- Meconium is a newborn's first intestinal discharge; it is composed of epithelial cells, fetal hair, mucus, and bile.
- Intrauterine stress may cause meconium to pass into the amniotic fluid before delivery.
- Meconium aspiration while in-utero due to fetal gasping or shortly after delivery can cause upper and lower airway obstruction and an inflammatory response (meconium-aspiration syndrome [MAS]).
- Full-term and post-date infants are at higher risk for meconium aspiration.
- Treatment is supportive and may include surfactant, inhaled nitric oxide, mechanical ventilation, high-frequency oscillatory ventilation, and extracorporeal membrane oxygenation (ECMO).

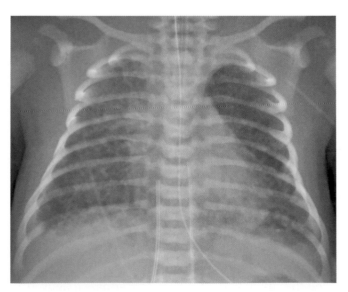

FIGURE 3-1. **Chest film demonstrating meconium aspiration syndrome.** (Reproduced, with permission, from Susan D. John, MD.)

Hypoxic Ischemic Encephalopathy

- Hypoxic ischemic encephalopathy is an important cause of neuronal damage due to hypoxia (decreased oxygen delivery) and/or ischemia (decreased blood flow) to the brain.
- Can be caused by maternal conditions (hypertension), placental insufficiency, placental abruption, severe neonatal blood loss, and overwhelming infection
- Neurologic manifestations may include hypotonia, absent or decreased primitive reflexes, coma, and seizures.
- Can result in cerebral palsy (CP), intellectual disability, and death
- Treatment includes support and selective head or whole-body cooling.

WARD TIP

Only 10% of patients with cerebral palsy have birth events associated with asphyxia. The cause of most cases of congenital CP remains unknown.

Hyperbilirubinemia

- Bilirubin is divided into direct (conjugated) and indirect (unconjugated) bilirubin.
- Bilirubin is conjugated in the liver.
- Bilirubin levels may be obtained through serum testing or a noninvasive transcutaneous bilirubinometer (TcB).
- Direct hyperbilirubinemia is defined as a direct bilirubin >1 or >20% of total bilirubin; it is never normal, and can be associated with liver disease and biliary atresia. (See GI chapter.)

EXAM TIP

A high direct serum bilirubin level and/or clinical jaundice in the first 24 hours of life are never physiologic.

INDIRECT HYPERBILIRUBINEMIA

- Common causes of indirect hyperbilirubinemia include:
  - ABO incompatibility or Rh isoimmunization—leads to increased hemolysis and increased bilirubin load.
  - Breast-feeding jaundice—related to relative dehydration in the first few days of life.
  - Breastmilk jaundice—theorized to be caused by an enzyme in some mothers' breast milk.
  - Physiologic jaundice—caused by decreased bilirubin uptake into the liver, decreased liver conjugation, and decreased bile-duct excretion, all immature processes in the neonate.
  - Infection.
- Physiologic hyperbilirubinemia is seen after the first 24 hours of life, usually peaking at 3 days in term infants, and resolves over 2 weeks.
- Bilirubin levels in premature infants tend to peak later than in term infants.
- Nomograms based on an infant's hour of life and risk factors allow bilirubin levels to be categorized into low, medium, or high-risk levels to help guide therapy.

TREATMENT

- Phototherapy: converts bilirubin in the skin to the more soluble lumirubin, which can be excreted without conjugation into bile and urine.
  - TcB measurements cannot be used during phototherapy, but they become reliable once the infant is off phototherapy for 24 hours.
  - Delivery of phototherapy can be with a fiber-optic "bili blanket" under or around the infant and/or "bili lights" arranged above the infant.
- Hydration usually can be achieved with oral feedings; IV hydration is rarely indicated.

- Significant hyperbilirubinemia may require an exchange transfusion, a process whereby small aliquots of "jaundiced" blood are removed and replaced with reconstituted blood.

BILIRUBIN-INDUCED NEUROLOGIC DYSFUNCTION (HENCE THE D IN BIND) (KERNICTERUS)

- BIND, also known as kernicterus, is due to irreversible bilirubin deposition in the basal ganglia. Only free bilirubin, not bound to albumin, can cross the blood–brain barrier.
- Symptoms of BIND can include subtle neurologic deficits, a high-pitched cry, severe back arching, hearing loss, profound encephalopathy, or death.

Prematurity

DEFINITIONS

- Premature infant: live-born newborn delivered prior to 37 weeks' gestation.
- Low birth weight (LBW): <2500 g.
- Very low birth weight (VLBW): <1500 g.
- Extremely low birth weight (ELBW): <1000 g.
- Extremely low gestational age neonate (ELGAN): <28 weeks' gestation.

ETIOLOGY

- Most premature births have no identifiable cause.
- Identifiable risk factors include maternal, fetal, and obstetric.
  - Maternal:
    - Previous history of premature delivery—most significant risk factor.
    - Maternal age below 17 or greater than 35.
    - Inadequate prenatal care.
    - Uterine malformations.
    - Maternal medical illness (preeclampsia, hypertension, renal disease, diabetes, cyanotic heart disease).
    - Maternal smoking or cocaine use.
  - Fetal:
    - Multiple gestation.
    - Congenital anomalies.
  - Obstetric:
    - Cervical insufficiency.
    - Polyhydramnios/oligohydramnios.
    - Chorioamnionitis.
    - Asymptomatic bacteriuria.
    - Vaginal bleeding due to placenta previa and abruptio placenta.

INCIDENCE

- About 10% of infants are born premature in the United States.
- The highest rate is among non-Hispanic Black mothers at 14.4%.
- The lowest rate is among non-Hispanic Asian mothers at 8.7%.

SURVIVAL OF PREMATURE NEONATES

- Disorders related to prematurity, low birth weight, chromosomal abnormalities, and congenital malformations are the leading causes of neonatal death.

- No worldwide, universally accepted gestational age defines viability.
- Survival rates in developed countries with intensive care is >90% for babies >27 weeks.
- Survival without significant impairment is substantially lower for infants born 25 weeks or less.

SPECIAL CONSIDERATIONS FOR PREMATURE NEONATES

- Thermoregulation: premature infants have increased susceptibility to heat loss (high body surface area-to-body weight ratio, decreased brown fat stores, nonkeratinized skin, and decreased glycogen supply).
- Glucose regulation: premature infants have increased susceptibility to hypo- and hyperglycemia.
- Fluid and electrolyte imbalances (renal proximal tubular dysfunction and nonkeratinized skin).
- Hyperbilirubinemia: more significant and peaks later than in term infants.
- Nutritional support: ex-preemies require a specialized high-calorie diet for optimized growth.
- Routine vaccination should be given based on postnatal (not gestational) age.
- Early identification and intervention are needed for infants with developmental problems.

Common Problems in Premature Newborns

RESPIRATORY DISTRESS SYNDROME (RDS)

ETIOLOGY/PATHOPHYSIOLOGY

- Immature lung structure: alveolar ducts form at ~25 weeks, alveoli between 32 and 36 weeks, and the neonatal rib cage is weak and highly compliant.
- Lung-surfactant deficiency due to immaturity of surfactant producing type 2 alveolar cells results in high alveolar surface tension and alveolar collapse. Alveolar collapse results in atelectasis, intrapulmonary shunting, hypoxemia, and cyanosis.
- Surfactant quality and quantity increases as fetus nears term.

SIGNS AND SYMPTOMS

- Usually seen within the first 4 hours of life.
- Tachypnea.
- Grunting and nasal flaring.
- Retractions.
- Cyanosis.

DIAGNOSIS

Diagnosis involves a chest x-ray with fine, diffuse reticulogranular or "ground glass" pattern with air bronchograms (see Figure 3-2).

TREATMENT

- Treatment involves respiratory support, including oxygen, continuous positive airway pressure (CPAP), intubation, and mechanical ventilation.
- Exogenous surfactant replacement can be administered via endotracheal tube.

WARD TIP

Breast milk with a fortifier is the best choice for enteral feeding for premature infants.

WARD TIP

If unable to use enteral feedings, optimal nutrition can be achieved by total parenteral nutrition (TPN)—a specialized solution consisting of amino acids, dextrose, minerals, and electrolytes.

EXAM TIP

Maternal steroid (betamethasone) administration can decrease incidence of RDS and IVH; it works best if given 24–48 hours prior to delivery. Every woman at increased risk of delivery before 34 weeks should be given betamethasone, if possible, and recent studies suggest improved outcomes with maternal steroids even in infants born between 34 and 36 weeks.

WARD TIP

These neonates may also receive antibiotics because clinically and radiographically RDS and congenital pneumonia are indistinguishable.

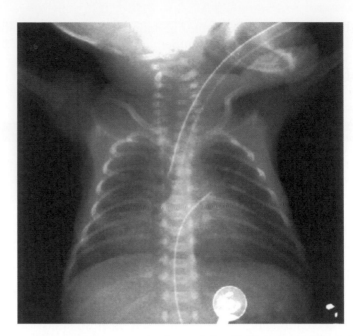

FIGURE 3-2. Chest x-ray demonstrating "ground glass" infiltrates consistent with respiratory distress syndrome (with a more focal area of infiltrate or atelectasis in the medial right lung base).

BRONCHOPULMONARY DYSPLASIA (BPD, CHRONIC LUNG DISEASE)

DEFINITION

- Characterized by the need for continued supplemental oxygen beyond 28 days of life or at 36 weeks postmenstrual age in a premature infant.
- Distortion of lung architecture with abnormal capillary development large cystic areas, interstitial fibrosis.

ETIOLOGY

- Multifactorial.
- Lung immaturity.
- Prolonged mechanical ventilation leading to barotrauma and volutrauma.
- Oxygen toxicity to the lungs.
- Infection (sepsis, chorioamnionitis).

SIGNS AND SYMPTOMS

- Tachypnea.
- Retractions.
- Wheezing or rales.

DIAGNOSIS

Chest x-ray shows air-trapping, atelectasis, and/or pulmonary edema. Hyperinflation may be seen in severe BPD.

TREATMENT

- Supportive care, adequate nutrition for growth.
- Bronchodilators.
- Diuretics.

WARD TIP

Infants with bronchopulmonary dysplasia can wheeze; remember, "not all that wheezes is asthma!"

EXAM TIP

BPD occurs most often in neonates born at less than 28 weeks.

WARD TIP

Ex-preemies can receive RSV prophylaxis with RSV monoclonal antibodies during RSV season (an IM injection once a month).

NECROTIZING ENTEROCOLITIS (NEC)

> An ex 28-week-gestation female infant was doing well and advanced to full enteral feeds at 14 days of life. At day 15 of life, she develops abdominal distention and bloody stools. An x-ray of the abdomen is shown (Figure 3-3). What is the likely diagnosis and management of the condition shown in this x-ray? *Think: NEC*
>
> The x-ray of this infant is consistent with NEC with evident pneumatosis intestinalis (free air within the bowel wall) in the descending colon area. Medical management includes NPO, IV nutrition, and IV antibiotics for 7–10 days. Serial x-rays are obtained to detect if bowel-wall perforation occurs, which would require immediate surgery.

NEC is the most common gastrointestinal emergency in premature infants.

ETIOLOGY

- NEC is seen primarily in premature infants, but it can occur in full-term neonates.
- The incidence and mortality are inversely related to gestational age and birth weight.
- Pathogenesis is unknown, but it is most likely a multifactorial etiology including bowel-wall ischemia and bacterial invasion.

SIGNS AND SYMPTOMS

- Intolerance of oral feeding (vomiting, bilious aspirates).
- Change in behavior (lethargy).
- Abdominal distention and/or tenderness, abdominal skin discoloration.
- Temperature instability.
- Respiratory distress; increased episodes of apnea and desaturation, respiratory failure.
- Metabolic acidosis, sepsis, shock.
- Abnormal lab values (low or high white blood count (WBC), thrombocytopenia, and glucose dysregulation).

DIAGNOSIS

- Abdominal x-ray with "pneumatosis intestinalis"—air bubbles within the bowel wall (see Figure 3-3) —is the hallmark radiographic finding for NEC.
- Air in portal vein.
- Free air in the abdomen (in case of perforation).
- Occult/frank blood per rectum.

TREATMENT

- NPO and bowel rest.
- Nasogastric decompression.
- Intravenous nutrition.
- Blood cultures and broad-spectrum antibiotics, with anaerobic coverage if pneumatosis present.
- Surgery if perforation occurs.

WARD TIP

Spontaneous intestinal perforation is different from NEC. It is more common in extremely premature infants treated with indomethacin for patent ductus arteriosus. It usually occurs early in life and requires surgical intervention.

WARD TIP

The most consistent risk factors for NEC are prematurity and formula feeding. Human milk, compared to formula, is protective against NEC.

WARD TIP

Serious sequelae of NEC include intestinal strictures, malabsorption, fistulae, and short-bowel syndrome (if a significant amount of bowel was removed surgically).

WARD TIP

An absolute indication for operative intervention in NEC is pneumoperitoneum, indicating bowel perforation.

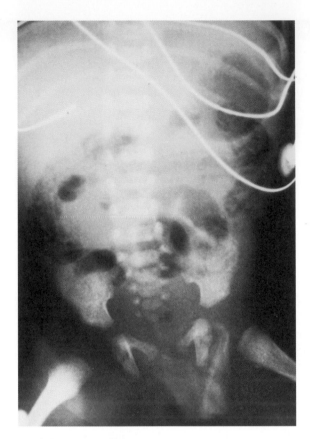

FIGURE 3-3. **Necrotizing enterocolitis.**

Currently, severe vision loss due to retinopathy of prematurity is rare due to judicious use of oxygen and treatment of retinopathy of prematurity (ROP).

EXAM TIP

All infants <1500 g birth weight or younger than 30 weeks' gestational age at birth are at risk of developing ROP.

RETINOPATHY OF PREMATURITY (ROP)

ROP is a potentially blinding disease of premature infants due to abnormal retinal vascularization.

ETIOLOGY

- Premature retinas are not fully vascularized. Vessels grow from macula outward.
- Vessels grow abnormally due to hyperoxia, hypoxia, or hypotension.
- Abnormally grown tortuous vessels can lead to retinal detachment and blindness.
- Incidence and severity are inversely related to gestational age and birth weight.

DIAGNOSIS

- An ophthalmology evaluation is necessary in all infants ≤1500 g or gestational age of <30 weeks, as well as for infants with birth weight 1500–2000 g and an unstable clinical course.
- First screening exam:
  - This exam occurs at postmenstrual age of 31 weeks or 5 weeks of age, whichever is later.

TREATMENT

- Treatment depends on severity.
- Multiple modalities are available, including laser photocoagulation, cryotherapy, and anti-vascular endothelial growth factor (anti-VEGF) agents.

INTRAVENTRICULAR HEMORRHAGE (IVH)

DEFINITION

- Rupture of germinal matrix blood vessels due to:
    - Germinal matrix fragility because of immaturity.
    - Fluctuations in cerebral blood flow: hypoxic-ischemic injury, increased arterial blood flow, or increased venous pressure.
- Most IVHs occur within 72 hours after birth.

PREDISPOSING FACTORS

- Prematurity.
- RDS.
- Hypo- or hypertension.
- Pneumothorax.

SIGNS AND SYMPTOMS

- May be asymptomatic.
- May present with fluctuating nonspecific findings over days: altered level of consciousness, hypotonia, decreased movements, changes in eye positioning or movement, disruption of respiratory function (apnea).
- Catastrophic presentation is least common and progresses rapidly with stupor, coma, respiratory failure, decerebrate posturing, seizures, flaccid weakness, cranial nerve abnormalities, bulging fontanelle, hypotension, bradycardia, falling hematocrit, metabolic acidosis and inappropriate ADH secretion.

DIAGNOSIS

- All infants <30 weeks of gestation should be screened at 7–14 days of chronological age and again at 36–40 weeks of postmenstrual age.
- Cranial ultrasound (through anterior fontanelle).
- Grade I: bleeding into the germinal matrix.
- Grade II: IVH in ≤ 50% of lateral-ventricle volume.
- Grade III: IVH in >50% of lateral-ventricle volume.
- Grade IV: large IVH with hemorrhagic infarction of periventricular white matter.

COMPLICATIONS

- Post-hemorrhagic hydrocephalus.
- Cerebral palsy.
- Seizures.
- Developmental delay.

TREATMENT

- The treatment is supportive care; a blood transfusion may be needed.
- For hydrocephalus a CSF reservoir or ventriculoperitoneal shunt placement may be required.
- Prognosis is dependent on the grade of IVH:
    - Grades I and II: good outcome, not at increased risk for developmental delay.
    - Grade III: may have cognitive impairment.
    - Grade IV (periventricular hemorrhage infarction): may have major neurologic problems, increased risk of mortality.

WARD TIP

All infants born before 30 weeks of gestation should have a cranial ultrasound in the first 7–14 days of life to look for intraventricular hemorrhage.

NOTES

HIGH-YIELD FACTS IN

Growth and Development

Growth

- Understanding normal growth patterns of childhood is important because they are an indication of a child's overall health.
- Growth is influenced by both genetics and environment.

GROWTH CHARTS

- Height, weight, and head circumference are plotted on growth curves to compare the patient to the population.
- Growth charts compare children to the 5th, 10th, 25th, 50th, 75th, 90th, and 95th percentiles.
- World Health Organization (WHO) vs Center for Disease Control (CDC) growth charts:
    - The WHO growth standard charts consider the effect of infant feeding on growth by using breastfeeding as the norm. These should be used for the first 24 months of life.
    - CDC growth reference charts were developed to represent all infants in the United States. Feeding criteria were not identified. Use these starting at 24 months.

The CDC growth charts may not adequately reflect the current growth patterns of infants in the United States, nor the growth pattern typically seen in breastfed infants.

- Serial plotting of growth allows for observation of growth patterns over time.
- Body mass index (BMI) is plotted on growth curves by gender from 2 to 20 years of age. BMI <5% is underweight; BMI >85% classifies as overweight and >95% as obese.
- Potential limitations of growth charts include development from small population sizes, ethnic differences, and if they represent growth potential versus proper care and feeding.
- Specialized charts exist for children who have specific genetic conditions (e.g., trisomy 21) or are premature (Fenton).

EARLY GROWTH TRENDS

- A term infant, who is breastfeeding, regains birth weight by 2 weeks. A formula-fed infant usually regains birthweight by 10 days.
- During the first 3 months, a child gains 20 to 30 g/day, or close to 1 kg/month.
- A child doubles birth weight by the fifth month of life and triples by the first birthday.
- Growth chart recording for premature infants is adjusted for gestational age until 2 years of age.
- Normal growth from birth to 6 months is 1.5–2.5 cm/month, and between 6 and 12 months, 1 cm/month.
- Children with genetic short stature may have normal length and weight at birth, but their growth percentiles decline within the first 2–3 years.
- Appetite normally decreases in the second year of life, coincident with the growth rate slowing.

INTRAUTERINE FACTORS

- Both insulin-like growth factor (IGF) -1 and -2 are important for fetal growth.
- Growth hormone and IGF are both important for postnatal growth.

WARD TIP

Having only one point on a growth chart is like having no point; the trend over time is what is important.

WARD TIP

How to calculate a BMI

BMI = mass(kg)/[height(m)]^2

BMI = mass (lb)/[height(in)]^2 × 703

Just like height and weight, BMI should be plotted on growth curves based on gender and age.

EXAM TIP

In the normal child, the greatest growth occurs in the first year of life.

EXAM TIP

Newborns may lose up to 10% of their birthweight in the first few days of life.

WARD TIP

Careful plotting on a growth chart is the most accurate method by which to follow a child's physical growth.

- Fetal weight gain is greatest during the third trimester.
- Teratogens, TORCH infections (toxoplasmosis, other [hepatitis B, syphilis, varicella-zoster virus], rubella, cytomegalovirus, herpes simplex virus/human immunodeficiency virus), and chromosomal abnormalities (trisomy 21, Turner syndrome) can impair fetal growth. Smoking during pregnancy can lead to a low birthweight.

TEETH

- Children should have all primary teeth, including second molars, by 30–33 months.
- Central incisors are first to erupt, between 6 and 12 months.
- Second molars are last to erupt, between 23 and 33 months.
- Secondary (permanent) teeth begin to erupt by age 6–7 years.
- Early or late tooth eruption may be normal, although it can be an indicator of a nutritional, genetic, or metabolic problem.
- Delayed eruption causes include:
    - endocrine disorders (hypothyroidism).
    - genetic abnormalities (trisomy 21).

Specific Growth Problems

MICROCEPHALY

DEFINITION

The definition of microcephaly is typically defined as a fronto-occipital circumference (FOC) more than 2 SD below the appropriate mean (in practice, less than the third percentile).

ETIOLOGY

- Genetic (familial, isolated).
- Syndromic:
    - Chromosomal: trisomy 21, 13, 18
    - Contiguous gene deletion: Cri-du-chat syndrome, Williams syndrome
    - Single-gene defects: Cornelia de Lange syndrome, Smith-Lemli-Opitz syndrome
- Prenatal insults (radiation, alcohol, hydantoin, TORCH infections, maternal phenylketonuria [PKU] and maternal diabetes, decreased placental blood flow), Zika virus
- Perinatal hypoxic-ischemic encephalopathy
- Structural malformation (e.g., lissencephaly)

IMPACT

Microcephaly is associated with abnormal brain growth. A small brain predisposes to impaired cognitive development, delayed motor functions and speech, and seizures.

MACROCEPHALY

DEFINITION

Head circumference is >2 standard deviations above the mean (in practice, >97%).

EXAM TIP

Measure parents' and siblings' head circumference to check for familial micro- or macrocephaly.

ETIOLOGY

- Increased brain parenchyma (megalencephaly, familial in majority of cases).
- Hydrocephalus.
- Other causes: cranioskeletal dysplasia, fragile X, achondroplasia, Sotos syndrome.

POOR WEIGHT GAIN / FAILURE TO THRIVE (FTT)

DEFINITION

FTT is caused by inadequate nutrition. It is defined as a weight below the third percentile with a decreased rate of weight gain, or a fall off the growth chart by two percentiles. Historically, FTT has been divided into "organic" causes (a physical problem, such as milk protein allergy) and "inorganic" causes (such as neglect or improper feeding), although this dichotomy is somewhat artificial and has fallen out of favor since the cause may be multifactorial.

ETIOLOGY

Many underlying problems can result in inadequate nutrition and poor weight gain (see Table 4-1).

SIGNS AND SYMPTOMS

- Expected age norms for height and weight not met.
- Hair loss.
- Loss of muscle mass.
- Subcutaneous fat loss.
- Dermatitis.
- Lethargy.
- Recurrent infection.
- Kwashiorkor: protein malnutrition.
- Marasmus: inadequate nutrition.

DIAGNOSIS

- Detailed history:
  - Gestation, labor, and delivery.
  - Neonatal problems (feeding or otherwise).
  - Breast-feeding mother's diet and medications.
  - Types and amounts of food, who prepares and how the formula or food is prepared, who feeds.
  - Vomiting, diarrhea, infection.
  - Sick parents or siblings.
  - Major family life events/chronic stressors.
  - Travel outside the United States.
  - Any injuries to child.
  - Abnormal newborn metabolic screen results.
- Observation of parent–child interactions, especially at feedings, is critical for diagnosis.
- The lack of weight gain after adequate caloric feedings suggests FTT is not solely due to inadequate intake, and further evaluation is required.
- Screening tests for common causes include complete blood count (CBC), electrolytes, blood urea nitrogen (BUN), creatinine, C-reactive protein, albumin, thyroid-stimulating hormone, and urinalysis.

EXAM TIP

Psychosocial reasons account for most cases of failure to thrive (FTT) in the United States.

EXAM TIP

With inadequate caloric intake weight is affected first, followed by height and head circumference.

TABLE 4-1. Etiology of FTT

Gastrointestinal	Pulmonary	Endocrine	Other
Nutritional	▪ Tonsillar hypertrophy	▪ Hypothyroidism	▪ Prematurity
▪ Kwashiorkor	▪ Cystic fibrosis	▪ Rickets	▪ Oncologic disease/treatment
▪ Marasmus	▪ Bronchopulmonary dysplasia	▪ Vitamin D resistance/deficiency	▪ Immunodeficiency
▪ Zinc/iron deficiency	▪ Asthma	▪ Hypophosphatemia	▪ Collagen vascular disease
Feeding Disorder	▪ Structural abnormalities	▪ Growth hormone resistance/	▪ Lead poisoning
▪ Oral-motor apraxia	▪ Obstructive sleep apnea	deficiency	**Nonorganic Causes**
▪ Cleft palate	**Renal**	▪ Adrenal insufficiency/excess	▪ Child neglect/abuse
▪ Dentition disorder	▪ Chronic pyelonephritis	▪ Parathyroid disorders	▪ Poverty
Vomiting	▪ Renal tubular acidosis	▪ Diabetes mellitus	▪ Lack of true caregivers
▪ Gastrointestinal reflux	▪ Fanconi syndrome	**Central Nervous System**	▪ Family mental illness
▪ Structural anomalies	▪ Chronic renal insufficiency	▪ Pituitary insufficiency	▪ Marital discord/spousal abuse in
▪ Pyloric stenosis	▪ Urinary tract infection	▪ Diencephalic syndrome	the home
▪ CNS lesions	▪ Diabetes insipidus	▪ Cerebral palsy	
▪ Hirschsprung disease	**Hepatic**	▪ Cerebral hemorrhages	
Diarrhea	▪ Chronic hepatitis	▪ Degenerative disorders	
▪ Chronic toddler diarrhea	▪ Glycogen storage disease	**Congenital**	
▪ Milk protein allergy/intolerance	**Infectious**	▪ Inborn errors of metabolism	
▪ Infectious	▪ Tuberculosis	▪ Trisomy 13, 18, 21	
▪ Bacterial	▪ HIV	▪ Russell-Silver syndrome	
▪ Parasitic	**Cardiac**	▪ Prader-Willi syndrome	
▪ Malabsorption	▪ Congenital heart malformations	▪ Cornelia de Lange syndrome	
		▪ Perinatal infection	
		▪ Fetal alcohol syndrome	

TREATMENT

▪ If the child is severely malnourished, hospitalization may be required.
▪ Treat the underlying cause of inadequate nutrition.

PROGNOSIS

Data are lacking, but little evidence supports the idea that isolated poor weight gain is directly associated with abnormal intellectual development.

Development

A child smiles spontaneously, babbles, sits without support, reaches, and feeds herself a cookie but has no pincer grasp. What is her approximate age? *Think: 8–9 months* (immature pincer grasp at 10 months). Fine pincer grasp of an object between the thumb and forefinger generally develops at 12 months of age.

▪ Developmental milestone attainment is an indicator of a child's overall neurologic function.

- Maturation of intellectual, social, and motor function should occur in a predictable manner.
- The clinician must recognize normal patterns to identify deviations early.

DEVELOPMENTAL MILESTONES

- Each new motor, language, and social skill should be acquired during an expected age range in a child's life.
- Each new skill is built on an earlier skill, and skills are rarely skipped (see Table 4-2).

TABLE 4-2. Developmental Milestones

AGE	MOTOR	LANGUAGE	SOCIAL	MEMORY AIDS
1 month	Reacts to pain	Responds to noise	Regards human face Establishes eye contact	
2 months	Eyes follow object to midline **Head up prone**	Vocalizes Coos by 3 months	Social **smile** Recognizes parent	
4 months	Eyes follow object past midline **Rolls over**	**Laughs and squeals**	**Regards hand**	
6 months	**Sits well unsupported** Transfers objects hand to hand (switches hands) **Rolls prone to supine**	**Babbles**	Recognizes strangers	6abbles (babbles) Six strangers switch sitting at six months
9 months	**Pincer grasp, immature (10 months)** **Crawls** Cruises (walks holding furniture)	Mama/dada, nonspecific Bye-bye	Starts to explore Stranger anxiety	Can crawl, therefore can explore It takes 9 months to be a "mama" Pinches furniture to walk
12 months	**Walks with one hand held** Throws object Fine pincer grasp	Mama/dada specific and knows **1–3 words** **Follows one-step command with gesture**		Walking away from mom causes anxiety Knows 1 word at 1 year
2 years	**Walks up and down stairs** Copies a line **Runs** **Kicks ball**	**2–3-word phrases** One half of speech is understood by strangers Refers to self by name **Pronouns**	Parallel play	Puts 2 words together at 2 At age 2, ¾ (½) of speech understood by strangers

TABLE 4-2. Developmental Milestones (*continued*)

AGE	MOTOR	LANGUAGE	SOCIAL	MEMORY AIDS
3 years	**Copies a circle** **Pedals a tricycle** Can build a bridge of 3 cubes Repeats 3 numbers	Speaks in sentences Three fourths of speech is understood by strangers Recognizes 3 colors	Group play **Plays simple games** Knows gender Knows first and last name	*Tricycle*, 3 cubes, 3 numbers, 3 colors, 3 kids make a group At age 3, ¾ of speech understood by strangers
4 years	Identifies body parts Copies a cross Copies a square (4.5 years) **Hops on one foot** **Throws overhand**	Speech is completely understood by strangers Uses past tense **Tells a story**	Plays with kids, social interaction	Song "head, shoulder, knees, and toes," 4 parts reminds you that at age 4, can identify 4 body parts At age 4, ¾ (all) of speech is understood by strangers When using past tense, speaks of things that happened *before* If a 2-year-old can copy one line, a 4-year-old can copy two lines to draw a cross and a square, which has 4 sides
5 years	Copies a triangle Catches a ball Skips with alternating feet Partially dresses self	Writes name Counts 10 objects		
6 years	Draws a person with 6 parts Ties shoes	Identifies left and right		At 6 years: skips, shoes, person with 6 parts

NEUROLOGIC DEVELOPMENT

- Nervous-system myelination begins mid-gestation and continues until 2 years of age.
- Myelination occurs in an orderly fashion, from head to toe (cephalo-caudal).
- The brain at birth weighs approximately 10% of the newborn's body weight; the adult brain weighs about 2% of body weight.
- Primitive reflexes are present after birth and most diminish by 6 months (see Table 4-3).

AGE ADJUSTMENT FOR PRETERM INFANTS

- Preterm infant development may differ from development for full-term infants.
- Age correction should be done until the child is 24 months old for children born more than 2 weeks early.
- Use the corrected age when assessing developmental progress and growth.

 WARD TIP

For age adjustment between birth and 2 years, subtract the number of weeks of prematurity from the chronological age. For an 18-month-old baby who is an ex-preemie at 30 weeks, the difference from full term at 40 weeks is 10 weeks. Therefore, the corrected age is 18 months minus 10 weeks = 15½ months.

TABLE 4-3. Primitive Reflexes

REFLEX	TIMING	ELICIT	RESPONSE
Moro	Birth to 5–6 months	While supine, allow head to suddenly fall back approximately 3 cm	Symmetric extension and adduction, then flexion, of limbs
Galant	Birth to 2 months	While prone, stroke the paravertebral region of the back	Pelvis will move in the direction of the stimulated side
Sucking	Becomes voluntary at 3 months	Stimulate lips	Sucks
Babinski	Birth to 4 months	Stroke from heel to anterior transverse arch (take care not to elicit a plantar grasp)	Extensor response / fanning of toes
Asymmetric tonic neck	Birth to 2–3 months	While supine, rotate head laterally	Extension of limbs on chin side, and flexion of limbs on opposite side (fencing posture)
Rooting	Less prominent after 1 month	Stroke finger from mouth to earlobe	Head turns toward stimulus and mouth opens
Palmar/plantar grasp	Birth to 3–4 months	Stimulation of palm or plantar surface of foot	Palmar grasp/plantar flexion
Parachute	Appears at 9 months remains throughout life	Horizontal suspension and quick thrusting movement toward surface	Extension of extremities

WARD TIP

Developmental Concerns

12 months: No babbling and no gesture
18 months: Less than 10 words
24 months: No two-word phrase, less that 30 words

EXAM TIP

At age 1 year, a child uses one word and follows a one-step command.

Developmental Delay

 An 18-month-old brought in for temper tantrums has normal gross and fine motor skills but lacks language development. He is cooperative and alert on exam. *Think: Hearing loss.*

Hearing screening in the newborn nursery has resulted in earlier detection of congenital hearing loss. Hearing impairment impacts language development. Inattention may be the initial presentation. It can also affect behavior and academic achievement.

DEFINITION

- A developmental delay is a condition in which a child is delayed in reaching early developmental milestones.
- A global developmental delay is a significant delay in two or more areas of development (gross or fine motor, speech and language, cognition, social and personal, and activities of daily living).
- Early delay detection is important since brain development is most malleable in the early years of life.

ETIOLOGY

Most developmental disabilities are thought to be caused by myriad factors including: genetics; parental health and behaviors (such as smoking and drinking) during pregnancy; birth complications; maternal or early childhood infections; and mother or child exposure to environmental toxins.

- Cerebral palsy.
- Learning disabilities.
- Hearing and vision deficits.
- Autism.
- Neglect.
- Lack of exposure.
- Genetic diseases (trisomy 21, fragile X).
- Fetal alcohol syndrome.

DIAGNOSIS

- The Denver Development Screening Test (Denver II, DDST) is a screening tool performed at well-child visits to identify children with developmental delay.
    - For children up to the age of 6 years.
    - Evaluates personal-social, fine motor, gross motor, and language skills.
    - Less commonly used now.
- Ages and Stages Questionnaire 3rd edition (ASQ-3).
    - Evaluates communication, gross motor, fine motor, personal-social, and problem-solving skills.
    - English, Spanish, and French versions available.
- Clinical Adaptive Test (CAT)/Clinical Linguistic Auditory and Milestone Scale (CLAMS) rates problem solving, visual motor ability, and language development from birth to 36 months of age.
- MCHAT (Modified Checklist for Autism in Toddlers)
    - This autism-screening tool is administered at 18 months and 2 years.
    - Early intervention is important; the younger a child is treated, the better the outcome.

Learning Disabilities (LDs)

- Learning disabilities are present in 3–10% of children.
- To make a diagnosis of learning disability, the child must have a normal IQ.
- These include difficulties with reading (dyslexia), arithmetic (dyscalculia), and writing (dysgraphia).
    - Dyslexia is one of the most common learning disabilities.
    - Consider when children fail to acquire reading skills in the usual time course.
    - These children may have excellent spoken language.
    - Learning disabilities present with different degrees of severity.

Sleep Patterns

- Two sleep stages are REM (irregular pulse and time when dreaming occurs) and non-REM (deep sleep).
- Newborns sleep 18 hours per day, with 50% rapid eye movement (REM) sleep, compared to an adult with 20% REM sleep.

EXAM TIP

Rule of Twos: At age 2 years, a child uses 2- to 3-word phrases and follows 2-step commands, and others can understand 1/2 of the child's speech.

EXAM TIP

Lead exposure in children can lead to learning disabilities and attention-deficit disorder (ADD).

EXAM TIP

Rule of 3: At age 3 years, a child uses 3-word sentences, and others can understand 3/4 of the child's speech.

EXAM TIP

Rule of 4s: At age 4 years, a child should be 40 lbs and 40 inches tall and be able to draw a 4-sided figure. Others should be able to understand 4/4, or all, of the child's speech.

- By age 4 months, nighttime sleep becomes consolidated (rather than the episodic sleep of newborns). (See Table 4.4.)
- Parasomnias (sleep disorders) begin near age 3 years.
- Nightmares occur during REM sleep: the child awakens in distress about a dream.
- Night terrors occur in non-REM sleep: the child appears awake and frightened but is not responsive, and then is amnestic about the event the next morning. These occur between ages 2 and 8 years.
- Somnambulism (sleepwalking) occurs in non-REM sleep, most commonly in ages 4–8 years.
- Somniloquy (sleeptalking) is common throughout life, and sometimes accompanies night terrors and sleepwalking.

SLEEP RECOMMENDATIONS FOR CHILDREN

TABLE 4-4. **Sleep Recommendations for Children**

AGE	RECOMMENDED SLEEPING HOURS
Newborn 0–2 months	10–19 hours
Infants 2–12 months	12–13 hours
Toddler 1–2 years	11–13 hours
Preschool 3–5 years	9–10 hours
School-aged children 6–13 years	9–11 hours
Adolescents 13–18 years	7-7.5 hours average 9–10 hours recommended

Nutrition and Fluid Management

Newborn Nutrition

NEWBORN FEEDING TIPS

- For term newborns, the caloric requirement is 100–120 kcal/kg/day (as compared to a 1-year-old with a 75 kcal/kg/day requirement).
- Newborns can be breastfed in the first hour of life.
- Infants typically lose weight for first 5–7 days and regain birth weight by 10–14 days.
- Newborns gain weight at a rate of about 30 g/day.
- Newborns typically want to breast- or formula-feed every 3–4 hours.
- Hunger is not the only reason infants cry, so they don't need to be fed every time they cry.
- *Supply = demand*—the more often the baby breastfeeds, the more milk will be produced.
- After a period of about 6 months of exclusive breastfeeding, begin to introduce solid foods into the infant's diet.
- Human milk is ideal for a term infant in the first year of life, but complementary foods must be added starting around six months for complete nutrition.
- Whole cow's milk is not suitable for infants because of low iron content and higher intake of sodium, potassium, and protein, leading to increased renal-solute load.
- Cow's milk (whole milk until age 2y unless the baby is overweight or a family history of dyslipidemia exists) can be introduced after the first birthday.

COLOSTRUM

- Colostrum is the first maternal milk produced after birth.
  - Usually a deep lemon color.
  - High in protein, minerals, immunologic factors, and antimicrobial peptides such as lactoferrin and lactoperoxidase; low in carbohydrates and fat.

BENEFITS OF BREASTFEEDING

- Infant:
  - Decreased incidence of infection (i.e., otitis media, pneumonia, bacteremia, diarrhea, urinary tract infection, necrotizing enterocolitis).
  - Higher levels of immunologic factors: immunoglobulins, complement, interferon, lactoferrin, lysozyme.
  - Decreased exposure to enteropathogens.
  - Decreased incidence of sudden infant death syndrome, type 1 and 2 diabetes, lymphoma, leukemia, childhood obesity, allergies, celiac disease, inflammatory bowel disease.
  - Other postulated benefits include higher IQ, better vision, less fussy eaters, but data are mixed.
- Maternal:
  - Increased maternal oxytocin levels.
  - Decreased postpartum bleeding and more rapid involution of uterus.
  - Less menstrual blood loss.
  - Delayed ovulation.
  - Decreased risk of ovarian and breast cancer.

WARD TIP

Term infants, due to loss of extracellular water and suboptimal caloric intake, may lose up to 10% of their birth weight in the first week of life. If breastfed, they should regain their birth weight by the end of the second week; if formula-fed, they should regain their birth weight by 10 days of life.

WARD TIP

Whole cow's milk is not recommended before 1 year of age because an infant's gastrointestinal (GI) tract is not developed enough to digest (poor absorption), predisposing to allergy, GI blood loss and iron deficiency.

WARD TIP

Don't put baby to sleep with a bottle; it increases the risk of dental caries.

WARD TIP

Breast milk's predominant protein is whey (whey-to-casein ratio: 70:30) early in lactation; it changes to ~50:50 in late lactation.

EXAM TIP

Immunoglobulin A (IgA) accounts for most of the immunoglobulins in breast milk.

- Psychological benefits: Increased maternal-child bonding.
- Other: Saves money for the family and for society, no risk of mixing errors, correct temperature, convenient, no preparation.

COMMON PROBLEMS WITH BREASTFEEDING

- Soreness of nipples: caused by improper feeding position or removal, not by prolonged feeding.
- Engorgement: unpleasant/painful swelling of the breasts when the feeding cycle is decreased suddenly (relieved by increased feeding on the affected breast).
- Maternal fatigue, stress, and anxiety, which affects hormones needed for lactation and reduction in milk production.
- Jaundice (see Table 5-1 and "Chapter 3: Prematurity and the Critically Ill Neonate" chapter).
- Mastitis: erythema, inflammation, and tenderness of an area of the breast caused by a blocked milk duct; can lead to infection with systemic symptoms.

CONTRAINDICATIONS TO BREASTFEEDING

- Cancer chemotherapy.
- Some medications (such as antimetabolites, chloramphenicol, methimazole, and tetracycline).
- Street drugs, unless enrolled in a methadone-maintenance program.
- Herpetic breast lesions (expressed milk acceptable).
- Untreated, active tuberculosis (expressed milk acceptable).
- Varicella 5 days before through 2 days after infection (expressed milk acceptable).
- Human immunodeficiency virus (HIV) infection, in developed countries; in developing countries, the benefits outweigh the risks.
- Infants with galactosemia should not ingest lactose-containing milk.

EXAM TIP

Cow's milk predominant protein is casein (~80%).

WARD TIP

Breastfed infant requires the following supplements:
- Vitamin D 400 IU/day
- Fluoride (after 6 months)
- Iron-rich foods or supplemental drops from 4 to 12 months

WARD TIP

Tip for the breastfeeding mother: If the baby doesn't let go, break the suction by inserting a finger into the corner of the baby's mouth; don't pull.

EXAM TIP

Breastfeeding jaundice (insufficient intake) occurs in the first week. Breast-milk jaundice (inhibitor of glucuronyl transferase or increased bilirubin absorption from the gut) starts after 1 week of life declining by 3 weeks of age.

EXAM TIP

An oral contraceptive is not a contraindication for breastfeeding.

WARD TIP

Not every woman will feel "milk letdown," despite proper breastfeeding.

TABLE 5-1. **Breastfeeding versus Breast Milk Jaundice**

BREASTFEEDING JAUNDICE	BREAST MILK JAUNDICE
Usually due to decreased or poor infant milk intake	Syndrome of prolonged unconjugated hyper-bilirubinemia thought to be due to an inhibitor to bilirubin conjugation in the breast milk of some mothers or increased absorption of bilirubin from the gut
Occurs *during* first week of life	Begins *after* first week of life; peaks usually after second to third week
Reduced enteral intake, → infrequent and small bowel movements and ↑ enterohepatic circulation of bilirubin	Transient unless severe unconjugated hyperbilirubinemia No treatment necessary

SIGNS OF INSUFFICIENT FEEDING OF INFANT

- Fewer than six wet diapers per day after age 1 week (before that, count one wet diaper per age in days for first week of life).
- Continual hunger, crying.
- Continually sleepy, lethargic baby.
- Fewer than eight feeds per day.
- Long intervals between feedings.
- Sleeping through the night without feeding.
- Loss of >10% of weight.
- Increased jaundice.

REASONS FOR FAILURE TO GROW AND GAIN WEIGHT

 An 18-month-old male is seen for a health evaluation. The family members are refugees. On examination, you find that he is below the 2nd percentile in height and weight and is thin looking. The parents deny childhood illnesses or severe illness. The complete blood count, chemistry, and liver function tests are within normal limits; the albumin is 2.3. *Think: Failure to thrive (FTT).* It is a condition when the physical growth of a child is below the third or fifth percentile. Nonorganic or psychosocial FTT is more common. The laboratory evaluation is usually normal and should be obtained judiciously. A detailed history is the most important part of evaluation, which helps to determine if the cause is organic or nonorganic.

- Improper formula preparation, especially diluted formula.
- Use of skim and 2% milk before age 2.
- Prolonged use of BRAT (bananas, rice, applesauce, toast) diet after illness.
- Excessive juice or water.
- Inappropriate feeding schedule.

FORMULA TYPES

- Cow's milk-based for healthy premature and term infants (Similac, Enfamil).
- Soy protein-based for galactosemia or lactose intolerance (Isomil, ProSobee).
- Protein hydrolysate for infants with malabsorption or food allergies (Nutramigen, Pregestimil, Alimentum).
- Free amino acid-based for food allergies, short gut (Neocate, EleCare).
- High medium-chain triglyceride oil for chylous ascites or chylothorax.
- Formulas for specific metabolic diseases, such as PKU (Lofenalac) or propionic academia (Propimex-1).
- Inappropriate formulas (see Table 5-2).

SOLID FOODS

- Solids should be introduced around 6 months; an earlier introduction does not contribute to a healthier child nor help the infant to sleep better.
- New foods should be introduced individually, about a week apart to identify any allergies and intolerance (rash, vomiting, diarrhea). The order of introduction is controversial with few data. Iron-fortified rice cereal is often recommended. New data suggest that for breastfed infants, initiation with meats may result in improved zinc intake and increased head circumference.

TABLE 5-2. Inappropriate Formulas

Cow's milk	↓ iron, essential fatty acids, vitamin E
	↑ sodium, potassium, chloride, and protein
Goat's milk (not goat milk-based formula)	Allergen potential
	Very high potential renal solute load
	High protein
	Low in folate and iron
	Questionable pasteurization
Rice milk	Very low in protein and fat
	Low in electrolytes and almost all vitamins and minerals
Commercial soy milk (not soy formula)	Soy induces L-thyroxine depletion through fecal waste, creating an ↑ requirement for iodine, potentially → goiter

READINESS FOR SOLID FOODS

- Demonstration of exploratory feeding behaviors.
- Decreased tongue-protrusion reflex.
- Sits with support.
- Lack of head lag.
- Opens mouth to spoon.

CALORIC REQUIREMENTS

Estimated average requirement:
- 0–12 months: 90–120 kcal/kg/day.
- 1–2 years: 75–90 kcal/kg/day.
- 2–18 years depends on gender and physical-activity level.
  - In general, males have a higher caloric need than females, and those who are physically active have a higher caloric requirement than those who are sedentary.

Fluid Management

PHYSIOLOGIC COMPARTMENTS

Total Body Water (TBW)

TBW makes up 50–75% of the total body mass depending on age, sex, and fat content.

Distribution

- Intracellular fluid accounts for two-thirds of TBW and 50% of total body mass.
- Extracellular fluid accounts for one-third of TBW and 25% of total body mass.

EXAM TIP

The predominant fat in preterm infant formula is medium-chain triglycerides.

WARD TIP

The formula for an infant who is allergic to both cow milk and soy protein is hydrolysate formula.

WARD TIP

Do not give an infant under 6 months of age water or juice. Water fills them up; juice contains empty calories, and excess sugar can cause diarrhea.

WARD TIP

Typical formulas contain 20 kcal/ounce.

WARD TIP

Avoid foods that are choking risks, including small fruits, raw vegetables, nuts, candy, and gum.

WARD TIP

Neonates have a greater percentage of TBW per weight than do adults (about 70–75%).

Extracellular Fluid (ECF)

ECF is composed of plasma (intravascular volume) and interstitial fluid (ISF).

MAINTENANCE FLUID THERAPY

Goals

Maintain normal perfusion of organs.

Methods

- Fluid requirements can be determined from caloric expenditure.
- For each 100 kcal metabolized in 24 hours, the average patient will require 100 mL of water, 2–4 mEq Na^+, and 2–3 mEq K^+.
- This method overestimates fluid requirements in neonates under 3 kg.

Maintenance

- Replacement of *normal* body fluid loss.
- Causes of water fluid loss per 100 calories metabolized/day include:
    - Urinary loss: 60%.
    - Insensible fluid loss (i.e., lungs and skin): 35%.
    - Stool loss: 5%.
- Example: For a 25-kg patient, 100 cc/kg for first 10 kg (=1000 cc) + 50 cc/kg for second 10 kg (=500 cc) + 20 cc/kg for remainder (=100 cc)→total 1600 mL/day or 65 mL/hr over 24 hours (see Table 5-3).
- Ongoing controversy around use of hypotonic fluids (e.g., D5½NS) versus isotonic fluids (D5NS) for maintenance.

DEHYDRATION FLUID THERAPY

Goals

Rapidly expand the ECF volume and restore tissue perfusion, replenish fluid and electrolyte deficits, meet the patient's nutritional needs, and replace ongoing losses.

For signs, symptoms and diagnosis, see Table 5-4.

ETIOLOGY

- Causes can be divided into two categories:
    - decreased intake.
    - increased loss (e.g., vomiting, diarrhea).
- Hypovolemia gradually affects each organ system.

TREATMENT

- Oral rehydration is preferred, especially for mild to moderate dehydration. Contraindications include severe dehydration with altered mental status, gastrointestinal obstruction, and intolerance of oral formulation.

WARD TIP

Neonates have a greater percentage of TBW per weight than do adults (about 70–75%).

WARD TIP

You know a patient is dehydrated when he or she is **PARCHED**:

Decreased **P**ee, low blood **P**ressure
Sunken **A**nterior fontanel
Slow capillary **R**efill
Crying
Increased **H**eart rate
Decreased **E**lasticity of skin
Dryness of mucous membranes

WARD TIP

For convenience, use the Holliday-Segar method to determine maintenance intravenous (IVF) requirements:

- Give 100 mL/kg of water for the first 10 kg.
- For a child >10 kg and <20 kg, give 1000 mL + 50 mL/kg for each kilogram >10 kg.
- For a child >20 kg, give 1500 mL + 20 mL/kg for each kilogram >20 kg.

WARD TIP

Calculations for fluid therapy are just estimates—you must monitor the success of fluid replacement by measuring ins and outs, body weight, and clinical picture (see Table 5-4).

T A B L E 5 - 3 .   Calculating Maintenance Fluids per Day

BODY WEIGHT (KG)	MILLILITERS PER DAY	MILLILITERS PER HOUR
0–10	100/kg	4/kg
11–20	1000 + 50/kg over 10	40 + 2/kg over 10
>20	1500 + 20/kg over 20	60 + 1/kg over 20

TABLE 5-4.   Signs and Symptoms of Normonatremic Dehydration

	MILD	MODERATE	SEVERE
% Body weight loss	3–5%	6–9%	> 10%
General	Consolable	Irritable	Lethargic/obtunded
Heart rate	Regular	Increased	More increased
Blood pressure	Normal	Normal/low	Low
Tears	Normal	Reduced	None
Urine	Normal	Reduced	Oliguric/anuric
Skin turgor	Normal	Tenting	None
Anterior fontanel	Flat	Soft	Sunken
Capillary refill	< 2 sec	2–3 sec	> 3 sec
Mucous membranes	Moist	Dry	Parched/cracked

- Parenteral:
  - During the urgent phase, restore intravascular volume to ensure vital organ perfusion with a bolus of 20 cc/kg normal saline or Ringer's lactate.
  - During the correction phase, gradually correct the water and electrolyte abnormalities. Isonatremic and acute hyponatremic dehydration are corrected over 24 hours. Chronic hyponatremic and hypernatremic dehydration are replenished over 48 hours.

ELECTROLYTE DISTURBANCE

Hyponatremia

In hyponatremia, serum Na^+ < 135 mEq/L.

ETIOLOGY

- Hypervolemic hyponatremia: relatively larger water than sodium retention.
  - Congestive heart failure.
  - Cirrhosis.
  - Nephrotic syndrome.
  - Acute or chronic renal failure.
- Hypovolemic hyponatremia: increased sodium loss along with water loss.
  - Due to renal loss:
    - Diuretic excess, osmotic diuresis, salt-wasting diuresis.
    - Adrenal insufficiency, pseudohypoaldosteronism.
    - Salt-losing nephropathies (interstitial nephritis, polycystic kidney disease).
  - Due to extra-renal loss:
    - Gastrointestinal (GI): vomiting, diarrhea.
    - Sweat, especially in patients with cystic fibrosis.
    - Third-spacing: pancreatitis, burns, muscle trauma, peritonitis, effusions, ascites.

WARD TIP

Percentage of dehydration can be estimated using (pre-illness weight – illness weight / pre-illness weight) × 100%.

WARD TIP

4-2-1 IVF RULE: To determine the **maintenance** rate in milliliters per hour, use 4 (for first 10 kg) × 10 kg + 2 (for second 10 kg) × 10 kg + 1 (for remainder) × remaining kg = mL/hr. Example: for a 16 kg patient, IVF rate is (4cc/hr × 10kg) + (2cc/hr × 6kg) = 52cc/hr

WARD TIP

Hyponatremia can be factitious in the presence of high plasma lipids or proteins; consider the presence of another osmotically active solute in the ECF, such as glucose or mannitol when hypotonicity is absent.

- Euvolemic hyponatremia:
  - Syndrome of inappropriate antidiuretic hormone secretion (SIADH)
    - Stress (such as hospitalization, pain, postoperative state)
    - Tumors.
    - Chest disorders.
    - Central nervous system (CNS) disorders: infection, trauma, shunt failure.
    - Drugs: vincristine, thiazide diuretics, carbamazepine, amitriptyline, opioids, isoproterenol, nicotine, nonsteroidal anti-inflammatory drugs, colchicine, ecstasy.
  - Glucocorticoid deficiency.
  - Hypothyroidism.
  - Water intoxication due to intravenous (IV) therapy, tap-water enema, or psychogenic (excess water drinking).

Signs and Symptoms

- Acute hyponatremia causes symptoms at higher sodium levels than chronic hyponatremia.
- Cerebral edema, apnea, and brainstem herniation occur, especially in acute hyponatremia.
- Signs include anorexia, nausea, headache, mental status changes, posturing, autonomic dysfunction, respiratory depression, seizures, and coma.
- Central-pontine myelinolysis can occur if hyponatremia is corrected too quickly.

Diagnosis

- Assess volume status.
- Determine if it is an acute or a chronic condition.
- Serum and urine osmolality and sodium concentration, blood urea nitrogen (BUN), creatinine, other labs (glucose, aldosterone, thyroid-stimulating hormone [TSH], etc.).

Treatment

- See "Dehydration Fluid Therapy" above.
- If serum Na^+ is low and CNS symptoms are present, a 3% NaCl solution may be given via an IV over 1 hour to raise the serum Na^+ and prevent further neurologic damage.

Hypernatremia

Serum $Na^+ > 145$ mEq/L.

Etiology

- Decreased water or increased sodium intake.
- Decreased sodium or increased water output.
- Diabetes insipidus (nephrogenic or central) due to urinary free-water losses.
- Hypovolemic hypernatremia:
  - Extrarenal (skin or GI) or renal fluid losses.
  - Decreased thirst (behavioral or hypothalamic thirst center damage).
- Hypervolemic hypernatremia:
  - Hypertonic saline infusion.
  - Sodium bicarbonate administration.
  - Accidental salt ingestion.
  - Mineralocorticoid excess (Cushing syndrome).
- Euvolemic hypernatremia:
  - Extrarenal losses: increased insensible loss.
  - Renal free water losses: central or nephrogenic diabetes insipidus (DI).

SIGNS AND SYMPTOMS

- Anorexia, nausea, irritability.
- Mental status changes.
- Muscle twitching, ataxia.

TREATMENT

- Reduction of elevated serum Na^+ is done gradually at a rate of no greater than 12 mEq/L/day.
- During the urgent phase, restore the intravascular volume to ensure vital-organ perfusion with a bolus of 20 cc/kg normal saline (not Ringer's lactate).
- During the correction phase, it varies, but typically, fluid might be D5½NS (with 20 mEq/L KCl if urinating) run at 1.25x to 1.5x the maintenance rate.
- Too rapidly correcting hypernatremia can result in cerebral edema.

Hypokalemia

Serum $K^+ < 3.5$ mEq/L, but generally asymptomatic until < 3.0 mEq/L

ETIOLOGY

Excess renin, excess mineralocorticoid, Cushing syndrome, renal tubular acidosis (RTA), Fanconi syndrome, Bartter syndrome, diuretic use/abuse, GI losses, skin losses, diabetic ketoacidosis (DKA), transcellular shifts (alkalemia, insulin, refeeding syndrome), anorexia.

SIGNS AND SYMPTOMS

Decreased peristalsis/ileus, hyporeflexia, paralysis, rhabdomyolysis, muscle weakness/cramps, and arrhythmias (premature ventricular contractions, atrial nodal or ventricular tachycardia, and ventricular fibrillation).

DIAGNOSIS

- Serum value.
- Electrocardiogram (ECG) may demonstrate flattened T waves, depressed ST segment, and U waves.

TREATMENT

- Cardiac monitor.
- If K^+ is dangerously low (< 2.5 mEq/L) and the patient is symptomatic, use IV potassium.
- Do not exceed the K^+ infusion rate of 0.5 to 1 mEq/kg/hr.
- Oral K^+ may be given to replenish stores over a longer period of time.

Hyperkalemia

- Mild to moderate: $K^+ = 5.5$–7.0.
- Severe: $K^+ > 7.0$.

ETIOLOGY

Renal failure, hypoaldosteronism, aldosterone insensitivity, K^+-sparing diuretics, cell breakdown (hemolysis, rhabdomyolysis, tumor lysis), metabolic acidosis, transfusion with aged blood, leukocytosis, exercise, malignant hyperthermia, lupus nephritis, NSAIDs, heparin.

EXAM TIP

A hypervolemic hypernatremic condition can be caused by the administration of improperly mixed formula, or this condition may present as a primary hyperaldosteronism. Review with parents the proper mixing of formula.

WARD TIP

If the serum Na^+ falls rapidly, cerebral edema, seizures, and cerebral injury may occur, secondary to fluid shifts from the ECF into the CNS.

WARD TIP

Hypokalemia can precipitate digitalis toxicity.

WARD TIP

For every 0.1-unit reduction in serum pH, there is an increase in serum K^+ of about 0.2–0.4 mEq/L.

SIGNS AND SYMPTOMS

Muscle weakness, paresthesias, tetany, ascending paralysis, and arrhythmias including sinus bradycardia, sinus arrest, atrioventricular block, nodal or idioventricular rhythms, and ventricular tachycardia and fibrillation.

DIAGNOSIS

- Serum value.
- ECG may demonstrate peaked T waves, prolonged PR interval, and wide QRS.

TREATMENT

- If hyperkalemia is severe or symptomatic, the priorities are to stabilize the cardiac membrane and remove K^+.
- Administer calcium chloride or gluconate solution to stabilize cardiac membranes.
- Sodium bicarbonate, nebulized albuterol, or glucose plus insulin can be given to shift K^+ to the intracellular compartment.
- Kayexalate resin can be given to bind K^+ in the gut (this treatment works slowly).
- Furosemide can be given to enhance urinary K^+ excretion.
- In extreme cases, hemo- or peritoneal dialysis may be necessary.

Vitamin and Mineral Supplements

FLUORIDE

- Supplement after age 6 months for nonfluoridated water (particularly well water).
- If <0.3 ppm in the family's water supply, supplement with 0.25 mg/day for children 6 months to 3 years.
- Deficiency: dental caries.
- Excess: fluorosis—mottling, staining, or hypoplasia of the enamel.
- Children <6 years should be supervised when brushing to avoid swallowing toothpaste. Children <2 years of age should use a "smear" of fluoridated toothpaste; children <6 years of age should use a pea-sized amount.

VITAMIN D

- Vitamin D is critical for skeletal development and cellular function because of its effect on calcium homeostasis (by promoting intestinal calcium absorption).
- Breast milk contains about 25 IU/L of vitamin D, which may be insufficient for rickets prevention.
- Deficiency can occur if exclusively or partially breastfed, or if the infant is fed on whole cow's milk.
- Supplementation is with 400 IU/day.
- With a deficiency, impaired mineralization of bone tissue (osteomalacia) and of growth plates (rickets) occurs.
- Vitamin D deficiency can cause hypocalcemia.

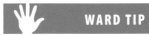

WARD TIP

Because of the increased risk for fluorosis, don't give fluoride supplements before age 6 months.

WARD TIP

Most bottled water is not fluoridated; check labels to be sure.

IRON

A 4-year-old female is seen for the sudden onset of diarrhea and vomiting. The mother reports blood in the vomitus. On examination, the child is very irritable. She is breathing rapidly, and her heart rate is 167 beats/min, with a blood pressure of 96/57 mm Hg. The mother states that the child is healthy with no recent illnesses; she is current on vaccinations. No travel is reported. Her 3-year-old brother is not ill. The child's diet has not changed. The mother states that she is very conscientious of the diets in the house because she is trying to get pregnant. *Think: Iron overdose.*

Iron poisoning is often fatal in children. Iron preparations are readily available due to their use in prenatal care. The brightly colored tablets appear similar to candy, and some are sucrose-coated to make them palatable and thus attractive to children. Iron poisoning should be considered in a child with acute onset of vomiting and hypoperfusion. Serum iron levels are helpful in predicting the patient's clinical course.

- Newborn iron stores are sufficient for 6 months in a term infant.
- Therefore, breastfed infants need iron supplementation 1 mg/kg/day (i.e., iron-fortified cereals and baby foods) beginning at 4 to 6 months.
- Preterm breastfed infants should receive 2 mg/kg/day starting at 2 months of age.
- Iron deficiency results in anemia (hypochromic, microcytic) and growth failure.
- Only iron-fortified formula should be used for weaning or for supplementing breast milk in children younger than 12 months; low iron formula is not appropriate.

VITAMIN K

- Vitamin K is necessary for the synthesis of clotting factors II, VII, IX, and X.
- Human breast milk is vitamin K deficient, and all infants have limited body stores.
- Thus, all infants require 1-mg vitamin K IM at birth.
- Vitamin K deficiency contributes to hemorrhagic disease of the newborn.
- Vitamin K is fat soluble and requires bile salts for absorption beyond the newborn period.

ZINC

- Serves as a catalyst for many enzymes.
- Deficiency-associated intestinal malabsorption, nutritional intake limited to breast milk beyond 4 to 6 months.
- Deficiency manifests as acrodermatitis, impaired immune system, growth failure.

VITAMIN A

A 14-month-old infant has anorexia, pruritus, and failure to gain weight; he has a bulging anterior fontanel and tender swelling over both tibias. The mother buys all the family's food at a natural foods store. *Think: Hypervitaminosis A.*

Acute vitamin A toxicity is not common. Symptoms include irritability, tiredness, and somnolence. A bulging fontanel due to increased intracranial pressure may be present in infants. Pain and tenderness, particularly in the long bones, may develop.

WARD TIP

Breast milk has less iron than cow's milk, but the iron in breast milk is more bioavailable.

- Hypovitaminosis A is associated with night blindness, hyperkeratosis of skin, poor growth, and increased infection.
- Hypervitaminosis A
  - Acute:
    - Pseudotumor cerebri: bulging fontanel, drowsiness, cranial nerve palsies.
    - Nausea, vomiting.
  - Chronic:
    - Poor weight gain.
    - Irritability.
    - Tender swelling of bones—hyperostosis of long bones, craniotabes; decreased mineralization of skull.
    - Pruritus, fissures, desquamation.

OTHER SUPPLEMENTS

- If a breastfeeding mother is a strict vegan, supplementation with B12 is recommended.
- Commercial formula is often modified from cow's milk and fortified with vitamins and minerals so that no additional supplements are needed for the full-term infant.
- Children maintaining strictly vegan diets require attention to adequate caloric, vitamin D, zinc, and iron intake. Supplementation with B12 is recommended.

Obesity

DEFINITION

- Pediatric definitions:
  - Overweight is a body mass index (BMI)-for-age in the 85th to 94th percentile.
  - Obese is a BMI-for-age >95th percentile.
- BMI is calculated by dividing weight (in kilograms) by height (in meters squared).
- Adults:
  - Normal BMI: 18.5–24.9 kg/m².
  - Overweight: 25.0–29.9 kg/m².
  - Obesity: 30.0–39.9 kg/m².
  - Extreme obesity: >40 kg/m².

RISK FACTORS

- Excessive intake of high-energy foods ("empty" calories).
- Inadequate exercise in relation to age and activity, sedentary lifestyle.
- Low metabolic rate relative to body composition and mass
- Cause: combination of socioeconomic status and genetics.
  - Higher incidence in children of obese parents.
  - Higher incidence in minorities and the economically disadvantaged.
- Certain genetic disorders (Cushing syndrome, hyperinsulinism, Laurence-Moon-Bardet-Biedl syndrome, muscular dystrophy, Down syndrome, Prader-Willi syndrome, hypothyroidism, pseudohypoparathyroidism, Turner syndrome).

COMPLICATIONS

- Negative social attitudes: embarrassment, harassment, low self-esteem.
- Behavioral: depression, anxiety, disordered eating, worsening school performance, social isolation.

- Respiratory: obstructive sleep apnea, snoring.
- Orthopedic: slipped capital femoral epiphysis (SCFE), back pain, joint pain.
- Endocrine: type 2 diabetes mellitus, metabolic syndrome.
- Cardiovascular: hypertension, hyperlipidemia.
- Gastrointestinal: gallbladder disease, nonalcoholic fatty liver disease.

PREVENTION

- Parent education regarding appropriate nutrition and feeding habits.
- Promote exercise (60 min/day) and limit screen time.
- Avoid overfeeding when children are upset.
- Newborns are fed on demand.
- Begin a feeding schedule in the first year; offer food only when the child is hungry.
- Have predictable eating schedules; offer child-sized portions using child-sized plates.
- Avoid using food as a reward or punishment.

DIAGNOSIS

BMI is the most useful index for screening for obesity. It correlates well with subcutaneous fat, total body fat, blood pressure, blood lipid levels, and lipoprotein concentrations in adolescents.

TREATMENT

- Adherence to a well-organized program, including a balanced diet *and* exercise.
- Behavioral modification.
- Involvement of family in therapy.
- Surgery and pharmacotherapy should be used judiciously in children.
- Very-low-calorie diets are detrimental to growth and development—all nutritional needs should be met.
- Avoid rapid decrease in weight.
- The goal of effective weight management in children is not so much to lose pounds but to maintain weight through growth spurts.
- If BMI is >97th percentile for age and sex, weight reduction may be recommended even prior to pubertal growth spurt.

WARD TIP

For risks associated with obesity, think
SHADE:
 SCFE
 Hypertension
 Apnea (sleep)
 Diabetes
 Embarrassment

NOTES

Health Supervision and Prevention of Illness and Injury in Children and Adolescents

Morbidity and Mortality

- The leading cause of death in children <1 year of age is the effect of congenital malformations, deformations, and chromosomal abnormalities. Rounding out the top five are:
  - Prematurity.
  - Unintentional injury.
  - Sudden infant death syndrome (SIDS).
  - Complications of pregnancy.
- From 1 year to 24 years of age, the leading cause of death is unintentional injuries. The most common injury leading to death is:
  - From 1 year to 4 years, drowning.
  - From 4 years to 24 years, motor vehicle crash.

Prevention

Prevention is of primary importance in caring for the pediatric patient and is promoted through:

- Parental guidance (anticipatory guidance and counseling).
- Screening tests.
- Immunization.

Parental Guidance

Age-appropriate anticipatory guidance is provided at various well-child visits.

1 WEEK–1 MONTH

 A 1-month-old infant is brought to the emergency department (ED) with poor feeding, weak suck, drooling, constipation, and decreased spontaneous movements. He is exclusively breastfed, and his mother has been giving him a home remedy for "colic." Physical exam shows hypotonia. *Consider: botulism* and its relationship to some home remedies prepared with honey. Treatment is with human botulism immune globulin (BIG-IV).

- Sudden infant death syndrome (SIDS) prevention includes:
  - Placing the infant to sleep on their back (not side or stomach).
  - No co-sleeping.
  - No soft objects, loose bedding (comforters, pillows, bumper pads), or stuffed animals in crib.
  - Maintaining a smoke-free environment.
- Use a car seat, rear facing in back seat and buckled in.
- Know the signs of illness.
- Use a rectal thermometer.
- Set water temperature at <120°F (48.8°C). Know that it takes 5 minutes for a baby to get a burn at this temperature, 10 seconds at 130°F, and 3 seconds at 140°F.
- Do not give honey to a child <1 year of age (botulism risk).

- Discuss normal crying behavior and give suggestions for infant calming, such as swaddling in a light blanket, rocking in a cradle, or using a windup swing/vibrating chair.
- Never shake your baby.
- Assess parental well-being using a validated tool (e.g., Edinburgh Postnatal Depression Scale). "Baby blues" are normal, but if they persist beyond 2 weeks, provide resources for postpartum depression.
- The AAP recommends supplemental vitamin D for breastfed babies.

2 MONTHS–1 YEAR

- Childproof the home to keep children safe from poisons, household cleaners, medications, water-filled buckets and tubs, plastic bags, electrical outlets, hot liquids, matches, small and sharp objects, guns, and knives.
- Syrup of ipecac is no longer recommended. Provide the poison-control hotline number.
- Do not introduce solid food until around 6 months.
- Introduce single-ingredient foods one at a time to assess for allergies.
- Do not introduce fruit juice until >1 year of age.
- Avoid using baby walkers.
- Do not put baby to bed with a bottle; milk can pool around the front teeth and cause dental caries ("baby bottle caries").
- Breastfeed or give iron-fortified formula; introduce whole milk <u>after</u> 1 year of age.
- Avoid choking hazards (coins, peanuts, popcorn, carrot sticks, hard candy, whole grapes, and hot dogs).
- May start using sippy cup at 6–9 months.
- Do not leave baby alone in a tub or high places.
- Do not drink hot liquids while holding your baby.
- Realize the importance of tummy time to meet milestones and decrease positional plagiocephaly.
- Visit the dentist after the first tooth erupts or by 12 months.

1–5 YEARS

- Use a toddler car seat (ages 1–4); switch to booster seat for older children of the appropriate weight and height. See the car seat section.
- Limit screen time in children <18 months to video chat, to supervised high-quality learning programs and apps for children 18–24 months, and to <1 hour daily for children 2–5 years old.
- Brush teeth twice daily with plain water and a soft toothbrush, and see the dentist twice a year.
- Limit juice to <4 ounces a day.
- Wean from bottle (start by 9 months of age with the introduction of a cup).
- Ensure home is childproof.
- Restrict the child's access to stairs.
- Allow the child to eat with their hands or utensils.
- Use sunscreen (can use as early as 6 months).
- Wear properly fitting bicycle helmet.
- Provide close supervision, especially near dogs, driveways, streets, and lawnmowers.
- Ensure the child is supervised when near water; build a fence with latched gate around all four sides of a swimming pool.
- Screen for amblyopia, strabismus, and visual acuity.
  - Strabismus: cover or use a Hirschberg corneal light-reflex test in children <3 years.
  - Visual acuity: >3 years with screening every 1–2 years thereafter.

EXAM TIP

Exposure to second-hand smoke increases:
- Incidence of SIDS.
- URI.
- Lower respiratory-tract infections (bronchiolitis, pneumonia).
- RAD and asthma.
- Ear infections.

EXAM TIP

Any child with a rectal temperature >100.4°F (38°C) in the first 2 months of life should be seen immediately and evaluated for sepsis. Top bacterial causes are Group B *Streptococcus, Listeria,* coagulase negative *Staphylococcus,* and *E. coli.*

WARD TIP

Assess head control before allowing baby to start solid foods to decrease the risk of choking.

EXAM TIP

Falls and drowning are major risks of injury and death in toddlers.

EXAM TIP

Most infants drown in their own bathtub.

- Early childhood caries (cavities) is the number 1 chronic disease affecting children.
- Early childhood caries is four times more common than asthma.

Water heater temperature should be kept below 120°F (49°C) to prevent accidental scalding injuries.

Adolescent HEEADDSSS assessment
Home
Education
Eating
Activities
Drugs and Alcohol
Depression
Safety
Sex
Suicide

6–10 YEARS

- Reinforce personal hygiene.
- Teach stranger safety.
- Provide healthy meals and snacks. Eat 5+ servings of fruits and vegetables a day; eat breakfast.
- Limit digital media before bedtime, and do not allow devices in the child's bedroom.
- Be physically active 60 minutes a day.
- Keep matches and guns out of reach.
- Use a booster seat until the child is 4 feet 9 inches in height, and then always use a seat belt.
- Brush teeth twice daily with pea-sized amount of fluoride toothpaste.
- Ensure adequate sleep (8–12 hours a day).
- Visit a dentist twice a year.
- Teach pedestrian safety.
- Teach children to swim.

11–21 YEARS

- Continue to support a healthy diet and exercise.
- Wear appropriate protective sports gear.
- Counsel on safe sex and avoiding alcohol and drugs.
- Promote a healthy social life, balanced diet, and at least 60 minutes of exercise every day, with 30 minutes of vigorous exercise 3 times per week.
- Ask about mood or eating disorders.
- Address school performance, homework, and bullying.

Screening

BLOOD PRESSURE

- High blood pressure (hypertension) is blood pressure (BP) that is the same as or higher than 95% of children who are the same sex, age, and height as your child.
- Annual BP monitoring should begin at age 3 years.
  - Children who are obese, have heart and kidney diseases, are taking medications that increase BP or have diabetes should have their BP checked at every visit.
- The most common cause of a high BP reading in children is inappropriate cuff size.
- High BP can be primary or secondary; the younger the child and the higher the BP, the higher the likelihood the high BP has an identifiable cause.
- Contributing factors include family history, race, excess weight, or obesity.

METABOLIC SCREENING

The specific diseases tested for in metabolic screening vary from state to state in the United States.

The newborn screen tests for disorders for which early management may prevent long-term poor health outcomes. At 24 hours of life, the neonate should receive screening for various metabolic disorders including hypothyroidism, phenylketonuria (PKU), sickle cell disease, and adrenal cortex abnormalities.

Some states mandate a second metabolic screening at around 1–2 weeks of age. (See Metabolic chapter.)

LEAD SCREENING

- Exposure is increased by:
  - Living in or visiting a house built before 1978 with peeling or chipped paint.
  - Plumbing with lead pipes or lead solder joints.
  - Living near a major highway where soil may be contaminated with lead.
  - Contact with someone who works with lead.
  - Living near an industrial site that may release lead into the environment.
  - Taking home remedies that may contain lead.
  - Playing with lead-containing toys.
  - Using traditional cosmetics (e.g., kohl, an ancient cosmetic sometimes made with lead sulfide, often used as eyeliner).
  - Having friends/relatives who have had lead poisoning.
- Screen for lead levels at age 12 months and 24 months.

HEMATOCRIT

- Screen for anemia at 9–12 months of age if the appropriate risk factors are present.
- Have a second test 6 months later in high-risk communities for iron deficiency.
- Annually screen children from ages 2–5 years with risk factors.
- Risk factors for anemia include low socioeconomic status, birth weight under 1500g, whole milk received before 6 months of age, low-iron formula given, and low intake of iron-rich foods.
- Adolescent females with low iron intake, heavy menstrual flow, or a history of iron deficiency anemia should be screened annually from ages 12–21.

HYPERLIPIDEMIA

- Screen for hyperlipidemia in children older than 2 years with appropriate risk factors, including:
  - Family history of coronary or peripheral vascular disease before the age of 55 years in parents or grandparents.
  - Parent with a total serum cholesterol level >240 mg/dL.
  - Obesity.
  - Hypertension.
  - Diabetes mellitus.
- Screening may also be considered in children with inactivity and in adolescents who smoke.
- All children should be screened between 9 and 11 years and again between 17 and 21 years.

VISION AND HEARING

- A hearing screen is recommended shortly after birth, ideally before discharge from the newborn nursery, using a screening auditory brainstem response (AABR) or an otoacoustic emissions (OAE) test.
- Vision screening may begin at age 3 years, sooner if concerns arise.

WARD TIP

Infants and young children are more likely to be exposed to lead than are older children. They may chew paint chips, and their hands may be contaminated with lead dust. Young children also absorb lead more easily and sustain more harm from it than do adults and older children.

- Suspect hearing loss earlier if speech is not developing appropriately.
- A child's cooperation is essential to obtaining an accurate result (possible at about 3 years).

MENTAL HEALTH

- Mental health screening should be part of all well-child visits.
- Validated screening questionnaires are used with the child, the parent, or both. Examples include:
  - Edinburgh Postnatal Depression Scale for new mother.
  - Pediatric Symptom Checklist (17 or 35 items) for general psychosocial screening.
  - Vanderbilt Diagnostic Rating Scales for ADHD, disruptive behavior, anxiety, and depression.
  - Modified Checklist for Autism in Toddlers (M-CHAT).

TUBERCULOSIS (TB)

- Asymptomatic children at high risk for TB should be screened with a purified protein derivative (PPD) test annually.
- The QuantiFERON®-TB Gold Plus test (QFT-Plus) is an Interferon-Gamma Release Assay (IRGA) alternative for TB detection.
  - Does not boost responses measured by subsequent tests, which can happen with tuberculin skin tests (TSTs).
  - Not subject to reader bias, which can occur with TSTs.
  - Not affected by prior BCG (bacille Calmette-Guérin) vaccination.

WARD TIP

Ask the following questions to determine the need for a PPD:
- Has a family member or contact had tuberculosis disease?
- Has a family member had a positive tuberculin skin test?
- Was your child born in a high-risk country (countries other than the United States, Canada, Australia, New Zealand, or Western European countries)?
- Has your child traveled (had contact with resident populations) to a high-risk country for more than one week?

AAP Car Seat Recommendations

- Infants and toddlers: rear facing only or rear facing convertible (until 2 years and 20 lbs).
- Toddlers and preschoolers: convertible or forward facing with harness (until 4 years and 40 lbs).
- School aged: booster seats (until 4 feet 9 inches tall).
- Older children: when large enough, use standard lap and shoulder belts. Younger than 13 should sit in backseat.
- Other car seat notes:
  - Never place a car seat in front of an air bag (front passenger-side and side-impact air bags).
  - The safest place for the infant is the middle portion of the rear seat.
  - Each car seat has different weight limits, so the above numbers are guides. Parents should follow the weight limits of their car seat.

WARD TIP

Newborns should not leave the hospital without a car seat.

Vaccines

- See latest CDC vaccine schedule which is updated annually (Figure 6-1).
- Site of injection
  - Infants: anterolateral thigh.
  - Children: deltoid.

These recommendations must be read with the notes that follow. For those who fall behind or start late, provide catch-up vaccination at the earliest opportunity as indicated by the green bars. To determine minimum intervals between doses, see the catch-up schedule (Table 2).

Vaccine	Birth	1 mo	2 mos	4 mos	6 mos	9 mos	12 mos	15 mos	18 mos	19–23 mos	2–3 yrs	4–6 yrs	7–10 yrs	11–12 yrs	13–15 yrs	16 yrs	17–18 yrs
Hepatitis B (HepB)	1st dose	←--- 2nd dose ---→					←--- 3rd dose ---→										
Rotavirus (RV): RV1 (2-dose series), RV5 (3-dose series)			1st dose	2nd dose	See Notes												
Diphtheria, tetanus, acellular pertussis (DTaP <7 yrs)			1st dose	2nd dose	3rd dose			←--- 4th dose ---→				5th dose					
***Haemophilus influenzae* type b (Hib)**			1st dose	2nd dose	See Notes		←3rd or 4th dose, See Notes→										
Pneumococcal conjugate (PCV13)			1st dose	2nd dose	3rd dose		←--- 4th dose ---→										
Inactivated poliovirus (IPV <18 yrs)			1st dose	2nd dose			←--- 3rd dose ---→					4th dose					
Influenza (IIV4)								Annual vaccination 1 or 2 doses							Annual vaccination 1 dose only		
or													or				
Influenza (LAIV4)											Annual vaccination 1 or 2 doses				Annual vaccination 1 dose only		
Measles, mumps, rubella (MMR)					See Notes		←--- 1st dose ---→					2nd dose					
Varicella (VAR)							←--- 1st dose ---→					2nd dose					
Hepatitis A (HepA)					See Notes			2-dose series, See Notes									
Tetanus, diphtheria, acellular pertussis (Tdap ≥7 yrs)														1 dose			
Human papillomavirus (HPV)														See Notes			
Meningococcal (MenACWY-D ≥9 mos, MenACWY-CRM ≥2 mos, MenACWY-TT ≥2years)								See Notes						1st dose		2nd dose	
Meningococcal B (MenB-4C, MenB-FHbp)															See Notes		
Pneumococcal polysaccharide (PPSV23)														See Notes			
Dengue (DEN4CYD; 9-16 yrs)															Seropositive in endemic areas only (See Notes)		

Range of recommended ages for all children

Range of recommended ages for catch-up vaccination

Range of recommended ages for certain high-risk groups

Recommended vaccination can begin in this age group

Recommended vaccination based on shared clinical decision-making

No recommendation/not applicable

FIGURE 6-1. Recommended Immunization Schedule for Children and Adolescents Aged 18 Years or Younger—United States, 2022. Source: Centers for Disease Control and Prevention. Immunization Schedules. https://www.cdc.gov/vaccines/schedules/index.html.

HEPATITIS B

 A 25-year-old female who is hepatitis B surface antigen positive is about to deliver a baby, and she asks the best way to keep the baby from having hepatitis B. *Think: Prevention.* Babies born to women who are hepatitis B surface antigen positive receive hepatitis B immunoglobulin and hepatitis B vaccine within 12 hours after birth. These infants then receive at 1 month and at 6 months a hepatitis B vaccine. At the 9-12 months well-child visit, after completing three doses of hepatitis B vaccine, the baby should be tested for hepatitis B surface antigen and the antibody.

- The first dose is given intramuscularly (IM) at birth or within first 2 months of life.
- The second dose is given at least 1 month after the first dose.
- The third dose is given at least 4 months after the first dose and at least 2 months after the second dose, but not before 6 months of age.
- If the baby is exposed to hepatitis B transplacentally or if the maternal status is unknown, a dose must be given at birth with hepatitis B immune globulin (HBIG).
- Infants born to mothers who are positive for hepatitis B surface antigen (HBsAg-positive) should be tested for HBsAg and for the antibody to HBsAg after completion of at least three doses of the HepB vaccine, at about age 9 months.

CONTENT

Recombinant noninfectious hepatitis B surface antigen proteins are produced in yeast cells.

SIDE EFFECTS

- Pain at injection site in 3 to 29%.
- Fever >99.9°F (37.7°C) in 1–6%.

CONTRAINDICATIONS

Anaphylactic reaction to vaccine, yeast, or another vaccine constituent.

PRECAUTIONS

For infants born <2 kg at birth to hepatitis B negative mothers, wait until one month of age or hospital discharge, whichever comes first.

DIPHTHERIA, TETANUS, AND ACELLULAR PERTUSSIS (DTaP)

- Minimum age: 6 weeks.
- DTaP is given IM at 2, 4, and 6 months, with a fourth dose given between 15 and 18 months of age.
- The fourth dose can be given as early as age 12 months provided 6 months occur between third and fourth doses.
- Administer the final dose at age 4–6 years.
- DT without the pertussis vaccine can be used in children <7 years of age if the pertussis vaccine is contraindicated.
- Tdap is administered at age 10–12.

CONTENT

- DTaP is diphtheria and tetanus toxoids with acellular pertussis.
- DTP contains a whole-cell pertussis.

WARD TIP

Fever is not a contraindication to receiving immunization. Moderate/severe illness is a precaution, not a contraindication. This holds true for all vaccines.

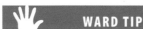
EXAM TIP

DTaP is used for children under 7 years of age. Td or Tdap is given after 7 years of age.

EXAM TIP

DTP (using the whole inactivated pertussis organism) has greater risks of side effects than DTaP (which uses an immunogenic portion of the pertussis organism, a = acellular). DTP is no longer used in the United States.

SIDE EFFECTS

- Erythema, pain, and swelling at the injection site.
- Fever >100.4°F (38°C).
- Crying ≥1 hour.
- Severe side effects (more common with DTP, very rare with DTaP): crying >3 hours; hypotonic-hyporesponsive episode; seizures; fever >40.5°C.

CONTRAINDICATIONS

- Severe allergic reaction (e.g., anaphylaxis) after a previous dose or to a vaccine component.
- Encephalopathy not attributable to another cause within 7 days of a prior dose of pertussis vaccine.

PRECAUTIONS

- Seizure disorder or seizures within 3 days of receiving a previous DTaP dose:
    - Precautions include poorly controlled or new-onset seizures. Defer pertussis immunization until the seizure disorder is well controlled and any progressive neurologic disorder is excluded.
    - Personal or family history of febrile seizures are other precautions to consider. Give DTaP and antipyretics around the clock for 24 hours after immunization.
- Temperature of 40.5°C (104.8°F) within 48 hours after immunization with previous dose of DTaP.
- Collapse or shock-like state (hypotonic-hyporesponsive episode within 48 hours of receiving a previous dose of DTaP).
- Persistent inconsolable crying lasting >3 hours within 48 hours of receiving a previous dose of DTaP.
- Guillain-Barré syndrome within 6 weeks after a prior dose.

EXAM TIP

DTaP is not a substitute for DTP if a contraindication to pertussis exists.

WARD TIP

A common misconception is that DTaP is contraindicated in patients with a family history of seizure or SIDS. This is NOT true.

HAEMOPHILUS INFLUENZAE TYPE B (HIB)

- Minimum age: 6 weeks.
- Given IM at 2, 4, and 6 months of age, and then again between 12 and 15 months of age.

CONTENT

Consists of a capsular polysaccharide antigen (polyribosylribitol phosphate, PRP) conjugated to a protein carrier.

SIDE EFFECTS

Erythema, pain, and swelling at the injection site in 25%; other side effects are extremely rare.

CONTRAINDICATIONS

Anaphylactic reaction to vaccine or vaccine components.

MEASLES, MUMPS, AND RUBELLA (MMR)

A 12-month-old boy is due for his vaccines in the middle of October. His mother mentions that he developed a skin rash as well as some respiratory problems the previous month after she fed him eggs for the first time. He is due for MMR, varicella, and influenza vaccines. *Think: Egg allergy.* Historically this has been a contraindication, but recommendations have evolved, and MMR can be given with caution to children with egg allergy.

- Minimum age: 12 months (9 months in countries with high measles incidence and mortality).
- First dose given subcutaneously (SC) at 12–15 months of age and second dose at 4–6 years of age.
- The second dose may be given at any time after 4 weeks from the first dose, if necessary.
- Must be at least 12 months old; repeat any dose before 12 months.

CONTENT

Composed of live attenuated viruses, neomycin, gelatin, and several other inactive ingredients.

SIDE EFFECTS

- Fever >102.9°F (39.4°C) 6–12 days after immunization can last up to 5 days in 10%.
- Transient rash in 5%; may occur 1–6 weeks after vaccination.
- Febrile seizures and encephalopathy with MMR vaccine are rare. Transient thrombocytopenia may occur 2–3 weeks after vaccine in 1/40,000.
- Swollen lymph nodes.
- Pain or stiffness in joints.

CONTRAINDICATIONS

- Anaphylactic reaction to prior vaccine.
- Anaphylactic reaction to neomycin or gelatin.
- Immunocompromised states, but <u>acceptable</u> for HIV+ without clinical manifestations and CD4 >200.
- Pregnant women.

PRECAUTIONS

- Recent intravenous immunoglobulin (IVIG) administration or blood transfusion requires delaying MMR vaccination.
- Thrombocytopenia or a history of thrombocytopenic purpura, however the benefits of the vaccine outweigh risks of low platelet count.

INACTIVATED POLIOVIRUS (IPV)

- Minimum age: 6 weeks.
- IPV is given IM or SQ at 2 and 4 months, then again between 6 and 18 months, and then a fourth between 4 and 6 years of age.
- The final dose should be administered on or after the fourth birthday and at least 6 months following the previous dose.
- Oral poliovirus vaccine (OPV) is a live attenuated vaccine and is given orally. It is no longer used in the United States.
- IPV is frequently given as part of a combination vaccine.

CONTENT

- IPV contains inactivated poliovirus types 1, 2, and 3.
- Live OPV contains live attenuated poliovirus types 1, 2, and 3.

SIDE EFFECTS

- Vaccine-associated paralytic polio (VAPP) with OPV in 1/760,000.
- Local reactions, fever.

CONTRAINDICATIONS

- Anaphylaxis to vaccine or vaccine component.
- Anaphylaxis to streptomycin, polymyxin B, or neomycin.

VARICELLA

- Minimum age: 12 months.
- Given SC between 12 and 18 months of age; second dose between 4 and 6 years (may be administered before age 4, provided at least 3 months have elapsed since the first dose).
- Susceptible persons >13 years of age must receive two doses at least 4 weeks apart.

CONTENT

Live attenuated varicella virus, neomycin, gelatin, and other inactive ingredients.

SIDE EFFECTS

- Erythema and swelling in 20–35%.
- Fever in 10%.
- Varicelliform rash in 1–4%.

CONTRAINDICATIONS

- Anaphylactic reaction to vaccine, neomycin, or gelatin.
- Patients with altered immunity, including corticosteroid use for > 14 days.
- Patients with active untreated tuberculosis.
- Moderate or severe febrile illness.
- Pregnant women.

PRECAUTIONS

- Recent blood product or IG administration (defer the vaccine).
- Patients on salicylate therapy; should avoid salicylates for 6 weeks after vaccine administration.

INFLUENZA VACCINE (SEASONAL)

- Minimum age:
  - 6 months for quadrivalent inactivated influenza vaccine (IIV).
  - 2 years for live attenuated influenza vaccine (LAIV).
  - 18 years for recombinant influenza vaccine (RIV).
  - Given IM to children >6 months of age yearly beginning in autumn, usually between October and mid-November (two doses 1 month apart for the first time).
  - All children should receive this vaccine, especially high-risk children.

CONTENT

- IIV contains four virus strains, usually both type A and type B based on the expected prevalent influenza strains for the coming winter.
- Children <9 years of age should receive the "split" vaccine only.
- Children receiving the vaccine for the first time should receive 2 doses 1 month apart to obtain a good response.

SIDE EFFECTS

- Pain, swelling, and erythema at injection site.
- Fever may occur, especially in children <24 months of age.
- In children >13 years of age, fever may occur in up to 10%.

CONTRAINDICATIONS

Severe allergic reaction (e.g., anaphylaxis) after a previous dose of any IIV or LAIV or to a vaccine component, including egg protein.

EXAM TIP

Varicella vaccine contains live virus.

WARD TIP

It is especially important to vaccinate for influenza those with asthma, chronic lung disease, cardiac defects, immunosuppressive disorders, sickle cell anemia, chronic renal disease, and chronic metabolic disease.

WARD TIP

Chemoprophylaxis against influenza is recommended as an alternative means of protection after exposure in those who cannot be vaccinated.

WARD TIP

Inactivated influenza vaccine does not cause the disease. Studies have been conducted evaluating the risk of GBS after influenza vaccine, and the CDC monitors this risk during each flu season. Where an increased risk of GBS has been noted, the incidence has been minimal, with 1–2 additional cases of GBS per million flu vaccine doses.

PRECAUTIONS

- Moderate or severe acute illness, with or without fever.
- History of Guillain-Barré Syndrome (GBS) within 6 weeks of previous influenza vaccination.
- Persons whose egg allergy reaction is limited to hives only may receive RIV (if age 18–49) or, with additional safety precautions, IIV.
- LAIV should not be given to children aged 2–4 years who have had wheezing in the past 12 months.

PNEUMOCOCCUS

- Two different inactivated vaccines:
    - Pneumococcal conjugate vaccine (PCV): 13 different serotypes, minimum age 6 weeks.
    - Pneumococcal polysaccharide vaccine (PPSV): 23 different serotypes, minimum age 2 years.
- Babies receive three PCV doses 2 months apart starting at 2 months, and a fourth dose when they are 12–15 months old.
- PCV is recommended for all children aged <5 years. Administer one dose of PCV to all healthy children aged 24–59 months who are not completely immunized for their age.
- Administer PPSV ≥2 months after last dose of PCV to children aged 2 years or older with certain underlying medical conditions, including a cochlear implant and sickle cell anemia.

CONTENT

- The older PPSV-23 vaccine (not indicated under age 2) contains the purified capsular polysaccharide antigens of 23 pneumococcal serotypes. The PPV-23 is usually reserved for high-risk children and adults 65 years and older.
- The PCV-13 vaccine includes 13 pneumococcal serotypes, including several strains that have developed significant antibiotic resistance.

SIDE EFFECTS

- Erythema and pain occur at the injection site.
- Anaphylaxis is reported rarely.
- Fever and myalgia are uncommon.

CONTRAINDICATIONS

- For PCV13, severe allergic reaction (e.g., anaphylaxis) after a previous dose of PCV7 or PCV13 or to a vaccine component, as well as to any vaccine containing diphtheria toxoid.
- For PPSV23, severe allergic reaction (e.g., anaphylaxis) after a previous dose or to a vaccine component.

HEPATITIS A

- Minimum age: 12 months.
- Administer to all children aged 1 year (12–23 months).
- Administer two doses at least 6 months apart.
- Recommended for adults who are at increased risk of hepatitis A (international travelers, men who have sex with men, people who will have close contact with international adoptees, those who are experiencing homelessness, and those with potential occupational exposure).

WARD TIP

The pneumococcal vaccine helps to protect against meningitis, bacteremia, pneumonia, and otitis media caused by serotypes of *Streptococcus pneumoniae*.

HUMAN PAPILLOMAVIRUS (HPV)

- First dose for boys and girls 11–12 years of age (can be given as early as 9) and up to 26 years.
- Two-dose series, with second dose given 6–12 months after the first dose.
- A three-dose series is recommended if the first dose is given after the 15ᵗʰ birthday and for immunocompromised patients.
- Contains nine strains of HPV: HPV 6 & 11 (genital warts) and HPV 16, 18, 31, 33, 45, 52, and 58 (cancers including cervical, oropharyngeal, anal, vulvar, and penile).

SIDE EFFECTS

Pain, swelling, dizziness, syncope

WARD TIP

Observation for syncope is recommended for 15 minutes after administration of HPV vaccine.

MENINGOCOCCUS

- Available against groups A, C, Y, W-135 (MenACWY).
- A second vaccine is available against just group B (MenB).
- All children receive tetravalent conjugate vaccine (MenACWY) between age 11 and 12, with a booster at age 16.
- Minimum age: as early as 2 months for immunocompromised or at-risk individuals:
  - Persistent complement component deficiency.
  - Anatomic or functional asplenia.
  - Travel to regions where meningococcal disease is endemic.

SIDE EFFECTS

- Localized erythema and pain.
- Fever.
- Headache.
- Fatigue.

CONTRAINDICATION

Severe allergic reaction (e.g., anaphylaxis) after a previous dose or to a vaccine component.

PRECAUTION

History of Guillain-Barré syndrome.

ROTAVIRUS

- Minimum age: 6 weeks.
- Administer the first dose at age 6–14 weeks (maximum age: 14 weeks 6 days). Vaccination should not be initiated for infants aged 15 weeks 0 days or older.
- The maximum age for the final dose in the series is 8 months 0 days.
- If Rotarix rotavirus vaccine is administered at ages 2 and 4 months, a dose at 6 months is not indicated.

CONTRAINDICATION

SCID, history of intussusception, and hypersensitivity to vaccine components.

PRECAUTIONS

Preexisting chronic gastrointestinal disease, spina bifida, or bladder exstrophy.

EXAM TIP

Live attenuated vaccines used in the United States include:

- Measles / Mumps / Rubella
- Varicella
- Nasal influenza vaccine
- Rotavirus

Other live attenuated vaccines not routinely used in the U.S. include:

- OPV (in contrast, IPV is inactivated, not live)
- Smallpox
- Typhoid (also an inactivated version)
- Yellow fever

These should be avoided in the immunocompromised.

SIDE EFFECTS

Diarrhea, vomiting, irritability

RESPIRATORY SYNCYTIAL VIRUS (RSV)

- Palivizumab (Synagis) is a monoclonal antibody used for prophylaxis against infections with respiratory syncytial virus (RSV). In contrast to the previous vaccines discussed, palivizumab provides *passive* immunity and does not generate an immune response.
- The vaccine is given IM monthly during RSV season, usually beginning in October and ending in March.
- The vaccine is expensive, and guidelines restrict its use to former premature infants in their first year of life and children <2years old with significant immunocompromise, significant congenital heart, or chronic lung diseases.

TUBERCULOSIS (TB)

- The BCG tuberculosis vaccine is not routinely used in the United States, but immigrants may have received it.
- BCG decreases the risk of tuberculous meningitis and miliary disease.
- The vaccine can cause a false-positive reaction to a tuberculin skin test; these patients should be screened for TB using IGRAs.

Medications

Historically, most medications used in children were "off label," i.e., studies had not been done in pediatric populations. The Best Pharmaceuticals for Children Act (BPCA) in 2002 and the Pediatric Research Equity Act (PREA) of 2003 provide additional patent protection to medications that were tested in children.

DIFFERENCES BETWEEN CHILDREN AND ADULTS

ABSORPTION

- Infants have thinner skin; topical substances are more likely to cause systemic toxicity.
- Children do not have the stomach acidity of adults until age 2, and gastric emptying time is slower and less predictable, potentially altering absorption of some medications.

DISTRIBUTION

- Less predictable in children.
- Total body water decreases from 90% in infants to 60% in adults.
- Fat stores are similar to adults in term infants, but much less in preterm infants.
- Newborns have lower protein concentration; therefore, less blood binding of substances occurs.
- Infants have an immature blood–brain barrier.

METABOLISM

Infants metabolize some drugs more slowly or rapidly than adults and may create a different proportion of active metabolites.

ELIMINATION

Kidney function changes with age, so younger children may clear drugs less efficiently.

DOSAGE

- Pediatric medications are generally dosed by milligrams per kilogram (mg/kg).
- In addition to injections and tablets, children's medication come in liquids, chewables, sub-lingual dissolvables, and sprinkles. Ensure you understand the form likely to work for your patient before prescribing.

Child Abuse

DEFINITION

Child maltreatment encompasses a spectrum of abusive actions and lack of action that result in morbidity or death. Forms of child abuse include:

- Physical abuse
- Psychological abuse
- Sexual abuse
- Neglect

RISK FACTORS

- Parental risk factors include:
  - Low socioeconomic status.
  - Young age, single parent.
  - History of abuse as a child.
  - Alcoholism, substance abuse, psychosis.
  - Transient caregivers in the home.
  - Social isolation.
- Child risk factors:
  - Children with special needs, handicapped children (chronic illness, congenital malformation, intellectual disability).
  - Prematurity.
  - Age <4 years.
  - Nonbiologic relationship to the caretaker.
  - "Difficult" children.
- Family and environmental factors:
  - Unemployment.
  - Intimate partner violence.
  - Poverty.

PHYSICAL ABUSE

Suspect physical abuse if:

- Injury is unexplained or unexplainable.
- Injury is inconsistent with mechanism suggested by history.
- History changes each time it is told.
- History of repeated "accidents."
- History of a delay in seeking care.

Bruises

- Bruises are the most common manifestation of physical abuse.
- Suspicious if:
  - Seen on nonambulatory infants.
  - Have geometric pattern (belt buckles, looped-cord marks).

WARD TIP

If the story doesn't make sense, suspect abuse.

WARD TIP

Congenital dermal melanocytosis (previously called Mongolian spots) spots can be confused with bruises.

EXAM TIP

A baby should never be shaken for any reason.

EXAM TIP

The most common reason for shaking a baby is inconsolable crying.

WARD TIP

Sometimes abusive parents "punish" their children for enuresis or resistance to toilet training by forcibly immersing their buttocks in hot water.

Burns

- Suspicious if:
  - Involve both hands or feet in stocking-glove distribution or buttocks with sharp demarcation line (forced immersion in hot water).
  - Cigarette burns—if nonaccidental, usually full-thickness, sharply circumscribed.
  - "Branding" injuries (inflicted by hot iron, radiator cover, etc).

Skeletal Injuries

Suspicious if:

- Spiral fractures of lower extremities in nonambulatory children (see Figure 6-2A and B).
- Posterior rib fractures (usually caused by squeezing the chest).
- Fractures of different ages.
- Metaphyseal "chip" fractures (usually caused by wrenching).
- Multiple fractures.
- Scapular and clavicle fractures.

Central Nervous System (CNS) Injuries

- The most common cause of death in child abuse is "Shaken Baby Syndrome." This may also be referred to as "Shaken Impact Syndrome" or "Abusive Head Trauma."
- It occurs due to violent shakes and slamming against a mattress or a wall while an infant is held by the trunk or upper extremities.
- Findings include:
  - Retinal hemorrhages.
  - Subdural hematoma (from rupturing of bridging veins between dura mater and brain cortex).
- Symptoms include:
  - Lethargy or irritability.
  - Vomiting.
  - Seizures.
  - Bulging fontanelle.

WARD TIP

In the absence of a motor vehicle collision, epiphyseal-metaphyseal injury is virtually diagnostic of physical abuse in an infant since an infant cannot generate enough force to fracture a bone at the epiphysis.

WARD TIP

Shaken baby syndrome can mimic meningitis or sepsis.

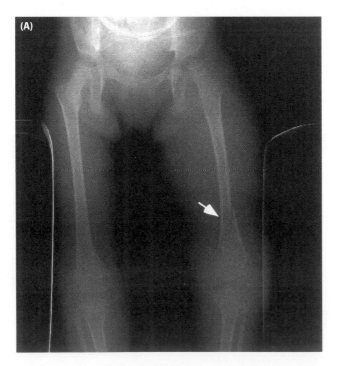
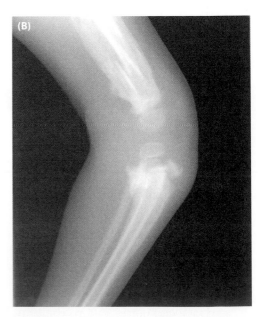

FIGURE 6-2.   **(A)** Spiral fracture (arrow) of the femur in a nonambulatory child, consistent with nonaccidental trauma. **(B)** Same child 2 months later. Note the exuberant callus formation at all the fracture sites in the femur and proximal tibia and fibula.

Abdominal Injuries

- These are the second most common cause of death in child abuse.
- Usually, there are no external marks. Most commonly, the liver or spleen is ruptured.
- Symptoms include vomiting, abdominal pain or distention, and shock.

SEXUAL ABUSE

- This abuse includes genital, anal, oral contact; fondling; and involvement in pornography.
- The most common perpetrators are fathers, stepfathers, the mother's boyfriend(s) (i.e., adults known to the child).
- Suspect if:
  - Genital trauma.
  - STDs in small children.
  - Sexualized behavior toward adults or children.
  - Unexplained decline in school performance.
  - Runaway or homeless patient.
  - Chronic somatic complaints (abdominal pain, headaches).
- Although exam findings are frequently absent, signs may include:
  - Tears/bleeding in female or male genitalia.
  - Anal tears or hymenal tears.

EVALUATION OF SUSPECTED ABUSE

Physical Abuse

- Bleeding disorders must be ruled out in case of multiple bruises.
- Perform an x-ray skeletal survey (skull, chest, long bones) in children <2 years of age (to find old/new fractures).
- Collect computed tomographic (CT) scans of the head/abdomen, as indicated.
- Obtain an ophthalmology consult.

Sexual Abuse

- Sexual abuse includes *any* sexual activity (nonconsensual and consensual) between an adult and a child.
- Conduct studies for STDs and test for sperm, if indicated (usually within 72 hours of assault).
- Some facilities may have RNs or APNs designated as "sexual assault nurse examiners" (SANE nurse) who have special training to evaluate sexual abuse victims.

MANAGEMENT

- If abuse is suspected, the event must be reported to child protective services (CPS) after any necessary medical stabilization.
- All siblings need to be evaluated for abuse, too (up to 20% of them might have signs of abuse).
- Disposition of the child (i.e., whether to discharge the patient to parents or to a foster family) is decided by CPS in conjunction with treating physician.
- The family must receive intensive intervention by social services and, if needed, legal authorities.
- *Remember*: If the child is sent back to an abusive family without intervention, up to 5% of children can be killed and up to 25% seriously reinjured.

WARD TIP

Children too young to talk about what has happened to them (generally younger than 2) should have a complete skeletal survey if abuse is suspected.

WARD TIP

A child who presents with multiple fractures at multiple sites and in various stages of healing should be considered abused until proven otherwise.

NEGLECT

DEFINITION

- Neglect is the most common form of reported abuse.
- Neglect to meet nutritional, medical, and/or developmental needs of a child can present as:
  - Failure to thrive.
  - Poor hygiene (severe diaper rash, unwashed clothing, uncut nails).
  - Developmental/speech delay.
  - Delayed immunizations.
  - Not giving treatment for chronic conditions.

MANAGEMENT

If nonorganic (i.e., due to insufficient feeding) failure to thrive is suspected:
- Patient should be hospitalized and given unlimited feedings for several days; rapid weight gain is expected.
- In severely malnourished children, monitor carefully for metabolic derangements associated with refeeding syndrome.
- Report all suspected cases of neglect to CPS.

MUNCHAUSEN SYNDROME BY PROXY

DEFINITION

- Also known as "factitious disorder imposed on another."
- The parent/caregiver either simulates illness, exaggerates actual illness, or induces illness in a child.
- Psychiatrically disturbed parent(s) gain satisfaction from attention and empathy from hospital personnel or their own family because of problems created.

EPIDEMIOLOGY

- Affected children are usually < 6 years old.
- The parent (usually the mother) has some medical knowledge.

SIGNS AND SYMPTOMS

- Vomiting (induced by ipecac).
- Chronic diarrhea (from laxatives).
- Recurrent abscesses or sepsis (usually polymicrobial, from injecting contaminated fluids).
- Apnea (from choking the child).
- Fever (from heating thermometers).
- Bloody vomiting or diarrhea (from adding blood to urine or stool specimens).

DIAGNOSIS

Diagnosis is difficult, but it is initiated by removing the child from the parent via hospitalization. Usually, the child without parent access will have all/most symptoms resolve; testing will also usually be normal.

MANAGEMENT

- Admit the child to the hospital for observation, possibly using hidden video cameras in cooperation with law enforcement.
- Report all cases of suspected Munchausen syndrome by proxy to CPS.

EXAM TIP

Baron von Munchausen was an 18th-century nobleman who became famous because of his incredible stories, which included travel to the moon and flying atop a cannonball over Constantinople, as well as visiting an island made of cheese. His name became a synonym for gross confabulations.

SUDDEN INFANT DEATH SYNDROME (SIDS)

DEFINITION

- SIDS is the sudden death of an infant (< 1 year old) that remains unexplained after thorough case investigation, autopsy, and review of the clinical history.
- SIDS is one of the leading causes of death of infants.

ETIOLOGY

Unknown; possible abnormality in respiratory control and arousal from sleep.

DIAGNOSIS

Difficult to differentiate from intentional harm.

PREVENTION

- Placing the infant to sleep on their back (not side or stomach).
- No co-sleeping.
- No soft objects, loose bedding (comforters, pillows, bumper pads), or stuffed animals in crib.
- Maintaining a smoke-free environment.

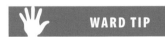 **WARD TIP**

Infants unable to roll over should be placed on their back while sleeping.

NOTES

Congenital Malformations, Chromosomal Anomalies, and Genetic Diagnoses

Recognizing the signs and symptoms of congenital disorders, including their associated phenotypic features, is critical. Involving medical genetics for appropriate screening, treatment, and guidance on genetic testing and counseling regarding siblings and possible future offspring is vital. About 2–4% of infants are born with a birth defect. While the etiology may be unknown, most birth defects are caused by genetic or environmental factors or a combination of the two (multifactorial) (Table 7-1).

Environmental Factors

 An infant born to a mother from Puerto Rico has microcephaly with ventriculomegaly and intracranial calcifications on a brain CT scan. Think **congenital ZIKA infection** if the mother is from an endemic area or has symptoms including fever, rash, conjunctivitis, or arthralgias during her pregnancy.

EXAM TIP

The most common complex birth defects are heart defects, neural tube defects, and cleft lip/palate.

- Maternal infection: most commonly TORCH (**t**oxoplasma, **o**ther [syphilis, Zika, varicella], **r**ubella, **c**ytomegalovirus, **h**erpes).
- Maternal nutritional status: iodine deficiency (congenital hypothyroidism), folate deficiencies (neural tube defects and clefting defects), and diabetes mellitus.
- Maternal teratogen exposure: phenytoin, valproic acid, warfarin and lithium, or exposures to alcohol, tobacco, and pesticides.

TABLE 7-1. Patterns of Inheritance

AUTOSOMAL-DOMINANT	AUTOSOMAL-RECESSIVE	X-LINKED
One of the two alleles carries a pathogenic variant.	Each of the two alleles carries a pathogenic variant.	The affected allele is on the X chromosome. Males have only one allele.
Proband may be first affected individual in pedigree (*de novo*), or multiple individuals in successive generations are affected.	Parents are obligate carriers and unaffected. May see multiple people in the same generation affected, without earlier generations being affected.	Pedigree will typically only show affected males, with affected males related through unaffected females.
If *de novo*, recurrence risk is <1%. If parent is affected, recurrence risk is 50% for each child.	Parents are typically unaffected. Risk to each is child is: 25% affected, 50% unaffected carrier (like parents), and 25% unaffected non-carriers.	Female carrier has a 50% chance that each daughter will be a carrier and 50% chance that each son will be affected. Affected males will have 100% of daughters be carriers and sons will be normal.
Typically related to gain-of-function or dominant negative mutations	Almost always loss-of-function mutations. Increased risk with consanguinity may cause pedigree to appear autosomal dominant.	Heterozygous females are typically normal but may have mild to full manifestations, depending on X-inactivation
Ex: Marfan syndrome, neurofibromatosis Type 1, Achondroplasia	Ex: Cystic fibrosis	Ex: Duchenne and Becker muscular dystrophy, hemophilia A and B, G6PD

Genetic Factors

Genetic factors can be divided into cytogenetic or molecular etiologies. Cytogenetic abnormalities are numerical or structural chromosomal aberrations. Molecular abnormalities include single gene defects, imprinting defects, and trinucleotide repeat expansions.

- Cytogenetic abnormalities
  - Numerical abnormalities
    - Trisomy: an extra chromosome as seen in Down syndrome (Trisomy 21;47,XY,+21).
    - Monosomy: a missing chromosome as in Turner syndrome (45,X).
  - Structural abnormalities:
    - Translocations: anomalies where a whole chromosome or part of a chromosome is joined or exchanged with another chromosome.
  - Microdeletions and duplications: variations where chromosome portions (hundreds to millions of base pairs) are duplicated or deleted affecting one to hundreds of genes.
- Molecular abnormalities:
  - Single gene defects: most commonly single base pair substitutions, deletions, or duplications that disrupt gene function.
  - Imprinting defects: derangements in the regulation or expression of genes, which leads to disease without altering the genetic code itself.
  - Triplet repeat expansions: arising from DNA slippage, the repeated segmental duplication of a three-nucleotide sequence leading to disease when the repeat number reaches a specific threshold.

WARD TIP

Except in a few rare situations, translocations in and of themselves rarely cause disease. However, they present significant problems during recombination and gametogenesis and can lead to unbalanced rearrangements in an individual's offspring.

Trisomy Syndromes

TRISOMY 21 (DOWN SYNDROME)

- Most common malformation syndrome.
- Most common chromosome disorder.
- Most common genetic cause of moderate intellectual disability.

ETIOLOGY

- Extra copy of the genetic material on chromosome 21 (47,XX or XY,+21).
- Ninety-five percent are complete trisomy (meiotic nondisjunction of homologous chromosomes).
- Four percent Robertsonian translocation (most commonly to chromosome 14).
- One percent mosaicism.

EPIDEMIOLOGY/RISK FACTORS

- One in 600 births.
- Advanced maternal age (≥35 years old).
- Carrier of a Robertsonian translocation.

SIGNS AND SYMPTOMS

- More than 100 different physical signs can be present (Figure 7-1).
- Hypertelorism, with upslanting palpebral fissures and epicanthal folds.
- Flat nasal bridge.

WARD TIP

A Robertsonian translocation is the fusion of two acrocentric chromosomes (13, 14, 15, 21, or 22).

WARD TIP

Knowing a patient's etiology of Down syndrome is important for assessing recurrence risk in their parents!

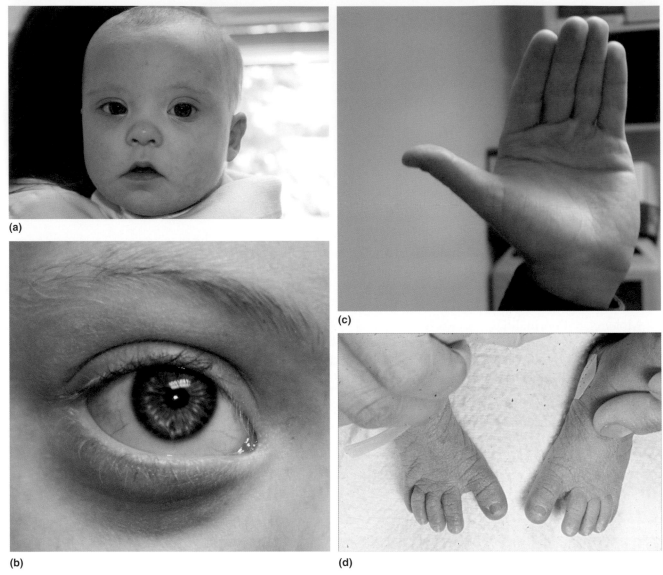

FIGURE 7-1. **Down syndrome.** (a) Typical facial features. (b) Eye showing Brushfield spots (small light-colored spots within the iris due to focal dysplasia of the connective tissue). (c) Single transverse palmar crease. (d) Sandal-gap deformity (wide gap between first and second toes). Reproduced, with permission, from Schaefer GB, Thompson JN Jr., eds. *Medical Genetics: An Integrated Approach.* New York, McGraw Hill, 2014, Figure 5-40.)

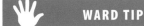

WARD TIP

Some of the features of Down syndrome, such as flattened nasal bridge or excess nuchal skin, may be interpreted on prenatal ultrasound as absent nasal bone and increased nuchal translucency or cystic hygroma.

- Protruding tongue/tongue thrusting.
- Small, low-set, boxed-shaped ears.
- Short neck with excess nuchal skin.
- Single transverse palmar creases.
- Short stature.
- Joint laxity.
- Brushfield spots on irises.
- Intellectual disability (mostly mild to moderate with IQs between 35 and 70).
- Generalized hypotonia (central nervous system origin).
- Global developmental delay, meeting major milestones at twice the normal age.
- Endocardial cushion defects including atrial septal (ASD) and ventricular septal (VSD) defects, atrioventricular (AV) canal, and tetralogy of Fallot.
- Duodenal atresia, Hirschsprung disease, and imperforate anus (Figure 7-2).

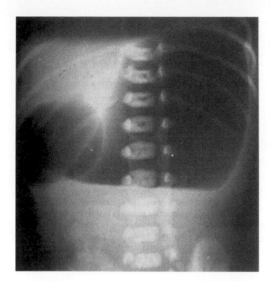

FIGURE 7-2. **Duodenal atresia.** Gas-filled and dilated stomach show the classic "double-bubble" appearance of duodenal atresia. Note the lack of distal gas. (Reproduced, with permission, from Rudolph CD, et al (eds). *Rudolph's Pediatrics*, 21st ed. New York: McGraw-Hill, 2002: 1403.)

- Hearing loss.
- Hypothyroidism.
- Increased risk of acute lymphocytic, myelogenous, or megakaryocytic leukemia and transient myeloproliferative disorder.
- Increased risk of neonatal leukemoid reactions.
- Atlantoaxial instability in later life.
- Amyloid plaques and neurofibrillary tangles in brain (early onset dementia).
- Most males with Down syndrome are infertile, but some females have been able to reproduce.

> A 36-week-gestation male infant born to a 40-year-old mother has a depressed nasal bridge, wide-spaced eyes, low hairline, and low-set ears. He also has bilateral single palmar creases. At 6 hours of life, he has bilious emesis. The abdominal x-ray is shown (Figure 7-3). What is the diagnosis and management of this infant?
>
> The infant was born to a mother with advanced maternal age (>35 years) and has features consistent with Trisomy 21 (Down syndrome). The x-ray has the classic double-bubble sign, which is pathognomonic for duodenal atresia. Management includes surgical repair of the abdominal defect and a chromosome analysis to confirm the Trisomy 21 diagnosis.

WARD TIP

Think of duodenal atresia in a newborn with Down syndrome presenting with bilious vomiting.

WARD TIP

The predisposition to early onset dementia and Alzheimer's in Down syndrome is believed to arise from the presence of the amyloid precursor protein gene (*APP*) on chromosome 21.

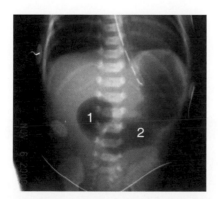

FIGURE 7-3. **Abdominal X-ray showing "double bubble" sign in a newborn infant with duodenal atresia.** The two "bubbles" are numbered. (Reproduced, with permission, from Brunicardi FC, Andersen DK, Billiar TR, et al (eds). *Schwartz's Principles of Surgery*, 11th ed. New York, McGraw Hill, 2019, Figure 39-13.

WARD TIP

Look for "double-bubble sign" in a plain abdominal radiograph (see Figure 7-3).

DIAGNOSIS

- Karyotype: prenatal diagnosis can be made via amniocentesis or chorionic villus sampling.
- See Prenatal Screening at the end of the section.

TREATMENT

- Early childhood intervention to maximize social and intellectual capacity.
- Life skills training.
- Surgery for cardiac and duodenal defects.
- Follow Health Supervision Guidelines for Children with Down Syndrome (https://pediatrics.aappublications.org/content/pediatrics/128/2/393.full.pdf).

TRISOMY 18 (EDWARDS SYNDROME)

ETIOLOGY

- This condition typically involves complete trisomy chromosome 18.
- Small percentage are due to mosaicism.

EPIDEMIOLOGY

- One in 6,000 live births; this is the second-most common trisomy.
- Fifty percent die within first week of life, most commonly from apnea.
- Five to ten percent survive beyond the first year.

SIGNS AND SYMPTOMS

- Intrauterine growth restriction or small for gestational age.
- Small facial features (small mouth, micrognathia, small palpebral fissures, microphthalmia).
- Clenched hands (second and fifth digits overlap third and fourth digits).
- Congenital heart defects (VSD, pulmonary stenosis, coarctation).
- Prominent occiput.
- Rocker-bottom feet.
- Low-set ears.
- Short sternum.
- Inguinal or umbilical hernia, omphalocele.
- Renal anomalies.
- Hypertonia.

DIAGNOSIS

- Karyotype: prenatal diagnosis can be made via amniocentesis or chorionic villus sampling.
- Fluorescence in situ hybridization (FISH) provides 24-hour turnaround.

TREATMENT

- Supportive treatment is recommended.
- Those who survive are severely intellectually disabled.

WARD TIP

Trisomies:
- Age 13, **P**uberty: **Patau syndrome**
- Age 18, can vote—"**E**lect": **Edwards syndrome**
- Age 21, can **D**rink: **Down syndrome**

TRISOMY 13 (PATAU SYNDROME)

Often results in stillbirths and spontaneous abortions.

ETIOLOGY

- Seventy-five percent complete trisomy.
- Twenty-three percent Robertsonian translocation (to chromosome 14).
- Four percent mosaicism.

EPIDEMIOLOGY

- One in 10,000 live births.
- Eighty percent die within first month; 5% survive past 6 months.

SIGNS AND SYMPTOMS

- Holoprosencephaly: the telencephalon fails to divide into two hemispheres, resulting in a large central ventricle; the brain assumes the configuration of a fluid-filled ball.
- Microphthalmia and other eye defects (coloboma, cyclopia) are other signs.
- Midline facial defects.
- Polydactyly.
- Scalp cutis aplasia.
- Cystic kidneys.
- VSD.

DIAGNOSIS

- Karyotype: prenatal diagnosis can be made via amniocentesis or chorionic villus sampling.
- FISH provides 24-hour turnaround.

TREATMENT

- Supportive.

PREGNANCY SCREENING

- Occurs in the late first or early second trimester.
- Maternal serum screening
    - Evaluates levels of specific analytes in maternal blood:
        - Beta-human chorionic gonadotropin (β-hCG).
        - Pregnancy associated plasma protein A (PAPP-A).
        - α-fetoprotein (AFP).
        - Estriol.
        - Inhibin A.
    - Specific pattern may suggest specific trisomy (Table 7-2).
- Non-invasive prenatal screening (NIPS)
    - Fetal cell-free DNA assessment in maternal circulation.
    - >99% sensitive and specific for trisomy 21 and 18.
    - About 90% sensitive for trisomy 13.
- Ultrasound findings can increase concern for trisomies:
    - Increased nuchal translucency.
    - Congenital heart defect.
    - Absent nasal bone.
    - Cleft lip/palate.
    - Omphalocele.

WARD TIP

Pregnancy screening results raise concern for trisomies and other genetic disorders, but they are not diagnostic of disease. They must always be evaluated postnatally with appropriate testing if the concern persists.

WARD TIP

Elevated AFP levels can indicate an open neural tube defect or abdominal wall defect, but they most commonly reflect inaccurate pregnancy dating.

TABLE 7-2. **Maternal Serum Screening**

	PAPP-A	β-hCG	AFP	ESTRIOL	INHIBIN A
Trisomy 21	↓	↑	↓	↓	↑
Trisomy 18	↓	↓↓	↓	↓	↓↓
Trisomy 13	↓	↓	↓	–	↓

Sex Chromosome and Related Anomalies

TURNER SYNDROME

 A newborn has lymphedema of the hands and feet, extra skin folds at a short neck, widely spaced nipples, and decreased femoral pulses. *Think: Gonadal dysgenesis and specifically 45,X (Turner syndrome).* Confirm the diagnosis with a chromosomal analysis.

Many infants with Turner syndrome are recognized at birth due to the features described. Coarctation of aorta may be present in up to 20% of cases.

ETIOLOGY

- 45,X: caused by a loss of part or all of an X chromosome.
- 50% are 45,X; 25% have a structurally abnormal second X; 25% are mosaic.

EPIDEMIOLOGY/ RISK FACTORS

- One in 2000–2500 live female births.
- High risk of spontaneous abortion.
- NOT related to advanced maternal age.

PATHOPHYSIOLOGY

Unknown. Not all X chromosome portions are subject to X-inactivation.

SIGNS AND SYMPTOMS

- Phenotypically female.
- Short stature.
- Short, webbed neck.
- Epicanthal folds.
- Narrow maxilla and high-arched palate.
- Small mandible.
- Broad shield-like chest with wide-spaced nipples.
- Coarctation of the aorta and/or bicuspid aortic valve.
- Congenital malformations of the renal/urinary system.
- Lymphedema of hands and feet.
- Impaired hearing (sensorineural).
- Normal intelligence with difficulty in spatial reasoning.
- Ovarian dysgenesis, infertility, amenorrhea.

DIAGNOSIS

Karyotype.

TREATMENT

- Growth hormone therapy administered in early childhood to maximize adult height.
- Hormone replacement therapy for puberty induction and secondary sex characteristic development.
- Monitor for autoimmune hypothyroidism.
- Lifelong hearing testing recommended every 1 to 5 years.

KLINEFELTER SYNDROME

ETIOLOGY

Presence of an extra X chromosome in males; 47, XXY.

WARD TIP

Turner syndrome is the most common cause of primary amenorrhea.

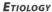

WARD TIP

A high association between Turner syndrome and coarctation of the aorta is found. Therefore, genetic testing for Turner syndrome should be performed in all girls diagnosed with coarctation.

WARD TIP

Noonan syndrome is an autosomal dominant disorder with significant phenotypic overlap with Turner syndrome: short stature, web neck, broad chest, and heart defects. Noonan syndrome is distinguished by the presence of hypertelorism, low-set ears, pectus excavatum, and typically, some degree of intellectual disability. Heart defects in Noonan syndrome tend to be on the right side (pulmonary stenosis) versus the left side (coarctation of the aorta) in Turner syndrome. It affects both males and females!

EPIDEMIOLOGY/ RISK FACTORS

- One in 500 males.
- Advanced maternal age.

DIAGNOSIS

- Karyotype.
- Diagnosis is rarely made before puberty (normal phenotype prepubertal).
- Most cases are diagnosed during infertility or gynecomastia evaluation.

SIGNS AND SYMPTOMS

- Most patients are phenotypically normal until puberty.
- Tall thin stature with long extremities.
- Small testes but puberty occurs at the normal age.
- Female hair distribution, gynecomastia.
- Learning disabilities.
- Delay of motor skill development.
- Hypogonadism.
- Azoospermia.

TREATMENT

- Testosterone during puberty to improve secondary sex characteristics.
- Interventions for developmental delays/learning disabilities.

Microdeletion and Microduplication Syndromes

22q11 MICRODELETION SYNDROME (DIGEORGE SYNDROME; VELOCARDIOFACIAL SYNDROME)

ETIOLOGY

Caused by the deletion of a small piece of the long arm of chromosome 22.

EPIDEMIOLOGY

Occurs in 1 in 4,000 births.

DIAGNOSIS

Chromosomal microarray.

SIGNS AND SYMPTOMS

- Congenital heart defects: VSD, tetralogy of Fallot, aortic arch anomalies.
- Palatal abnormalities (velopharyngeal insufficiency to clefting): feeding difficulties.
- Thymic aplasia: immune deficiency due to defective T-cell function.
- Hypocalcemia: parathyroid underdevelopment.
- Characteristic facial features: prominent nasal bridge, bulbous nose, micrognathia, asymmetric crying facies.
- Developmental delay/learning disability.

TREATMENT

- Developmental therapies (speech, occupational, physical).
- Screening CBC, thyroid studies, and calcium levels at birth.
- Subspecialists follow-up depending on clinic findings.

 EXAM TIP

The most common cause of hypogonadism and infertility in males is Klinefelter Syndrome.

 EXAM TIP

Microdeletion/duplication syndromes occur recurrently in the population because of repetitive genetic elements in these regions leading to nonhomologous recombination.

 WARD TIP

The reciprocal gain of 22q11 causes 22q11 microduplication syndrome, which has significant phenotypic overlap with the deletion syndrome but is generally milder.

 WARD TIP

About 7% of cases of 22q11 microdeletion are inherited from an affected parent, who may be undiagnosed.

 EXAM TIP

Chromosomal microarray is the diagnostic test of choice for all microdeletion/ duplication syndromes. Karyotype does not have a high enough resolution to detect all of them. FISH is a screening test and should only be used to test family members after the breakpoints of the deletion have already been determined.

DiGeorge syndrome should not be confused with **CHARGE** syndrome.

C: Coloboma
H: Heart defects
A: Atresia choanae
R: Retarded growth and development
G: Genitourinary (GU) anomalies
E: Ear anomalies

The eye, ear, and GU anomalies are distinctive to CHARGE, which is caused by pathogenic variants in the *CHD7* gene.

WARD TIP

Cri du chat translates as "cat's cry." The distinctive cry is the source of the common name of the condition.

WARD TIP

If the chromosomal microarray demonstrates a terminal gain in addition to the 4p loss diagnostic of Wolf-Hirschhorn, a karyotype should be evaluated for a translocation event. This would increase the recurrence risk in the family if a parent carries the balanced form of the translocation.

EXAM TIP

Children with Williams syndrome will typically be described as very friendly and outgoing, and they are loquacious with a good concrete (but not conceptual) vocabulary.

5p- SYNDROME (Cri du Chat)

ETIOLOGY

Caused by the deletion of a piece of the short arm of chromosome 5.

EPIDEMIOLOGY

Occurs in 1 in 15,000–50,000 births.

DIAGNOSIS

Chromosomal microarray or karyotype.

SIGNS AND SYMPTOMS

- Congenital heart defects: VSD or ASD.
- Pre- and postnatal growth failure including microcephaly.
- Characteristic facial features: round face, hypertelorism with down-slanting palpebral fissures and epicanthal folds, small down-turned mouth and chin, abnormal ears.
- Distinctive cat-like cry and hypotonia in infancy.
- Global delay with significant intellectual disability.

TREATMENT

Supportive therapies.

4p- SYNDROME (WOLF-HIRSCHHORN SYNDROME)

ETIOLOGY

- Caused by the deletion of a piece of the short arm of chromosome 4.
- About 40% arise due to a parental balanced translocation.

EPIDEMIOLOGY

Occurs in 1 in 50,000 births.

DIAGNOSIS

Chromosomal microarray.

SIGNS AND SYMPTOMS

- Pre- and postnatal growth failure, including microcephaly.
- Characteristic facial features: "Greek warrior helmet appearance," i.e., hypertelorism with high forehead and prominent glabella, epicanthal folds, cleft lip/palate.
- Hypotonia.
- Seizures.
- Severe global developmental delay with intellectual disability.

TREATMENT

Supportive, therapies.

WILLIAMS SYNDROME

ETIOLOGY

Caused by the deletion of a piece of the short arm of chromosome 7 (7q11.23).

EPIDEMIOLOGY

Occurs in 1 in 7,500 births.

DIAGNOSIS

Chromosomal microarray.

SIGNS AND SYMPTOMS

- Prenatal and infantile growth failure, and eventual short stature.
- Congenital heart defects: classically supravalvular aortic stenosis.
- Characteristic facial features: "elfin facies," i.e., broad forehead with bitemporal narrowing, periorbital fullness, stellate irises, short nose with broad tip, malar flattening, thick upper and lower lip, and small wide-spaced teeth. Older children may have a longer thin face and neck.
- Hypermobility with loose joints and lax skin.
- Distinctive personality of overfriendliness with lack of stranger anxiety.
- Global developmental delay.
- Severe intellectual disability to normal intelligence with particular strengths of verbal short-term memory and language.
- Idiopathic hypercalcemia/hypercalciuria.

TREATMENT

- Supportive therapies.
- Monitoring calcium levels and risk of subsequent kidney stones.
- Cardiology surveillance for life.

Imprinting Disorders

Genomic imprinting is a normal state of genetic expression where only one of the two parental alleles is expressed and the other is suppressed. Changes in this expression pattern can lead to disease.

ANGELMAN SYNDROME

ETIOLOGY

Loss of **maternal** expression of chromosome 15q11q13, specifically *UBE3A*; usually a maternal deletion.

EPIDEMIOLOGY

One in 20,000

DIAGNOSIS

Methylation studies and chromosomal microarray.

SIGNS AND SYMPTOMS

- Normal prenatal and birth history and normal brain imaging.
- Happy disposition with inappropriate laughter and ataxia.
- Can have lighter pigmentation than expected, often blond-haired, blue-eyed.
- Profound intellectual disability with absent speech.
- Post-natally acquired microcephaly.
- Hypotonia.
- 80% have epilepsy.
- Unusual faces: a large mandible and open-mouthed expression revealing the tongue.

TREATMENT

- Supportive: development therapies, some may communicate with technology devices.
- Seizures are often refractory to anticonvulsant therapy.
- Normal life span.

 WARD TIP

Angelman syndrome was previously described as the "happy puppet" ("marionette joyeuse") syndrome because of the happy disposition and ataxic gait, resembling that of a marionette.

 EXAM TIP

Angelman syndrome patients present at ~18 months of age on average with speech delay, motor problems, and possible onset of seizures.

 EXAM TIP

The same chromosomal deletion causes the majority of Angelman syndrome and Prader-Willi syndrome cases. The difference is the parent of origin of the defect:
Angel**m**an syndrome = missing **M**aternal genetic material
Prader-Willi = missing **P**aternal genetic material

PRADER-WILLI SYNDROME

ETIOLOGY

Loss of **paternal** expression of chromosome 15q11q13, usually a **paternal** deletion.

EPIDEMIOLOGY

One in 20,000

DIAGNOSIS

Methylation studies and chromosomal microarray.

SIGNS AND SYMPTOMS

- Infantile hypotonia and poor feeding, followed by childhood hyperphagia and obesity.
- Dysmorphic features: almond-shaped eyes, thin upper lip, bitemporal narrowing, small hands and feet.
- Short stature.
- Lighter pigmentation than expected.
- Hypogonadism.
- Males: micropenis, cryptorchidism, small testis.
- Sleep disturbances, central/obstructive apnea.
- Mild to moderate intellectual disability.
- Significant behavioral problems.
- Obsessive/compulsive traits.

TREATMENT

- Strict diet and behavioral interventions are used to prevent obesity.
- Growth hormone is used to promote stature, and other timely hormone supplementation promotes secondary sex characteristics.
- Obesity may limit the patient's quality of life and life span.

> **EXAM TIP**
>
> Neonatal hypotonia and poor feeding is one of the hallmarks of Prader-Willi syndrome and is a clue to initiate testing.

> **EXAM TIP**
>
> Prader-Willi syndrome is the most common cause of syndromic obesity.

BECKWITH-WIEDEMANN SYNDROME (BWS)

ETIOLOGY

- About 55% arise from methylation defects on **maternal** 11p15.5.
- Although it can be inherited, most cases are *de novo*.

EPIDEMIOLOGY

1 in 10,000

DIAGNOSIS

Methylation studies will identify many; the remainder of diagnoses are clinical.

SIGNS AND SYMPTOMS

- BWS is an overgrowth syndrome.
- Major findings include: macrosomia, visceromegaly, omphalocele, macroglossia, hemihyperplasia (asymmetric overgrowth of one side of the body), renal anomalies, anterior ear lobe creases, neonatal hypoglycemia, and polyhydramnios.
- A predisposition to embryonal tumors during the first 8 years of life includes Wilms, hepatoblastoma, neuroblastoma, and rhabdomyosarcoma (Figure 7-4).

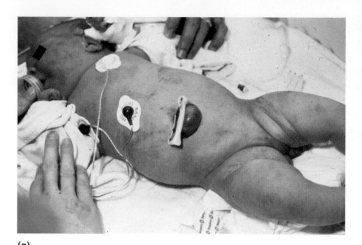

(a)

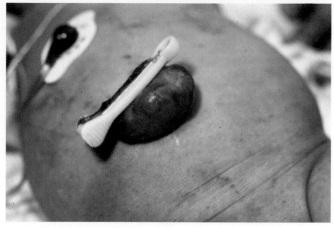

(b)

FIGURE 7-4.   (a) Newborn female with Beckwith-Wiedemann syndrome. (b) Close-up view of the child's omphalocoele. (Reproduced, with permission, from Schaefer GB, Thompson JN Jr. *Medical Genetics: An Integrated Approach*. New York, McGraw Hill, 2014, Figure 12-23AB.)

TREATMENT

- Monitoring for and correcting hypoglycemic episodes are the early treatment for this syndrome.
- Ultrasound of the kidneys.
- Surgical correction of omphalocele, if present.
- Screening for tumors: checking AFP levels every 3 months until age 4 years and performing abdominal ultrasounds every 3 months until age 8 years.

RUSSEL-SILVER SYNDROME (RSS)

ETIOLOGY

- 50% arise from loss of **paternal** methylation at 11p15.5.
- About 40% have no identified genetic etiology.

EPIDEMIOLOGY

1 in 30,000–100,000

DIAGNOSIS

Methylation studies will identify many, with remainder made by clinical findings.

SIGNS AND SYMPTOMS

- RSS is an undergrowth syndrome.
- Patients must have four of the following:
  - Birth weight and/or length ≤ 2 standard deviations from the mean.
  - Postnatal growth failure.
  - Relative macrocephaly at birth.
  - Frontal bossing or prominent forehead.
  - Body asymmetry.
- Classically described as having a triangular face with micrognathia, high-pitched voice, and fifth finger clinodactyly.

TREATMENT

- RSS is treated by monitoring for and correcting hypoglycemic episodes.
- Monitoring growth.
- Growth hormone may improve height in some individuals.

WARD TIP

Like Angelman and Prader-Willi syndrome, Beckwith-Wiedemann syndrome and Russel-Silver syndrome are imprinting disorders arising from the same genetic locus. Beckwith-Wiedemann is an overgrowth syndrome of **maternal** origin, while Russel-Silver is an undergrowth syndrome of **paternal** origin.

WARD TIP

Neither BWS nor RSS are associated with cognitive deficits, although an increased risk of learning difficulties has been suggested in RSS.

Triplet Repeat Disorders

FRAGILE X SYNDROME

ETIOLOGY

This syndrome is caused by repeat expansion of the existing trinucleotide repeat sequence CGG in the *FMR1* gene on the X chromosome to >200 repeats, most commonly during maternal transmission.

EPIDEMIOLOGY/ RISK FACTORS

- One in 2000 births.
- The male-to-female ratio is 2:1.
- Family history is a risk factor.

SIGNS AND SYMPTOMS

- Moderate intellectual disability.
- Autism and/or behavior problems (ADHD, anxiety, stereotypies).
- Characteristic features: protruding ears, prominent forehead, long face, flat malar bones, and prominent jaw becoming more evident with age.
- Characteristic macroorchidism in boys is not present until after puberty.

TREATMENT

Treatment includes cognitive and behavioral therapies.

Congenital Anomalies

POLYDACTYLY

DEFINITION

- Polydactyly is the presence of more than five fingers or toes, which may be rudimentary to fully developed.
  - Pre-axial: occurring on the radial side of the hand or medial side of the foot.
  - Post-axial: occurring on the ulnar side of the hand or lateral side of the foot.
- Incidence: 2 per 1000 live births.

ETIOLOGY

This condition may occur as an isolated defect or as part of a syndrome.

DIAGNOSIS

Clinical examination

TREATMENT

Surgery, usually in the first year of life

SYNDACTYLY

DEFINITION

Syndactyly is the webbing or fusing of two or more fingers or toes, which may be bony and/or cutaneous. It is often identified between the second and third toes.

PATHOPHYSIOLOGY

The cause is failure of cell apoptosis between digits during development.

TREATMENT

Surgery

CRANIOSYNOSTOSIS

DEFINITION

- Premature closing of one or more cranial sutures due to skull development abnormalities.
- Can be a primary skull/bone defect or the result of failure of brain growth
- Syndromic craniosynostosis is seen in 20% of cases.
- The most common syndromes are Apert syndrome and Crouzon syndrome.

ETIOLOGY

May occur alone or in conjunction with syndromes.

SIGNS AND SYMPTOMS

Early closure of fontanels and sutures with decreased head growth.

COMPLICATIONS

- Hydrocephalus.
- Increased intracranial pressure (ICP).
- Developmental delay.

TREATMENT

- A craniotomy is done to prevent intracranial and ophthalmologic complications.
- Multidisciplinary approach includes genetics, psychology, pediatrics, surgery, and neurology.
- Treatment includes long-term follow-up.

Normocephaly

 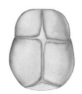 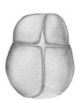

Scaphocephaly Trigonocephaly Anterior plagiocephaly Brachycephaly Posterior plagiocephaly

FIGURE 7-5. **Patterns of single suture craniosynostosis.** Scaphocephaly results from sagittal synostosis. Trigonocephaly results from metopic synostosis. Anterior plagiocephaly results from unilateral coronal synostosis. Brachycephaly results from bilateral coronal synostosis. Posterior plagiocephaly results from unilateral lambdoidal synostosis. Reproduced, with permission, from Brunicardi FC, Andersen DK, Billiar TR, et al (eds). *Schwartz's Principles of Surgery*, 11th ed. New York, McGraw Hill, 2019, Figure 45-39.

AMNIOTIC BAND SEQUENCE

DEFINITION

- Fibrous strands of membrane stretching across the chorionic cavity are indicative of this sequence.
- In this form of disruption, normal tissue is acted upon by another force, leading to a change.

EPIDEMIOLOGY

It is not associated with problems in future pregnancies.

ETIOLOGY

- Spontaneous.
- Associated with abdominal trauma, including chorionic villus sampling.

PATHOPHYSIOLOGY

This sequence is caused by early amnion rupture and chorionic fluid leakage.

SIGNS AND SYMPTOMS

- May be innocent and not cause any fetal harm.
- Can cause limb or other body part constriction or amputation (amniotic band syndrome).
- May be associated with oligohydramnios and decreased fetal movement.

DIAGNOSIS

Ultrasound or clinical examination.

TREATMENT

- Most prenatal bands disappear spontaneously, resolving on a follow-up ultrasound.
- Necrosis distal to vascular occlusion might necessitate surgical release.

CLEFT PALATE/LIP

DEFINITION

- This condition includes a spectrum of defects of the upper lip, philtrum, and hard and soft palates.
- Cleft lip, cleft palate, or both.
- Unilateral or bilateral.

EPIDEMIOLOGY

- This is the third most common complex birth defect.
- Incidence of orofacial clefting is 1 in 700 live births.
- Occurs more often in Asian, Latino, or Native American infants.
- More common in males.

ETIOLOGY

- Teratogens: ethanol, anticonvulsants, steroids, chemotherapy, maternal vitamin A excess.
- Gestational factors: maternal diabetes, maternal folate deficiency.

- Syndromic: chromosomal abnormalities, single gene disorders.
- Idiopathic (majority).

PATHOPHYSIOLOGY

- Clefting of the lip and anterior (primary) palate due to a defect in fusing of both maxillary processes with the frontonasal process during embryologic weeks 5 and 6.
- Clefting of the posterior (secondary) palate due to defect in fusion of palatal shelves during embryologic weeks 7 and 8.

SIGNS AND SYMPTOMS

- Feeding difficulties.
- Speech impediments.
- Increased incidence of middle-ear infection and associated hearing loss.
- Dental malalignment.

DIAGNOSIS

Physical exam of lips, palate, and oropharynx.

TREATMENT

- May require assistance with feeding.
- Surgical lip repair within first months of life, palate around 1 year of life; final repairs and scar revisions in adolescence.
- The cleft team can include plastic and oral surgeons; geneticist; otolaryngologist; dentist; speech pathologist; audiologist; social worker or psychologist; and nurse coordinator.

OMPHALOCELE

DEFINITION

This condition is an abdominal content herniation (usually only involving the intestine, but it can include the liver and/or spleen) through the umbilical root, which is covered only by the peritoneum.

EPIDEMIOLOGY

- May be associated with other congenital defects, including chromosomal anomalies, heart defects, and diaphragmatic hernia.
- Associated with Beckwith-Wiedemann syndrome and trisomies 13 and 18.

DIAGNOSIS

Some may be detected on prenatal ultrasounds.

TREATMENT

- Cover the extruded abdominal contents while managing more urgent conditions.
- Abdominal contents are placed in a holding sack of dressing material; typically called a "silo"
- Serial reductions of the silo, pushing intestines into the abdomen, are performed until skin closure is possible.

EXAM TIP

Pierre-Robin sequence is a genetic sequence that can lead to cleft lip and/or cleft palate. It arises from jaw underdevelopment (micrognathia). The underdeveloped jaw leads to posterior tongue displacement, which physically hinders the fusion of the processes and shelves and leads to clefting. However, not all clefting is caused by Pierre-Robin sequence.

EXAM TIP

The presence of an omphalocele should always prompt consideration of Beckwith-Wiedemann syndrome as a possible diagnosis.

WARD TIP

Omphalocele is differentiated from gastroschisis, where the abdominal contents herniate lateral to the umbilical root and have no covering. Omphalocele is more typically associated with genetic abnormalities, whereas gastroschisis is typically not genetic.

WARD TIP

Abdominal wall defects can lead to elevation in alpha-fetoprotein during pregnancy, similar to neural tube defects

POTTER SEQUENCE

- This sequence includes bilateral renal agenesis and the subsequent deformities arising from this defect.
- Renal agenesis causes severe oligo- or anhydramnios leading to pulmonary hypoplasia, skeletal anomalies, and characteristic facies (sloping forehead; flattened nose; recessed chin; and low-set, floppy ears).
- It is incompatible with neonatal life; death occurs due to pulmonary hypoplasia.

DIAGNOSIS

- Very low amniotic fluid index on ultrasound.
- Failure to visualize the kidneys on ultrasound.

TREATMENT

None.

WARD TIP

Suspect bilateral renal agenesis if the maternal ultrasonography shows oligohydramnios, non-visualization of the bladder, and absent kidneys.

Metabolic Disease

Inborn Errors of Metabolism

DEFINITION

These rare inherited biochemical disorders arise largely from enzyme deficiencies that lead to defective or abnormal breakdown, buildup, and/or storage of metabolites.

EPIDEMIOLOGY

Individually inborn errors of metabolism are rare, but collectively, they have an estimated incidence as high as ~1 in 800 individuals.

SIGNS AND SYMPTOMS

- Typically infants appear normal at birth, but some can show signs within hours, including metabolic acidosis, poor feeding, vomiting, lethargy, and convulsion
- Most inborn errors of metabolism are without dysmorphic features.
- Left untreated, many can lead to intellectual disability, organomegaly and/or end organ damage, and episodic metabolic decompensation.
- Most commonly present in the first year of life but can present at any age.

DIAGNOSIS

- **Newborn metabolic screening (NBS):**
  - State-regulated programs provide early detection of treatable disorders to preclude or reduce disease complications.
  - The disorders screened for and the testing modalities employed varies by state.
  - Tandem mass spectrometry is the usual screening method, but molecular testing via genetic sequencing and direct enzymatic assays are also employed.
- Classification:
  - Amino acid disorders
    - Phenylketonuria.
    - Homocystinuria.
    - Maple syrup urine disease.
    - Tyrosinemia.
  - Urea cycle disorders
    - Arginase deficiency.
    - Argininosuccinic academia.
    - Citrullinemia.
    - Ornithine transport defect.
  - Fatty acid oxidation disorders
    - Carnitine transport defect.
    - Medium-chain acyl-CoA dehydrogenase deficiency.
    - Very long chain acyl-CoA dehydrogenase deficiency.
    - Glutaric acidemia type 2.
  - Organic acid disorders
    - 3-hydroxy-3-methylglutaryl-CoA lyase deficiency.
    - Glutaric acidemia type I.
    - Isovaleric acidemia.
    - Methylmalonic acidemia.
    - Propionic acidemia.

WARD TIP

Newborn screening was initiated to identify newborns with phenylketonuria, but it has now expanded to include more than 50 conditions in some states.

WARD TIP

Newborn screening does not cover just inborn errors of metabolism. Hemoglobinopathies, endocrinologic, and immunologic diseases are also included, depending on the state.

WARD TIP

Medium-chain acyl-CoA dehydrogenase deficiency is the most common fatty acid oxidation disorder, and it may be associated with intermittent severe metabolic crises or sudden death.

EXAM TIP

Ornithine transcarbamylase deficiency is the most common urea cycle defect (UCD). It is X-linked and classically affects males. The hallmark of UCDs is hyperammonemia.

WARD TIP

Asking about the pregnancy is important when evaluating any neonate. In nonketotic hyperglycinemia, the mother may report that the baby was periodically very active or that they seemed to have hiccups frequently.

TREATMENT

- Treatment frequently includes dietary modifications.
- Can consist of administration of cofactors (such as vitamins).
- Enzyme replacement or gene therapy is increasingly available.

PHENYLKETONURIA (PKU)

DEFINITION

PKU is an inherited amino acid metabolism disorder with an impaired ability to metabolize the essential amino acid phenylalanine.

ETIOLOGY

A deficiency of phenylalanine hydroxylase which converts phenylalanine to tyrosine.

PATHOPHYSIOLOGY

- Accumulation of phenylalanine and its metabolites through alternate metabolic pathways disrupt normal metabolism and cause brain damage.
- Tyrosine becomes an essential amino acid.

EPIDEMIOLOGY

- Autosomal recessive.
- One in 10,000–20,000 live births.
- More common in the Caucasian population.

SIGNS AND SYMPTOMS

- Normal at birth.
- Hypopigmentation due to low tyrosine (fair hair and skin, blue eyes).
- If untreated, intellectual disability, developmental delay, seizures, eczema, and spasticity develop in the first few months of life.
- If a patient stops treatment, neurologic features including difficulty concentrating, psychiatric problems, and fatigue can develop. More severe features result the earlier therapy is discontinued.

DIAGNOSIS

- Screened in all states.
- If not screened neonatally, diagnosis is made at 4–6 months of age with symptom onset.
- Plasma amino acid analysis shows phenylalanine elevations and low tyrosine levels.
- Molecular confirmation can be made with genetic sequencing of the *PAH* gene. This also allows for prenatal and carrier testing.

TREATMENT

- Limiting dietary phenylalanine results in significant natural protein restriction.
- Protein is replaced through a medical formula containing protein without phenylalanine and additional supplemental tyrosine.
- Because of dietary restrictions, patients are at risk for micronutrient deficiencies.
- Some patients will respond to tetrahydrobiopterin (Kuvan) because this enzymatic cofactor can augment residual enzyme activity.
- Enzyme substitution therapy (Pegvaliase) is now available in adults.

EXAM TIP

Glutaric aciduria/acidemia type I (GAI) can be mistaken for child abuse with the presence of subdural hematomas. If other signs of abuse are absent (retinal hemorrhages, patterned bruising, characteristic fractures), think about GAI.

WARD TIP

Most fatty acid oxidation disorders present with nonketotic hypoglycemia.

WARD TIP

Hyperphenylalaninemia can also be caused by a deficiency in the synthesis or recycling of the phenylalanine hydroxylase cofactor tetrahydrobiopterin. This accounts for ~2% of cases of hyperphenylalaninemia. Differentiation of the two disorders is important for treatment because a cofactor deficiency will not respond to dietary restriction.

WARD TIP

Tyrosine is important because it is a precursor of L-dopa and dopamine, important neurotransmitters.

EXAM TIP

Phenylketonuria is the most common inborn error of metabolism.

WARD TIP

Lethargy, anorexia, anemia, rashes, and diarrhea are signs of tyrosine deficiency.

WARD TIP

Based on the level of residual enzyme activity, some people with hyperphenylalaninemia will not reach phenylalanine levels high enough to require treatment, but infants must be monitored throughout early life during growth and dietary changes to ensure phenylalanine levels do not reach levels requiring treatment. This is referred to as "benign hyperphe."

EXAM TIP

The artificial sugar aspartame contains phenylalanine, and it must be avoided by patients with PKU.

WARD TIP

Tetrahydrobiopterin can rarely be a sufficient management of classic PKU, but it can liberalize the patient's dietary restrictions. Enzyme substitution can completely treat PKU and remove dietary restriction.

EXAM TIP

Pregnant women with uncontrolled PKU can give birth to children with Maternal PKU syndrome. Thus, strict dietary control and PKU monitoring during pregnancy in affected women is important (phenylalanine is concentrated in the fetus ~1.5 times higher than in the mother). Maternal PKU syndrome presents with intellectual disability, microcephaly, congenital heart disease, intrauterine growth restriction, and low birth weight. Following birth, phenylalanine levels in the infant will normalize, but in utero damage is permanent.

EXAM TIP

Elevations of homocysteine can be seen in other disorders, including defects in vitamin B12 metabolism (cobalamin) and disorders of folate metabolism, which will typically have low or normal methionine levels.

HOMOCYSTINEMIA/HOMOCYSTINURIA

DEFINITION

Inherited amino acid metabolism disorder in which homocysteine is not broken down and leads to its elevation in plasma and urine, as well as increases in levels of methionine.

ETIOLOGY

Deficiency of cystathionine β-synthase (CBS).

PATHOPHYSIOLOGY

CBS deficiency prevents homocysteine to cystathione conversion, and it increases remethylation to methionine. Homocysteine is thought to directly damage the vasculature.

EPIDEMIOLOGY

Autosomal recessive: 1 in 200,000 live births.

SIGNS AND SYMPTOMS

- Symptoms are highly variable, primarily affecting the eye, skeleton, brain, and vascular systems.
- Eye problems can include progressive myopia and possible ectopia lentis.
- Skeletal features are primarily seen after puberty with a marfanoid body habitus and joint stiffness.
- Brain problems include early childhood learning difficulties, developmental delay or intellectual disability, and progressive dystonia, seizures, or psychiatric problems into adulthood.
- Vascular problems include increased risk of thromboembolism and atherosclerosis.

DIAGNOSIS

- Normal at birth; diagnosis usually made after 3 years of age.
- Elevated methionine and homocysteine in body fluids.
- Biallelic pathogenic variants in the *CBS* gene.

TREATMENT

- Pyridoxine responsive form: 50% are this form and are easily missed in the neonatal period. Treatment includes high-dose vitamin B_6.
- Pyridoxine unresponsive form: methionine restriction and cysteine supplementation are used. (Concurrent folic acid may be needed to show response.) Betaine can also play a role in this group.
- Other types may require vitamin B_{12} or methionine supplementation.

MAPLE SYRUP URINE DISEASE (MSUD)

DEFINITION

MSUD is an inherited disorder of branched-chain amino acid metabolism in which elevated quantities of leucine, isoleucine, and valine accumulate.

ETIOLOGY

Deficiency of branched-chain alpha-ketoacid dehydrogenase complex (BCKD), which is responsible for the second step of catabolism of all three branched chain amino acids.

PATHOPHYSIOLOGY

A defect in the decarboxylation of leucine, isoleucine, and valine by BCKD leads to subsequent elevations in all three amino acids.

EPIDEMIOLOGY

One in 185,000 live births in the general population.

SIGNS AND SYMPTOMS

- Significant clinical variability with neonatal period through adulthood onset, with chronic progressive and intermittent forms.
- Neonatal: poor feeding, vomiting, apnea, irritability, stereotyped "fencing" or "bicycling" movements, encephalopathy/lethargy and coma/death.
- Milder/intermittent: developmental delay, poor growth, anorexia, irritability.
- Acute crises: hypoglycemia, acidosis, encephalopathy.
- Odor of maple syrup in urine, sweat, and/or cerumen.

DIAGNOSIS

- Elevated plasma and urine levels of leucine, isoleucine, valine, and alloisoleucine.
- Biallelic pathogenic variants in the *BCKDHA*, *BCKDHB*, or *DBT*.

TREATMENT

- Treatment includes the dietary restriction of branched-chain amino acids in the diet.
- Valine and isoleucine supplementation can lower damaging leucine levels.
- Increased caloric support during acute illness can help.
- Liver transplant may be considered, but early identification and dietary treatment can limit neurological sequelae.

Lysosomal Storage Diseases (LSD)

See Table 8-1.

DEFINITION/ETIOLOGY/PATHOPHYSIOLOGY

Inherited deficiencies of lysosomal hydrolases lead to the buildup of specific products in lysosomes, leading to end organ damage.

EPIDEMIOLOGY

Most are autosomal recessive.

SIGNS AND SYMPTOMS

Depends on site of abnormal accumulations:

- Nervous system: neurodegeneration, ocular findings.
- Viscera: organomegaly, skeletal abnormalities, pulmonary infiltration.

DIAGNOSIS

- Measurement of specific enzymatic activity in leukocytes or cultured fibroblasts.
- Molecular testing with clinical suspicion.

WARD TIP

Ectopia lentis is subluxation of the lens, signaled by iridodonesis (quivering of iris) and myopia. Downward ectopia lentis is seen in homocystinuria, while upward ectopia lentis is seen in Marfan syndrome.

WARD TIP

Homocysteine and methionine each must be tested for specifically and then tested together to help differentiate etiologies of the elevation. Methylmalonic acid levels can help in this aspect as well.

EXAM TIP

Marfanoid habitus = tall and thin, with thin extremities, enlarged epiphyses, and arachnodactyly.

- Differential diagnosis:
    - Homocystinuria: marfanoid habitus, ectopia lentis, intellectual disability.
    - Ehlers-Danlos syndrome types 1 and 3: marked joint hypermobility, mitral valve prolapse, large scars of the skin, skin hyperextensibility.
    - Stickler syndrome (hereditary arthro-ophthalmopathy): tall stature, retrognathia, mitral valve prolapse, midfacial hypoplasia, retinal detachment.
    - Klinefelter syndrome: marfanoid habitus, small testes and genitalia, learning difficulty.

EXAM TIP

Branched-chain amino acids are leucine, isoleucine, and valine.

WARD TIP

In MSUD, plasma leucine levels are usually higher than those of the other accumulating branched amino acids.

TABLE 8-1. **Lysosomal Storage Diseases—Lipidoses**

DISEASE	DEFICIENCY/ACCUMULATION	FEATURE	INHERITANCE/TREATMENT
GM1 gangliosidoses	■ Deficiency of β-galactosidase ■ Accumulation of GM1 ganglioside	■ Infantile, juvenile, adult-onset forms ■ 50% have cherry red spot located on macula ■ Hepatosplenomegaly ■ Edema, hypotonia, developmental regression, seizures ■ Blind and deaf by 1 year, death by 3–4 years of age (infantile) ■ Vacuolated lymphocytes and foamy histiocytes	■ Autosomal recessive ■ No treatment available
GM2 gangliosidoses	*Tay-Sachs disease:* ■ Deficiency of α subunit hexosaminidase A ■ Results in accumulation of GM2 ganglioside in brain *Sandhoff disease:* ■ Defect of β subunit hexosaminidases A and B ■ Accumulation of GM2 ganglioside in brain and peripheral organs	■ Infantile, juvenile, adult forms (multiple forms) ■ Onset at 5–6 months, death by 3–5 years of age ■ Cherry red spot located on macula ■ Hyperacusis (exaggerated startle response) ■ No organomegaly in Tay-Sachs ■ Hepatosplenomegaly in Sandhoff disease	■ Autosomal recessive ■ Ashkenazi Jews (Tay-Sachs) ■ No treatment available
Niemann-Pick disease (Types A, B, and C)	■ Deficiency of sphingomyelinase ■ Accumulation of sphingomyelin and cholesterol in reticuloendothelial and parenchymal cells	■ 50% have cherry red spot located on macula in type A and normal in B and C types ■ Hepatosplenomegaly, neonatal jaundice ■ Type A: early onset with neurologic deterioration, early death ■ Type B: later onset without neurologic signs, may involve lungs ■ Type C: variable onset with neurologic deterioration/psychiatric symptoms, death in childhood to early adulthood ■ Foam cells in bone marrow aspirates	■ Autosomal recessive ■ Ashkenazi Jews ■ Types A and B have no treatment. ■ Type C may have some response to the same substrate reduction therapy as Gaucher disease.
Gaucher disease (three types)	■ Deficiency of β-glucosidase ■ Accumulation of glucocerebroside in reticuloendothelial system	■ Type I is most common ■ Affects bone, liver, spleen, bone marrow ■ Pancytopenia ■ Bone fractures, pain, avascular necrosis ■ Gaucher cells in bone marrow —"crinkled paper" cytoplasm ■ Type 2 and 3 also have brain involvement and neurologic deterioration, distinguished by age of onset	■ Autosomal recessive ■ Ashkenazi Jews ■ Treated with enzyme replacement or substrate reduction therapy
Fabry disease	■ Deficiency of α-galactosidase A ■ Accumulation of glycosphingolipids in vascular endothelium, nerves, and organs ■ Clinical onset in childhood and adolescence with highly variable presentation	■ Angiokeratomas (dark red punctate macules that do not blanch) occur in clusters mostly between the umbilicus and knees ■ Acroparesthesias—episodic severe neuropathic limb pain ■ Corneal verticillata and lenticular changes—visible only on slit lamp that do not affect vision ■ Progressive kidney disease ■ Cardiomyopathy ■ Small vessel disease leading to TIA/stroke ■ Hypohidrosis/anhidrosis and GI pain/symptoms	■ **X-linked recessive** ■ Treated with enzyme replacement therapy ■ Women can be affected as well with varying severity and symptoms.

TABLE 8-1. Lysosomal Storage Diseases—Lipidoses *(continued)*

DISEASE	DEFICIENCY/ACCUMULATION	FEATURE	INHERITANCE/TREATMENT
Krabbe disease (globoid cell leukodystrophy)	■ Deficiency galactocerebrosidase ■ Accumulation of galactosylceramide within lysosomes of brain white matter	■ Progressive central nervous system degeneration; symptoms present within first 6 months of life ■ Increasing irritability, vomiting, feeding problems, tonic spasms induced by stimulation (visual or auditory), signs of peripheral neuropathy. ■ Late disease with blindness hyperpyrexia, opisthotonic posturing and death. ■ Globoid cells (multinucleated macrophages) in areas of demyelination	■ Autosomal recessive ■ Hematopoietic stem cell transplant may ameliorate disease in asymptomatic patients identified on NBS transplanted before 1 month of life.

TREATMENT

- Usually there is no specific treatment; therapy is primarily supportive/symptomatic.
- Gaucher Type I disease: enzyme replacement and substrate-reduction therapy.
- Fabry disease: enzyme-replacement therapy.
- Others: hematopoietic stem cell transplant has met with limited success.

MUCOPOLYSACCHARIDOSES (MPS)

DEFINITION/ETIOLOGY/PATHOPHYSIOLOGY

Inherited deficiencies of lysosomal enzymes needed for glycosaminoglycan (GAG)/mucopolysaccharide (MPS) degradation that result in widespread lysosomal storage of dermatan, heparan, keratan, or chondroitin sulfates and clinical abnormalities. Presentations are variable, but classical presentations are discussed below. See Table 8-2.

EPIDEMIOLOGY

Most are autosomal recessive.

SIGNS AND SYMPTOMS

- Most children are normal at birth with diagnosis at greater than a year.
- Severe forms may present with hydrops fetalis.
- Progressive mental and/or physical deterioration.
- Coarse facial features, with facial features appearing larger than expected.
- Corneal clouding in some but not all.
- Organomegaly.
- Skeletal abnormalities include short stature, dysostosis multiplex, joint pain, and stiffness.
- Hearing loss.

DIAGNOSIS

- Urinary excretion of GAGs: specific patterns can differentiate diagnosis.
- Detection of enzyme deficiency in leukocytes or cultured fibroblasts.
- Radiographic changes consistent with dysostosis multiplex.
- Molecular testing.

TREATMENT

- Enzyme-replacement therapy (ERT) is used for most, but it does not cross the blood-brain barrier and has no effect on CNS manifestations.
- Disease progression monitoring, hearing aids, and physical accommodations are used for support.

 WARD TIP

Correcting the serum glucose level in MSUD does not improve the clinical state.

 EXAM TIP

BCKD is made up of three subunits. Defects in the E1 or E2 subunit lead to MSUD. The E1 subunit is made of two alpha subunits and two beta subunits. Therefore, biallelic defects in three different genes can cause MSUD.

EXAM TIP

Due to a founder variant, prevalence in some Old Order Mennonite populations can reach as high as 1 in 380.

 WARD TIP

Suspect MSUD:
- Intermittent symptoms (feeding difficulties and apnea) related to protein ingestion
- Sweet-smelling cerumen

EXAM TIP

It is largely the elevation of leucine that causes the neurologic phenotype in untreated MSUD patients.

TABLE 8-2.   Lysosomal Storage Diseases—Mucopolysaccharidoses

SYNDROME	DEFICIENCY	DISTINCTIVE FEATURES	INHERITANCE
MPS Type I Hurler syndrome (severe) Hurler-Scheie syndrome (intermediate) Scheie syndrome (mild)	α-L-iduronidase	■ **Corneal clouding** ■ Detection after 1 year of age with coarsening of facial features, growth problems, and delays ■ Hurler-Scheie and Scheie syndromes are more mildly affected, with little CNS involvement and likely normal stature and lifespan	■ Autosomal recessive ■ ERT available
MPS Type II Hunter syndrome	Iduronate 2-sulfatase	■ Mild to severe; clinical onset 1–2 year of age and death before 15 years in severe form ■ More gradual onset of symptoms than MPS 1 ■ **Clear cornea** but associated with retinopathy and papilledema in severe cases	■ **X-linked recessive** ■ No affected females ■ ERT Available
MPS Type III Sanfilippo syndrome Types A,B,C, and D	4 different enzymes, one for each type	■ Later onset and predominated with neurological presentation—autism, behavior problems, intellectual disability, developmental delay ■ Other MPS features are less prominent	■ Autosomal recessive ■ No treatment available
MPS Type IV Morquio syndrome Type A and Type B	Iduronate 2-sulfatase	■ No neurological involvement ■ Severe skeletal involvement	■ Autosomal recessive ■ ERT Available

EXAM TIP

Detection of alloisoleucine on plasma amino acids is pathognomonic for MSUD.

EXAM TIP

The smells of metabolic disorders:
PKU: mousy or musty odor
MSUD: sweet smelling
Isovaleric acidemia: sweaty feet odor

WARD TIP

Gaucher disease is the most common lysosomal storage disease (1 in 75,000). Splenomegaly is the most common presenting sign.

EXAM TIP

Fabry disease is X-linked.

POMPE DISEASE—GLYCOGEN STORAGE DISEASE II

DEFINITION

Inherited disorder of glycogen metabolism characterized by the deposition of glycogen in cardiac and skeletal muscle.

ETIOLOGY

Deficiency of lysosomal acid α-1,4-glucosidase (acid maltase).

PATHOPHYSIOLOGY

■ Glycogen within the lysosome cannot be broken down, leading to cellular damage and autophagy and subsequent tissue damage primarily in the muscle and heart.

EPIDEMIOLOGY

Autosomal recessive

SIGNS AND SYMPTOMS

INFANTILE

■ Presents in the first months of life with poor feeding, hypotonia, hypertrophic cardiomyopathy, motor delay, and hepatomegaly.
■ Rapid, progressive cardiomyopathy with massive cardiomegaly, macroglossia, hypotonia, hepatomegaly; death by 1–2 years.
■ The juvenile form is milder, with slowly progressive myopathy and little to no cardiac abnormality. Death is usually secondary to respiratory failure.

DIAGNOSIS

- Electrocardiogram (ECG) may show shortened PR interval.
- Electromyogram (EMG) is used, too.

TREATMENT

Recombinant α-glucosidase enzyme replacement delays disease progression.

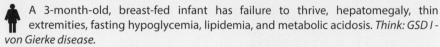

Defects of Carbohydrate Metabolism—Glycogen Storage Diseases (GSD)

GSD 1—VON GIERKE DISEASE

 A 3-month-old, breast-fed infant has failure to thrive, hepatomegaly, thin extremities, fasting hypoglycemia, lipidemia, and metabolic acidosis. *Think: GSD I - von Gierke disease.*

GSD I is an inherited disorder of glycogen metabolism. The glucose-6-phosphatase deficiency results in accumulation of glucose-6-phosphate, which in turn causes increased glycolysis and lactic acidosis. It is characterized by growth retardation, hypoglycemia, hepatomegaly, hyperlipidemia, hyperuricemia, lactic acidemia, and seizure. In the neonatal period, hypoglycemia and lactic acidosis are common. Hepatomegaly becomes evident by 3–4 months of age.

DEFINITION

Inherited disorder of glycogen metabolism characterized by deposition of glycogen in the liver, kidney, and intestine.

ETIOLOGY

Deficiency of glucose-6-phosphatase (GSD Ia) or glucose-6-phosphate exchanger (GSD Ib).

PATHOPHYSIOLOGY

Enzymes catalyze the first step of glycolysis and the last step of glycogenolysis. Patients are unable to utilize carbohydrate stores during fasting.

EPIDEMIOLOGY

Autosomal recessive

SIGNS AND SYMPTOMS

- Fasting hypoglycemia leads to possible lethargy or seizures.
- Significant hepatomegaly.
- Elevated serum levels of lactate, uric acid, cholesterol, triglycerides secondary to activation of alternate metabolic pathways.
- Renal complications (Fanconi syndrome, nephrocalcinosis, focal segmental glomerulosclerosis).
- Poor growth, bleeding diathesis, and gout.
- Untreated patients are at an increased risk for hepatic adenoma and possible hepatocellular carcinoma.
- Untreated patients will have a doll-like facial appearance with full cheeks, thin extremities, and protuberant abdomens.
- GSD Ib patients have a risk of neutropenia, inflammatory bowel disease.

EXAM TIP

A cherry red spot on the macula is seen in 50% of cases of GM1 Gangliosidoses and Niemann-Pick compared to most cases of GM2 Gangliosidoses (Tay-Sachs/Sandhoff disease).

EXAM TIP

Hepatosplenomegaly occurs in the GM1 gangliosidoses and Sandhoff disease, but not in Tay-Sachs disease.

EXAM TIP

Gaucher disease is the most common LSD and has the highest carrier frequency of any disease in the Ashkenazi Jewish population.

EXAM TIP

Hunter syndrome is X-linked and does not have corneal clouding.
"The Hunter must see his spot and X marks the spot."

WARD TIP

Dysostosis Multiplex
- Large dolichocephalic skull
- Thickened calvarium
- Ovoid vertebral bodies
- Flared iliac bones
- Shallow acetabula
- Thickened clavicles
- Irregular widening of long bones

WARD TIP

MPS VI = Maroteaux Lamy syndrome, which includes mild to severe problems, more skeletal phenotype, clouded corneas, and joint laxity. ERT is available.
MPS VII = Sly syndrome, which is severe and rare, has no treatment available.

WARD TIP

Pompe affects the "**P**ump."

WARD TIP

Pompe disease is a lysosomal storage disorder and a glycogen storage disorder. In Pompe disease glycogen stores build up in the lysosome.

EXAM TIP

Lactose = galactose + glucose.

WARD TIP

The typical age of presentation for GSD I is around 4 months of age when infants begin to sleep through the night. Prior to this event, regular feedings supply a regular glucose source. Prolonged sleep periods are fasting periods and lead to significant hypoglycemic events, which will bring patients to attention.

WARD TIP

McArdle disease affects the **m**uscles.

DIAGNOSIS

- Normal at birth.
- Administration of epinephrine, glucagon, galactose, fructose, or glycerol does not provoke normal hyperglycemic response (may precipitate acidosis).
- Genetic sequencing.
- Enzymatic testing.
- A liver biopsy demonstrates accumulation of glycogen in the cells.
- Hypoglycemia will develop within three hours of eating.

TREATMENT

- Avoid fasting and simple sugars.
- Supportive therapy aimed at maintaining normal glucose levels.
- Complex carbohydrate meals and uncooked cornstarch administration allow for prolonged fasting times. Smaller children may require nocturnal gastric infusions.
- A high-protein diet is not effective.
- Granulocyte colony–stimulating factors for neutropenia and inflammation in GSD Ib.
- Allopurinol to lower urate levels, bicarbonate or potassium citrate for lactic acidosis.
- With improved dietary management, liver transplant is rarely needed.

GSD V—MCARDLE DISEASE

DEFINITION

Inherited disorder of glycogen metabolism characterized by the deposition of glycogen in skeletal muscle.

ETIOLOGY

Deficiency of muscle glycogen phosphorylase (myophosphorylase).

EPIDEMIOLOGY

Autosomal recessive

SIGNS AND SYMPTOMS

- Involves only skeletal muscles (glycogen accumulations predominant in subsarcolemmal location).
- Characterized by exercise intolerance: weakness and cramping during or after exercise.
- Characteristic "second wind" phenomenon with fatty acid metabolism initiation.
- No rise in blood lactate during exercise.
- Severe episodes can lead to rhabdomyolysis, myoglobinuria, and concomitant renal failure.

DIAGNOSIS

- Asymptomatic during infancy, presents in adolescence/early childhood.
- Muscle biopsy and enzyme assay show deficiency of enzyme.
- Myoglobinuria and serum creatine kinase are always elevated (elevated CK at rest).
- Genetic sequencing.

TREATMENT

- Dietary modification: high fat and protein.
- Simple sugar consumption prior to exercise.
- Moderate intensity aerobic training.

GALACTOSEMIA

A 2-week-old neonate presents in septic shock. He has jaundice, hepatomegaly, and positive urinary reducing substance. Odor of urine is normal. Blood culture returns positive for gram negative rods. *Think: Galactosemia.*

Since galactosemia is included in the newborn screening, it is usually diagnosed before the symptoms develop. Jaundice, hepatomegaly, vomiting, lethargy, and feeding difficulties are the common initial presentation. The presence of urine reducing substances in infants ingesting lactose establishes the diagnosis.

DEFINITION

Inborn error of carbohydrate metabolism that results in elevated galactose and metabolite levels in blood and urine.

ETIOLOGY

- Three types: classic, clinical variant, and Duarte.
- All types arise from the absence or reduction of galactose-1-phosphate uridyltransferase (GALT) activity.
- Classic and clinical variant galactosemia can present similarly in the neonate and require treatment, but clinical variant patients do not bear long-term complication risks.
- Duarte galactosemia has a similar biochemical profile, has sufficient enzyme activity (not at risk of complications), and does not require treatment.

PATHOPHYSIOLOGY

- Inability to break down galactose leads to increased concentration of galactose and toxic byproducts in the blood.
- Toxic substances, galactitol, cause organ damage.

EPIDEMIOLOGY

- Autosomal recessive.
- Clinical variant galactosemia is most commonly seen in the native African and African American populations.

SIGNS AND SYMPTOMS

- Infants present early with cataracts (with oil-spot appearance), hepatosplenomegaly, jaundice, FTT, lethargy, and possible sepsis (*E. coli*).
- Later complications include learning difficulties and intellectual disability.
- Triad: **Liver failure** (jaundice and coagulation disorder), **renal tubular dysfunction** (glucosuria, aminoaciduria, and acidosis), and **cataract** (galactitol deposition in the lens).
- Most females with galactosemia suffer from ovarian failure.

DIAGNOSIS

- All three forms are detected by NBS, but illness may occur before results are available.
- Diagnosis includes checking for the presence of a reducing substance in urine after the ingestion of milk or formula.
- Elevated red blood cell galactose-1-phosphate level and decreased galactose-1-phosphate uridyltransferase enzyme function occurs.
- Multiple common genetic variants are known to cause specific forms of the disease.

WARD TIP

When diagnosis of galactosemia is not made at birth, damage to the liver and brain become irreversible.

WARD TIP

Deficiencies of galactokinase or uridine diphosphate galactose-4-epimerase can lead to disease similar to galactosemia, but they are much rarer.

WARD TIP

Neonates with galactosemia are at ↑ risk for *Escherichia coli* sepsis.

TREATMENT

- Restriction of galactose (thus lactose) in diet (example: dairy and breast milk).
- Soy-based formula.
- Due to endogenous galactose production, treatment ameliorates but does not completely alleviate long-term classic galactosemia complications.

Defects in Purine Metabolism

LESCH-NYHAN SYNDROME

DEFINITION

An X-linked-recessive disorder of purine metabolism results in the deposition of purines in tissues and subsequent clinical abnormalities.

ETIOLOGY

Deficiency of hypoxanthine–guanine phosphoribosyl transferase (HGPRT) leads to an increased *de novo* synthesis or uric acid and the terminus of purine degradation.

SIGNS AND SYMPTOMS

- Normal until 3–6 months of age when delayed motor development begins.
- Hypotonia, choreoathetosis, spasticity, dystonia, hyperreflexia.
- Self-injurious behavior.
- Intellectual disability and possible seizures.
- Hyperuricemia, urinary tract calculi, urate nephropathy, tophi, gouty arthritis.

DIAGNOSIS

- Around 3–6 months when motor delay becomes apparent.
- Uric acid crystalluria may first be noted as orange crystals in the diaper.
- Serum uric acid levels are elevated.
- Enzymatic or molecular testing is also used.

TREATMENT

- No specific treatment; supportive therapy.
- Allopurinol to reduce serum uric acid levels.
- Prevention of self-injury.
- Death (infection, respiratory failure, or renal failure) in the second or third decade.

Fatty Acid Oxidation Disorders (FAODS)

GENERAL

DEFINITION

These disorders impede or prohibit oxidation of fats in the mitochondria for use in energy production during fasting.

ETIOLOGY

Multiple disorders are differentiated by the fat length that can be broken down.

EXAM TIP

Self-injurious behavior in Lesch-Nyhan syndrome can include banging the head against a wall and biting/mutilating the fingers and lips.

WARD TIP

Think Lesch-Nyhan syndrome in the presence of self-mutilation and characteristic choreoathetosis and intellectual disability in a male.

SIGNS AND SYMPTOMS

- Onset and severity vary between disorders and within the same disorder, ranging from sudden neonatal death to exercise intolerance.
- All share some combination of:
  - Hypoketotic hypoglycemia.
  - Heart: hypertrophic cardiomyopathy, arrhythmias.
  - Myopathy: muscle weakness or rhabdomyolysis.
  - Transaminitis.

DIAGNOSIS

- Most detected on NBS.
- Lack of ketones during acute hypoglycemic episode.
- Elevations in CK, transaminases, and lactic acid.
- Defining elevation or deficiency on plasma acylcarnitine profile.
- Enzymatic and molecular testing.

TREATMENT

- *Avoid fasting.* Fasting times increase with age and glycogen store development.
- IV glucose during acute decompensation.
- Dietary fat restriction with supplementation of usable length fats in diet, primarily medium chain triglycerides.

General Concepts and Other Disorders

- Sudden infant death syndrome (SIDS), apparent life-threatening event (ALTE), or brief resolved unexplained event (BRUE) may be the initial presentation of an inborn error of metabolism.
- Unexplained developmental delay may indicate an underlying metabolic disease.

EXAM TIP

These are the most common fatty acid oxidation disorders:

    VLCAD—very long chain acyl-CoA dehydrogenase deficiency

    CPTI/CPTII—Carnitine Palmitoyl Transferase I/II deficiency

    MCAD—medium-chain acyl-CoA dehydrogenase deficiency

    Primary Carnitine Deficiency

WARD TIP

Lipid metabolism is the primary source of energy during a fasting state after glucose stores are exhausted. Neonates have little to no glycogen stores. Lipid metabolism is what produces ketones.

WARD TIP

MCAD is the most common fatty acid oxidation defect in North America.

WARD TIP

FAODs were a likely cause of sudden infant death syndrome before their detection on newborn screening.

NOTES

Immunologic Disease

Transplacental antibodies protect neonates against chickenpox, measles, mumps, and rubella, but not chlamydia, gonorrhea, or group B *Streptococcus*.

- First immunoglobulin to appear in the bloodstream after the initial exposure to an antigen (primary antibody response): IgM
- Secretory antibody response: IgA
- Major antibody to protein antigens: IgG

WARD TIP

Transient hypogammaglobulinemia of infancy

- Prolongation of physiologic hypogammaglobulinemia of infancy
- Generally resolves by 2–4 years of age
- Recurrent sinopulmonary infections
- Normal B and T cell counts
- Atopy a common finding

WARD TIP

Anaphylactoid Reaction
- Clinically similar to anaphylaxis
- Not IgE mediated
- Caused by direct, nonimmune-mediated release from mast cells and/or basophils
- Does not require previous exposure

Immune System

- Primary lymphoid organs—development of lymphocytes: bone marrow, fetal liver, and spleen; thymus: maturation of T cells.
- Secondary lymphoid tissue—sites of antigen recognition: lymph nodes, spleen, mucosal-associated lymphoid tissues, and gut-associated lymphoid tissues.
- Maternal serum antibodies (transplacental immunoglobulin G [IgG]) protect the infant until about 3 to 4 months of age, and they disappear by 12–18 months of age. A physiologic nadir of serum antibodies occurs at 6 months.
- Maternal antibodies (IgA) are transferred to the child's intestinal tract through breast milk.
- A child's IgG antibodies begin developing between 6 months and 1 year of age.
- Children <2 years develop strong immune response to vaccine polysaccharide antigens (*Haemophilus influenzae*, pneumococcal) when conjugated to a protein carrier.

Hypersensitivity Reactions

See Table 9-1 for types of hypersensitivity reactions.

- Urticaria (hives): pale or reddened irregular, elevated itchy skin patches.
- Angioedema: giant wheals caused by localized dilation and increased capillary permeability in the deep dermis.
- Vesicle: a fluid collection below epidermis <5 mm in diameter.
- Bulla: blister >5 mm in diameter with thin walls.

ANAPHYLAXIS

DEFINITION

A severe, potentially life-threatening systemic IgE-mediated reaction caused by release of mediators from tissue mast cells and blood basophils

TABLE 9-1. Types of Hypersensitivity Reactions

HYPERSENSITIVITY	ANTIBODY	EFFECT	EXAMPLES
Type I	IgE	Mast cells mediated	Anaphylaxis; Allergic rhinitis
Type II	IgM, IgG	Cytotoxic: cell lysis	Goodpasture's syndrome
Type III	IgM, IgG	AG-AB complex triggers complement	Serum sickness
Type IV	None	T cells infiltrate	Poison ivy dermatitis, PPD positivity

ETIOLOGY

- Foods: peanuts, milk, egg, shellfish.
- Drugs: β-lactam antibiotics, ibuprofen, radiocontrast agents.
- Vaccine, immune globulin, blood products.
- Latex (gloves, Foley catheters, and endotracheal tubes).
- Insect stings, venom.

SIGNS AND SYMPTOMS

- Abrupt onset and rapid progression within 5–30 minutes.
- Generalized pruritus, urticaria, tearing, angioedema.
- Warmth, flushing, dizziness.
- Vomiting, abdominal cramps, esp. for ingested allergens.
- Respiratory symptoms: upper-airway obstruction (laryngeal angioedema), bronchospasm.
- Hypotension, shock.

DIAGNOSIS

- History of exposure and clinical presentation.
- Less commonly confirm with serum tryptase (at 1, 4, and 8 hours).

TREATMENT

- Airway, breathing, circulation (ABC).
- Epinephrine within 30 minutes of symptoms.
- Inhaled β-agonist.
- Diphenhydramine.
- Cimetidine.
- Corticosteroids to attenuate late-phase inflammatory response.
- Observe in emergency department for at least four hours before discharge.

WARD TIP

Risk factors for severe anaphylactic reaction:
- Asthma
- β-blockade or α-adrenergic antagonist
- Angiotensin-converting enzyme inhibitors

WARD TIP

Prophylaxis:
- Avoid allergen
- ID bracelet
- Self-injectable epinephrine (EpiPen® or Auvi-Q®)

URTICARIA (HIVES)

See Dermatology Chapter

SERUM SICKNESS

> For the past two weeks, a 6-year-old boy has had puffy eyelids on awakening and swelling of the feet and abdomen in the afternoon. He complains of joint aches and intermittent fever. His history includes a recent sting by a yellow jacket. Physical examination is significant for generalized lymphadenopathy. Urinalysis shows protein 3+ and ESR is 35. *Think: Serum sickness.*

DEFINITION

This type III hypersensitivity reaction does not require prior sensitization.

PATHOPHYSIOLOGY

Antigen-antibody complexes form blood vessel deposits, particularly in joints and glomeruli, where they activate the classical complement pathway, resulting in vasculitis.

ETIOLOGY

- Serum/blood products from other species, anti-venoms.
- Antimicrobials: cefaclor, penicillin, griseofulvin, sulfonamides.
- Neurologics: phenytoin, sulfonamides, barbiturates, carbamazepine.

SIGNS AND SYMPTOMS

- Onset 1–3 weeks after initial exposure to an offending agent.
- Fever, arthralgia, lymphadenopathy, and rash (serpiginous and urticarial or polymorphous).
- Facial edema.
- Rarely arthritis, carditis, glomerulonephritis, peripheral neuritis (Guillain-Barré).
- Symptoms persist 7–14 days and resolve spontaneously.

DIAGNOSIS

- Clinical.
- Thrombocytopenia, elevated ESR and C-reactive protein, proteinuria, hematuria.
- Low levels of C3, C4 (complement components), and CH50.

TREATMENT

- Withdrawal of the offending agent.
- Occasionally, antihistamines, analgesics, antipyretics, and for severe disease steroids.

DRUG REACTION

DEFINITION

- Abnormal immunologically-mediated hypersensitivity responses.
- Relatively rare.

ETIOLOGY

Potentially any drug can cause a drug reaction.

PATHOPHYSIOLOGY

- Type I (IgE mediated): penicillin, cephalosporin.
- Type II (cytotoxic antibody mediated): penicillin—hemolytic anemia; quinidine—thrombocytopenia.
- Type III (immune complex mediated): penicillin, sulfonamides, cephalosporin.
- Type IV (cell mediated): contact dermatitis—neomycin.

CLINICAL CRITERIA

- Reactions do not resemble a pharmacologic action of the drug.
- Similar to those that may occur with other allergens.
- Timing: 7–10 days.
- Reproduced by minute doses.
- Discontinuation may result in resolution.

SIGNS AND SYMPTOMS

- Mild rash to anaphylaxis.
- Fixed drug eruptions: recur at the same site after each administration of causative drug (sulfonamides are the most common).

DIAGNOSIS

- Eosinophilia is a clue, but it is not diagnostic, especially with drug rash with eosinophilia and systemic symptoms (DRESS) syndrome.
- A skin test is available for penicillin but not most other drugs. It is indicated for patients who have a history of penicillin-associated anaphylaxis, urticaria, or serum sickness.
- Direct Coombs test for drug-induced hemolytic anemia.

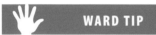

WARD TIP

The most common causes of drug reactions are penicillin and sulfonamides.

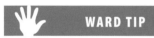

WARD TIP

Drug Reactions
- Most are afebrile.
- Eruption may worsen before improving after discontinuation of the drug.

WARD TIP

The most common site for the manifestation of drug reactions is the skin.

DISPOSITION

- Discontinue likely offending agent.
- Admit if:
  - Stevens-Johnson syndrome.
  - Toxic epidermal necrolysis.
  - Severe drug reaction, such as DRESS.

PENICILLIN ALLERGY

TYPES

Wide variety of allergic reactions:
- Type I: anaphylaxis.
- Type II: hemolytic anemia.
- Type III: serum sickness.

FOOD ALLERGY/SENSITIVITY

PATHOPHYSIOLOGY

- Most of the true hypersensitivities to food products are IgE mediated. IgE binds to mast cells, resulting in histamine and other mediator release. Most common triggers are peanuts, shellfish, and eggs.
- It presents early in life. Only ~5% of children <4 years have food hypersensitivity. It is seen even less frequently in older children.
- Most adverse reactions to food do not have an immunologic basis.
- Nonimmunologic food intolerances are common, such as enzyme deficiencies (e.g., lactase deficiency, which causes vomiting and diarrhea).

SIGNS AND SYMPTOMS

- IgE-mediated hypersensitivity reactions can begin within minutes of the responsible food intake, often with urticaria, edema, and anaphylaxis.
- Allergic enterocolitis of infancy with vomiting and diarrhea (becomes bloody) is a cow's milk protein hypersensitivity, but it is not IgE mediated. It causes failure to thrive. Half of these infants also react to soy protein. Presentation is in the first 2 months of life.
- Gluten-sensitive enteropathy is a non-IgE-mediated food hypersensitivity (celiac disease) that causes failure to thrive. Gradual onset of symptoms at 4 to 6 months of life, when the child starts to eat grains containing gluten protein.

TREATMENT

Avoidance of offending agent.

 WARD TIP

Most common food allergies:
- Peanut
- Shellfish
- Eggs

Immunodeficiencies

- A constellation of infection types and frequencies are concerning for primary immunodeficiencies (see Table 9-2).
- Primary (congenital) immune deficiencies (PIs) (Table 9-3) can be differentiated by presentation.
- PIs are characterized by recurrent or unusually hard-to-cure infections, or two or more of the warning signs listed in the Table 9-2.
  - Age of onset: neutrophil defects present in the first few months of life. Innate immunity and T-cell defects present in the first 3–4 months

TABLE 9-2. **Warning Signs of Primary Immunodeficiency**

1. One or more systemic bacterial infections (sepsis, meningitis)
2. Recurrent serious respiratory (pneumonia, sinusitis, draining otitis media) or other bacterial infections (cellulitis, lymphadenitis) in a year
3. Serious infections at unanticipated sites (brain or liver abscess)
4. Infections with unusual pathogens or unusually severe presentation of common childhood pathogens
5. Failure of an infant to gain weight or grow normally
6. Recurrent, deep skin or organ abscesses
7. Persistent thrush or fungal infection on skin
8. Need for unanticipated, prolonged intravenous antibiotics to clear infections
9. Diagnosis of autoimmune disease
10. A family history of PI

TABLE 9-3. **Phagocytic and Chemotactic Disorder**

Disorder	Inheritance	Defect	Clinical	Infections	Diagnosis
Chronic granulomatous disease	X-linked	Pyruvate deficiency in PMNs and macrophages	Gingivitis, seborrheic dermatitis, retinitis pigmentosa	Deep soft tissue abscesses, lymphadenitis, *Staphylococcus*, *Aspergillus*	Neutrophil oxidation test NBT = old Leukocytosis
Chédiak-Higashi	Autosomal recessive	Abnormal chemotaxis and fusion of intracellular granules	Partial albinism, progressive neuropathy, HSM	Skin and lung, *Staphylococcus*	Chemotaxis test, leukopenia
Job (hyper-IgE) syndrome	Autosomal dominant	Connective tissue and chemotaxis disorder	Coarse features, eczema, lax joints	Skin and lung, *Staphylococcus*, *Aspergillus*	IgE > 10,000, eosinophilia
Leukocyte adhesion deficiency	Autosomal recessive	Impaired phagocyte recruitment from blood due to impaired adhesion	Delayed separation of umbilical cord, poor wound healing	Severe gingivitis, bacterial infections without pus	Neutrophilia, flow cytometry for CD18

HSM, hepatosplenomegaly; NBT, nitroblue tetrazolium; PMN, polymorphonuclear neutrophil.

of life, whereas B-cell disorders present after 6 months of age, when maternal antibodies disappear.

- X-linked inheritance: similar case in a male relative (Bruton's, Wiskott-Aldrich, chronic granulomatous disease [CGD]).
- Sites of infection:
  - Phagocytes (CGD): sinopulmonary and soft tissues.
  - Immunoglobulin deficiencies: sinopulmonary and gastrointestinal (*Giardia*).
  - T cells: disseminated (mycobacteria, varicella-zoster virus).

- Types of microorganisms
  - Intracellular infections in T-cell disorders (viruses, mycobacteria, *Pneumocystis*).
  - Extracellular encapsulated organisms (*Streptococcus pneumoniae*, *Haemophilus influenzae* type B, and group A streptococcus) and *Giardia* in B-cell disorders.
  - Extracellular encapsulated organisms (*Streptococcus pneumoniae*, *Haemophilus influenza*) and *Neisseria* infections in late-complement deficiency.
  - *Staphylococcus, Pseudomonas, Escherichia coli*, and *Aspergillus* in neutrophil disorders.
- Associated problems
  - Malignancies tend to accompany T-cell defects; congenital heart disease and hypocalcemia indicates DiGeorge syndrome; atopic dermatitis indicates hyper-IgE syndrome; abnormal gait and telangiectasia indicate ataxia-telangiectasia; and an easy bruising/bleeding disorder suggests Wiskott-Aldrich syndrome.
- Workup
  - Complete blood count (CBC) with differential white blood cell count and morphology, hemoglobin, and platelet count (B and T lymphocyte disorders, phagocytic disorders), quantitative immunoglobulins (B lymphocyte disorders), CH50 (complement disorders).
  - Radiograph of area of infection (chest, sinus, mastoids, or long bones).
  - Cultures, if appropriate.

CHRONIC GRANULOMATOUS DISEASE (CGD)

A 10-month-old male presents with a temperature of 101.6°F (38.7°C) and a 3 × 4-cm abscess of the left buttock. His WBC count is 19.9/mm³, 77% neutrophils. At the age of 5 months, he had staphylococcal cervical lymphadenitis that required drainage. His uncle also had recurrent abscesses. *Think: CGD.*

DEFINITION

- Most common inherited phagocyte disorder.
- 70% X-linked, 30% autosomal recessive.

PATHOPHYSIOLOGY

- NADPH oxidase complex defect leads to defective production of reactive oxygen species in neutrophils and macrophages.
- Susceptibility to catalase-positive microorganisms: *Aspergillus species*, *Staphylococcus aureus, Burkholderia, Serratia, Nocardia*.
- Granulomatous inflammatory responses occur due to macrophage functional impairment.

SIGNS AND SYMPTOMS

- Recurrent bacterial and fungal infections that begin in the first year of life: pneumonia, abscesses of the skin, soft tissue, organs (perianal/perirectal, liver, lung), lymphadenitis, osteomyelitis, bacteremia/fungemia, superficial skin infections (cellulitis/impetigo).
- Growth failure, abnormal wound healing, diarrhea.
- Hepatomegaly, splenomegaly, lymphadenopathy (enlarged by granulomas).

DIAGNOSIS

- Dihydrorhodamine oxidation test (preferred) or Nitroblue tetrazolium test (classic).
- Genetic testing confirms diagnosis.

WARD TIP

Catalase-positive infections in CGD include: *Aspergillus, S. aureus, Burkholderia, Serratia, Nocardia, Candida, Salmonella.*

TREATMENT

- Aggressive, early treatment of infection.
- Surgical excision of abscesses.
- Antimicrobial prophylaxis: TMP-SMX, itraconazole, and interferon-gamma.
- Hematopoietic cell transplantation is effective for refractory infection.

CHEDIAK-HIGASHI SYNDROME

DEFINITION

This autosomal-recessive disease is caused by a lysosomal-trafficking regulator gene mutation, resulting in fusion of intracellular granules and dysfunctional neutrophil degranulation.

SIGNS AND SYMPTOMS

- Recurrent skin infections and pneumonias, esp. *Staphylococcus aureus*.
- Partial oculocutaneous albinism.
- Mild bleeding diathesis.
- Progressive peripheral neuropathy.

DIAGNOSIS

- Giant gray granules in the cytoplasm of nucleated cells.
- Leukopenia, neutropenia.
- Chemotaxis test.

TREATMENT

- Benefit of high-dose ascorbic acid controversial.
- Antibiotics for acute infections.
- Bone marrow transplant (does not prevent nor cure peripheral neuropathy).

JOB SYNDROME (HYPER-IGE)

 A 10-year-old boy has a history of severe pneumonia with empyema at the age of 5 years. He is allergic to pollens and animal dander. Now he has fever of 102.3°F (39.1°C). On examination, he has coarse facial features, eczematous patches on the extremities, and a tender 4 × 3-cm right anterior cervical lymph node. WBC is 24.7/mm³. *Think: Job syndrome.*

DEFINITION

- This autosomal dominant neutrophil chemotactic disorder is caused by STAT3 gene mutation.
- Hyperimmunoglobulinemia E with impaired chemotaxis.
- Characteristic findings include eczema, recurrent "cold," staphylococcal skin abscesses, sinusitis, and otitis media.

SIGNS AND SYMPTOMS

- Recurrent sinopulmonary staphylococcal infections.
- Eczema.
- Lax (hyper-extensible) joints.
- Osteopenia with fractures, coarse facial features, retention of baby teeth.

DIAGNOSIS

- IgE >2,000 IU/mL.
- Eosinophilia.

TREATMENT

- Skin hydration and management of pruritus.
- TMP-SMX prophylaxis for patients with frequent infections.
- Hematopoietic cell transplant variably successful.

LEUKOCYTE ADHESION DEFICIENCY (LAD TYPE 1)

 A 2-month-old male has a temperature of 103°F, HR 200 beats/min, RR 50 breaths/min, and appears lethargic. His umbilical cord has not separated; the surrounding skin is erythematous and indurated. He is admitted for sepsis. His white blood cell count is 22,000/mm³ with 90% neutrophils. *Think: defective neutrophil migration.*

DEFINITION

LAD type 1 is an autosomal recessive condition of neutrophil migration with impaired chemotaxis, tight adhesion of neutrophils to endothelium, and phagocytosis.

SIGNS AND SYMPTOMS

- Failure of separation of umbilical cord, with secondary omphalitis and sepsis.
- Poor wound healing.
- Bacterial infections without pus.
- Severe gingivitis.

DIAGNOSIS

- Neutrophilia without infection; during infection, count can range >50,000/mm³.
- Flow cytometry testing for CD 11b/CD18.

TREATMENT

- Oral hygiene.
- Aggressive antibiotic management of infections.
- Hematopoietic cell transplant for severe cases.

COMPLEMENT DEFICIENCY

 A 16-year-old female presents with a second episode of meningococcal meningitis. Her CH50 is 78%. *Think: C5–C9 deficiency.*

Deficiency of complement proteins leads to severe immunodeficiency; different deficiencies are associated with specific infections, as noted below.

COMPLEMENT

Complex system of nine serum proteins (C1–C9).

FUNCTIONS OF COMPLEMENT

- Opsonization.
- Bacteria cell lysis.
- Facilitating chemotaxis.

ASSOCIATED DISEASES

- C1q and C4 deficiency: systemic lupus erythematosus (SLE).
- C1 esterase inhibitor (C1 INH) deficiency: hereditary angioedema.

EXAM TIP

Hypocomplementemia occurs in patients with lupus nephritis and poststreptococcal glomerulonephritis, but not in Henoch-Schönlein purpura or minimal change disease.

Vaccination is the best way to protect a patient with complement deficiency. For meningococcus, both quadrivalent (covers A, C, Y, W-135 strains) and MenB vaccines are recommended. While the pneumococcal vaccine PCV-13 is recommended for all children, PPSV23 is also recommended for children with complement deficiency.

Onset of SCID at 3 months of age:
- No palpable lymph nodes
- Opportunistic infections
- Failure to thrive

Measures to be taken in SCID:
- Protective isolation
- Irradiation of all blood products
- Avoidance of live vaccines

- C2 and C3 deficiency: pneumococcal (majority), *Haemophilus influenzae* and meningococci infections.
- C5–C9 terminal complement deficiency: *Neisseria* infection.

DIAGNOSIS

- CH50 screening test.

SEVERE COMBINED IMMUNODEFICIENCY (SCID)

A 4-month-old female with failure to thrive (FTT) presents with respiratory distress. She has a temperature of 101°F (38.3°C), RR 70 breaths/min, and oxygen saturation of 91% (on room air). Thrush and bilateral rhonchi are present but no lymphadenopathy. Her white blood cell count is 16.2/mm³, 83% neutrophils, 11% monocytes. Chest x-ray shows diffuse bilateral interstitial infiltrates. *Think: Pneumocystis jirovecii pneumonia (PCP)*.

Infection with opportunistic organisms such as PCP is common in infants with SCID. Absence of lymph nodes in an infant with FTT is suggestive of SCID. Thrush, extensive diaper rash, and FTT are the prominent features.

DEFINITION

Abnormalities of both humoral and cellular immunity.

ETIOLOGY

- A group of genetic abnormalities that result in severe T-cell depletion (or dysfunction) and B-cell dysfunction (e.g., enzyme deficiencies cause defects in stem cell maturation).
- X-linked SCID most common form.
- Adenosine deaminase deficiency: about 15% of all SCID cases.

SIGNS AND SYMPTOMS

- Presents within first 3 months with diarrhea, pneumonia, otitis, sepsis, FTT, and skin rashes.
- Increased frequency and/or severity of infections.
- Persistent infection with opportunistic organisms (*Candida*, mycobacteria, herpes viruses, CMV, PCP).
- Absent lymph nodes, hypoplastic thymus.

DIAGNOSIS

- Lymphopenia: absolute lymphocyte count <500.
- Decreased serum IgG, IgA, and IgM.
- Low or no T and B cells.
- SCID part of newborn screening in most states.

TREATMENT

- Aggressive antimicrobial treatment of even mild infections.
- Palivizumab for RSV prophylaxis during appropriate season.
- Recombinant adenosine deaminase replacement for X-linked SCID.
- Stem cell transplantation or gene therapy.

PROGNOSIS

Death within first year if untreated.

X-LINKED HYPER-IGM SYNDROME

DEFINITION

- Defect in CD40 ligand, leading to impaired T-cell "help" to B cells.
- Characterized by failure of isotype switching from IgM to IgA, IgG, and IgE.

SIGNS AND SYMPTOMS

- Presentation during first or second year of life
- Recurrent sinopulmonary infections with pyogenic bacteria.
- Severe intracellular infections due to impaired cellular immunity (*Pneumocystis jirovecii*).
- Malignancies.

DIAGNOSIS

- Serum Ig analysis: markedly high IgM, low IgG, IgA, and IgE.

TREATMENT

- IVIG.
- Stem cell transplantation.
- High mortality rate.

T-Cell Disorders

LANGERHANS CELL HISTIOCYTOSIS (LCH)

 A 2-year-old girl presents with two "bumps on the head." Physical examination shows weight below third percentile; two palpable scalp masses; and scaly, greasy patches over the scalp, eyebrows, neck, and in the ear canals; generalized lymphadenopathy; and hepatosplenomegaly. WBC: 5.6/mm³, Hb 8.4 g/dL, platelet count 76/mm³. Lateral skull radiograph shows two well-defined lytic lesions. *Think: Langerhans cell histiocytosis.*

Patients with this disease typically present with a scaly seborrhea and eczematous rash involving the scalp, ear canals, abdomen, and intertriginous areas of the neck and face. Typical presentation age is under 2 years. There is a potential for pancytopenia because of hematopoietic involvement.

DEFINITION

- CD207+ cell proliferation in multiple tissues triggering granulomatous inflammation.
- Manifestation of immune dysregulation that is incompletely understood.

SIGNS AND SYMPTOMS

- Bone (80%): skull, vertebrae (eosinophilic granuloma, lytic lesions).
- Skin (50%): seborrheic dermatitis in a child of <2 years of age.
- Lymphadenopathy (33%).
- Hepatosplenomegaly (20%).
- Exophthalmos due to retro-orbital accumulation of granulomatous tissue.
- Pituitary dysfunction: growth retardation, diabetes insipidus.
- Systemic manifestations: fever, anorexia, weight loss, irritability, FTT.
- Bone marrow suppression: anemia, thrombocytopenia, neutropenia.

EXAM TIP

Langerhans Cell Histiocytosis
- Lytic lesions
- Lymphadenopathy
- Seborrheic dermatitis

LAB

- Complete blood count (CBC), liver function tests (LFTs), coagulation profile.
- Chest x-ray.
- Skeletal survey.
- Urine osmolality.
- Tissue biopsy of any skin or bone lesions.

TREATMENT

- Single-system disease: arrest the progression of lesions (low-dose local radiation, steroid injection).
- Multisystem disease: multi-agent chemotherapy.

DIGEORGE SYNDROME (THYMIC HYPOPLASIA)

> A 2-month-old infant with a heart defect and cleft palate has cough and tachypnea. He has a history of seizures. Chest x-ray shows diffuse infiltrates and no thymic shadow. Serum calcium is 6.5 mg/dL. *Think: DiGeorge syndrome.*
>
> DiGeorge syndrome is a T-cell deficiency that results from failure of development of the third and fourth pharyngeal pouches, which are responsible for thymus and parathyroid gland development. These result in lack of T-cell-mediated immunity, tetany, and congenital defects of the heart and great vessels. Without treatment, the condition is fatal.

PATHOPHYSIOLOGY

- Deletion in chromosome 22, resulting in a defect of development of the third and fourth pharyngeal pouches.
- Phenotypical translation into midline defects of the heart, head, parathyroids, and thymus.

SIGNS AND SYMPTOMS

- Dysmorphic features: hypertelorism, cleft palate.
- Congenital heart disease: truncus arteriosus, interrupted aortic arch.
- Hypoparathyroidism presents as hypocalcemic seizures ("tetany").
- Recurrent infections: opportunistic infections when T-lymphocyte counts are low.

DIAGNOSIS

- Calcium level and parathyroid hormone.
- T-cell count (variable).
- Chest x-ray: no thymic shadow.
- Echocardiogram.
- Fluorescent *in-situ* hybridization (FiSH) test detects the 22q11.2 deletion.

TREATMENT

- Evaluation for hearing difficulties.
- Cultured thymic transplant.
- Hematopoietic cell transplant improves immune function but not T-cell production (no thymus); risk of graft-versus-host disease unless donor is HLA-identical.
- Use irradiated blood products only.

ATAXIA-TELANGIECTASIA

DEFINITION

This autosomal-recessive disorder of DNA repair presents as telangiectasias, ataxia, and variable extent of T-cell deficiency, with progressive loss of T helpers. Both humoral and cellular immunodeficiency occur.

SIGNS AND SYMPTOMS

- Usually presents soon after walking initiates, wheelchair confinement by 10–12 years.
- Earliest sign: telangiectasias on the sclerae (misdiagnosed as "pink eye").
- Progressive cerebellar ataxia.
- Chronic sinusitis, bronchiectases.
- Opportunistic infections (OIs).
- Increased risk of malignancy (lymphomas, leukemia).

LAB

- Absence of antibodies after vaccination.
- Low IgA, IgE, and IgG.
- T4 lymphocytes decline over time.
- Increased serum α-fetoprotein.

TREATMENT

- Supportive therapy.
- Improve pulmonary function.
- Prophylaxis of OIs.
- Avoidance of ionizing radiation.
- Immunoglobulin replacement if recurrent infections.

EXAM TIP

Ataxia-telangiectasia:
- Telangiectasias of conjunctivae and exposed areas
- Ataxia
- Lymphoma

WARD TIP

Thymic hypo- or aplasia results in a deficiency of functional T cells.

CHRONIC MUCOCUTANEOUS CANDIDIASIS

DEFINITION

- This T-cell dysfunction results in an inability to recognize candidal antigens.
- This heterogeneous group of disorders is characterized by recurrent or persistent superficial candidal infections of the skin, nails, and mucous membranes.

SIGNS AND SYMPTOMS

- Refractory thrush may extend to the esophagus.
- Refractory severe diaper rash occurs.
- Nails thicken, and significant edema and erythema of the surrounding periungual tissue occurs.
- Often associated with endocrinopathy: hypo/hyperthyroidism and polyendocrinopathy.

TREATMENT

- Systemic antifungals.
- Skin care.

WISKOTT-ALDRICH SYNDROME

A 10-month-old boy presents with thrush despite 10 days of nystatin. He had four episodes of otitis media. Physical examination shows thrush and multiple eczema patches. Both tympanic membranes are dull. His WBC is 7.6/mm³, Hb 11.3 g/dL, platelet count 97/mm³. His uncle died in infancy of infection. *Think: Wiskott-Aldrich syndrome.*

Wiskott-Aldrich syndrome is an X-linked recessive syndrome characterized by the classic presentation of eczema, thrombocytopenia, and otitis media (immunodeficiency). The initial manifestation usually is petechiae or bleeding in the first few months of life.

EXAM TIP

Wiskott-Aldrich syndrome:
- Eczema
- Thrombocytopenia
- ↑ IgA/IgE

WARD TIP

Oral candidiasis at >6 months of age should arouse suspicion for the presence of an immunodeficiency.

DEFINITION

X-linked-recessive disorder of cell cytoskeleton, presents as eczema, thrombocytopenia, and increased susceptibility to infection.

SIGNS AND SYMPTOMS

- Atopic dermatitis/eczema (see Table 9-4).
- Thrombocytopenic purpura, mucosal bleeding, bloody diarrhea, cerebral hemorrhage.
- Recurrent infections in infancy: pneumococcal (otitis, pneumonia), persistent thrush.
- OIs: *Pneumocystis jirovecii* pneumonia (PCP).
- Lymphoma.

LABS

- Decreased IgM.
- Increased IgA and IgE.
- Absence of antibodies after vaccination.

TREATMENT

- Prophylaxis: TMP-SMX for PCP; acyclovir prophylaxis for recurrent HSV.
- IVIG.
- Hematopoietic cell transplant.
- Elective splenectomy for thrombocytopenia/bleeding if not bone marrow transplant candidate; increased risk for sepsis.

TABLE 9-4. Combined and Primary T-Cell Immune Deficiencies

DISORDER	DEFECT	LYMPHOCYTES	IMMUNOGLOBULINS	CLINICAL	INFECTIONS	TREATMENT
SCID group (ADA = 15%)	Variable enzyme deficiencies	Low/no T, some/no B	Low/no titers	0–3 months FTT, thrush, ALC < 500	PCP, sepsis, severe VZV	BMT, gene therapy, ADA replacement
DiGeorge	22q11gene mutation Midline defects No thymus	Low/no T	Low/no titers	Low Ca, truncus arteriosus, aortic arch interruption	Same as SCID	Thymus transplant
Wiskott-Aldrich	X-linked, defective cytoskeleton of the cells	Normal #	High IgA, IgE Low IgM, titers	Eczema, TCP	OIs (PCP), severe HSV and VZV	BMT, IVIG
Ataxia-telangiectasia	AR, defect in DNA repair	Progressive loss of T4	Low IgA, IgE, and titers	Wobbly gait, red sclerae, lymphomas	OIs, sinopulmonary	Antibiotics
Chronic mucocutaneous candidiasis	T cells do not respond to candidal antigens	Normal #	Normal	Endocrinopathy (thyroid)	Persistent thrush, thickened nails	Systemic antifungal

ADA, adenosine deaminase; ALC, absolute lymphocyte count; AR, autosomal recessive; BMT, bone marrow transplantation; FTT, failure to thrive; HSV, herpes simplex virus; OIs, opportunistic infections; PCP, *Pneumocystis jirovecii* pneumonia; SCID, severe combined immunodeficiency; TCP, thrombocytopenia; VZV, varicella-zoster virus.

Common Variable Immunodeficiency (CVID)

DEFINITION

- A group of B-cell disorders results in low IgA and IgG, and sometimes IgM levels (see Table 9-5). An absence of protective antibody titers occurs.
- Can be familial.

SIGNS AND SYMPTOMS

- Most commonly presents in second decade of life.
- Lymphadenopathy, splenomegaly.
- Association with autoimmune diseases: rheumatoid arthritis, lupus, idiopathic thrombocytopenia.
- Lymphoid interstitial pneumonitis, granulomas on various organs.
- Increased risk of malignancies: lymphoma.
- Sinopulmonary infections: encapsulated organisms.
- Gastrointestinal (GI) infections: *Giardia*.
- Patients with CVID have normal numbers of B-lymphocytes as compared to patients with X-linked agammaglobulinemia and autosomal recessive agammaglobulinemia.

BRUTON'S X-LINKED AGAMMAGLOBULINEMIA

DEFINITION

- X-linked tyrosine kinase deficiency resulting in arrest of B-cell maturation (see Table 9-6).
- Severe hypogammaglobulinemia.

SIGNS AND SYMPTOMS

- No tonsils.
- No palpable lymphatic nodes.
- Recurrent/chronic sinopulmonary infections with encapsulated organisms (*Haemophilus influenzae, Streptococcus pneumoniae*).
- Severe/chronic gastrointestinal infections due to lack of IgA (*Giardia*).
- Increased susceptibility to enteroviral meningoencephalitis.

 EXAM TIP

Bruton's agammaglobulinemia:
- Male
- No palpable lymph nodes
- No tonsil
- Respiratory and gastrointestinal infections

TABLE 9-5. B-Cell Disorders and Immunoglobulin Deficiencies

DISORDER	DEFECT	LYMPHOCYTES	IMMUNOGLOBULINS	CLINICAL	INFECTIONS	TREATMENT
Bruton's agamma-globulinemia	X-linked arrest of B-cell maturation	No B Normal T	Low/no titers	No tonsils, no palpable lymph nodes	Pneumococcal, Rotaviral, *Giardia*	IVIG
Selective IgA deficiency	No switch to IgA	Normal #	No IgA Normal IgM, IgG, and titers	Allergies, celiac disease	Mostly respiratory or gastrointestinal	IVIG is contraindicated
CVID (a group of disorders)	Dysfunctional B-cells Can be familial	Normal #	Low IgA, IgG, and/or IgM. Low titers	Lymphadenopathy, autoimmune lymphomas	Pneumococcal, *Giardia*, sinusitis	IVIG

CVID, common variable immunodeficiency; IBD, inflammatory bowel disease; IVIG, intravenous immunoglobulin.

TABLE 9-6. **Immunoglobulin Disorders**

DISORDER	B CELLS	IgM	IgG	IgA	IgE
Hyper-IgE (Job) Syndrome	Normal	Normal	Normal	Normal	↑
Selective IgA Deficiency	Normal	Normal	Normal	↓	Normal
Transient Hypogammaglobulinemia of Infancy	Normal	Normal	↓	Normal	Normal
Wiskott-Aldrich	Normal	↓	↓	↑	↑
Hyper-IgM Syndrome	Normal	↑	↓	↓	↓
Common Variable Immunodeficiency	Normal	↓	↓	↓	↓
Bruton's X-Linked Agammaglobulinemia	↓	↓	↓	↓	↓
Severe Combined Immunodeficiency	↓	↓	↓	↓	↓

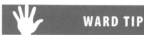

Infants with Bruton's agammaglobulinemia remain well for the first 6 months due to the presence of maternal IgG antibodies.

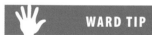

Immunoglobulin infusions confer passive immunity.

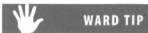

Patients with selective IgA deficiency can develop anti-IgA antibodies with blood product exposure that may lead to fatal anaphylaxis with blood or IVIG infusion. IVIG should be used with caution in patients with IgA deficiency.

DIAGNOSIS

Look for very low or absent mature B lymphocytes and all immunoglobulin classes. No production of protective antibodies occurs. Genetic testing is available for B-cell-specific gene mutation.

TREATMENT

- Monthly intravenous immunoglobulin.
- Prophylactic antibiotics if immunoglobulin treatment alone fails.
- Live vaccines are contraindicated; other vaccines lack an appreciable antibody response.

SELECTIVE IGA DEFICIENCY

DEFINITION

Deficiency of IgA-predominant immunoglobulin on mucosal surfaces due to failure of B cells to differentiate into IgA-secreting plasma cells.

EPIDEMIOLOGY

This is the most common of the primary antibody deficiencies, occurring in 1 in 600 persons.

SIGNS AND SYMPTOMS

- Usually asymptomatic, but may have recurrent respiratory or GI infections.
- Allergies.
- Associated with autoimmune diseases: celiac disease.

DIAGNOSIS

- IgA <10 mg/dL.

- Normal levels of other immunoglobulins and normal response to vaccination.
- Normal cell-mediated immunity.

ASPLENIA

 A 7-year-old African-American girl who immigrated from Togo presents with fever of 104°F (40°C). Physical examination did not reveal any source of fever. The spleen is not palpable. Her WBC count is 28.2/mm³, Hct 27.1/mm³ and Howell-Jolly bodies are noted. Blood culture grew *Streptococcus pneumoniae. Think: Sickle cell disease.*

Patients with asplenia are at increased risk for the development of sepsis, most commonly due to *S. pneumoniae*. Patients with sickle cell disease develop functional asplenia. Howell-Jolly bodies indicate hyposplenism.

DEFINITION

Absence of the functional spleen.

ETIOLOGY

- Congenital asplenia is suspected when a newborn has abnormalities of abdominal viscera and complex cyanotic congenital heart disease (heterotaxia syndrome).
- Functional asplenia may be secondary to sickle cell disease (SCD) or other hemoglobinopathies.
- Hyposplenia may be secondary to SLE, rheumatoid arthritis, IBD, GVHD, nephrotic syndrome, or prematurity.
- Splenectomy may result due to trauma, Hodgkin's lymphoma, chronic ITP, and hereditary spherocytosis.

DIAGNOSIS

Howell-Jolly bodies in erythrocytes.

COMPLICATIONS

Sepsis with encapsulated organisms: *S. pneumoniae, Haemophilus influenzae* type B, *Neisseria meningitides, Bartonella bacilliformis.*

TREATMENT

- Penicillin prophylaxis through at least first 5 years of life.
- Immunizations: pneumococcal (PCV-13 and PPSV23), *H. influenzae* and meningococcal (quadrivalent and MenB).

GRAFT-VERSUS-HOST DISEASE (GVHD)

DEFINITION

- Donor lymphocytes detect the host as foreign.
- Complication of hematopoietic cell transplantation.

ETIOLOGY

Engraftment of immunocompetent donor lymphocytes into immunologically compromised host.

PATHOPHYSIOLOGY

Donor T-cell activation by antibodies against host results in major histocompatibility and complex antigens.

WARD TIP

IgA is the major immunoglobulin within the upper airway.

EXAM TIP

Asplenia:
- Howell-Jolly bodies
- Increased risk of infection from encapsulated organisms

WARD TIP

Children with sickle cell anemia develop functional asplenia during the first year of life, and overwhelming sepsis is the leading cause of early death in the disease.

SIGNS AND SYMPTOMS

- Acute (<100 days) typical findings include:
  - Erythroderma.
  - Cholestatic hepatitis: abnormal LFTs.
  - Enteritis: diarrhea and cramps.
  - Increased susceptibility to infections.
- Chronic (>100 days) typical findings include:
  - Localized or general skin involvement including scleroderma.
  - Hepatic dysfunction with abnormal LFTs and positive liver biopsy.
  - Involvement of the eye ("keratoconjunctivitis sicca" = dry eye).
  - Involvement of minor salivary glands or oral mucosa (dryness).
  - Involvement of any other target organ, such as fasciitis, bronchiolitis obliterans.

TREATMENT

- High-dose glucocorticoids.
- Immunosuppressive therapy.

Infectious Disease

Occult Bacteremia

DEFINITION

- Defined as a fever without an obvious source of infection in a well-appearing child with a positive blood culture for a bacterial pathogen.
- The incidence has significantly decreased with effective pneumococcal immunization.
- Recent management guidelines suggest that the previous standards of routine blood cultures and empiric parenteral antibiotics are not required in fully immunized well-appearing children

ETIOLOGY

- *Streptococcus pneumoniae* (previously most common).
- *Salmonella sp.*
- *Staphylococcus aureus.*
- *Streptococci pyogenes.*

SIGNS AND SYMPTOMS

- Fever >38°C (100.4°F).
- Leukocytosis—WBC is often elevated, but it is not a reliable indicator of infection (neither sensitive nor specific).

PREDISPOSING FACTORS

- Prematurity.
- Loss of external defenses (burns, ulceration, indwelling catheter).
- Inadequate immune function.
- Non-immunized or under-immunized.
- Impaired reticuloendothelial function (asplenia, underlying condition like sickle cell disease).

DIAGNOSTIC WORKUP

- Urinalysis and culture in children at increased risk.
- Consider blood cultures, particularly with very high fever or unclear immunization status.
- Complete blood count (CBC): normal WBC count is $5.0–15.0 \times 10^3$ cells/µL.
- Lumbar puncture if <60 days old.

TREATMENT

- Febrile well-appearing immunized children with either no risk factors for a UTI or a negative urinalysis can be managed prospectively at home without antibiotics.
- Close follow-up is required.

Urinary Tract Infection

A 3-week-old male infant presents with fever, vomiting, and decreased fluid intake. A UA reveals 100 WBCs. *Think: E. coli UTI. Next step—urine culture.* Neonates with UTI are more likely to develop nonspecific symptoms (irritability, fever, and vomiting). *E. coli* is the most common organism in children of all ages. Urinalysis may show positive urinary leukocyte esterase, positive urinary nitrite, pyuria, and/or bacteruria.

DEFINITION

Growth of a single pathogen in the urine of >100,000 colony forming units (CFU)/mL in a clean catch specimen, >50,000 CFU/mL in catheterized urine samples, or >1000 CFU/mL in suprapubic bladder aspiration samples.

ETIOLOGY

Most common organisms:

- *Escherichia coli.*
- *Klebsiella.*
- *Proteus.*
- *Staphylococcus saprophyticus.*
- *Enterococcus* spp.

SIGNS AND SYMPTOMS

- Fever >38°C (100.4°F) without a source in females under 2 years, circumcised males under 6 months, and uncircumcised males under 1 year.
- Dysuria or frequency in older children.
- Pyuria.

PREDISPOSING FACTORS

- Age—boys younger than 1 year and girls younger than 2 years; female infants are at four times higher risk than males.
- Uncircumcised penis.
- GU abnormalities—structural or functional (neurogenic bladder or vesicoureteral reflux).

DIAGNOSTIC WORKUP

- Urinalysis demonstrating leukocyte esterase (more sensitive) or nitrites (more specific).
- Pyuria on microscopic evaluation (>10 wbc/hpf).
- Urine culture.
- Renal ultrasound should be performed on all first-time febrile UTIs in children <24 months to evaluate for hydronephrosis.
- Voiding cystourethrography (VCUG) should be performed on all patients with an abnormal ultrasound. Reflux of urine increases the risk of renal scarring.
- Imaging guidelines for children diagnosed with febrile UTI are controversial; check for updated practice guidelines.

TREATMENT

- Empiric treatment with antibiotics should begin as soon as a diagnosis is made. Cephalosporins are a good first-line agent; the most common UTI-causing organisms are susceptible.
- Hospitalize infants under 2 months and all ill-appearing children.

WARD TIP

Urinary tract infections are the most common occult serious bacterial illness in infants and young children.

Neonatal Sepsis

DEFINITION

- Early-onset infection—onset before 7 days of life
  - Organisms typically acquired before or during delivery from mother.
- Late-onset infection—onset at 7 days of life or later
  - Organisms are typically acquired in the hospital or the community.

ETIOLOGY

- Group B streptococci.
- *Escherichia coli.*
- *Listeria monocytogenes.*
- Viridans streptococci.
- Coagulase-negative *Staphylococcus* (preterm infants, catheter-related).

SIGNS AND SYMPTOMS

- Nonspecific signs of infection, including:
  - Temperature instability (newborns may not develop fever in response to infection).
  - Poor perfusion.
  - Tachycardia or bradycardia.
  - Apnea or respiratory distress.
  - Jaundice.
  - Feeding intolerance.
  - Bleeding.

TREATMENT

- Early-onset sepsis: ampicillin + aminoglycoside.
- Late-onset sepsis: vancomycin + aminoglycoside.

WARD TIP

Escherichia coli is now the most common overall cause of early-onset sepsis (EOS), supplanting group B streptococcus. GBS is still the most common cause of EOS in term infants.

Sepsis Beyond the Newborn Period

DEFINITION

- This "systemic inflammatory response syndrome" (SIRS) to infection results in hemodynamic and metabolic compromise.
- Hypoperfusion abnormalities in sepsis result in lactic acidosis, oliguria, altered mental status, and increased oxygen utilization (oxygen dissociation curve moves to the right).

DIAGNOSTIC CRITERIA

Pediatric SIRS criteria are met by ≥2 conditions, one of which must be abnormal temperature or leukocyte count:

- Hyper- or hypothermia (≥101.3°F [38.5°C] or <96.8°F [36°C]).
- Tachycardia or bradycardia.
- Tachypnea (respiratory rate >2 SD above age normal) or need for mechanical ventilation.
- WBC count >15,000 or <5000 cells/µL or >10% bandemia.
- Sepsis = SIRS + source of infection.
- Recent literature emphasizes that sepsis is characterized by life-threatening organ dysfunction due to the host's response to infection.
- SIRS criteria may not adequately predict mortality.

ETIOLOGY

Same as for occult bacteremia above.

SIGNS AND SYMPTOMS

- May be nonspecific and include ill-appearance, listlessness, hyperthermia, or hypothermia.
- Vomiting and poor feeding are common, nonspecific findings in any infant with fever.

DIAGNOSIS

- This is a presumed infection with systemic inflammatory response leading to compromised perfusion states.
- Sepsis is a clinical condition and can be caused by viral as well as bacterial causes.
- Ten percent will have negative blood cultures.

RISK FACTORS

- Age (younger children at greater risk).
- Prematurity.
- Immunodeficiency (may be underlying condition or medication related — i.e., steroids).
- Indwelling catheters.
- Contact with known *N. meningitidis* or *Haemophilus influenzae* infection.

SEPTIC SHOCK

DEFINITION

Clinical evidence of infection plus persistent hypotension despite adequate fluid resuscitation, along with evidence of hypoperfusion abnormalities or end organ dysfunction.

DIAGNOSTIC CRITERIA

Meets sepsis criteria, plus one of the following:

- Hypoperfusion requiring >40 mL/kg isotonic fluid (crystalloid or colloid) and/or inotropic support.
- Hypotension (age-based).
- More than one manifestation of organ hypoperfusion (e.g., oliguria, elevated hepatic enzymes, altered mental status, prolonged capillary refill).

A 3-month-old female is brought to the ED with fever, vomiting, decreased activity, and poor breast-feeding for one day. Previous history is unremarkable. Physical examination shows an ill-appearing girl with a temperature of 101.1°F (38.4°C), HR 196 beats/min, and no identifiable "focus" of infection. *Think: Sepsis.*

Young infants are at increased risk for serious infection. They may present with nonspecific "signs" and symptoms, and they often lack focal signs of infection.

TREATMENT

- IV broad-spectrum antibiotics.
- Manage shock with aggressive IV fluid resuscitation and vasopressors as needed to maintain blood pressure, perfusion, and oxygenation.

MENINGOCOCCEMIA

A 5-year-old boy presents with sudden onset of chills, fever, and listlessness. Physical examination shows a temperature of 103.5°F (39.7°C) and palpable, reddish-purple, nonblanching spots (purpura). He is rapidly progressing to shock. *Think: Meningococcemia.*

Typical presentation is sudden onset of fever, vomiting, headache, and lethargy. Most patients have petechiae on presentation. The infection can progress rapidly to profound shock and DIC.

WARD TIP

Rule of thumb for hypotension: lowest acceptable systolic blood pressure is 70 + 2× (age in years).

EXAM TIP

Meningococcemia
- Fever
- Purpura
- Rapid progression to shock

- This condition presents nonspecifically with petechiae, then purpura, and finally eschar (skin breakdown in areas of profound hypoperfusion).
- Typical rash distribution: trunk and extremities.
- Progresses rapidly (within hours) to septic shock due to endotoxin.
- Diagnosed by blood, cerebrospinal fluid (CSF), and skin lesion cultures.
- Adrenal hemorrhage (Waterhouse-Friedrichsen syndrome) and insufficiency are classic complications.

Treatment

- IV ceftriaxone or cefotaxime are initial treatments of choice.
- Fluid resuscitation and vasopressor support as discussed above.

Fever and Rash

- Enanthem: lesion on mucosal surface (mouth).
- Exanthem: lesion on the skin (rash).
- Polymorphous rash: consists of various primary elements.

TABLE 10-1. Fever and Rash

Infection	Sequence of Events	Primary Element(s) of Rash	Distribution, Pattern	Hallmarks
Measles (rubeola)	Fever and "3Cs" × 3–4 days precede rash: **C**oryza, **C**onjunctivitis, **C**ough (barking)	Maculopapular	"Shower" from the top down Becomes confluent, also from the top	Koplik's spots on buccal mucosa
Rubella	Low-grade fever may start 1–2 days prior to rash	Maculopapular	"Shower" from the top down	Suboccipital lymphatic nodes
Roseola (HHV 6,7) (exanthem subitum)	High fever 4–5 days; rash appears after fever has resolved	Maculopapular	Discrete, may last just for a few hours	Febrile seizures, suboccipital lymphatic nodes, red eardrums
Erythema infectiosum (Parvovirus B19) (Fifth disease)	Fever and malaise prodrome, then red ("slapped") cheeks	Maculopapular	Lacelike, fluctuates over time with room temperature changes	Rare arthritis, knee; aplastic crisis in sickle cell disease; hydrops fetalis in pregnancy
Scarlet fever (erythrotoxin of group A *Streptococcus*)	Exactly "red fever," often with sore throat, × 7 days; desquamation (peeling) in week 2	Sandpaper-feeling confluent redness of the skin (erythroderma)	Accentuated in folds, where darker Pastia's lines are seen	Nasolabial triangle and chin are spared ("circumoral pallor"); high anti-streptolysin O, positive throat culture
Varicella	Crops of "dew drops on a rose petal" appear over 3–7 days, with fever	Evolution from papule to vesicle to pustule to excoriation	Rash in the different stages of evolution; palms and soles spared	May be associated with meningitis or encephalitis
Hand-foot-mouth disease (Coxsackievirus A16)	Fever, rash, with or without sore throat, upper respiratory/gastrointestinal infection symptoms	Macules, papules, vesicles	Palms and soles involved	Enanthem: Erosions on the pharynx, palate, tongue

- Primary rash elements (see Dermatologic Disease chapter for specifics):
  - Macule: flat, discolored, blanching spot.
  - Papule: small, raised bump.
  - Vesicle: small, round fluid-filled lesion.
  - Pustule: small, round pus-filled lesion.
  - Petechia: pinpoint nonblanching purplish spot (extravasation).
  - Purpura: small, raised, purplish nonblanching lesion (extravasation).
  - Erythroderma: confluent redness of the skin.
  - Excoriation: scratches, abrasions.
  - Eschar: Dead tissue (or ulcer) covered by dry, dark scab.
- To recognize infection, keep in mind:
  - Primary element(s) of rash.
  - Distribution and/or pattern of the rash.
  - Sequence (timeline) of events.
  - Associated hallmarks of infection.
  - Vaccine-preventable infection is most likely to develop in an unvaccinated child (for example, in a new immigrant or in an adoptee).
- Remember: Any rash may be itchy.

WARD TIP

The most common cause of fever and rash is nonspecific viral exanthem. No workup is generally needed in well-appearing child with classic blanching, maculopapular rash.

Viral Infections

RUBEOLA (MEASLES)

 A 6-year-old girl has a one-day history of a rash that started on her face and spread to her trunk. Prior to developing the rash, she had a four-day history of runny nose, pink eyes with crusting, barking cough, and high fever. She was never immunized because of her parents' beliefs. On exam, her temperature is 103°F (39.4ºC), and a maculopapular rash is seen most prominently on the trunk. Three tiny, whitish, round spots are present on her buccal mucosa. *Think: Measles.*

Measles is characterized by high fever, an enanthem (Koplik's spots), cough, coryza, conjunctivitis, and a maculopapular rash (exanthem). The rash usually begins on the face and appears several days after the initial symptoms. Koplik's spots precede the onset of rash.

EXAM TIP

Rubeola (Measles) classic findings:
- Coryza
- Cough
- Conjunctivitis
- Koplik spots

ETIOLOGY

Paramyxovirus (RNA virus)

SIGNS AND SYMPTOMS

- A high fever and the "3Cs" (see Table 10-1) precede the rash (3–5 days).
- Conjunctivitis is exudative (yellow discharge).
- Cough is croupy (barking, or "seal-like").
- Rash starts as faint macules on the upper-lateral neck, behind the ears, along the hairline, and on the cheeks.
- Lesions become maculopapular and spread quickly downward ("shower distribution"), while the rash becomes confluent (erythroderma) starting from the top.
- Lymphadenopathy or splenomegaly may be present.
- Koplik spots (pathognomonic) appear: irregularly shaped spots with grayish, whitish, or bluish centers on buccal mucosa (see Figure 10-1).

DIAGNOSIS

- Clinical.
- Laboratory evaluation is rarely necessary for diagnosis but is important for confirmation and surveillance.

EXAM TIP

Children under the age of 6 months do not usually get measles due to passive immunity from mother.

FIGURE 10-1. **Koplik spots (rubeola).** (Reproduced, with permission, from Nester EW, Anderson DG, Roberts CE Jr, et al. *Microbiology: A Human Perspective*, 6th ed. New York: McGraw Hill, 2008.)

COMPLICATIONS

- It is highly contagious; R_0 reported to be 12–18, meaning one infected person would infect between 12 and 18 susceptible individuals.
- Diarrhea (most common).
- Otitis media.
- Pneumonia (may be fatal in HIV patients).
- Encephalitis is the most feared complication; 1:1000 cases can result in permanent brain damage.

TREATMENT

- Supportive.
- The World Health Organization recommends vitamin A supplementation for all children with measles, regardless of their country of residence.
- Ribavirin has been used in severe cases, but it has not been well studied.

EXAM TIP

Always give vitamin A for measles.

VACCINE

- A live attenuated vaccine is included in measles-mumps-rubella (MMR) vaccine; it does NOT have an association with autism.
- Generally given at 12–15 months with a booster given at 4–6 years.

RUBELLA

A 3-year-old girl develops a rash. She was recently adopted from Romania, and her immunization history is unknown. She has a fever for one day. On physical examination, she is not ill-appearing, her temperature is 100.4°F (38.0°C), and she has a confluent maculopapular rash on her face and a discrete rash on her trunk. Suboccipital and posterior cervical lymph nodes are palpable. WBC 7.2×10^3 cells/µL. *Think: Rubella.*

Rubella has a prodrome of low-grade fever, sore throat, red eyes, headache, malaise, and anorexia. Suboccipital or postauricular lymphadenopathy is common. Rash is usually the first symptom, which appears on the face and spreads centrifugally to the extremities.

- Also known as "German" or "three-day" measles.
- Rubella is contagious from 1 week before the rash appears to 1 week after it fades.

ETIOLOGY

Togavirus (RNA virus).

SIGNS AND SYMPTOMS

- Mild fever prodrome for 1–2 days.
- The rash begins on the face and spreads quickly to the trunk ("shower distribution"). As it spreads to the trunk, it clears from the face.
- Lymphadenopathy (retroauricular, posterior cervical, and suboccipital).
- Conjunctivitis may be present.
- Polyarthritis is common in adolescent females.

COMPLICATIONS

- Progressive panencephalitis (very rare):
    - Insidious behavior changes.
    - Deteriorating school performance.
    - Later appearance of dementia and multifocal neurologic deficits.
- Thrombocytopenia (rare).

TREATMENT

Supportive; usually lasts about 3 days.

VACCINE

- A live attenuated vaccine is included in the MMR vaccine.
- Generally given at 12–15 months with a booster given at 4–6 years.

CONGENITAL RUBELLA SYNDROME

- Maternal rubella infection during pregnancy can lead to miscarriage, fetal death, or a live-born infant with congenital anomalies.
- Rubella immunization primarily exists to prevent this syndrome. The earlier in gestation rubella occurs, the higher the complication risk—more than 80% in the first trimester and 25% at the end of the second trimester.
- Neonatal manifestations are often severe:
    - Intrauterine growth retardation.
    - Pneumonitis.
    - Radiolucent bone lesions.
    - Hepatosplenomegaly.
    - Thrombocytopenia and "Blueberry muffin" rash (extramedullary erythropoiesis).
- Eye: cataracts, congenital glaucoma, pigmentary retinopathy, microphthalmos.
- Heart: patent ductus arteriosus (PDA), peripheral pulmonary artery stenosis.
- Sensorineural hearing impairment.
- Neurologic: meningoencephalitis, intellectual disability.

ROSEOLA

An 11-month-old boy has had a fever of 103–104°F (39.4–40ºC) for four days and was seen in ED because of febrile seizures. He had no vomiting, did not look sick, and his neurologic examination was normal. The only finding at the time was small suboccipital lymph nodes. No workup was done. One day later, the child's fever has resolved, but now he has a maculopapular rash. *Think: Roseola.*

Roseola is associated with high fever for 3–5 days. A high association with febrile seizures is noted. The rash appears when the fever disappears. Mild cervical or occipital lymphadenopathy may be present.

ETIOLOGY

- Human herpesvirus types 6 and 7.
- By the age of 4 years, almost all children are immune.

SIGNS AND SYMPTOMS

- High fever (may exceed 104°F; 40°C).
- Mild upper respiratory symptoms or (commonly) no symptoms other than fever.
- Cervical and suboccipital lymphadenopathy.
- Maculopapular rash that spreads to the neck, face, and proximal extremities.

TREATMENT

Supportive (antipyretics, increased oral fluid intake, rest).

ERYTHEMA INFECTIOSUM (FIFTH DISEASE)

> An 8-year-old girl has a four-day history of fever and bright red cheeks. Now she has rash everywhere and complains of knee pain. On examination, she is not sick-appearing, her temperature is 100.8°F (38.2°C), and she has "slapped"-looking cheeks and a discrete macular rash on the trunk and extremities that looks lacy. Her joints are intact with a full range of motion. *Think: Erythema infectiosum, Parvovirus B19.*
>
> Erythema infectiosum is a self-limiting exanthematous illness in children. A slapped-cheek appearance is the classic presentation. In addition, a lacy, reticulated appearance on the extremities is often present.

ETIOLOGY

Parvovirus B19

PATHOPHYSIOLOGY

- Attacks red blood cell precursors.
- Transmitted in respiratory secretions.

SIGNS AND SYMPTOMS

- Prodrome: one week of low-grade fever, headache, malaise, myalgia, and mild upper respiratory symptoms.
- "Slapped cheeks," circumoral pallor.
- Rash spreads rapidly to trunk and extremities in ornamental "lacelike" pattern.
- Arthritis (knee), rare in children.
- Papular-purpuric gloves-and-socks-syndrome (PPGSS)—painful pruritic papules, purpura, and petechiae of the distal extremities.

DIAGNOSIS

- Clinical (serum parvovirus B19 immunoglobulin M assay is available, e.g., for arthritis cases).
- Parvovirus B19 serology may be offered to women of childbearing age in frequent contact with children to determine their susceptibility to infection (e.g., teachers).

COMPLICATIONS

- Transient aplastic crisis in patients with chronic hemolysis including sickle cell disease (SCD), thalassemia, hereditary spherocytosis, and pyruvate kinase deficiency.
- Chronic anemia/pure red cell aplasia in immunocompromised hosts.
- Infection during pregnancy may lead to hydrops fetalis: generalized edema due to fetal congestive heart failure caused by fetal anemia.

EXAM TIP

The high fever seen with roseola often triggers febrile seizures.

WARD TIP

The name "Fifth Disease" comes from a classification of childhood exanthems proposed in 1905 by Dr. Léon Cheinisse, a French physician of Russian descent. Others on the list include measles (first), scarlet fever (second), rubella (third), and roseola (sixth). Dukes' disease, or fourth disease, is now thought to be a variant of scarlet fever.

TREATMENT

- Supportive (antipyretics, increased oral fluid intake, rest).
- Intravenous immune globulin (IVIG) should be considered for immuno-compromised patients.

VARICELLA (CHICKENPOX)

> A 5-year-old boy has had a fever for three days and an itchy rash that started yesterday. He is a recent immigrant. On examination, his temperature is 101.8°F (38.8°C), and he does not look sick. He has crops of papules, vesicles, pustules, and crusts on his face, trunk, and extremities. *Think: Varicella.*
>
> Varicella is a highly contagious disease characterized classically by a prodrome of URI symptoms followed by a generalized, vesicular, pruritic rash with a centripetal distribution. In a patient with chickenpox, erythematous macules, papules, vesicles, and scabbed lesions are present in various stages simultaneously.

DEFINITION

This highly contagious ($R_0 = 10\text{-}12$), self-limited viral infection is characterized by multiple pruritic vesicles (Figure 10-2).

ETIOLOGY

Varicella-zoster virus (VZV), group of herpesviruses.

EPIDEMIOLOGY

- Ninety percent of patients are <10 years old.
- A history of exposure to an infected individual is often found.
- The incidence is significantly decreased since varicella vaccine was introduced.

PATHOPHYSIOLOGY

- Transmitted by respiratory secretions and fluid from the skin lesions.
- Replicates in the respiratory tract.
- Establishes lifelong infection in sensory ganglia cells.

SIGNS AND SYMPTOMS

- May have a prodrome of fever, with URI symptoms or with malaise, anorexia, headache, and abdominal pain 24–48 hours before the onset of the rash.
- "Dew drops on a rose petal" (vesicles with an erythematous base) initially appear on the face and spread to the trunk and extremities, sparing the palms and soles.
- Within days, vesicles become turbid and then crusted.
- Vesicles occur in "crops." At any given time, new, turbid, and crusted vesicles may be present.

DIAGNOSIS

- Clinical; Tzanck preparation is no longer used to diagnose varicella.
- PCR can be performed on a swab from the vesicle.

COMPLICATIONS

- Skin lesions may be superinfected by bacteria (*Streptococcus pyogenes* or *Staphylococcus aureus*). For unknown reasons, these skin superinfections may lead to severe complications such as necrotizing fasciitis.
- Pneumonia in immunocompromised or pregnant patients.
- Encephalitis.
- Reye syndrome (associated with aspirin use).

WARD TIP

Herpes zoster (shingles) is the reactivation of VZV from nerve ganglia and occurs in dermatomal distributions.

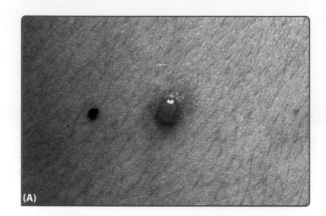

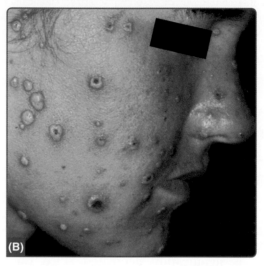

FIGURE 10-2. **Varicella (chickenpox).** Note dewdrop appearance of lesion. (Part A: From Usatine RP, Smith MA, Mayeaux EJ Jr, Chumley HS. *The Color Atlas and Synopsis of Family Medicine*, 3rd ed. New York, McGraw Hill, 2019, Figure 129-5. Reproduced, with permission, from Richard P. Usatine, MD. Part B: Reproduced, with permission, from Kang S, Amagai M, Bruckner AL, et al., eds. *Fitzpatrick's Dermatology*, 9th ed. New York, McGraw Hill, 2019, Figure 165-2E.

 WARD TIP

Smallpox generally presents with all lesions in the same stage (compared with chickenpox with lesions at various stages).

TREATMENT

- For most immunocompetent children: symptomatic for fever and pruritus.
- For VZV pneumonia and for immunocompromised individuals: acyclovir.
- Infants born to mothers with varicella in the peripartum period should receive varicella zoster immune globulin (VZIG); such infants are at high risk of morbidity and mortality.

VACCINE

Live attenuated vaccine; first dose given between 12 and 18 months of age, second dose age >4 years.

CONGENITAL VARICELLA SYNDROME

Caused by maternal varicella infection in first 20 weeks of pregnancy

WARD TIP

Varicella-zoster immune globulin (VZIG) is used for post-exposure prophylaxis in immunocompromised or newborns exposed to maternal varicella.

SYMPTOMS

- Cicatricial skin lesions (cutaneous scarring).
- Limb hypoplasia.
- Neurologic deficits.
- Eye abnormalities.

HAND-FOOT-MOUTH DISEASE

ETIOLOGY

Enteroviruses—specifically coxsackie virus.

EPIDEMIOLOGY

- Fecal-oral and respiratory routes of infection.
- Summer and fall seasonal peaks exist against a background of year-round disease.

SIGNS AND SYMPTOMS

- GI discomfort.
- Ulcerative mouth lesions (small, superficial, round erosions) (see Figure 10-3a).
- Hand and foot lesions are tender and vesicular (see Figure 10-3b and c).

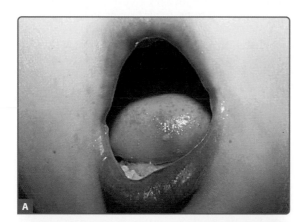

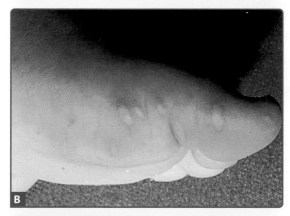

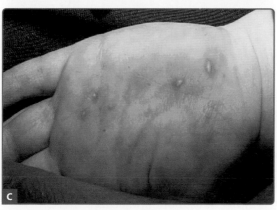

FIGURE 10-3. **Hand Foot Mouth Disease.** (Reproduced, with permission, from Kang S, Amagai M, Bruckner AL, et al, eds. *Fitzpatrick's Dermatology*, 9th ed. New York, McGraw Hill, 2019, Figure 163-12A-C.)

- Hands are more commonly involved than feet. May be ONLY oral.
- May occur on palms and soles.

COMPLICATIONS

- Aseptic meningitis.
- Encephalitis.

MUMPS

An unvaccinated 14-year-old boy presented with fever of 100.9°F (38.3°C), bilateral facial swelling, and inability to eat normally because of pain when he tried to chew. On examination, he was active and had trismus (inability to open mouth wide) and swelling in front of the earlobes. There was no redness or purulent discharge at Stenson duct openings. At a follow-up visit eight days later, his parotid swelling has resolved, but now he has a swollen, tender left testis. *Think: Mumps orchitis.*

Parotid swelling is the classic feature of mumps. Parotitis is often accompanied by a prodrome of low-grade fever, myalgias, and anorexia. Epididymo-orchitis is a common extra–salivary gland complication of mumps in postpubertal males. It is characterized by marked testicular swelling and severe pain and may be associated with fever, nausea, and headache. Testicular atrophy may follow, although sterility is not common.

ETIOLOGY

Paramyxovirus (RNA virus).

PATHOPHYSIOLOGY

- Spread via respiratory secretions.
- Incubation period of 14–24 days.

SIGNS AND SYMPTOMS

- Rare viral prodrome.
- Swelling and tenderness in one or both parotid glands.
- Difficulty opening the mouth (trismus).

COMPLICATIONS

- Meningoencephalomyelitis (rare).
- Orchitis/oophoritis common after puberty.
- Pancreatitis.
- Arthritis.
- Thyroiditis.
- Deafness.

VACCINE

- Live attenuated vaccine is included in the MMR vaccine.
- The vaccine is generally given at 12–15 months with a booster given at 4–6 years.

EPSTEIN-BARR VIRUS (EBV)

ETIOLOGY

- Herpesvirus.
- Spread through intimate contact.
- Primary cause of infectious mononucleosis ("mono").
- Associated with B and T cell lymphomas, Hodgkin lymphoma.
- May cause lymphoproliferative disorder in transplant recipients.

EPIDEMIOLOGY

- Widely disseminated; 90 to 95% of adults are seropositive.
- Infection frequently occurs in the first few years of life, but occurs later in developed countries.

SIGNS AND SYMPTOMS

- May be asymptomatic in infants and young children.
- Infectious mononucleosis
  - Fatigue, headache, low grade fever.
  - Pharyngitis; tonsillitis with exudate.
  - Cervical lymphadenopathy.
  - GI findings may include nausea, vomiting, anorexia, and mildly elevated LFTs.
  - Splenomegaly in 50% of cases, risk of splenic rupture (see below).
  - Peripheral smear may have lymphocytosis with elevated atypical lymphocytes.

DIAGNOSIS

- Monospot for children 5 years old and up (frequent false negative in younger children).
- EBV specific antibodies against viral capsid antigen (VCA), nuclear antigen (EBNA), and early antigen (EA) for young children and to clarify clinical diagnosis with a negative monospot.

TREATMENT

- Symptomatic care—fluids, acetaminophen/ibuprofen.
- Steroids are controversial. They do not seem to shorten the course, but they are warranted for impending airway compromise and may be useful in severe disease.
- Acyclovir decreases viral shedding but it does not demonstrate clinical benefit and does not affect latent infection.
- Student athletes should wait at least three to four weeks before resuming practice. The highest risk of splenic rupture occurs within 21 days of onset of symptoms.

COMPLICATIONS

- Splenic rupture is rare but potentially life threatening.
- Tonsillar enlargement may be prominent and cause airway concerns.
- Rash—morbilliform (measles-like), commonly in response to administration of ampicillin.
- Fatigue can last for months.

Bacterial Infections

SCARLET FEVER

A 7-year-old boy has a sore throat, fever, and rash. His classmate had similar symptoms one week ago. On examination, his temperature is 102°F (38.9°C). He has red tonsils, swollen, tender bilateral anterior cervical lymphatic nodes (2.5 cm), and a confluent red rash that feels "sandpaper-like." He has circumoral pallor (nasolabial triangle and chin are spared). *Think: Scarlet fever.*

Scarlet fever has an abrupt onset of fever, chills, malaise, and sore throat with a distinctive rash that begins on the chest. Circumoral pallor is often present. The rash has a rough, sandpaper-like texture.

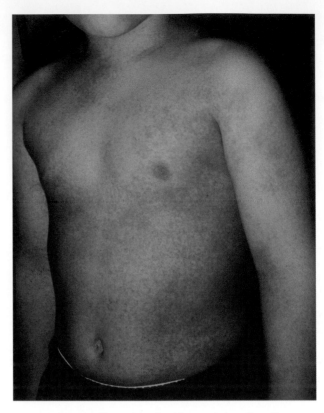

FIGURE 10-4. **Scarlet Fever.** (Reproduced, with permission, from Lawrence B. Stack, MD.)

ETIOLOGY

Erythrogenic exotoxins of group A β-hemolytic *Streptococcus* (GAS).

SIGNS AND SYMPTOMS

- Fever, often with sore throat.
- Confluent erythematous (erythroderma) sandpaper-like rash.
- Rash spares nasolabial triangle and chin (circumoral pallor).
- Accentuation of rash in a linear pattern in skin creases (Pastia lines).
- Desquamation (peeling), starting with fingers, in the second week.

DIAGNOSIS

- Clinical.
- Throat culture, anti-streptolysin O (ASO), and deoxyribonuclease B titers.

COMPLICATIONS

Rheumatic fever

TREATMENT

Penicillin

EXAM TIP

Scarlet fever common findings:
- Sandpaper rash
- Pastia lines (lines in skin creases formed by confluent petechiae)
- Desquamation

RHEUMATIC FEVER (SEE CARDIOVASCULAR DISEASE CHAPTER)

A 14-year-old girl presents after recently immigrating from Central America with fatigue, a swollen, painful knee, and a truncal rash. She has no known medical history but indicates that she had a sore throat for a few weeks prior to leaving her home country. *Think: Rheumatic fever.*

Rheumatic fever is a diagnosis based on Jones criteria (see Cardiovascular Disease chapter).

TOXIC SHOCK SYNDROME (TSS)

DEFINITION

This syndrome is an acute, febrile, exanthematous illness that involves multiple systems with potential complications that include shock, renal and myocardial failure, and acute respiratory distress syndrome (ARDS).

PATHOPHYSIOLOGY

- Hematogenous dissemination of an endotoxin.
- Toxins from *Staphylococcus* or *Streptococcus* act as superantigens activating T cells nonspecifically, resulting in massive release of cytokines with profound physiologic consequences (i.e., fever, vasodilation, hypotension, and multisystem organ involvement).

SIGNS AND SYMPTOMS

- Ill-appearing patient.
- Diffuse erythroderma is classic.
- Staphylococcal TSS (*S. aureus*): associated with high absorbancy tampons in the early 80s, less so now. The source may be nasal or wound packing, or an abscess.
- Streptococcal TSS (group A *Streptococcus*): usually, there is evidence of soft tissue infection, classically necrotizing fasciitis in a patient with varicella.
- Nikolsky sign (see Dermatologic Disease chapter) is present in staphylococcal scalded skin syndrome and is characterized by sloughing of intact skin with minor shearing force.

TREATMENT

- Aggressive fluid replacement.
- Eradication of infectious source.
- Parenteral β-lactamase-resistant antibiotic plus clindamycin (reduces toxin synthesis).
- Recovery in 7–10 days with appropriate treatment.

TABLE 10-2. Diagnostic Criteria of Toxic Shock Syndrome (TSS)

STREPTOCOCCAL **TSS**	STAPHYLOCOCCAL **TSS**
Isolation of GAS (throat, wound, blood) and hypotension	- Temp > 102°F
	- Diffuse erythroderma
And ≥ 2 signs:	- Desquamation in week 2 (hands)
- Soft tissue necrosis (fasciitis, gangrene)	- Hypotension
- ARDS	And ≥ 3 signs:
- Erythroderma, desquamation	- Vomiting/diarrhea at onset
- Renal (creatinine)	- Myalgia or elevated CPK
- Liver (transaminases)	- Red mucosae (oropharyngeal, vaginal, conjunctival)
- Coagulopathy (thrombocytopenia, DIC)	- CNS: altered mental status
	- Renal (creatinine)
	- Liver (transaminases)
	- Thrombocytopenia

ARDS, adult respiratory distress syndrome; CPK, creatine phosphokinase; DIC, disseminated intravascular coagulation; GAS, group A *Streptococcus*.

TYPHOID (ENTERIC) FEVER

 An 8-year-old boy develops a fever five days after returning from Africa. The fever escalates in the next seven days. He develops abdominal pain and refuses to eat. His last bowel movement occurred prior to the onset of fever and was normal. On examination, his temperature is 103°F (39.4°C), HR 68 beats/min. The abdomen has fine pink spots and a palpable spleen (2.5 cm). Abdomen is soft, with mild, inconsistent tenderness and no guarding or rebound. WBC is 2.9 × 10³ cells/μL and blood smear shows no parasites. *Think: Typhoid fever.*

Typhoid fever is characterized by a prolonged fever, relative bradycardia, splenomegaly, rose spots, and leukopenia. It is caused by infection with *Salmonella typhi*.

ETIOLOGY

Salmonella typhi

PATHOPHYSIOLOGY

- Fecal-oral transmission.
- Incubation period of 7–14 days.
- Time of incubation is dependent on the inoculum size.

SIGNS AND SYMPTOMS

- Fever: gradual rise in the first week, gradual decrease in the third week.
- Malaise.
- Anorexia.
- Myalgia.
- Headache.
- Abdominal pain.
- Diarrhea is a late sign.
- Transient rose-colored spots on trunk.
- Hepatosplenomegaly.

COMPLICATIONS

- Intestinal hemorrhage.
- Intestinal perforation.
- Sepsis.

DIAGNOSIS

- Blood, urine, and stool cultures.
- Blood culture sensitivity is ~60%.

TREATMENT

- Ceftriaxone.
- Consider dexamethasone for severe cases with altered mental status.

VACCINE

Available for travelers to endemic areas (not routinely recommended in United States).

Tick-Borne Infections

LYME DISEASE

An afebrile 6-year-old boy develops limping, swelling, and pain in his right knee. Physical examination shows temperature of 98.6°F (37.4°C) and no distress. No rash, murmur, or organomegaly are noted. The right knee is swollen and warm, but not red, with decreased range of motion due to pain on passive movement. *Think: Lyme disease vs. reactive or post-viral arthritis.*

> 🚺 An 11-year-old girl presents with an enlarging erythematous, non-itchy spot on her left shoulder. She was camping in upstate New York two weeks ago. On examination, her temperature is 100.3°F (37.9°C), she is not sick-appearing, and she has a flat annular lesion 7 cm in diameter on the left shoulder. No regional lymphadenopathy is noted. *Think: Lyme disease.*
>
> Lyme disease is a tick-borne, inflammatory disorder due to the spirochete *Borrelia burgdorferi*. The most common manifestation of Lyme disease in children is erythema migrans rash and arthritis. Most cases of Lyme disease are from the Mid-Atlantic states and upper Midwest.

DEFINITION

This multisystem disease is transmitted by the bite of an *Ixodes scapularis* tick infected with spirochetes.

ETIOLOGY

- *Borrelia burgdorferi (North America, Europe)*.
- *Borrelia mayonii* (North American upper midwest, newly identified).
- *Borrelia afzelii, Borrelia garinii* (Europe, Asia).

EPIDEMIOLOGY

- Patients are often unaware of the tick bite.
- Incubation period: 2–31 days.
- Keep in mind geography (presence of a vector) and season (see Table 10-3).

PATHOPHYSIOLOGY

Disseminated Lyme is due to spirochetemia.

SIGNS AND SYMPTOMS

- Acute onset of fever, chills, myalgia, arthralgia, weakness, headache, and photophobia.
- Erythema migrans (EM):
  - Begins as a red macule or papule that gradually (over days to weeks) turns into an annular, erythematous lesion of 5–15 cm in diameter (Figure 10-5).
  - Sometimes associated with partial central clearing ("bull's eye" appearance).
  - May have vesicular or necrotic areas in its center and can be confused with cellulitis.
  - Usually is painless and not pruritic.
  - May be located at the axilla or in the groin; not necessarily found at the site of the bite.

TABLE 10-3. **Epidemiology of Tick-Borne Infections**

INFECTION	GEOGRAPHY (UNITED STATES)	TICK (VECTOR)	SEASON
Lyme borreliosis	Upper East Coast: New Hampshire to Virginia	*Ixodes scapularis*	April–October
	Upper Midwest: Wisconsin, Minnesota	*Ixodes scapularis*	
	West Coast: California	*Ixodes pacificus*	
Rocky Mountain spotted fever	Western states	*Dermacentor andersoni (wood tick)*	May–September
	Southeast: North Carolina, South Carolina	*Dermacentor variabilis (American dog tick)*	
	South central: Tennessee, Oklahoma Arizona	*Rhipicephalus sanguineus (brown dog tick)*	

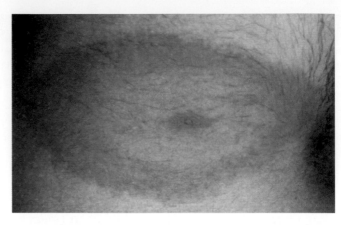

FIGURE 10-5. **Erythema migrans rash characteristic of Lyme disease.** (Reproduced, with permission, from Vijay Sikand, MD.)

- Isolated facial palsy (CN VII, Bell palsy): develops 3–5 weeks after exposure
    - Treatment of Lyme does not affect resolution of facial palsy, but it prevents late events (arthritis).
    - Self-limited and may be bilateral.

DIAGNOSIS

- Confirmed by serology.
- During the first four weeks of infection, serologic tests are negative and not recommended.
- Immunoglobulins M and G (IgM and IgG) peak 4–6 weeks after exposure and are detected by ELISA (screening, may be false positive) with reflex Western immunoblot for confirmation.
- False-positive results with other spirochetal infections (syphilis, leptospirosis) and in patients with some autoimmune disorders (lupus, rheumatoid arthritis).
- An elevated IgG titer in the absence of an elevated IgM indicates prior exposure as opposed to recent infection.
- PCR can detect spirochete DNA in CSF and synovial fluid, but it has high false-negative results (poor sensitivity) and is not a first-line test.

COMPLICATIONS

- Arthritis—will develop in 60% of patients if left untreated.
- Carditis—can be evidenced by heart block (most common).
- Meningitis—requires prolonged period of parenteral treatment.

TREATMENT

- Oral Amoxicillin, cefuroxime, or doxycycline:
    - EM lesions: 14–21 days.
    - Multiple EM lesions: 21 days.
    - Isolated facial palsy: 21–28 days.
    - Arthritis: 28 days.
- Ceftriaxone IV: carditis, meningitis, persistent/recurrent arthritis: 14–28 days; when stabilized, may be discharged to complete therapy with oral options above.

WARD TIP

If untreated, lesions fade within 28 days. If diagnosis is delayed, may have permanent neurologic or joint disabilities.

WARD TIP

If treated adequately, Lyme-related lesions fade within days and the late manifestations are prevented.

ROCKY MOUNTAIN SPOTTED FEVER (RMSF)

An 8-year-old girl from North Carolina presents in July with three days of fever, severe headache, and myalgia. On examination, she has a temperature of 102.9°F (39.4°C), HR 134 beats/min. She is complaining of headache and has a macular rash on her wrists, palms, ankles, and soles. She has no other significant findings. Her platelets are 68×10^3 cells/µL and serum sodium is 129 mEq/L. *Think: Rocky Mountain spotted fever.*

RMSF is a systemic tick-borne illness caused by *Rickettsia rickettsii*. Rash is considered the hallmark of this disease, which characteristically involves the palms and soles. Severe frontal headache is common. Abdominal pain, splenomegaly, and conjunctivitis may also be present. Highest incidence rates for RMSF are in North Carolina, Oklahoma, Arkansas, Tennessee, and Missouri. Classic laboratory abnormalities include thrombocytopenia, hyponatremia, and elevated liver enzymes.

DEFINITION

This potentially life-threatening disease is transmitted by the bite of a *Dermacentor* tick infected with bacteria.

ETIOLOGY

Rickettsia rickettsii.

EPIDEMIOLOGY

Keep in mind geography (presence of a vector) and season (see Table 10-3).

PATHOPHYSIOLOGY

- An intracellular infection of the endothelial cells lining the small blood vessels, resulting in vascular necrosis and extravasation of blood.
- Only 60% of patients report a history of a tick bite.
- The incubation period is 2–14 days.
- It rarely occurs in the Rocky Mountains.
- The highest incidence occurs in children 5–10 years old.

SIGNS AND SYMPTOMS

- Sudden onset of high fever, myalgia, severe headache, rigors, nausea, and photophobia.
- Fifty percent develop rash within three days, another 30% within six days.
- Rash consists of 2- to 6-mm pink initially blanchable macules that first appear peripherally on wrists, forearms, ankles, palms, and soles.
- Within 6–18 hours, the exanthem spreads centrally to the trunk, proximal extremities, and face (centrifugal).
- Within 1–3 days, the macules evolve to deep-red papules, and within 2–4 days, the exanthem is hemorrhagic, petechial, and no longer blanchable.
- Up to 15% have no rash ("spotless").
- Many patients have exquisite tenderness of the gastrocnemius muscle.
- Meningitis is common.
- If untreated, myocarditis, disseminated intravascular coagulation (DIC), and shock can result, with fatality rate up to 25%.

DIAGNOSIS

- Clinical.
- Rash biopsy would demonstrate necrotizing vasculitis.
- Indirect fluorescent antibody (IFA) assay: titer >1:64 is diagnostic.

WARD TIP

RMSF is a clinical diagnosis. It is important not to delay treatment while awaiting serologic confirmation.

WARD TIP

Typical RMSF:
- Ill appearing with fever, myalgia, and headache
- Hyponatremia and thrombocytopenia
- Rash on palms and soles

TREATMENT

Doxycycline, regardless of patient's age.

COMPLICATIONS

- Noncardiogenic pulmonary edema.
- Meningoencephalitis.
- Multiorgan damage due to vasculitis.

Fungal Infections

See Table 10-4 for a comparison of endemic fungal infections.

TABLE 10-4. **Comparison of Endemic Fungal Infections**

	HISTOPLASMOSIS	COCCIDIOIDOMYCOSIS
Geography	Mississippi, Ohio, and Missouri River valleys	Utah, Arizona, New Mexico, Texas, California
Setting	Gardening, demolition, visiting caves (bat droppings); playing in barns, hollow trees with bird roosts	Dust storms, earthquakes, archeologic digging, picnic in a desert
Focal infection	Pulmonary infiltrates, hilar adenopathy In adolescents: Erythema nodosum[a]	Influenza-like or pneumonia: Fever, cough, headache, malaise, myalgia, and chest pain Erythema multiforme Erythema nodosum[a]
Disseminated infection	Prolonged fever, pneumonitis, lymphadenopathy, hepatosplenomegaly, failure to thrive or weight loss, meningitis, pancytopenia	Rare Skin: Papules, nodules osteomyelitis, arthritis Meningitis, pneumonitis
Diagnosis	Culture of sputum, blood, bone marrow Histology: Intracellular yeast with silver stain	Serology: IgM and IgG Histology. Spherules in pleural fluid bronchoalveolar lavage, and skin biopsy specimens
Treatment Focal infection Disseminated infection	 Itraconazole Amphotericin B	 Fluconazole or itraconazole Amphotericin B

[a]Erythema nodosum is an inflammatory exanthem, an area of tender, red and shiny induration, usually on the shins.

COCCIDIOIDOMYCOSIS

A 13-year-old girl develops fever, cough, and chest pain. On examination, her temperature is 102.5°F (39.2°C), RR 44 breaths/min, no hypoxemia, and rales are heard over her left lower lobe. She has symmetrical tender, red, shiny indurations on both shins. WBC: 16.8×10^3 cells/μL. Chest radiograph shows left lower-lobe consolidation. Further history-taking reveals a recent trip to Arizona. *Think: Coccidioidomycosis.*

Coccidioidomycosis is an infectious disease caused by the fungus *Coccidioides immitis*. Also known as San Joaquin Valley fever, coccidioidomycosis should be considered in southwestern U.S. states (Arizona, California, Nevada, New Mexico, Utah, and Texas). Symptoms usually develop 1–3 weeks after exposure. Clinical features include dry cough, chest pain, myalgia, arthralgia, fever, anorexia, and weakness. Infection is often subclinical.

ETIOLOGY

Coccidioides immitis or *Coccidioides posadasii* (no clinical distinction).

EPIDEMIOLOGY

- Southwestern United States.
- Black and Filipino, pregnant women, neonates, and immunocompromised people have higher risk of disseminated disease.
- Incubation period: 1–3 weeks.
- Transmission: inhalation of airborne spores.
- Person-to-person transmission does not occur.
- Infection produces lifelong immunity.

SIGNS AND SYMPTOMS

- Usually asymptomatic or self-limited: influenza-like or pneumonia, with fever, cough, headache, malaise, myalgia, and chest pain; may also have night sweats and anorexia.
- Maculopapular rash, erythema multiforme, or erythema nodosum may be the only manifestations.
- Dissemination is rare, mostly in infants or immunocompromised patients: skin, bones and joints, central nervous system (CNS), and lungs.
- Meningitis almost invariably is fatal if untreated.

DIAGNOSIS

- Coin-like pulmonary lesions may be present on the chest x-ray.
- Spherules with endospores in tissue or body fluid is pathognomonic.
- Laboratory diagnosis with serology (IgG and IgM) or fungal cultures (may be infectious—notify lab *Coccidioides* infection being considered).
- Elevated erythrocyte sedimentation rate (ESR) and alkaline phosphatase.
- Eosinophilia.

TREATMENT

- Fluconazole or itraconazole.
- Surgical resection for chronic pulmonary coccidioidal disease that is unresponsive to IV azole or amphotericin B therapy.

HISTOPLASMOSIS

A 6-year-old boy from Indiana develops fever, chest pain, and cough. He was playing in a cave 10 days ago and got scared by bats. A physical exam shows no distress, temperature of 100.7°F (38.2°C), RR 28 breaths/min, oxygen saturation 95%. Rhonchi are heard over the lung fields bilaterally. WBC: 14.9×10^3 cells/μL. Chest x-ray shows bilateral diffuse reticulonodular infiltrates and hilar lymphadenopathy. *Think: Histoplasmosis.*

Histoplasmosis is the most common endemic mycosis causing human infection. Pneumonia is the most common presentation, and atypical pneumonia is usually the initial diagnosis. An initial chest x-ray may show patchy infiltrates, while diffuse reticulonodular infiltrates are present in progressive disease. The presence of hilar or mediastinal lymphadenopathy increases the suspicion for fungal pneumonia.

ETIOLOGY

Histoplasma capsulatum

EPIDEMIOLOGY

- Endemic infection: Ohio and Mississippi River valleys.
- History of exposure to bird or bat droppings.
- Incubation period: 1–3 weeks.
- Transmission: inhalation of airborne spores.
- Reinfection can occur with large inoculum.

SIGNS AND SYMPTOMS

- Generally asymptomatic.
- Flulike prodrome.
- The more spores are inhaled, the more symptoms are present.
- Severe acute pulmonary infection: diffuse nodular infiltrates, prolonged fever, fatigue, and weight loss.
- Progressive disseminated histoplasmosis: in infants <2 years of age and in the immunosuppressed, it often begins as "fever of unknown origin."

DIAGNOSIS

- Mediastinal adenitis or granuloma may be seen on a chest x-ray.
- *Histoplasma* antigen assay: urine or serum; cross-reaction with other endemic fungi.
- Cultures: sputum, blood, bone marrow; may be negative.

TREATMENT

- Uncomplicated infection in an immunocompetent child is self-limited and does not require treatment.
- Oral itraconazole is used for serious focal (pulmonary) infection.
- IV amphotericin B is used for progressive disseminated disease.

Parasitic Infections

SCHISTOSOMIASIS

 A 16-year-old presents with fever, arthralgia, cough, abdominal pain, and rash for five days. He went to Puerto Rico for a river rafting trip three weeks ago. On examination, his temperature is 102°F (38.9°C), scattered urticaria on his trunk and extremities wax and wane, and his spleen is palpable 3 cm below the costal margin. WBC count is 6.1×10^3 cells/μL, with 23% eosinophils. *Think: Schistosomiasis.*

Schistosomiasis is transmitted in tropical and subtropical areas. Clinical presentation includes fever, chills, cough, abdominal pain, diarrhea, nausea, vomiting, headache, rash, and lymphadenopathy. Physical examination may show an enlarged, nontender liver and an enlarged spleen. Eosinophilia is often prominent.

ETIOLOGY

Caused by blood trematodes (flukes):

- *Schistosoma mansoni* (Africa, South America).
- *Schistosoma japonicum* (East Asia).
- *Schistosoma haematobium* (Africa, Middle East).

EPIDEMIOLOGY

- Ova from urine or feces hatch to release miracidia, which penetrate snail tissue and grow into larvae (cercaria).
- Larvae leave the snail into fresh water and penetrate the skin.
- After skin penetration, larvae travel to particular organs and tissues, and there develop into mature forms.

SIGNS AND SYMPTOMS

- "Swimmer's itch" (cercarial dermatitis)—transient, a few hours after water exposure, followed in 1–2 weeks by an intermittent pruritic, papular rash; caused by species of schistosomes that parasitize birds but larvae die in the human dermis.
- Invasive stage: within weeks to months of exposure—fever, malaise, cough, abdominal pain, and nonspecific rash (Katayama syndrome).
- Ulceration of intestine and colon, abdominal pain, and bloody diarrhea (*Schistosoma intercalatum* and *Schistosoma mekongi*).
- Eggs can embolize to the lungs or central nervous system.
- *S. haematobium* infection can occur in the urogenital tract and cause dysuria, hematuria, hydronephrosis, pelvic pain, prostatitis, and bladder cancer.

DIAGNOSIS

- Eggs in stool or urine.
- Peripheral eosinophilia.

TREATMENT

Praziquantel

WARD TIP

Pay attention to travel history and timing from return (incubation period from weeks to months).

WARD TIP

Risk is exposure to fresh water (lake, river) in an endemic area through swimming, fishing, and playing.

TOXOCARIASIS

ETIOLOGY

Toxocara canis and *Toxocara cati* (roundworms of puppies or kittens).

EPIDEMIOLOGY

- Fecal-oral transmission: eggs in soil enter the mouth via hands or toys.
- Role of pica (eating soil): ingested eggs hatch and penetrate the GI tract, migrating to the liver, lung, eye, central nervous system, and heart, where they die and calcify.

SIGNS AND SYMPTOMS

- Most individuals are asymptomatic.
- Symptomatic in young children (under 4 years of age).
- The more larvae, the more symptoms occur.
- Visceral: fever, cough, wheezing (pneumonitis), hepatomegaly.
- Rare: myocarditis, encephalitis (seizures).
- Ocular: endophthalmitis or retinal granulomas, usually in older children or adolescents.

> A 4-year-old boy presents with fever and cough for 10 days. On exam, he has a temperature of 101.8°F (38.8°C) and hepatomegaly. He has leukocytosis with 45% eosinophils. He likes to play with his puppy in a sandbox. What is the diagnosis? *Think: Visceral larva migrans.*

DIAGNOSIS

- Leukocytosis and hypereosinophilia.
- ELISA for *Toxocara* antibodies. ELISA is more sensitive in visceral than in the ocular form of infection.

TREATMENT

Albendazole

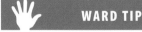

Traumatic Infections

ANIMAL BITES/SCRATCHES

- Cleaning, debridement, and irrigation are the most important treatment.
- Antibiotic prophylaxis for all human bites ("fight bites" on hands are particularly susceptible to infection and may require surgical debridement for tenosynovitis).
- Cat bites more likely to get infected than dog bites (cat puncture wounds deposit bacteria deeply). Prophylaxis is recommended for wounds on the hands, feet, or face. For other wounds, base prophylaxis on the degree of tissue damage.
- X-ray to check for bone involvement or foreign body if the wound is deep.
- Most bite wounds on extremities should not be sutured; if wounds are deep, surgical consult should be considered.
- Assess risk for rabies using local epidemiological information.
- Antibiotic of choice is typically amoxicillin/clavulanic acid.
- Ensure tetanus immunization is up to date.

CAT SCRATCH DISEASE

ETIOLOGY

- *Bartonella henselae* infection.

EPIDEMIOLOGY

- Cats are a natural reservoir for *B henselae*.
- Present in 30–40% of domestic and adopted shelter cats in the United States
- Cat-to-cat transmission occurs via the cat flea (*Ctenocephalides felis*); persistent asymptomatic bacteremia is present in affected cats.
- Humans are inoculated through a bite, scratch, or lick (especially from kittens).

SIGNS AND SYMPTOMS

- The incubation period in humans is 3–12 days.
- Skin papule or pustule appears at inoculum site in the majority of cases.
- Regional lymphadenopathy develops in 1–2 weeks after lesion.

DIAGNOSIS

- Enzyme immunoassay (EIA) and indirect immunofluorescent antibody (IFA) for antibodies.
- PCR for tissue or body fluids; not recommended for testing blood.

TREATMENT

- Typically self-limited, resolving in 2 to 4 months.
- For patients with lymphadenitis, azithromycin usually results in rapid improvement.

COMPLICATIONS

- Ocular complications in 5–10%
  - Parinaud oculoglandular syndrome.
  - Neuroretinitis.
- Endocarditis.
- Encephalitis.
- Pneumonia.
- Prolonged fever with hepatic and splenic granulomas.

ABRASIONS AND LACERATIONS

A 10-year-old boy steps on a dirty nail that punctures his foot through his sneaker. Two days later, he presents with pain, swelling, and redness of the heel, with purulent drainage from a central pinpoint opening. He has no fever. WBC is 14.6×10^3 cells/µL. X-ray shows no foreign body, no fracture, and no gas in the soft tissue. *Think: Wound likely to become infected with* Pseudomonas. *The organism has an affinity for rubber and plastic, and the association of* Pseudomonas *with plantar puncture wounds through a shoe is well recognized.*

- Cleaning, debridement, and irrigation are most important initial treatment. Suturing should be considered, but it increases risk of infection so must be weighed against cosmetic outcome.
- If secondarily infected, debride and drain.
- Antibiotic prophylaxis generally is not indicated unless the wound is heavily soiled or a large amount of tissue damage is present; gram stain and culture to determine the best antibiotic in chronic or complex wounds.

- *Staphylococcus* and *Streptococcus* are the most common pathogens, so a first-generation cephalosporin such as cephalexin or clindamycin is commonly given as empiric treatment.
- *Pseudomonal* coverage must be added for a puncture wound through the shoe.
- Ensure tetanus immunization is up to date.

Human Immunodeficiency Virus (HIV) in the Child

ETIOLOGY

- Infants: vertical transmission from mothers either perinatally or through breast milk (preventable with antiretroviral prophylaxis)
- Adolescents: sexual transmission or IV drug use.

CLINICAL PRESENTATION

- Suspect HIV infection in a child with failure to thrive, thrush after 12 months of age, generalized nontender lymphadenopathy, hepatosplenomegaly, and thrombocytopenia.
- Consider acute HIV syndrome in a sexually active adolescent with mononucleosis-like illness with fever, lymphadenopathy, and hepatosplenomegaly.

DIAGNOSIS

- HIV screening is part of prenatal care.
- In non-breast-feeding infants <18 months of age and born to HIV-infected mothers, exclusion of HIV-1 is based on:
  - Negative HIV PCR at 2–3 weeks, 1–2 months and again at 4–6 months
    - For high-risk infants (high maternal viral load), additional testing is recommended.
  - No other laboratory or clinical evidence of HIV-1 infection, including no AIDS-defining illness for which there is no other underlying immunosuppression.
- In adolescents >13 years of age, rapid oral swab enzyme immunoassay (EIA) is an alternative diagnostic method. If it is positive, confirmatory enzyme-linked immunosorbent assay (ELISA) and Western blot are required.

TREATMENT

- Multiple classes:
  - Nucleoside reverse transcriptase inhibitors (NRTIs).
  - Non-nucleoside reverse transcriptase inhibitors (NNRTIs).
  - Protease inhibitors.
  - Entry and fusion inhibitors.
  - Integrase inhibitors.
  - Pharmacokinetic enhancers for protease inhibitors.
- HIV rapidly becomes resistant; therefore, multidrug therapy is necessary.

Common Opportunistic Infections in HIV

TOXOPLASMOSIS

ETIOLOGY

- *Toxoplasma gondii* (intracellular protozoan).
- Toxoplasma oocysts are classically present in cat feces.

EXAM TIP

Perinatal HIV
- Generalized lymphadenopathy
- Hepatosplenomegaly
- Persistent oral and diaper candidiasis
- Failure to thrive

SIGNS AND SYMPTOMS

- Mononucleosis-like syndrome including fever, lymphadenopathy, and hepatosplenomegaly.
- Disseminated infection with T-cell deficiency.

DIAGNOSIS

Serologic antibody tests, biopsy, visualization of parasites in CSF.

TREATMENT

Pyrimethamine and sulfadiazine used concurrently (both inhibit folic acid synthesis, so replace folic acid).

CRYPTOCOCCOSIS

DEFINITION

- Fungal infection.
- Primary infection in lungs.
- The fungus disseminates to brain, meninges, skin, eyes, and skeletal system in immune compromised individuals.

SIGNS AND SYMPTOMS

- Subacute or chronic meningitis is the most common presentation in AIDS.
- Typically presents with fever, headache, and malaise.
- Postinfectious sequelae is common, including:
  - Hydrocephalus.
  - Change in visual acuity.
  - Deafness.
  - Cranial nerve palsies.
  - Seizures.
  - Ataxia.

DIAGNOSIS

- A definitive diagnosis requires isolation of the organism from body fluid or tissue specimens: sputum, bronchopulmonary lavage (BAL), or CSF.
- Bird Seed agar (Staib's medium) can increase detection in sputum and urine.
- The latex agglutination test and EIA for detection of cryptococcal capsular polysaccharide antigen in serum or CSF specimens are excellent rapid diagnostic tests.
- Microscopy: encapsulated yeast is seen as white halos when CSF is mixed with India ink.
- It can be grown in a culture (takes up to three weeks).
- May also see cryptococcomas on head CT.

TREATMENT

- Treat with combination therapy using amphotericin B and flucytosine.
- Relapse rate is very high. This is a reason for subsequent maintenance therapy with oral fluconazole.

PNEUMOCYSTIS JIROVECII PNEUMONIA

Formerly *P. carinii*, now classified as an atypical fungus.

EPIDEMIOLOGY

- Peak incidence: 3–6 months of age.
- Highest mortality rate in infants.

SIGNS AND SYMPTOMS

- Acute onset of fever, tachypnea, dyspnea, dry cough, and progressive hypoxemia.
- Chest x-ray—diffuse bilateral interstitial infiltrates or alveolar disease may have characteristic "ground glass" appearance.

DIAGNOSIS

- Diagnosis by methenamine silver staining of bronchoalveolar lavage (BAL) to identify cyst walls or Giemsa staining to identify nuclei of trophozoites; LDH > 500.
- PCR becoming more widely available.

TREATMENT

- First-line treatment with prednisone is trimethoprim-sulfamethoxazole (TMP-SMX) for 5–7 days.
- Alternative regimens include: pentamidine, TMP-SMX plus dapsone, atovaquone.
- Resistant to most antifungals.

PROPHYLAXIS

Starting at 6 weeks of age, TMP-SMX if CD4 < 15%, or <200/mm^3 for age 6–12 years and <500/mm^3 for age 1–5 years. Risk displacement of bilirubin exists in neonate.

ATYPICAL MYCOBACTERIAL INFECTIONS

ETIOLOGY

- *Mycobacterium avium* complex (MAC).
- Considered an AIDS-defining illness. Patients with CD4 counts <50/mm^3 are at highest risk.

SIGNS AND SYMPTOMS

Disseminated disease:

- Fever.
- Malaise.
- Weight loss.
- Night sweats.
- May have gastrointestinal (GI) symptoms.

DIAGNOSIS

Diagnosis by culture from blood, bone marrow, or tissue.

TREATMENT

Two-drug regimen:

- Either clarithromycin *or* azithromycin.
- *Plus* ethambutol, rifabutin, rifampin, ciprofloxacin, *or* amikacin.

PROPHYLAXIS

For CD4 < 50 × 10^3 cells/μL: Give azithromycin once a week.

EXAM TIP

Rifabutin decreases serum levels of zidovudine (ZDV) and clarithromycin.

WARD TIP

Fluconazole can decrease the level of rifabutin by 80%.

WARD TIP

Rifabutin can color body secretions such as urine, sweat, and tears a bright orange.

CYTOMEGALOVIRUS (CMV)

ETIOLOGY

Member of herpesvirus family

PATHOPHYSIOLOGY

- In immunocompetent individuals, initial infection is typically asymptomatic.
- Infection is lifelong, as with any other herpesvirus. It may be acquired early in life and stay latent until the host becomes immunocompromised, years later. Lung, liver, kidney, GI tract, and salivary glands are the most common organs infected.

SIGNS AND SYMPTOMS

- Pneumonitis.
- Esophagitis.
- Retinitis (can cause blindness).

DIAGNOSIS

- Reactivation may be associated with the appearance of IgM in serum.
- The pp65 antigen in white blood cells is used to detect infection in immunocompromised hosts. Quantitative polymerase chain reaction (PCR) as a measure of viral load in blood is available.
- Urine shedding of virus is lifelong. Positive urine CMV culture does not indicate association with current disease.

TREATMENT

- Ganciclovir; systemic plus intraocular treatment for retinitis.
- IV foscarnet in ganciclovir-resistant infection.

WARD TIP

CMV is the most common congenital viral infection, the most common infectious cause of birth defects in the United States, and the most common cause of non-hereditary sensorineural hearing loss in childhood.

NOTES

Gastrointestinal Disease

Esophageal Atresia

WARD TIP

Esophageal atresia can be associated with the **VACTERL** sequence with anomalies in the following areas:

Vertebral
Anorectal
Cardiac
Tracheal
Esophageal
Renal
Limb

WARD TIP

Suspect esophageal atresia in a neonate with drooling and excessive oral secretions.

WARD TIP

An inability to pass a 10 French NGT from the mouth to the stomach suggests esophageal atresia.

A full-term infant has copious oral secretions requiring frequent suctioning to prevent choking. Attempts to place a nasogastric tube (NGT) were unsuccessful, with the tube curling in the esophagus. What is the likely diagnosis?

The NGT with the tip in the proximal esophagus and failure to advance further signifies an esophageal atresia. The most common type is blind-proximal esophageal pouch with a distal tracheoesophageal fistula. Esophageal atresia is often associated with VACTERL sequence.

DEFINITION

- The esophagus ends blindly ~10–12 cm from the nares.
- Occurs in 1/2500–1/3500 live births.
- In 85% of cases, the distal esophagus communicates with the posterior trachea (distal tracheoesophageal fistula [TEF]; Figure 11-1).

SIGNS AND SYMPTOMS

- History of maternal polyhydramnios.
- Newborn with increased oral secretions.
- Choking, cyanosis, coughing during feeding, aspiration of pharyngeal secretions.
- Aspiration of gastric contents via distal fistula—life threatening (chemical pneumonitis).
- Recurrent coughing with aspiration pneumonia (delayed diagnosis); (See Chapter 12 [Respiratory Disease] for further discussion).

DIAGNOSIS

- Usually made soon after delivery.
- Unable to pass NGT into stomach (see coiled NGT on chest x-ray [Figure 11-2]).
- May also use contrast radiology, video esophagram, or bronchoscopy.
- Chest x-ray (CXR) demonstrates air in upper esophagus.
- Abdominal film shows no air in TEF Types B and D.

TREATMENT

- Maintain airway.
- Decompress upper pouch.
- Surgical repair (may be done in stages).

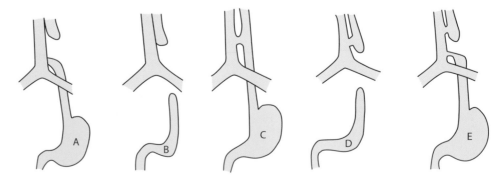

FIGURE 11-1. Types of tracheoesophageal fistulas (TEFs). Type A, esophageal atresia (EA) with distal TEF (87%). Type B, isolated EA (8%). Type C, isolated TEF (4%). Type D, EA with proximal TEF (<1%). Type E, EA with double TEF (<1%).

Esophageal Foreign Body

- Most commonly coins, but also pins, screws, batteries.
- Common ages 6 to 36 months or older children with developmental delay.
- Preexisting abnormalities (i.e., tracheoesophageal repair) result in higher risk of foreign-body impaction at abnormality site.
- Site of impaction:
  - Upper esophageal sphincter at the cricopharyngeus muscle (between clavicles on CXR).
  - Mid-esophagus where aortic arch and left main stem bronchus indent esophagus.
  - Lower esophageal sphincter.

SIGNS AND SYMPTOMS

- 40% asymptomatic; high index of suspicion required for suspected ingestion.
- Gagging/choking.
- Difficulty with secretions.
- Dysphagia/food refusal.
- Throat pain or chest pain.
- Emesis/hematemesis.

DIAGNOSIS

- History, sometime witnessed event.
- X-ray (AP/lateral CXR; see Figure 11-3).

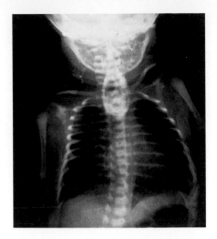

FIGURE 11-2.   Esophageal atresia. Radiograph demonstrating coiled tube in the upper esophagus. (Reproduced, with permission, from Brunicardi FC, Andersen DK, Billiar TR, et al, eds: *Schwartz's Principles of Surgery*, 11th ed. New York, McGraw Hill, 2019, Fig. 39-10.)

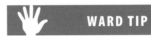

WARD TIP

The most common site of esophageal impaction is at the thoracic inlet.

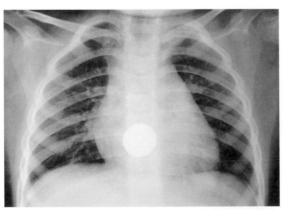

A

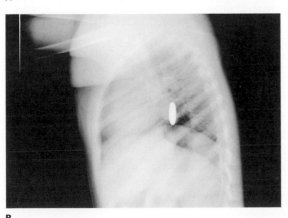

B

FIGURE 11-3.   Esophageal foreign body. A coin in the esophagus will be seen flat or en face on an AP radiograph, and on its edge on a lateral view. (Reproduced, with permission, from Stone CK, Humphries RL, eds: *Current Diagnosis & Treatment: Emergency Medicine*, 8th ed. New York, McGraw Hill, 2017, Fig. 50-6.)

TREATMENT

- Generally requires endoscopic treatment if symptomatic or fails to pass to stomach (below diaphragm on x-ray) within a few hours.
- Impacted objects, pointed objects, and batteries must be removed immediately.
- Ingestion for longer than 24 hours can cause erosion or necrosis of esophageal wall.

Gastroesophageal Reflux Disease (GERD)

DEFINITION

- Passive reflux of gastric contents across the lower esophageal sphincter (LES) is gastroesophageal reflux, a condition affecting most children and adults.
- GER increases through the first 4 to 6 months of life, decreasing by about 8 months of life. Affected children are called "happy spitters."
- GERD is defined as GER **with** failure of normal protective measures, resulting in damage to the aerodigestive tract.

RISK FACTORS

- Prematurity.
- Neurologic disorders.
- Strong family history.

SIGNS AND SYMPTOMS

- Excessive spitting up in the first week of life.
- Symptoms resolve in most GER cases without treatment by age 2.
- Forceful vomiting (occasional).
- Aspiration pneumonia.
- Chronic cough, wheezing, and recurrent pneumonia (later childhood).
- Rarely may cause laryngospasm, apnea, and bradycardia.

DIAGNOSIS

- Clinical assessment alone suffices in most cases.
- Esophageal pH probe, barium esophagography, or gastric emptying studies in severe cases.
- Esophagoscopy with biopsy; findings typically distal.

TREATMENT

- Positioning following feeds: keep infant upright up to an hour after feeds.
- Avoid placing infants with GER in a car seat (increases abdominal pressure).
- In older children, have mealtime more than 2 hours before sleep and have child sleep with head elevated.
- Thicken commercial formula or add rice cereal to traditional formula.
- Medications:
    - Antacids, histamine-2 (H_2) blockers (famotidine), and proton pump inhibitors (PPIs; omeprazole).
    - Gastric motility agents (metoclopramide, erythromycin).
    - Surgery: Nissen fundoplication.

Eosinophilic Esophagitis

DEFINITION

- Eosinophilic infiltrate of the esophageal wall.
- Four times more common in boys.
- Biphasic: ages 1 to 4 and 10 to 14 years.

SIGNS AND SYMPTOMS

- Younger children: food aversion, failure to thrive, vomiting.
- Older children: vomiting, dysphagia, food impaction.

DIAGNOSIS

- Esophagoscopy with adherent white plaques throughout; biopsy with elevated eosinophils.

TREATMENT

- Elimination diet of potential allergen or trial of hypoallergenic formula.
- Systemic or topical (swallowing of inhaled) corticosteroids.

Peptic Ulcer

DEFINITION

Includes primary and secondary.

SIGNS AND SYMPTOMS

- Primary
  - Neonates: GI hemorrhage and perforation.
  - Infants and young children: vomiting, pain, feeding problems, and GI hemorrhage.
  - School age and adolescents: periumbilical and postprandial pain (with vomiting and hemorrhage), anemia.
  - Epigastric pain relieved by food ingestion seen in adults but is less common in children.
  - Infectious—*Helicobacter pylori*.
- Secondary
  - Stress ulcer due to sepsis, respiratory or cardiac insufficiency, or dehydration.
  - Stress ulcers associated with burns, surgery or head trauma (Curling ulcers).
  - Drug related—nonsteroidal anti-inflammatory drugs (NSAIDs) or steroids.

DIAGNOSIS

- Upper GI endoscopy.
- Upper GI barium studies not sensitive and not utilized.
- *H. pylori* testing (hydrogen breath test, stool antigen).

TREATMENT

- Antibiotics for eradication of *H. pylori*: triple therapy—PPI + 2 antibiotics (amoxicillin, clarithromycin, PPI).
- Antacids, sucralfate, and misoprostol.

 WARD TIP

Antimicrobials: 14 days
PPIs: 1 month

- H_2 blockers and PPIs.
- Peptic-ulcer prophylaxis when child is NPO or is receiving steroids.
- Surgery (vagotomy, pyloroplasty, or antrectomy) for extreme cases.

Colic

 The parents of a 5-week-old infant report she has nightly bouts of inconsolable crying. During the day, the child seems happy; each evening, she begins to have crying spells during which she draws up her legs, clinches her fists, has a facial expression of pain, and begins to pass gas. Interventions do not resolve the episodes; the episodes resolve spontaneously after several hours. *Think: Colic.*

Colic is described in an otherwise normal child who has late afternoon or early evening episodes of crying, motor behaviors such as drawing up the legs or clinching the fists, facial expression of pain, passing of gas, inability to console and spontaneous resolution.

DEFINITION

- Rule of 3's: crying >3 hours/day, >3 days/week for >3 weeks between the ages of 3 weeks and 3 months.
- Frequent complex paroxysmal abdominal pain, severe crying.
- Etiology unknown.
- Colic is a diagnosis of exclusion. First look for other causes (hair in eye, corneal abrasion, strangulated hernia, otitis media, fracture, sepsis).

SIGNS AND SYMPTOMS

- Sudden-onset loud crying (paroxysms may persist for several hours).
- Facial flushing.
- Circumoral pallor.
- Distended, tense abdomen.
- Legs drawn up on abdomen.
- Passage of feces or flatus.

TREATMENT

- No single treatment provides satisfactory relief.
- Careful examination is critical to rule out other causes.
- Avoid overstimulation.
- Avoid over- or underfeeding.
- Resolves spontaneously with time.

> **WARD TIP**
>
> A head-to-toe examination is essential. Physical examination *must* be normal.

> **WARD TIP**
>
> Parents and caretakers of children with colic are often very stressed, putting the child at risk for child abuse.

Pyloric Stenosis

A 4-week-old male infant has a 5-day history of vomiting after feedings. Physical examination shows a hungry infant with an epigastric peristaltic wave. Laboratory evaluation shows: Na 129, Cl 92, HCO_3 28, K 3.1, BUN 24. *Think: Hypertrophic pyloric stenosis.*

Pyloric stenosis is the most common surgical cause of non-bilious emesis in infants. It is more common in males (M:F 4:1). It usually presents during the third to eighth week of life. Initial symptom is forceful, nonbilious vomiting. Classic findings of an olive mass are pathognomonic but sometimes hard to feel. Ultrasound criteria for diagnosis include pyloric muscle thickness >3 mm and length of pyloric canal >14 mm. Hypochloremic, hypokalemic metabolic alkalosis is the classic electrolyte abnormality.

DEFINITION

- The most common etiology is idiopathic.
- It is associated with exogenous administration of erythromycin, eosinophilic gastroenteritis, epidermolysis bullosa, trisomy 18, and Turner syndrome.
- First-born males are affected more often.

SIGNS AND SYMPTOMS

- Typical: projectile vomiting, palpable mass, and peristalsis—not always present.
- Nonbilious vomiting (projectile or not).
- Usually progressive, after feeding.
- Usually after 3 weeks of age, may be as late as 5 months.
- Palpable pyloric olive-shaped mass in mid-epigastrium (difficult to find).
- Visible peristalsis: left to right.
- Hypochloremic, hypokalemic metabolic alkalosis.

DIAGNOSIS

- Ultrasound (90% sensitivity)
  - Elongated pyloric channel (>14 mm).
  - Thickened pyloric wall (>3 mm).
- Radiographic contrast series
  - String sign: from elongated pyloric channel.
  - Shoulder sign: bulge of pyloric muscle into the antrum.
  - Double tract sign: parallel barium streaks in the narrow channel.

TREATMENT

- Correct dehydration and acid-base abnormalities before surgery.
- Surgery: pyloromyotomy is curative. Infants may eat as soon as they awake from anesthesia.

Duodenal Atresia

DEFINITION

- Failure to recanalize lumen after solid phase of intestinal development.
- Can be complete (most common), stenotic, or fenestrated web.

SIGNS AND SYMPTOMS

- Bilious vomiting without abdominal distention, typically within hours of birth.
- Scaphoid abdomen if obstruction complete.
- Placement of orogastric tube typically yields a significant amount of bile-stained fluid.
- History of polyhydramnios occurs in 50% of pregnancies.
- It is commonly seen with trisomy 21.
- Associated anomalies include congenital heart disease, malrotation, annular pancreas, renal anomalies, and esophageal atresia.

DIAGNOSIS

- Clinical.
- X-ray findings: double-bubble sign (air in the stomach and duodenum) proximal to the site of atresia (Figure 11-4).

TREATMENT

- Naso- or orogastric decompression and intravenous fluids
- Treat life-threatening anomalies if found
- Surgery: duodenoduodenostomy

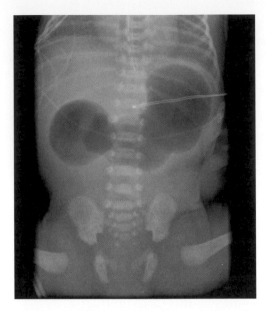

FIGURE 11-4. Duodenal atresia. Gas-filled and dilated stomach shows the classic "double-bubble" appearance of duodenal atresia. Note no distal gas is present. (Reproduced, with permission, from Elsayes KM, Oldham SAA: *Introduction to Diagnostic Radiology.* McGraw-Hill, New York, 2014, Fig. c6.1.)

Malrotation and Volvulus

DEFINITION

- Malrotation includes a group of disorders of incomplete rotation and fixation of the bowel during fetal development.
- Volvulus occurs when midgut axial rotation around the superior mesenteric artery causes intestinal obstruction, ischemia, and potentially bowel necrosis (Figure 11-5).
- More than 50% of cases present in the first month of life and 85% in the first year.
- It is often associated with other GI, respiratory, cardiac, and genitourinary system abnormalities.

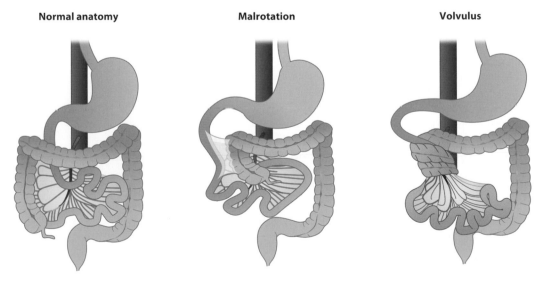

Normal anatomy   Malrotation   Volvulus

FIGURE 11-5. Volvulus. First AP view done 6 weeks prior to the second AP and corresponding lateral view. Note the markedly dilated stomach above the normal level of the left hemidiaphragm in the thoracic cavity. Also present is a large left-sided diaphragmatic hernia. (Reproduced, with permission, from Dr. Julia Rosekrans.)

SIGNS AND SYMPTOMS

- Vomiting, especially bilious, in infancy is the most common presentation.
- Abdominal pain results in acute abdomen.
- Early satiety in older children.
- Blood-stained stools.
- Distention.

DIAGNOSIS

- Abdominal films with contrast: characteristic "bird-beak" or "cork screw" finding.

TREATMENT

- Fluid and electrolyte stabilization.
- Treatment:
  - Malrotation with volvulus is emergent surgical correction.
  - Malrotation without volvulus may be laparoscopic correction.

COMPLICATIONS

- Perforation with peritonitis.
- Short gut syndrome occurs if bowel loss extensive.

Intussusception

 A 9-month-old female infant has vomiting and is crying. She had a "cold" three days ago. On arrival, she was sleepy but arousable. When she woke up, she cried and vomited. Between episodes of pain, she is playful. Physical examination revealed distended abdomen with an ill-defined mass in the right upper abdomen. What is the cause of her symptoms? *Think: Intussusception.*

How she should be treated? A contrast enema is diagnostic and may be therapeutic to reduce the intussusception. Pediatric surgery is on standby if the contrast enema fails. Intussusception is the most common cause of intestinal obstruction between 5 months and 3 years of age. Most children with intussusception are under 1 year of age. The classic triad of intermittent, colicky abdominal pain; vomiting; and bloody, mucous stools is not always present.

DEFINITION

This condition is the invagination of one portion of the bowel into itself. The proximal portion is usually drawn into the distal portion by peristalsis.

EPIDEMIOLOGY

- Incidence: 1–4 in 1000 live births.
- Male-to-female ratio: 3:1.
- Most commonly seen 3 months to 3 years; peak incidence: 4–10 months.
- Most common site is ileocolic (90%) Figure 11-6.

ETIOLOGY

- The most common etiology is idiopathic.
- Other causes:
  - Viral associated, possibly due to swollen Peyer patches.
  - A "lead point" (or focus) more common in 2–8% of children. Lead points include Meckel's diverticulum, polyp, lymphoma, Henoch-Schönlein purpuric lesions, and cystic fibrosis.

 EXAM TIP

Intussusception is the most common cause of bowel obstruction in children ages 5 months to 3 years.

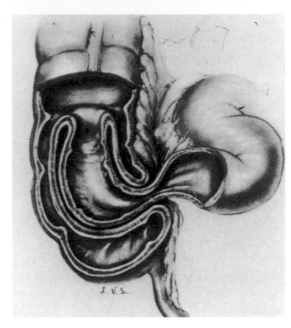

FIGURE 11-6. Intussusception. Note the telescoping of a segment of bowel (intussusceptum) into the adjacent segment (intussuscipiens). (Reproduced, with permission, from Doherty GM, ed: *Current Diagnosis & Treatment: Surgery*, 15th ed. New York, McGraw Hill, 2020, Fig. 45-20.)

EXAM TIP

Intussusception

- Classic triad of intermittent colicky abdominal pain, bilious vomiting, and currant jelly stool not always present.
- Absence of currant jelly stool does not exclude the diagnosis.

WARD TIP

A contrast enema for intussusception can be both diagnostic and therapeutic. Rule of threes:

- Barium column should not exceed a height of 3 feet.
- No more than 3 attempts
- Only 3 minutes/attempt

SIGNS AND SYMPTOMS

- Classic triad (not always present):
  - Intermittent colicky abdominal pain.
  - Bilious vomiting.
  - Currant jelly stool (late finding).
- Early in course, period of normal activity between bouts of abdominal pain.
- Neurologic signs:
  - Increasing lethargy.
  - Shock-like state.
- Right upper quadrant mass:
  - Ill-defined or sausage-shaped mass typically in right upper abdomen.

DIAGNOSIS

- Abdominal x-ray:
  - X-ray is neither specific nor sensitive; it can be completely normal.
- Ultrasound:
  - Typically, this is the first test of choice.
  - "Target" or "donut" sign: concentric layers of serosa and mucosa.
- Air or hydrostatic enema:
  - Air or hydrostatic enema is preferred (safe, with a lower absorbed radiation).
  - There is a coiled spring appearance on the evacuation film.
  - It provides the diagnostic and therapeutic benefit of a barium enema without the barium.
- Barium enema (less commonly used):
  - Contraindications: peritonitis, perforation, profound shock/hemodynamic instability.

TREATMENT

- Correct dehydration.
- NG tube for decompression.
- Hydrostatic reduction.
- Air or hydrostatic enema.
- Surgical reduction:
  - Failed reduction by enema.
  - Clinical signs of perforation or peritonitis.
- Recurrence:
  - With radiologic reduction: 3–15%; less common with surgical reduction.

Meckel Diverticulum

DEFINITION

Persistence of the omphalomesenteric (vitelline) duct (should normally disappear by seventh week of gestation).

SIGNS AND SYMPTOMS

- Usually in first 2 years:
  - Intermittent painless rectal bleeding most commonly.
  - Intestinal obstruction.
  - Diverticulitis.

DIAGNOSIS

- Meckel's scan (scintigraphy) has 85% sensitivity and 95% specificity. Uptake can be enhanced with cimetidine, glucagons, or gastrin.
- Most common heterotopic mucosa is gastric.

TREATMENT

Surgical: diverticular resection with transverse closure of the enterotomy.

Appendicitis

DEFINITION

- Acute inflammation and infection of the vermiform appendix.
- Most common cause for emergent surgery in childhood.
- Perforation rates higher in young children (cannot localize symptoms).
- Three phases:
  1. Luminal obstruction and venous congestion progressing to mucosal necrosis.
  2. Bacterial invasion with inflammatory infiltrate through all layers.
  3. Necrosis of wall results in perforation and contamination.

SIGNS AND SYMPTOMS

- Classically: pain, vomiting, and fever.
- Initially, periumbilical pain, especially with movement; emesis infrequent.
- Anorexia and malaise.
- Diarrhea infrequent unless perforated.
- Pain classically radiates to right lower quadrant (McBurney's point).
- Rigidity over the rectus muscles.

 WARD TIP

Meckel Rules of 2
- 2% of population
- 2 times more common in girls
- 2 inches long
- 2 feet from the ileocecal valve
- Patient is usually under 2 years of age
- 2% are symptomatic
- 2 types of ectopic tissue (pancreatic or gastric)

 WARD TIP

Meckel's diverticulum may mimic acute appendicitis and also act as lead point for intussusception.

- Rebound and referred tenderness (Rovsing sign) common.
- Psoas and obturator sign (pain with stretching of these muscles) common.
- Perforation rate >65% after 36–48 hours.

DIAGNOSIS

- History and a physical exam are key to rule out alternatives first.
- Pain usually occurs before vomiting, diarrhea, or anorexia.
- Atypical presentations are common—and cause a risk for misdiagnosis.
- The most common misdiagnosis is gastroenteritis.
- Labs are helpful to rule out other diagnoses; no laboratory test is specific for appendicitis.
    - A complete blood count might have an elevated white count with left shift.
    - Urinalysis might demonstrate a few white and red cells.
- The Pediatric Appendicitis Score, combining history, physical, and laboratory data, may aid in diagnosis.
- Ultrasound has replaced the computed tomographic scan, especially in experienced centers.
- CT has risk of radiation exposure, need for IV contrast, and higher cost.

TREATMENT

- Surgery, often laparoscopic for non-perforated, is considered upon diagnosis.
- Non-operative management with antibiotics and drainage is sometimes considered.
- Broad-spectrum antibiotics are needed for cases of perforation (ampicillin, gentamicin, clindamycin, or metronidazole × 7 days).

Constipation

A 4-year-old girl has not had a bowel movement for a week. Various laxatives and enemas have been tried in the past for this recurrent problem. Prior to toilet training, she had a daily bowel movement. Physical examination is normal except for a mass in the lower left quadrant and hard stool on rectal examination. *Think: Functional constipation.*

Constipation is a common problem in children, often presenting with abdominal pain. Functional constipation is more common in children; organic causes are common in neonates. The physical examination often reveals palpable stool in the suprapubic region. The finding of rectal impaction may establish the diagnosis. After removing the impaction, the next appropriate step is prolonged administration of stool softeners.

DEFINITION/SIGNS AND SYMPTOMS

- Common complaint in general pediatrics.
- Involuntary or intentional stooling into inappropriate places (e.g., clothing or floor).
- Passage of bulky or hard stool at infrequent intervals.
- Most commonly "functional" or "idiopathic" peaking at 2 to 4 years
    - In neonates, higher case of organic cause (Hirschsprung, cow's milk protein).
    - In toddlers, over-rigorous potty training.
    - In adolescents, avoidance of public restrooms.

- Prolonged constipation may result in overflow incontinence whereby the liquid part of stool oozes around the impaction, causing occasional confusion with diarrhea.
- "Organic" causes include medications, anatomic abnormalities, hypothyroidism, oppositional-defiant syndrome, and neurologic conditions such as spina bifida.
- A diagnosis is usually made with good history and a physical exam.
- A plain abdominal film will show a fecal mass; a barium enema can show Hirschsprung.

TREATMENT

- Clear fecal mass with oral laxatives such as polyethylene glycol.
- For functional constipation, develop a bowel regimen including increased oral fluid and fiber, prolonged laxative use (ensures soft stool), and dedicated "potty time" (prevent recurrence).

Hirschsprung Disease (congenital aganglionic megacolon)

 A 2-day-old term male has progressive abdominal distention and no stool since birth. He has been feeding well and appears to be fine otherwise. An abdominal x-ray shows distended loops of bowel without free air. A contrast enema has a narrowed segment of the colon leading to a distended loop.

The diagnosis is likely Hirschsprung disease. This condition results from absence of ganglion cells in the bowel wall, causing a narrowed segment of the bowel. The proximal normal bowel progressively dilates as food accumulates. A definitive diagnosis is made by a rectal biopsy, which demonstrates absent ganglion cells.

DEFINITION

- Abnormal innervation of bowel (i.e., absence of ganglion cells in bowel).
- Increased familial incidence.
- Occurs four times more commonly in males.
- Associated with Down syndrome.

SIGNS AND SYMPTOMS

- Delayed passage of meconium at birth.
- Increased abdominal distention may lead to decreased blood flow and deterioration of the mucosal barrier. Bacterial proliferation ensues, leading to enterocolitis.
- Chronic constipation and abdominal distention occur less commonly in older children.

DIAGNOSIS

- A rectal-suction biopsy includes submucosa to evaluate for ganglionic cells.
- Normal rectal manometry excludes disease; abnormal findings require a rectal biopsy.
- A barium enema shows dilated proximal loops with a contracted distal segment; findings are confirmed with a biopsy.

TREATMENT

Surgery is definitive (usually staged procedures).

Imperforate Anus

DEFINITION

- Absence of normal anal opening.
- Rectum is blind pouch; located 2 cm from perineal skin
  - Rectum may open into lower part of the vagina in females.
- Sacrum and sphincter mechanism are well developed.
- Prognosis good.
- Can be associated with VACTERL anomalies.

SIGNS AND SYMPTOMS

- Should be noted during first newborn examination in nursery.
- Failure to pass meconium.
- Abdominal distention.

DIAGNOSIS

- Physical examination.
- Abdominal ultrasonography to examine the genitourinary tract.
- Sacral radiography.
- Spinal ultrasound: association with spinal cord abnormalities, particularly spinal cord tethering.

TREATMENT

Surgery (colostomy in newborn period).

WARD TIP

Imperforate anus is frequently associated with Down syndrome and VACTERL.

Anal Fissure

 A normal 3-month-old infant is seen for constipation, blood-streaked stools, and excessive crying on defecation. *Think: Anal fissure.*
An anal fissure is a painful linear tear or crack in the distal anal canal. A diagnosis often can be made based on history and a physical examination.

DEFINITION

- Painful linear tears in the anal mucosa below the dentate line are often induced by constipation and stool withholding.
- Common age: 6–24 months.

SIGNS AND SYMPTOMS

- Pain with defecation/crying during bowel movement.
- Visible tear upon gentle lateral retraction of anal tissue.

DIAGNOSIS

Anal inspection

TREATMENT

Sitz baths, stool softeners, increased fluid intake.

Inflammatory Bowel Disease

DEFINITION

Idiopathic chronic diseases include Crohn disease and ulcerative colitis (UC).

TABLE 11-1. **Crohn Disease versus Ulcerative Colitis**

Feature	Crohn Disease	Ulcerative Colitis (UC)
Depth of involvement	Transmural	Mucosal
Ileal involvement	Common	Unusual
Mouth ulcers	Common	Unusual
Cancer risk	Increased	Greatly increased
Pyoderma gangrenosum	Rare	Present
Skip lesions	Common	Unusual
Fistula	Common	Unusual
Rectal bleeding	Sometimes	Common
Perianal disease	Common	Unusual

EPIDEMIOLOGY

- Common onset in late childhood and young adulthood.
- Bimodal pattern in patients 15–25 and 50–80 years of age.
- In children, Crohn disease is more common; equal distribution occurs in adults.
- Genetics: increased incidence in family members, especially Crohn disease.

SIGNS AND SYMPTOMS (TABLE 11-1)

- Crampy abdominal pain.
- Extraintestinal manifestations slightly greater in Crohn than UC.
- Crohn: perianal fistula, strictures, chronic active hepatitis, delayed puberty, ankylosing spondylitis, granuloma, erythema nodosum.
- UC: bloody diarrhea, toxic megacolon, pyoderma gangrenosum, sclerosing cholangitis, crypt abscesses, uveitis, marked by flare-ups.

TREATMENT

- Crohn disease: corticosteroids, aminosalicylates, methotrexate, azathioprine, cyclosporine, metronidazole (for perianal disease), sitz baths, antitumor necrosis factor-α, surgery for complications.
- UC: aminosalicylates, oral corticosteroids, colectomy.

Irritable Bowel Syndrome (IBS)

DEFINITION

Abdominal pain associated with intermittent diarrhea and constipation without organic basis; about 10% in adolescents.

SIGNS AND SYMPTOMS

- Abdominal pain.
- Diarrhea alternating with constipation.

DIAGNOSIS

- Difficult to make, exclude other pathology.
- Obtain CBC, ESR, stool occult blood to help evaluate for other conditions.

TREATMENT

- No specific treatments.
- Supportive with reinforcement and reassurance; address psychosocial stressors.
- Consider probiotics for diarrhea-predominant IBS.

Acute Gastroenteritis and Diarrhea

DEFINITION

- Diarrhea is the excessive stool loss of fluid and electrolytes, technically limited to the lower GI tract.
- Gastroenteritis is an inflammation of the entire GI tract, and it may involve vomiting and diarrhea.

EPIDEMIOLOGY

- Higher incidence seen in the young, immunodeficiency, malnutrition, travel, lack of breast-feeding, and contamination of food or water.
- The most common causes of diarrhea are viral, especially rotavirus. Norwalk agent is seen in foodborne outbreaks in schools, hospitals, and cruise ships.
- Bacterial agents include *Campylobacter*, *Salmonella* and *Shigella* species and various *Escherichia coli*.
- Parasitic pathogens include *Giardia* and *Cryptosporidium*.
- Consider pseudomembranous colitis (*C. difficile*) if antibiotics have been used recently.

SIGNS AND SYMPTOMS

- Obtain information regarding the frequency and volume.
- Determine if the patient is well appearing versus ill appearing.
- Associated findings include cramps, emesis, malaise, and fever.
- Systemic manifestations include fever, malaise, and seizures.
- Inflammatory diarrhea: fever, severe abdominal pain, tenesmus; may have blood/mucus in stool.
- Noninflammatory diarrhea: emesis, rarely fever, crampy abdominal pain, watery diarrhea.

DIAGNOSIS

- Examine stool for mucus, blood, and leukocytes (colitis).
- Stool culture for bloody diarrhea.
- Fecal leukocytes can suggest the presence of inflammation or infection.
- Patients with enterohemorrhagic *E. coli* and *Entamoeba histolytica*: minimal to no fecal leukocytes.
- Stool rotavirus assays (treatment rarely affected by results).
- *Clostridium difficile* toxins: test if antibiotics have been used recently.
- Serum electrolytes to assess dehydration or disturbance.

TREATMENT

- Rehydration (see also Chapter 5).
- Oral electrolyte solutions (e.g., Pedialyte®) are preferred.

WARD TIP

Acute diarrhea is usually caused by infectious agents (especially viral), whereas chronic persistent diarrhea may be secondary to infectious agents, infection of immunocompromised host, or residual symptoms due to intestinal damage.

WARD TIP

- Diarrhea and emesis—noninflammatory
- Diarrhea and fever—inflammatory process
- Diarrhea and tenesmus—large colon involvement

WARD TIP

Diarrhea is a characteristic finding in children with bacterial toxin of *Escherichia coli*, *Salmonella*, *Staphylococcus aureus*, and *Vibrio parahaemolyticus*, but not *Clostridium botulinum*.

TABLE 11-2.   Antimicrobial Treatment for Bacterial Enteropathogens

Bacteria	Treatment	Comments
Campylobacter	Erythromycin	Early in course of illness
Clostridium difficile	Metronidazole or vancomycin	Moderate to severe diagnosis
Escherichia coli		
Enterotoxigenic	TMP-SMZ	Severe or prolonged illness
Enteropathogenic	TMP-SMZ	Nursery epidemics
Enterohemorrhagic	Avoid antibiotics	Increased risk of hemolytic uremic syndrome if strain O157:H7 present
Salmonella	Ampicillin or chloramphenicol or TMP-SMZ	Infants < 3 months, immunodeficient patients, bacteremia otherwise no treatment
Shigella	TMP-SMZ, ceftriaxone	All susceptible organisms
Vibrio cholerae	Macrolides, fluoroquinolones, tetracycline	All cases

- Intravenous treatment may be required for severe dehydration.
- Rehydrate rapidly with replacement of ongoing losses during first 4–6 hours.
- High osmolality of soda, fruit juices, gelatin and tea may exacerbate diarrhea.
- Initiate a normal diet; the BRAT (bananas, rice, applesauce, toast) diet is outdated.
- Antidiarrheal compounds are not indicated.
- See Table 11-2 for antibiotic treatment of identified enteropathogens.

PREVENTION

- Hospitalized patients should be placed under contact precautions.
- Education.
- Exclude infected children from child-care centers.
- Report cases of bacterial diarrhea to the local health department.

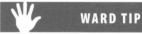 **WARD TIP**

Treatment of *E. coli* O157:H7 with antibiotics is associated with a higher incidence of hemolytic uremic syndrome.

Intestinal Worms

See Table 11-3 for common intestinal-worm infestations.

Abdominal Hernias

UMBILICAL

DEFINITION

- Occurs because of an incomplete closure of the umbilical ring.
- Common in low-birth weight, premature, and African-American infants.
- Soft swelling covered by skin that protrudes while crying, straining, or coughing.
- Usually 1–5 cm.

 EXAM TIP

The most frequent symptom of infestation with *Enterobius vermicularis* is perineal pruritus. Infection can be diagnosed with placing transparent adhesive tape to the perianal area overnight or first thing in the morning and then reviewing the tape under a microscope for eggs or worms.

TABLE 11-3. Common Intestinal Worms

Intestinal Nematodes	Mode of Transmission	Disease, Symptoms and Signs	Treatment
Enterobius vermicularis (pinworm)	Hand to mouth	Perianal itching, especially at night	Albendazole, mebendazole or pyrantel pamoate
Trichuris trichiura (whipworm)	Fecal-oral	■ Usually asymptomatic ■ Mild anemia ■ Abdominal pain ■ Diarrhea, tenesmus ■ Perianal itching	Albendazole or mebendazole
Ascaris lumbricoides	Fecal-oral	■ Pneumonia ■ Loeffler pneumonitis ■ Intestinal infection/obstruction ■ Liver failure	Albendazole or mebendazole
Necator americanus (New World hookworm) and *Ancylostoma duodenale* (Old World hookworm)	Skin penetration	■ Intense dermatitis ■ Loeffler pneumonitis ■ Significant anemia ■ GI symptoms ■ Developmental delay in children (irreversible)	Albendazole or mebendazole
Strongyloides stercoralis	Skin penetration	Same as for Necator, plus: ■ Diarrhea × 3–6 weeks ■ Superimposed bacterial sepsis	Ivermectin
Trichinella spiralis	Infected pork	Trichinosis ■ Myalgias ■ Facial and periorbital edema ■ Conjunctivitis ■ Pneumonia, myocarditis, encephalitis, nephritis, meningitis	Albendazole + prednisone

(Adapted, with permission, from Stead L. BRS Emergency Medicine. Lippincott Williams & Wilkins, 2000.)

TREATMENT

- Most disappear spontaneously by 1 year of age.
- Incarceration and strangulation rare.
- "Strapping" with coin or "belly band" ineffective.
- Surgery if symptomatic, incarcerated, strangulated, or grows larger after age 1 or 2.

EXAM TIP

In an inguinal hernia, the processus vaginalis herniates through the abdominal wall with hydrocele into the canal.

INGUINAL

DEFINITION

- Three types: indirect (99%), direct (0.5%), femoral (<0.5%).
- Embryology for indirect: patent processus vaginalis.
- Common, especially in preterm infants.

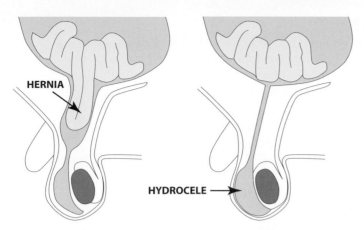

FIGURE 11-7. **Inguinal hernia (slippage of bowel through inguinal ring) vs. hydrocele (collection of fluid in scrotum adjacent to testes).**

- Males > females 8–10:1.
- Sixty percent right (delayed descent of the right testicle), 30% left, 10% bilateral.
- Increased incidence with positive family history.

SIGNS AND SYMPTOMS

- Infant with scrotal/inguinal bulge on straining or crying.
- Perform careful exam to distinguish from hydrocele (see Figure 11-7).

TREATMENT

- Elective surgery unless incarcerated.
- Avoid trusses or supports.
- Contralateral exploration for unilateral hernia not indicated.
- Prognosis excellent unless incarcerated.
- Therapy for incarceration—sedation and manipulation to reduce; immediate operation if not reduced; repair 24 to 48 hours if reduced.

 WARD TIP

An inguinal hernia increases with straining; a hydrocele remains unchanged.

Omphalocele

DEFINITION

- Failure of the lateral embryonic folds at the umbilical ring to fuse (Figure 11-8).
- Associated with other anomalies (heart, kidneys, limbs, face) in about 60% of cases.
- Found with trisomies 13, 14, 15, 18, and 21 and Beckwith-Wiedemann syndrome.

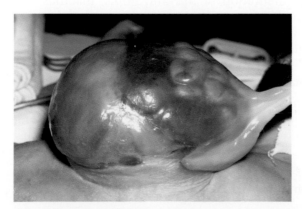

FIGURE 11-8. **An omphalocele results from a midline abdominal wall defect that allows herniation of abdominal contents into the base of the umbilical cord. The membrane consists of peritoneum, amnion, and Wharton's jelly.** (Reproduced, with permission, from Craig W. Lillehei, MD.)

SIGNS AND SYMPTOMS

- Extruded abdominal organs covered by a thin membrane.
- Elevated maternal α-fetoprotein.
- Normal acetyl-cholinesterase level in amniotic fluid.
- Prenatal ultrasound shows defect.

TREATMENT

- Evaluation for other congenital anomalies.
- Small lesions surgically closed primarily; larger lesions require staged approach.

Gastroschisis

DEFINITION

- Abdominal wall defect with protruding intestinal contents without an overlying protective membrane.

SIGNS AND SYMPTOMS

- Elevated maternal α-fetoprotein and amniotic acetyl-cholinesterase levels.
- Prenatal ultrasound shows defect.

TREATMENT

- Maintain temperature and fluid balance (high losses from exposed viscera).
- Surgical closure.

Peutz-Jeghers Syndrome

 A 15-year-old girl with spots on her lips has crampy abdominal pain associated with bleeding. *Think: Peutz-Jeghers syndrome.*

Peutz-Jeghers syndrome is the presence of multiple GI hamartomatous polyps and mucocutaneous hyperpigmentation. These patients have an elevated risk of intestinal and extraintestinal malignancies.

DEFINITION

- Mucosal pigmentation of lips and gums, macules on the hands and feet, and hamartomas most commonly of stomach, small intestine, and colon.
- High malignant potential.

SIGNS AND SYMPTOMS

- Deeply pigmented macules on lips and buccal mucosa at birth.
- Blue-black macules on the hands and feet; lesions may fade.
- Bleeding, crampy abdominal pain, and intussusception.

DIAGNOSIS

Genetic and family studies may reveal history.

TREATMENT

Excise intestinal lesions if they are significantly symptomatic.

Gardner Syndrome

DEFINITION

Multiple intestinal polyps, tumors of soft tissue and bone (especially mandible).

SIGNS AND SYMPTOMS

- Colonic polyps (usually early adulthood) with high malignant potential.
- Dental abnormalities.
- Pigmented lesions in ocular fundus.
- Colonic polyps (usually early adulthood) with high malignant potential.

DIAGNOSIS

- Autosomal dominant; genetic counseling.
- Colon surveillance in at-risk children.

TREATMENT

Aggressive surgical removal of polyps.

Carcinoid Tumors

DEFINITION

Tumors of enterochromaffin cells in intestine—usually appendix.

SIGNS AND SYMPTOMS

- May cause appendicitis.
- If metastasis to liver, may cause carcinoid syndrome (increased serotonin, vasomotor disturbances, cramping, or bronchoconstriction).

DIAGNOSIS

- Incidental finding at appendectomy.
- Elevated urinary 5-hydroxyindoloacetic acid (5-HIAA).

TREATMENT

Surgical excision.

Familial Adenomatous Polyposis

DEFINITION/ETIOLOGY

- Autosomal dominant (strong family history).
- Large number of adenomatous lesions, especially in colon.
- Secondary to germ-line mutations in adenopolyposis coli (APC) gene.
- High malignant potential.

SIGNS AND SYMPTOMS

- May see hematochezia, cramps, or diarrhea.
- Extracolonic manifestations (osteoma, thyroid cancer) possible.

DIAGNOSIS

- Routine colonoscopy with biopsy.

TREATMENT

Surgical resection of affected colonic mucosa.

Juvenile Polyposis Syndrome

DEFINITION/ETIOLOGY

- Polyps in the large and small intestine, and stomach.
- Autosomal dominant.
- Presents in the first decade of life.
- Increased risk of malignancy, especially colorectal.

SIGNS AND SYMPTOMS

- Bright-red painless bleeding with bowel movement.
- Iron deficiency anemia.
- Intussusception.

DIAGNOSIS

- Esophagogastroduodenoscopy.

TREATMENT

Surgical removal of polyp.

Malabsorption

SHORT BOWEL SYNDROME

DEFINITION/ETIOLOGY

- Occurs with loss of at least 50% of small bowel (with or without loss of large bowel).
- Decreased absorptive surface and bowel function.
- May be congenital (malrotation, atresia, etc.).
- Most commonly secondary to surgical resection.

SIGNS AND SYMPTOMS

- Malabsorption and diarrhea.
- Steatorrhea (fatty stools): voluminous foul-smelling stools that float.
- Dehydration.
- Hyponatremia, hypokalemia.
- Acidosis (secondary to loss of bicarbonate).

TREATMENT

- Total parenteral nutrition (TPN).
- Bowel rehabilitation with hydrolyzed protein and medium chain triglyceride-enriched feeds.
- Metronidazole empirically to treat bacterial overgrowth.

CELIAC DISEASE

 A 5-year-old girl presents with a protuberant abdomen and wasted extremities. *Think: Gluten-induced enteropathy.*

Celiac disease is an autoimmune disorder that primarily affects the small intestine. Gluten is the single major factor that triggers celiac disease. *Gluten-containing foods include* rye, wheat, and barley. The common presentation is diarrhea, borborygmus, abdominal pain, and weight loss. *Serologic marker:* Serum immunoglobulin A (IgA) endomysial antibodies and IgA tissue transglutaminase (tTG) antibodies.

DEFINITION/ETIOLOGY

- Sensitivity to gluten in diet.
- Classically described to be recognized in first 2 years of life.
- Increasingly recognized in teens and young adults.
- Gluten exposure in the genetically predisposed patient.
- Associated with HLA-DQ2.

SIGNS AND SYMPTOMS

- Diarrhea and vomiting leading to muscle wasting and failure to thrive.
- Abdominal distention.
- Large bulky stools.
- Delayed puberty.
- CNS changes including behavioral changes, epilepsy, and dementia.
- Anemia, thrombocytopenia.
- Osteopenia.

DIAGNOSIS

- Characteristic biopsy findings and symptom resolution with gluten-free diet.
- Anti-endomysial and anti-tissue transglutaminase antibodies.

TREATMENT

- Dietary restriction of gluten (must avoid barley, ryes, and wheat).

TROPICAL SPRUE

DEFINITION

- Generalized malabsorption associated with diffuse small-bowel mucosal lesions.
- Seen in people who live or have traveled to certain tropical regions.

SIGNS AND SYMPTOMS

- Fever, malaise, and watery diarrhea, acutely.
- After about a week, chronic malabsorption and signs of malnutrition occur, including night blindness, glossitis, stomatitis, cheilosis, and muscle wasting.

DIAGNOSIS

Small-bowel biopsy shows villous flattening, crypt hyperplasia, and chronic inflammatory cells in lamina propria.

TREATMENT

- Doxycycline or sulfamethoxazole/trimethoprim.
- Folate and vitamin B_{12} supplementation for 6 months.

LACTASE DEFICIENCY

DEFINITION

Decreased or absent lactase in the intestinal brush border.

ETIOLOGY

- Congenital absence rare.
- Commonly develops upon weaning in most mammals.
- Autosomal recessive.
- Affects about 85% of Black Americans.
- Can be transient secondary to diffuse mucosal disease (i.e., post-viral gastroenteritis).

SIGNS AND SYMPTOMS

- Seen in response to lactose ingestion.
- Watery diarrhea, abdominal distention, borborygmi, and flatulence.
- Recurrent, vague abdominal pain.

DIAGNOSIS

- H_2 breath test.
- Lactose elimination from diet.

TREATMENT

- Eliminate milk from diet.
- Oral lactase supplement (Lactaid) or lactose-free milk.

Cholecystitis

DEFINITION

- Inflammation of the gall bladder.
- Most commonly caused by stone (calculous cholecystitis).
- Acalculous cholecystitis is seen with systemic disease (parasites, gram-negative enteritis, hemolytic uremic syndrome, Kawasaki disease, cystic fibrosis).

SIGNS AND SYMPTOMS

- Right upper-quadrant pain with Murphy sign (pain with inspiration).
- Nausea and vomiting.
- Jaundice.
- Fever.

DIAGNOSIS

- Elevated white count.
- Elevated aminotransferases and GGT.
- Ultrasound findings of sludge or stones in the gall bladder.

TREATMENT

- Pain control.
- Maintain hydration status.
- Antibiotics if sepsis suspected.
- Definitive therapy is open or laparoscopic cholecystectomy.

Acute Pancreatitis

DEFINITION

- After an inciting event, an autodigestive process of pancreatic damage ensues.
- It may be related to trauma, systemic disease, medications, stones, or idiopathic reasons.

SIGNS AND SYMPTOMS

- Severe abdominal pain.
- Nausea and vomiting.
- Abdominal pain and guarding.

DIAGNOSIS

- Elevated serum lipase.
- Ultrasound (increased size, dilated ducts, cysts).
- Endoscopic retrograde cholangiopancreatography (ERCP) or magnetic resonance cholangiopancreatography (MRCP), if surgery is contemplated.

TREATMENT

- Hydration and pain control.
- Slow introduction of food when emesis resolves.
- Occasionally radiologic or surgical drainage of cysts or abscesses.

Indirect Hyperbilirubinemia

Neonatal Hyperbilirubinemia: See Gestation and Birth chapter.

GILBERT SYNDROME

Common, benign condition of unconjugated hyperbilirubinemia, often presenting after puberty, resulting in mild jaundice with stress or illness. No treatment is required.

CRIGLER-NAJJAR I SYNDROME

DEFINITION

- Rare autosomal recessive condition due to glucuronyl-transferase gene mutation resulting in the absence of the enzyme uridine diphosphate glycosyltransferase.
- Parents of affected children have partial defects but normal serum bilirubin.

SIGNS AND SYMPTOMS

- In homozygous infants, unconjugated hyperbilirubinemia in first three days of life.
- Kernicterus common in early neonatal period.
- Stools pale yellow.
- Indirect bilirubinemia >20 mg/dL after first week of life in absence of hemolysis suggests this syndrome.

DIAGNOSIS

- Early age of onset and extreme level of bilirubin without hemolysis.
- Definitive diagnosis: liver biopsy with glucuronyl-transferase activity measurement.
- DNA diagnosis available.

TREATMENT

- Maintain serum bilirubin <20 mg/dL for first 2–4 weeks of life.
- Repeated exchange transfusion.
- Phototherapy.
- Treat intercurrent infections.
- Hepatic transplant.

WARD TIP

- Indirect hyperbilirubinemia, reticulosis, and red cell destruction suggest hemolysis.
- Direct hyperbilirubinemia may indicate hepatitis, cholestasis, inborn errors of metabolism, cystic fibrosis, or sepsis.
- If reticulocyte count, Coombs', and direct bilirubin are normal, then physiologic or pathologic indirect hyperbilirubinemia is suggested.

EXAM TIP

Children with cholestatic hepatic disease require replacement of vitamins A, D, E, and K (fat soluble).

CRIGLER-NAJJAR II SYNDROME

DEFINITION

- Autosomal recessive condition due to glucuronyl-transferase gene mutation resulting in reduced enzyme uridine-diphosphate glycosyltransferase activity.

SIGNS AND SYMPTOMS

- Unconjugated hyperbilirubinemia in first three days of life.
- Concentration remains high after third week of life.
- Kernicterus unusual.
- Stool normal.
- Infants asymptomatic.

DIAGNOSIS

- Decrease in bilirubin upon administration of phenobarbital (induces enzyme activity).

TREATMENT

Phenobarbital

Direct Hyperbilirubinemia

ALAGILLE SYNDROME

DEFINITION

- Cholestasis due to absence or reduction in number of bile ducts.

SIGNS AND SYMPTOMS

- Unusual facies (broad forehead, wide-set eyes, underdeveloped mandible).
- Ocular abnormalities.
- Cardiovascular abnormalities (peripheral pulmonic stenosis).
- Tubulointerstitial nephropathy.
- Vertebral defect (butterfly vertebrae).

PROGNOSIS

Long-term survival can be good, but pruritis, xanthomas, hypercholesterolemia, and neurologic complications may occur, possibly requiring transplantation.

EXTRAHEPATIC BILIARY ATRESIA

DEFINITION

Noncystic obliterative cholangiopathy.

EPIDEMIOLOGY

- Most common, non-syndromic form (85%): obliteration of entire extrahepatic biliary tree at/above porta.
- Occurs in 1 in 10,000 to 1 in 15,000 live births.

SIGNS AND SYMPTOMS

- Prolonged neonatal jaundice.
- Acholic stools (very light, almost beige in color).
- Syndromic form: increased incidence of polysplenia syndrome (heterotaxia, malrotation, levocardia, and intra-abdominal vascular anomalies).

DIAGNOSIS

- Elevated conjugated bilirubin, GGT, alkaline phosphatase, and aminotransferase levels.
- Ultrasound demonstrating lack of gall bladder.
- Hepatobiliary scintigraphy with phenobarbital priming (less common).
- Liver biopsy is gold standard.

TREATMENT

- Kasai hepatoportoenterostomy, ideally less than 45 days of age.
- Liver transplant.

CHOLEDOCHAL CYSTS

DEFINITION

- Congenital cystic bile duct dilation causing obstruction and possible liver cirrhosis.

EPIDEMIOLOGY

- Four times more common in girls and in Asians.
- About 75% present in childhood.

SIGNS AND SYMPTOMS

- Jaundice in infants.
- In an older child, the classic triad is abdominal pain, jaundice, and abdominal mass.

DIAGNOSIS

- Ultrasound.

TREATMENT

- Surgical repair.

DUBIN JOHNSON SYNDROME

DEFINITION

- Autosomal recessive condition whereby conjugated bilirubin fails to be moved from the liver into the bile and stool.

EPIDEMIOLOGY

- Increased incidence in Iranian, Iraqi, and Moroccan Jews.

SIGNS AND SYMPTOMS

- Intermittent jaundice.
- Dark urine.
- Occasionally fatigue and fever.
- Black liver.

DIAGNOSIS

- Direct hyperbilirubinemia.
- Normal liver-function tests.
- HIDA scan fails to demonstrate gall bladder.
- Normal total urinary coproporphyrin levels, but elevated isomer 1.

TREATMENT

- None; caution when administering liver-metabolized medications.

ROTOR SYNDROME

DEFINITION

- Autosomal recessive condition of impaired storage of conjugated bilirubin in the liver.

SIGNS AND SYMPTOMS

- Intermittent jaundice.
- Dark urine.
- Normal color of liver cells.

DIAGNOSIS

- Direct hyperbilirubinemia.
- Normal or slightly elevated liver function tests.
- HIDA scan demonstrates gall bladder.
- Elevated total urinary coproporphyrin levels.

TREATMENT

- None; caution when administering liver-metabolized medications.

Hepatitis

- Major problem worldwide.
- Six known viruses cause hepatitis as their primary manifestation—A (HAV), B (HBV), C (HCV), D (HDV), E (HEV), and G (HGV).
- Other viruses cause hepatitis as part of their clinical spectrum—herpes simplex virus, cytomegalovirus, Epstein-Barr virus, rubella, enteroviruses, and parvovirus.
- HBV is a DNA virus; HAV, HCV, HDV, HEV, and HGV are RNA viruses.
- HAV and HEV are not known to cause chronic illness; HBV, HCV, and HDV cause morbidity and mortality through chronic infection.
- HAV causes most cases of hepatitis in children.
- HBV causes one-third of all cases; HCV is found in 20%.

HEPATITIS A

DEFINITION

- RNA-containing member of the Picornavirus family.
- Found mostly in developing countries.
- Causes acute hepatitis only.
- Increased risk in child-care centers, contaminated food or water, or travel to endemic areas.
- Asymptomatic cases common, especially in children.
- Transmission by person-to-person contact; spread by fecal-oral route.
- Mean incubation four weeks (15–50 days).

SIGNS AND SYMPTOMS

- Abrupt onset with fever, malaise, nausea, emesis, anorexia, and abdominal discomfort.
- Diarrhea common.

- Almost all recover but may have relapsing course over several months.
- Jaundice, although often anicteric, especially in children.

DIAGNOSIS

- Jaundice history in family contacts, child-care playmates, or travel to endemic region.
- Increased liver-function studies.
- Serologic criteria:
  - Immunoglobulin M (IgM) anti-HAV at illness onset, disappearing by 4–6 months; IgG is detectable by about 2 months.

TREATMENT

- Supportive.
- Intramuscular immunoglobulin prophylaxis in select cases.

PREVENTION

- Careful hand washing.
- Vaccines available.

HEPATITIS B

DEFINITION

- DNA virus from the Hepadnaviridae family.
- Infant risk factor is perinatal exposure to hepatitis B surface antigen (HBsAg)-positive mother.

SIGNS AND SYMPTOMS

- Many cases in children who are asymptomatic.
- Increased ALT prior to lethargy, anorexia, and malaise (6–7 weeks post exposure).
- May be preceded by arthralgias or skin lesions (Gianotti-Crosti syndrome).
- May see extrahepatic conditions, polyarteritis, glomerulonephritis, aplastic anemia.
- Jaundice.

DIAGNOSIS

- HBsAg (all infected persons, increased levels when symptomatic) and hepatitis B core antigen (HBcAg) (present during acute, highly infectious phase).
- HBsAg falls prior to symptom resolution; IgM Ab to HBcAg increases early after infectivity persisting for months before replacement by IgG Ab to HBcAg.
- HBcAg presents as early as HBsAg; it is present when HBsAg disappears.
- Only anti-HBsAg is detected in persons receiving hepatitis B vaccine; anti-HBsAb and anti-HBcAg are seen with resolved infection.
- HBeAg is present in acute and chronic infection; it is a marker for infectivity.

PREVENTION

- Screening blood donors.
- Screening pregnant women and treatment with HBIG and vaccination within 12 hours of life for all infants born to positive mothers (prevents vertical transmission).
- Routine vaccination of children in the first year of life.

EXAM TIP

Chronic hepatitis B is a risk factor for hepatocellular carcinoma. Vaccination prior to infection can eliminate this risk.

TREATMENT

- Interferon-α, lamivudine, adefovir, entecavir, and tenofovir are approved treatments in children, depending on their age.
- Liver transplant is the treatment for patients with end-stage HBV.

HEPATITIS C

DEFINITION

- Single-stranded RNA virus.
- Perinatal transmission rare except with high-titer HCV.
- High-risk behavior, including shared needles, including tattoos.

SIGNS AND SYMPTOMS

- Acute infection similar to other hepatitis viruses.
- After 20–30 years, 25% progress to cirrhosis, liver failure, or primary hepatocellular carcinoma.
- May see cryoglobulinemia (rare in children), vasculitides, and peripheral neuropathy.

DIAGNOSIS

- Increased ALT.
- Detection of antibodies to HCV.
- Polymerase chain reaction (PCR) for viral RNA detection.
- Confirmed by liver biopsy prior to starting treatment or unclear diagnosis.

PREVENTION

- Screening blood donors and avoidance of high-risk behaviors.
- No vaccine currently available.

TREATMENT

- Treat to prevent progression to future complications.
- Sofosbuvir/velpatasvir, glecaprevir/pibrentasvir, or sofosbuvir plus ribavirin, depending on the age of the patient and the genotype of the infection.

HEPATITIS D (DELTA AGENT)

DEFINITION

- Cannot produce infection without HBV infection
  - Coinfection at the same time as HBV infection.
  - Infection in someone with HBV (superinfection).
- Transmission by intimate contact.

SIGNS AND SYMPTOMS

- Similar to, but more severe than, other hepatitis viruses.
- In coinfection, acute hepatitis is more severe, risk of developing chronic hepatitis is low; in superinfection, acute illness is uncommon, but the risk of fulminant hepatitis is highest.

DIAGNOSIS

Detect IgM antibody to HDV (2–4 weeks after coinfection, 10 weeks after superinfection).

PREVENTION

No vaccine for hepatitis D

TREATMENT

No specific treatment for HDV, rather control and treatment of concurrent HBV.

AUTOIMMUNE (CHRONIC) HEPATITIS

DEFINITION

- Hepatic inflammatory process manifested by increased serum aminotransferase and liver-associated autoantibodies.
- Variable severity.
- Clinical constellation that suggests immune-mediated disease process responsive to immunosuppressive treatment.

SIGNS AND SYMPTOMS

- Variable.
- May mimic acute viral hepatitis.
- Onset frequently insidious.
- May be asymptomatic or may have fatigue, malaise, anorexia, or amenorrhea.
- Extrahepatic signs, including splenomegaly, arthritis, vasculitis, and nephritis.
- Mild to moderate jaundice.

DIAGNOSIS

- Mild elevation of bilirubin and transaminase common.
- Detection of autoantibodies (anti-smooth muscle, anti-liver-kidney-microsome, anti-soluble live antigen).
- Liver biopsy.
- Exclude other disease, such as viral hepatitis, drugs, and alcohol.

TREATMENT

- Corticosteroid.
- Azathioprine.
- 6-mercaptopurine.

Reye Syndrome

DEFINITION

- Acute encephalopathy and liver dysfunction.
- No other explanation for cerebral edema or hepatic abnormality.
- Decreased incidence in part due to reduced aspirin use for viral infections.
- Many other "Reye-like" syndromes exist (medium-chain fatty-acid oxidation defect or urea-cycle defects).

SIGNS AND SYMPTOMS

- Stereotypic, biphasic course.
- Usually seen after prodromal illness (classically influenza or varicella), followed by a 3–5 day period of recovery, then abrupt onset of progressive hepatic failure and encephalopathy.
- First neurologic manifestations: vomiting and lethargy.
- Neurologic symptoms including seizures, coma, or death.

DIAGNOSIS

- Elevated liver transaminases, hypoglycemia, hyperammonemia, prolonged INR, normal bilirubin level.
- Liver biopsy may show microvesicular steatosis.

TREATMENT

- Airway, breathing, circulation (ABC).
- Maintain glucose homeostasis.
- Control intracranial pressure (ICP) secondary to cerebral edema.
- Supportive management depending on clinical stage.

α_1-Antitrypsin Deficiency

DEFINITION

- α_1-Antitrypsin is a major protease inhibitor (PI).
- A small number of homozygous patients have neonatal cholestasis, and later cirrhosis.
- PiZZ phenotype causes clinical deficiency (<20% develop neonatal cholestasis).

EXAM TIP

The most likely clinical manifestation of α_1-antitrypsin deficiency in the newborn is jaundice (neonatal cholestasis).

SIGNS AND SYMPTOMS

- Jaundice, acholic stools, and hepatomegaly may occur in the first week of life; jaundice clears by the second to fourth month.
- Patient may have complete resolution, persistent liver disease, or cirrhosis.
- Older children may present with chronic liver disease.
- Emphysema is typically not seen in children.

DIAGNOSIS

- Determination of phenotype by serum α_1-antitrypsin level.
- Confirmed by liver biopsy.

TREATMENT

- Liver transplant curative.

Wilson Disease

DEFINITION

- Autosomal-recessive disease of excessive copper deposition in brain and liver.

SIGNS AND SYMPTOMS

- Asymptomatic in early stages.
- Jaundice, abdominal pain.
- Hepatomegaly, subacute/chronic hepatitis, or fulminant liver failure.
- Portal hypertension, ascites, edema, esophageal bleeding.
- Delayed puberty, amenorrhea, hemolytic anemia, or coagulation defect.
- Psychosis.
- Tremors.
- Kayser-Fleischer rings associated with Wilson disease:
    - Greenish-brown rings of pigment seen at the limbus of the cornea.
    - May not be present in younger children.
    - May require slit lamp in patients, especially in patients with dark eyes.
    - About 90% of Wilson Disease patients with neurologic involvement have Kayser-Fleischer rings.

DIAGNOSIS

Copper indices reveal:

- Low serum ceruloplasmin.
- High serum and urine copper level.
- Liver biopsy for histochemistry and copper quantification.
- Genetic testing, including siblings.

TREATMENT

- Disease is always fatal if left untreated.
- Restrict copper intake. Myriad foods are high in copper content; a consultation with the dietician is required.
- Copper-chelating agents to decrease deposition (e.g., penicillamine, trientine).
- Zinc: blocks copper absorption in GI tract.
- Patients with hepatic failure require liver transplant.

Hepatic Neoplasms (see Chapter 16 [oncology])

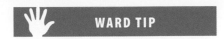

 WARD TIP

Consider ordering serum ceruloplasmin for any patient with an unexplained elevation of liver function tests (LFTs), neurologic symptoms, behavior changes, and psychiatric illness.

Amebic Liver Abscesses

DEFINITION

A serious manifestation of disseminated *Entamoeba histolytica* infection.

SIGNS AND SYMPTOMS

- A history of dysentery may be helpful.
- Abdominal pain, distention, and liver enlargement with tenderness are present.

DIAGNOSIS

- Leukocytosis.
- Increased ESR.
- Nonspecific ALT elevations.
- Stool exam may reveal trophozoites or cysts.
- Serologic testing for antibody.
- CT or MRI.

TREATMENT

- Metronidazole followed by paromomycin or iodoquinol.
- Aspiration of abscesses if rupture is imminent.

NOTES

Respiratory Disease

EXAM TIP

Infants and young children have smaller airways, proportionally larger tongues, a floppy epiglottis, and a higher and more anterior larynx leading to more acute respiratory illnesses.

WARD TIP

Respiratory arrest is the most common cause of cardiac arrest in children.

WARD TIP

- **Stertor** is a low-pitched sound like nasal congestion experienced with a cold or the sound made with snoring.
- **Stridor** is a higher-pitched noise that occurs with obstruction in the extra-thoracic airway.
- **Wheezing** is a high-pitched noise that occurs during expiration due to narrowing, spasm, or obstruction of the smaller airways in the lungs.

EXAM TIP

- Inspiratory stridor suggests a laryngeal obstruction.
- Expiratory stridor suggests tracheo-bronchial obstruction.
- Biphasic stridor suggests a subglottic or glottic anomaly.

Respiratory Disease in Children

- Pediatric respiratory disorders are responsible for acute and chronic health conditions, and they are a leading cause of emergency room visits and hospitalizations.
- Anatomic and physiologic differences in children versus adults predispose pediatric patients to more severe presentations.

Signs and Symptoms of Respiratory Distress

- Tachypnea (see Table 12-1 for normal respiratory rates by age).
- Intercostal retractions.
- Nasal flaring (indicates increased effort is needed to breathe).
- Use of accessory muscles for breathing (e.g., abdominals, sternocleidomastoids).
- Restlessness, agitation.
- Somnolence or lethargy, which may be due to severe hypoxia or hypercarbia.
- Pallor, cyanosis.
- Wheezing.
- Stridor, an inspiratory and/or expiratory sound that localizes respiratory distress to the upper airway.
- Grunting, a form of auto-PEEP (positive end expiratory pressure).
  - Due to exhalation against a partially closed glottis.
  - Occurs during expiration.

Upper Respiratory Infection (the Common Cold)

 A 7-year-old girl is well when she leaves for school but arrives home afterward with a sore throat and runny nose. She is also coughing and sneezing. *Think: Rhinovirus.* Rhinovirus colds frequently start as a sore or "scratchy" throat with a runny nose.

 A 17-year-old male has acute onset of fever, cough, conjunctivitis, and pharyngitis. *Think: Adenovirus.* Characteristic presentation: pharyngitis, rhinitis, and conjunctivitis (also known as pharyngoconjunctival fever).

DEFINITION

This multi-etiology illness has symptoms including cough, congestion, and rhinorrhea. Upper respiratory infections (URIs) are the most common pediatric ED presentation.

TABLE 12-1. **Normal Respiratory Rates in Children**

AGE	Birth–6 Weeks	6 Weeks–2 Years	2–6 Years	6–10 Years	Over 10 Years
RESPIRATORY RATE	45–60/min	22–37/min	20–30/min	18–25/min	12–20/min

ETIOLOGY

- >200 viruses—especially rhinoviruses (30–50%), coronavirus (10–15%), influenza (5–15%), parainfluenza, respiratory syncytial virus (RSV), adenovirus, metapneumovirus.
- Risk factors: child-care facilities, smoking, passive exposure to smoke, low income, crowding, and psychological stress.

EPIDEMIOLOGY

- Most frequent illness of childhood (three to eight episodes per year).
- Most common medical reason to miss school.
- Typically occurs in fall and winter.

SIGNS AND SYMPTOMS

- Nasal and throat irritation.
- Sneezing, nasal congestion, rhinorrhea.
- Sore throat, postnasal drip.
- Low-grade fever, headache, malaise, and myalgia.
- Possible complications, including otitis media, sinusitis; may trigger asthma.
- Infants have a variable presentation: congestion causes feeding and sleeping difficulties, vomiting may occur after coughing, and diarrhea may occur.

TREATMENT

- Supportive treatment includes oral hydration, humidified air, and topical nasal saline drops.
- Avoid aspirin and over-the-counter (OTC) cough suppressants or decongestants.
  - OTC medications lack documented efficacy.

Influenza

DEFINITION

This is a viral respiratory illness.

ETIOLOGY

- Influenza A and B—with varying epidemics associated with certain subtypes (e.g., H1N1).
- Influenza C—sporadic.

EPIDEMIOLOGY

Influenza is common over the winter months.

SIGNS AND SYMPTOMS

- Incubation period: 1–3 days.
- Sudden onset of fever, frequently with chills, headache, malaise, diffuse myalgia, and nonproductive cough.
- Pharyngitis; occasionally conjunctivitis (more common with H7 subtype).
- Typical duration of febrile illness: 2–4 days.
- Complications include otitis media, pneumonia, myositis, and myocarditis.
- Diarrhea and vomiting.

WARD TIP

Mucopurulent rhinitis may accompany a common cold and does not necessarily indicate sinusitis; it is not by itself an indication for antibiotics.

WARD TIP

The best treatment for the common cold is to increase oral fluids, *not* pharmacologic treatment.

WARD TIP

Infants typically breathe through their nose; the common cold can trigger respiratory distress in the young infant due to mucous obstruction of the nares. Judicious use of nasal saline drops and suctioning is important to relieve the obstruction.

WARD TIP

Avoid aspirin in young children due to the theoretical risk of Reye syndrome.

WARD TIP

Diagnosis of influenza depends on epidemiologic and clinical considerations.

WARD TIP

There is an increased risk for bacterial superinfection; most common organisms are *Staphylococcus aureus* and *Streptococcus pneumoniae*.

WARD TIP

Influenza can be severe in children with congenital heart disease, bronchopulmonary dysplasia (BPD), asthma, cystic fibrosis, and neuromuscular disease; if influenza vaccination is contraindicated, these high-risk patients would be candidates for influenza postexposure prophylaxis.

EXAM TIP

Initial treatment should begin as soon as possible (ideally within 48 hours of illness onset) with a single neuraminidase inhibitor such as oral oseltamivir or inhaled zanamivir; intravenous peramivir and oral baloxavir are alternatives.

DIAGNOSIS

- Nasal swab or nasal washing.
- During an epidemic, clinical signs can be used to reduce test costs.

TREATMENT

- Symptomatic treatment for healthy children—fluids, rest, acetaminophen, or ibuprofen.
- For children at risk, see Table 12-2 for drug options.
- Pregnant patients with H1N1 should receive a 5-day course of antiviral treatment.
- Oseltamivir is preferred during pregnancy.

VACCINE

Intramuscular (IIV)

- Vaccination is recommended for children >6 months, with priority to high-risk groups during vaccine shortage.
- High-risk groups include children with chronic diseases such as asthma, renal disease, diabetes, and other forms of immunosuppression.
- The best time to administer is mid-September to mid-November since the peak of the flu season is late December to early March.
- Antibodies take up to 6 weeks to develop in children. Consider prophylaxis in high-risk children during this period.
- Mutations gradually occur to the hemagglutinin (HA) and neuraminidase (NA) surface proteins (antigenic drift). The vaccine is modified annually

TABLE 12-2. Drug Treatments for Influenza

	INDICATIONS	AGE GROUPS	RX DOSE	ADVERSE EFFECTS
Baloxavir oral	For types A and B Treatment and prophylaxis	≥ 12 years (post-exposure)	<80kg 40mg × 1 >80kg 80mg × 1 For Px, same dosing	None more common than placebo

Oseltamivir oral	For types A and B
	Treatment and prophylaxis
		Tx: any age
		Px: ≥3 months
			<1yo 3mg/kg BID × 5 days
			>1yo:
			  <15kg 30mg BID
			  15–23kg 45mg BID × 5d
			  23–40kg 60mg BID × 5d
			  >40kg 75mg BID × 5d
			For Px, same above dose
			once a day for 7 days
				Nausea, vomiting, diarrhea, abdominal pain, bronchitis, dizziness, headache

Peramivir IV	For Type A and B Treatment only	Tx: age >2 years	12mg/kg up to max of 600 mg IV × 1 dose given over 15 minutes	Diarrhea, skin reactions, transient neuropsychiatric disorders
Zanamivir inhaled	For types A and B Treatment and prophylaxis	Tx: ≥7years Px: ≥5 years Not for use in patients with underlying respiratory disease	Tx: two inhalations (10 mg) bid × 5 days Px: two inhalations (10 mg) once daily × 5 days	Bronchospasm in patients with asthma; sinusitis, dizziness, skin reactions, transient neuropsychiatric events

Px, prophylaxis; Tx, treatment.

to accommodate these mutations; thus, the vaccine needs to be administered every year.

- IIV uses a killed virus and therefore cannot cause the flu.
- This vaccines is not approved for children <6 months of age.
- Recombinant vaccine (RIV) is available, but it is not approved for children.

Intranasal

- Live, attenuated vaccine (LAIV) is available for children ≥2 years old.
- It was not recommended for the 2016 and 2017 flu seasons due to concerns regarding efficacy.
- The Advisory Committee on Immunization Practices (ACIP) has now recommended a reformulated version.
- It is contraindicated in patients with anaphylaxis to egg protein or concomitant aspirin therapy.
- Use with caution in patients with wheezing.

Parainfluenza

Etiology

- Type 1 and 2—seasonal, less common
- Type 3—endemic, more prevalent
- See Table 12-3.

Pathogenesis

- It infects epithelial cells of the nose and oropharynx first.
- Parainfluenza moves distally to ciliated/alveolar cells of large and small airway epithelium.

Signs and Symptoms

- Incubation period: 2–6 days.
- Can be severe in immunocompromised patients.

Treatment

Specific antiviral therapy is not available.

EXAM TIP

Parainfluenza is a paramyxovirus.

WARD TIP

Parainfluenza types 1 (more common) and 2 cause croup; types 3 and 4 cause bronchiolitis, pneumonia, and upper respiratory tract infections.

TABLE 12-3. Respiratory Infections and Pathogens

RESPIRATORY INFECTION	MOST COMMON PATHOGEN	PARTICULAR SIGNS AND SYMPTOMS
Croup	Parainfluenza virus	Barking cough, steeple sign
Epiglottitis	*H. influenzae* type B	Tripod position, thumb sign
Tracheitis	*S. aureus, H. influenzae* type B	Rapidly progressive, biphasic stridor
Bronchiolitis	Respiratory syncytial virus	Paroxysmal wheezing
Bronchitis	Viral	Productive cough
Pharyngitis	Viral, group A strep	Sore throat, tonsillar involvement
Bacterial pneumonia	*S. pneumoniae*	Productive cough, lobar consolidation
Pulmonary abscess	*S. aureus,* group A strep, anaerobes	Cavity with air-fluid level

COVID/Coronavirus Infections

DEFINITION

Viral respiratory illness.

ETIOLOGY

- Single-stranded RNA viruses with crown-like (Latin: corona) surface projections.
- **S**evere **A**cute **R**espiratory **S**yndrome **co**ronavirus **2** (SARS-CoV-2)—emerged from China in late 2019, causes novel coronavirus disease 2019 (COVID-19).
- **S**evere **A**cute **R**espiratory **S**yndrome **co**ronavirus **1** (SARS-CoV-1) –caused a limited epidemic in 2002–2003, with last reported human infection in 2004.
- **M**iddle **E**ast **r**espiratory **s**yndrome coronavirus (MERS-CoV); causes MERS.
- Other human coronaviruses are found worldwide, and they typically cause a self-limited upper respiratory tract infection with rhinorrhea, sneezing, cough, and nasal congestion.

SIGNS AND SYMPTOMS

- Incubation period
  - SARS-CoV-2 and MERS-CoV: 2 to 14 days, with a median of 5 days.
  - Other coronaviruses may have shorter incubation periods, but more study is required.
- The most common presenting symptoms for COVID-19 in pediatric patients are fever and cough.
- Other symptoms include:
  - Shortness of breath, myalgia, fatigue, sore throat, and headache.
  - GI symptoms such as nausea, vomiting, diarrhea, and poor appetite.
- Loss of smell (anosmia) and loss of taste (ageusia) may occur.

DIAGNOSIS

- SARS-CoV-2 viral RNA may be identified through PCR from nasopharyngeal, nasal, oropharynx, trachea, or saliva swab, or direct antigen testing of nasopharyngeal or nasal swab.
- Serological testing can be useful in the diagnosis of MIS-C (see below), but it is not useful for the diagnosis of acute infection.

COMPLICATIONS

- **M**ultisystem **i**nflammatory **s**yndrome in **c**hildren (MIS-C).
- Presenting symptoms include fever, laboratory evidence of inflammation, and compromise of 2 or more organ systems.
  - May present with severe abdominal pain.
  - No other identifiable cause.
  - Evidence of SARS-CoV-2 infection, or exposure.
  - Features are similar to Kawasaki disease.
  - This condition is still being defined.

TREATMENT

- At the time of writing, treatment of SARS-CoV-2 is evolving.
  - Remdesivir is approved for use in hospitalized pediatric patients over one month of age; it inhibits viral replication.
  - Nirmatrelvir-ritonavir and molnupiravir are oral medications available for patients 12y and up. These medications also interfere with viral replication.

- Convalescent plasma and monoclonal antibodies are under investigation.
  - Steroids seem helpful in adults and are under investigation in children.
- No controlled trials have been performed for treatments of MERS-CoV or SARS-CoV-1.
- Other coronavirus infections are treated with supportive care.

VACCINE

Intramuscular

- Vaccines against SARS-CoV-2 first became available in late 2020.
- Initial vaccines used mRNA technology.
- An international effort is ongoing, but access to vaccines remains limited in many countries a year after their initial release.

Croup

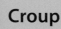 An 18-month-old boy awakens at night with sudden onset of inspiratory stridor and a barking cough with difficulty breathing that subsides on route to the emergency department. He has had a runny nose and cough for 2 days. On examination, he has a barky cough and inspiratory stridor only with agitation. *Think: Croup.*

DEFINITION

- Viral upper respiratory tract infection with inflammation and narrowing in the subglottic airway.
- A subset of patients will have recurrent, noninfectious spasmodic croup, occurring suddenly at night with very mild or no antecedent URI symptoms.

ETIOLOGY

Parainfluenza virus types 1 and 2 account for two-thirds of cases.

EPIDEMIOLOGY

It occurs in children 3 months to 3 years of age in fall and winter months, with an increased risk in males.

SIGNS AND SYMPTOMS

- Inspiratory stridor.
- Seal-like, barking cough with retractions and nasal flaring.
- May have coryza, fever, and congestion.
- Can include agitation, hypoxemia, hypercapnia, tachypnea, and tachycardia.
- Most cases are mild and last 3–7 days.
- Symptoms are worse at night, with sudden onset of symptoms.

DIAGNOSIS

- Diagnosis is made clinically.
- X-rays are usually not necessary. Consider an x-ray only if the diagnosis is in doubt.
- Steeple sign—narrowing of tracheal air column just below the vocal cords (see Figure 12-1).
- Ballooning distention of hypopharynx during inspiration.
- Differentiate croup from epiglottitis.

 WARD TIP

Croup is the most common cause of stridor in a febrile child.

 WARD TIP

Croup is the most common infectious cause of acute upper airway obstruction.

 WARD TIP

The most common cause of stridor in children is croup.

 EXAM TIP

Stridor and distress at home but calm and free of stridor in ED: *Think croup.*

 WARD TIP

Stridor at rest that is unresponsive to racemic epinephrine suggests that hospital admission is needed.

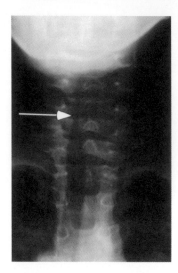

FIGURE 12-1. **Radiograph demonstrating steeple sign of croup.** Note narrowing of airway (arrow). (Used with permission from Dr. Gregory J. Schears.)

WARD TIP

Minutes count in acute epiglottitis.

WARD TIP

Primary source of pathogens in epiglottitis is from the posterior nasopharynx.

WARD TIP

Epiglottitis is an acute airway emergency, and treatment should not be delayed to obtain confirmatory radiographs.

WARD TIP

Epiglottitis is a true medical emergency. If suspected, DO NOT:
- Examine the throat
- Use narcotics or sedatives, including antihistamines
- Attempt venipuncture or other tests
- Place patient supine

TREATMENT

- A position of comfort is the treatment. Few data support the oft-used cool-mist humidification.
- Mild—dexamethasone (PO, IV, IM); may send home if no stridor occurs at rest.
- Moderate—dexamethasone, racemic epinephrine neb; observe 3–4 hours. If improved, consider discharge; if symptoms persist or worsen, repeat racemic epinephrine neb, and admit.
- Severe—racemic epinephrine, early use of corticosteroids, admit to intensive care unit (ICU), consider heliox.
- Admission criteria include:
  - Persistent stridor (especially at rest).
  - Respiratory distress.
  - Multiple doses of racemic epinephrine.
  - Possibility of alternate diagnosis.

CORTICOSTEROIDS IN RESPIRATORY PROBLEMS

- Dexamethasone (IM, IV, or PO 0.6 mg/kg).
- Side effects associated with short-term steroid use are minimal.

Epiglottitis

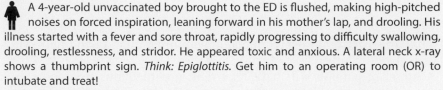

 A 4-year-old unvaccinated boy brought to the ED is flushed, making high-pitched noises on forced inspiration, leaning forward in his mother's lap, and drooling. His illness started with a fever and sore throat, rapidly progressing to difficulty swallowing, drooling, restlessness, and stridor. He appeared toxic and anxious. A lateral neck x-ray shows a thumbprint sign. *Think: Epiglottitis.* Get him to an operating room (OR) to intubate and treat!

The classic presentation is the "three Ds" (drooling, dysphagia, and distress).

See Figure 12-2.

DEFINITION

This condition is an acute, life-threatening bacterial infection of epiglottic and supraglottic tissues due to direct invasion of the epithelial layer by the organism.

ETIOLOGY

- *Haemophilus influenzae* type B.
- Other possible pathogens—*Streptococcus pyogenes, Streptococcus pneumoniae, and Staphylococcus aureus.*

PATHOPHYSIOLOGY

Acute inflammation and edema of epiglottis, aryepiglottic folds, and arytenoids

EPIDEMIOLOGY

- Decreased incidence due to *H. influenzae* type B vaccine (HiB).
- Usually occurs between 2–6 years of age, but it can occur at any age.
- Suspect in unvaccinated children and immunodeficient children.
- *H. influenzae* immunization has nearly eliminated epiglottitis in young children.

SIGNS AND SYMPTOMS

- Sudden onset of inspiratory stridor and respiratory distress.

- Three Ds: dysphagia, drooling, and distress.
- Tripod position—hyperextended neck, leaning forward, mouth open.
- Muffled voice ("hot potato" voice).
- High fever (usually the first symptom).
- Tachycardia is a constant feature.
- Cough is typically absent.
- The child will appear toxic.
- Severe respiratory distress develops within minutes to hours.
- May progress to restlessness, pallor/cyanosis, coma, and death.

DIAGNOSIS

- Laryngoscopy—swollen, cherry-red epiglottis.
- Lateral neck x-ray to confirm (obtain portable x-ray)
    - Swollen epiglottis (thumbprint sign).
    - Thickened aryepiglottic fold.
    - Obliteration of vallecula.

TREATMENT

- Engage the parents in comforting the child.
- Anticipate an airway compromise.
- Secure the airway (endotracheal intubation in OR).
- Administer ceftriaxone for 7–10 days.
- Use rifampin prophylaxis for close family contacts with incompletely immunized or immunocompromised children.

Bacterial Tracheitis

DEFINITION

- Rapidly progressive upper airway obstruction due to an invasive exudative bacterial infection of the soft tissues of the trachea.
- The larynx of healthy individuals is often colonized normally with bacteria and some potential pathogens. These pathogens can extend, at least transiently, into the trachea.

ETIOLOGY

- *S. aureus* and *H. influenzae* type b.
- Less commonly: *Moraxella catarrhalis*.
- High association with preceding viral infections, especially influenza A.

SIGNS AND SYMPTOMS

- Tracheitis often presents with croup symptoms. Differentiating factors include:
    - High fever.
    - Toxicity.
    - Expiratory or biphasic (inspiratory AND expiratory) stridor.
    - Purulent sputum.
- Tracheitis has features of croup (stridor and croupy cough) and epiglottitis (high fever and toxic appearance).

DIAGNOSIS

- X-ray—may be normal or identical to croup:
    - Epiglottis size normal.
    - Tracheal narrowing.
    - Pseudomembrane on lateral view may be seen.

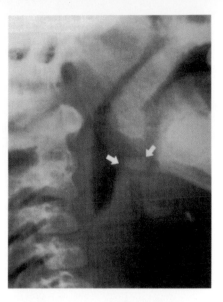

FIGURE 12-2. Radiograph of lateral soft tissue of neck demonstrating epiglottitis. Note the thickening of the epiglottic and aryepiglottic folds (arrows). (Reproduced, with permission, from Schwartz DT, Reisdorff BJ. *Emergency Radiology.* New York: McGraw-Hill, 2000: 608.)

EXAM TIP

Treat epiglottitis with third-generation cephalosporin and anti-staphylococcal agents (clindamycin, vancomycin) against MRSA. Ideally, a blood or epiglottic culture will clarify the causative organism and allow monotherapy.

WARD TIP

Bacterial tracheitis generally occurs in the setting of prior airway mucosal damage, as occurs with a preceding viral infection, especially an influenza A infection.

EXAM TIP

If croup symptoms persist for more than 2–3 days with a sudden worsening of symptoms with high fever and ill-appearance: *Think bacterial tracheitis.*

- Bronchoscopy shows inflamed and exudate-covered trachea.
- Copious purulent secretion is distal to glottis.
- Secretions should be obtained for Gram stain and culture.

TREATMENT

- Secure an adequate airway (endotracheal intubation):
    - Perform in an operating room under anesthesia.
    - Use suction of the endotracheal tube of purulent material to reduce the obstruction.
- Specialty consultation: otolaryngology (ENT), and anesthesia.
- Vancomycin PLUS either ceftriaxone or ampicillin-sulbactam.
- ICU admission for all to monitor disease progression.

Bronchiolitis

A previously healthy 4-month-old has rhinorrhea, cough, and a low-grade fever. The child then develops tachypnea, mild hypoxemia, and hyperinflation of lungs. *Think: Bronchiolitis.*

Classic presentation: acute onset of cough, wheezing, and increased respiratory effort after an upper respiratory tract prodrome (fever and runny nose), during winter months

DEFINITION

This is a viral infection of the lower respiratory tract (medium and small airways), which occurs after upper respiratory symptoms.

ETIOLOGY

- RSV—most common cause.
- Rhinovirus.
- Adenovirus.
- Parainfluenza 3 & 4.
- Influenza.
- Human metapneumovirus (hMPV): increasingly implicated.
- Two or more viruses are found in one-third of children hospitalized with bronchiolitis.

PATHOPHYSIOLOGY

- Inflammatory bronchiole obstruction (edema and mucus) is due to viral infection.
- Alterations in gas exchange are most frequently the result of mismatching of pulmonary ventilation and perfusion.
- Can lead to atelectasis.

EPIDEMIOLOGY

- Occurs in first 2 years of life.
- Reinfection is common.
- Occurs in winter and early spring.
- Risks include crowded conditions, not breast-fed, mothers who smoke, male gender, day care.
- Infants at higher risk include those with:
    - Cardiac disease.
    - Pulmonary disease and bronchopulmonary dysplasia.
    - Neuromuscular disease.
    - Prematurity.
    - Immunocompromise.

Signs and Symptoms

- Starts with mild upper respiratory symptoms: often profuse nasal discharge and congestion with or without fever.
- Respiratory distress gradually develops.
- Paroxysmal wheezing (common but may be absent), cough, dyspnea.
- Apneic spells—monitor young infants.
- Complications include atelectasis, respiratory failure, secondary infection (particularly otitis media and pneumonia).
- Most common complication is hypoxia.
- Dehydration is a common secondary complication and can lead to electrolyte disturbances.

Diagnosis

- The diagnosis is mostly clinical, but if other differential diagnoses are suspected, consider additional testing.
- Detect viruses in nasopharyngeal secretions via polymerase chain reaction or antigen detection; viral culture is less sensitive, and serology is typically only used in research.
- Use a chest x-ray (rule out pneumonia or foreign body) to identify hyperinflation of lungs or increased anteroposterior (AP) diameter of the rib cage.

Treatment

- Maintain a low threshold for hospitalization for high-risk infants.
- Humidified oxygen, high-flow nasal canula, or continuous positive airway pressure.
- Nasal suctioning.
- Trial of nebulized albuterol although no long-term benefit is shown (only 20–50% are responders; discontinue if no objective benefit).
- Hypertonic saline nebulizer treatments have the potential to reduce airway edema and mucous plugging.
- Steroids are not indicated in the first episode of bronchiolitis.
- Respiratory isolation.
- Ribavirin (aerosol form) is expensive, difficult to deliver and of uncertain efficacy; it is no longer routinely recommended.

Prevention

Palivizumab (RSV-specific monoclonal antibody) is given monthly before and during RSV season in high-risk infants (typically premature infants, infants with chronic lung disease, and patients with congenital heart disease and cardiac compromise).

Bronchiectasis

 A 7-year-old boy has an upper respiratory infection (URI) with productive cough (with purulent sputum). On examination, localized rales on the right side of his chest were noted. An x-ray shows two discrete densities located in the right upper lobe of the lungs. *Think: Bronchiectasis.* Predisposition: Cystic fibrosis (CF) and ciliary dyskinesia.

Definition

Abnormal and permanent dilatation of bronchi

Etiology

- Viruses: adenovirus, influenza virus.
- Bacteria: *S. aureus*, *Klebsiella*, anaerobes.

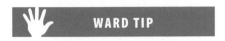

WARD TIP

Symptoms of asthma can be identical to bronchiolitis. Suspect asthma instead with:

- Family history of asthma or atopy
- Prior episodes of wheezing
- Response to bronchodilator

EXAM TIP

Cystic fibrosis is the #1 cause of bronchiectasis in children.

- Primary ciliary dyskinesia.
- Kartagener syndrome.
- Cystic fibrosis: *Pseudomonas aeruginosa*.
- α_1-antitrypsin deficiency.

PATHOPHYSIOLOGY

This condition is the consequence of inflammation and destruction of structural components of weak, easily collapsible bronchial walls and increased mucous plugs.

SIGNS AND SYMPTOMS

- The physical exam is quite variable and may reveal:
    - Persistent or recurrent wet cough.
    - Purulent sputum.
    - Hemoptysis is not as prevalent in children as it is in adults.
    - Dyspnea.
    - Crackles, rhonchi, less commonly wheezing.
    - Clubbing.

DIAGNOSIS

- Chest x-ray.
- Bronchography.
- Computed tomographic (CT) scan (using the most sensitive imaging method).
- Sputum culture.

TREATMENT

- Elimination of underlying cause.
- Clearance of secretions in airway with chest physiotherapy.
- Mucolytic agents.
- Control of infection—antibiotics.
- Reversal of airflow obstruction—bronchodilators and anti-inflammatory meds.

Pharyngitis

DEFINITION

Infection of the tonsils and/or the pharynx

ETIOLOGY

- Bacterial: streptococcal pharyngitis (*Streptococcus pyogenes*, also known as groups A β-hemolytic streptococcus [GABHS]); *Corynebacterium diphtheriae* (diphtheria, rare with vaccine).
- Viruses: rhinovirus, adenovirus, coxsackievirus, Epstein-Barr virus (mononucleosis).

SIGNS AND SYMPTOMS

- Symptoms of viral pharyngitis include:
    - Gradual onset.
    - Fever, malaise, throat pain.
    - Conjunctivitis, rhinitis, coryza, viral exanthem, and diarrhea.
    - EBV specific findings—enlarged posterior cervical nodes, hepatosplenomegaly.
    - Coxsackievirus specific findings—painful vesicles or ulcers on the palate or the posterior oropharynx.
- Symptoms of streptococcal pharyngitis (>2 years) (see Figure 12-3) include:
    - Headache, abdominal pain, and vomiting.
    - Fever, typically high.
    - Tonsillar enlargement with exudates.

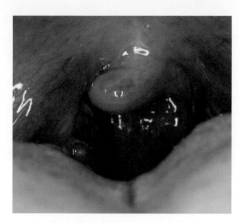

FIGURE 12-3. **Streptococcal pharyngitis.** Note white exudates on top of erythematous swollen tonsils. (Reproduced, with permission, from Knoop KJ, Stack LB, Storrow AB, et al. *Atlas of Emergency Medicine*, 3rd ed. New York: McGraw-Hill, 2010: 115.)

- Fetid odor.
- Cervical adenopathy.
- Palatal petechiae and uvular edema.
- Confluent erythematous sandpaper-like rash caused by exotoxins (scarlet fever).
- Clinically distinguishing viral from bacterial pharyngitis is not possible with certainty, although high fever, cervical adenopathy, and absence of URI symptoms suggest bacterial etiology.

DIAGNOSIS

Rapid antigen detection test (specificity 95%, sensitivity 70 – 90%)

- Culture if negative.
- Treat if positive.

TREATMENT

- Use oral penicillin for 10 days.
- Alternatively, intramuscular benzathine or procaine penicillin can be used.
- Use macrolides or clindamycin for penicillin-allergic patients for 10 days.
- Tetracycline and sulfonamides are not used to treat GABHS (high resistance).
- Antibiotics are not indicated for pharyngitis negative for GABHS.

COMPLICATIONS

- Suppurative complications include:
  - Peritonsillar abscess.
  - Retropharyngeal abscess.
  - Cervical adenitis.
  - Otitis media.
  - Sinusitis.
- Nonsuppurative complications include:
  - Acute glomerulonephritis.
  - Acute rheumatic fever.

WARD TIP

Use the modified Centor Score for pharyngitis: for ages <15, check for the presence of tonsillar exudates, tender anterior cervical lymphadenopathy, fever, and the absence of cough. Score one point per finding; patients with a score ≥3 should be tested for group A streptococcus.

WARD TIP

Penicillin remains the drug of choice for GABHS.

WARD TIP

The more mucous membranes involved, the more likely an infection is viral.

Pneumonia

A 2-month-old with fever, tachypnea, and mottled skin has a chest x-ray showing infiltrate of the right upper lung lobe, a pneumatocele, and a pleural effusion. *Think: S. aureus pneumonia.*

> A previously healthy 9-year-old boy has a 7-day history of increasing cough, low-grade fever, and fatigue on exertion. The chest x-ray shows widespread diffuse perihilar infiltrates. *Think: Mycoplasma pneumonia.*
>
> Initially, the child has a nonproductive cough and no fever. Later, a productive cough with fever, headache, coryza, otitis media, and malaise occur.

DEFINITION

Lower respiratory tract infection resulting in lung parenchyma inflammation

ETIOLOGY

- Viruses: RSV, influenza, parainfluenza, and adenovirus.
- Bacteria: less common, but more severe—S. *pneumoniae,* S. *pyogenes,* S. *aureus,* H. *influenzae* type B, M. *pneumoniae.*
- Fungi: *Pneumocystis jirovecii* (usually underlying a weakened immune system).

SIGNS AND SYMPTOMS

- Respiratory distress, including tachypnea, hypoxemia, and increased work of breathing.
- Fever, productive cough, and difficult feeding in infants.
- Afebrile pneumonia seen with *Chlamydia trachomatis* (pneumonitis syndrome) in infants.

DIAGNOSIS

- The classic lung exam reveals crackles, decreased breath sounds, and dullness to percussion.
- Use a chest x-ray to diagnose:
  - Viral (hyperinflation, perihilar infiltrate, hilar adenopathy, and atelectasis).
  - Bacterial (alveolar consolidation).
  - *Mycoplasma* (interstitial infiltrates).
  - Tuberculosis (hilar adenopathy; miliary pattern with disseminated TB).
  - *Pneumocystis* (reticulonodular infiltrates).
- CBC and blood culture (utility is debatable since only 2–3% of blood cultures in uncomplicated pediatric pneumonia are positive).

TREATMENT

- Inpatient:
  - IV ampicillin is first line in a fully immunized child. Consider second- or third-generation cephalosporin with or without vancomycin, depending on the degree of illness. Consider macrolide in 1- to 3–month-olds if chlamydia is suspected.
- Outpatient:
  - Patients should have normal O_2 saturation and take oral fluids well to be treated as an outpatient.
  - First line: high-dose amoxicillin; alternative, second- or third-generation cephalosporin or azithromycin.

Pertussis

DEFINITION

- "Whooping cough."
- Highly infectious acute respiratory illness.

ETIOLOGY

- *Bordetella pertussis* gram-negative coccobacilli with exotoxin.
- Humans are the only known host.
- Whooping cough syndrome also may be caused by:
  - *Bordetella parapertussis.*
  - *M. pneumoniae.*
  - *C. trachomatis.*
  - *C. pneumoniae.*
  - Adenoviruses.

PATHOPHYSIOLOGY

- Pertussis toxin is a virulence protein that causes lymphocytosis, inflammation of the respiratory tract, and systemic manifestations.
- Aerosol droplet transmission may occur.

EPIDEMIOLOGY

- Endemic, but epidemic every 3–4 years.
- About 151,000 cases and 89,000 deaths globally in 2018 (WHO data).
- Typically seen July to October.
- Occurs in 1- to 5-year-olds worldwide, 50% <1-year-olds in the U.S.

SIGNS AND SYMPTOMS

- Classic symptoms: inspiratory whoop, paroxysmal cough, post-tussive emesis.
- Incubation period 1–2 weeks.
- Three stages: catarrhal, paroxysmal, and convalescent.
- Duration: 6 weeks.
- Catarrhal stage (1–2 weeks): congestion, rhinorrhea, mild persistent cough.
- For the paroxysmal stage (2–4 weeks):
  - Paroxysmal cough, with characteristic whoop following (chin forward, tongue out, watery, bulging eyes, purple face).
  - Fever is typically absent.
  - Post-tussive emesis and exhaustion.
- Convalescent stage: number and severity of paroxysms plateaus.
- Complications include apnea, physical sequelae of forceful coughing, brain hypoxia/hemorrhage, secondary infections (bacterial pneumonia can lead to death).

DIAGNOSIS

- Diagnosis is primarily clinical involving:
  - Inspiratory whoop.
  - Post-tussive emesis.
  - Significant lymphocytosis.
- Chest x-ray—perihilar infiltrate or edema (butterfly pattern).
- Positive immunofluorescence test or PCR on nasopharyngeal secretions.

TREATMENT

- The goal is to decrease organism spread. Antibiotics do not affect illness in paroxysmal stage, which is toxin mediated.
- A macrolide antibiotic is used for patient and household contacts.
- Isolate until 5 days of therapy.
- Admit if patient is:
  - Infant <3 months.
  - Apneic.
  - Cyanotic.
  - Demonstrates respiratory distress.
- DTaP (diphtheria, tetanus, acellular pertussis) vaccine if not previously vaccinated.

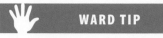

Despite having "whooping cough," most patients with pertussis do not whoop. Infants almost never whoop.

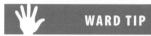

With pertussis, a fever may be absent or minimal; a cough may be the only complaint.

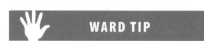

Apnea is common in infants with pertussis.

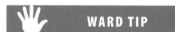

Suspect pertussis if a paroxysmal cough with skin-color change occurs.

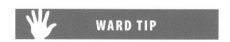

No single serologic test is diagnostic for pertussis.

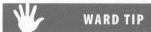

There is a risk of hypertrophic pyloric stenosis in infants younger than 6 weeks treated with oral macrolide antibiotics.

Diphtheria

DEFINITION

Membranous nasopharyngitis or obstructive laryngotracheitis

ETIOLOGY

- *Corynebacterium diphtheriae*, gram-positive bacillus.
- Humans are the only reservoir.

SIGNS AND SYMPTOMS

- Incubation period: 2–7 days.
- Erosive rhinitis with membrane formation and low-grade fever.
- Tonsillopharyngeal—sore throat, membranous exudate.
- Cardiac symptoms: myocarditis, arrythmias.
- Tachycardia out of proportion to fever.

DIAGNOSIS

- Perform a culture (nose, throat, mucosal, or cutaneous lesion).
- Material is obtained from beneath the membrane or a portion of membrane.
- All *C. diphtheriae* isolates should be sent to a diphtheria-familiar laboratory.

TREATMENT

- Antitoxin (obtained directly from CDC)—dose depends on:
  - Site of membrane.
  - Degree of toxic effects.
  - Duration of illness.
- Antibiotics:
  - Use erythromycin or penicillin G for 14 days.
  - Organism elimination is documented by two consecutive cultures.

Tuberculosis (TB)

DEFINITION

- Signs and symptoms and/or radiographic manifestations caused by *M. tuberculosis* are apparent.
- It may be pulmonary, extrapulmonary, or both.

ETIOLOGY

Mycobacterium tuberculosis—acid fast bacilli

PATHOPHYSIOLOGY

The primary portal of entry into children is the lung.

EPIDEMIOLOGY

- Children are never the primary source (look for adult contacts).
- Risk factors include:
  - Urban living.
  - Low income.
  - Recent immigrants.
  - HIV.

SIGNS AND SYMPTOMS

- Chronic cough (nonproductive) for more than 3 weeks.
- Hemoptysis.
- Fever.
- Night sweats.
- Weight loss or failure to thrive.
- Anorexia.
- Lymphadenopathy.
- Present to ED with:
  - Primary pneumonia.
  - Slow decline in mental status for CNS disease.
  - Miliary TB (may mimic sepsis).

DIAGNOSIS

- Suspect TB when symptoms occur including:
  - Hilar adenopathy.
  - Pulmonary calcification or caseating granulomas.
  - Pneumonia with infiltrate and adenopathy.
  - Pneumonia with pleural effusion.
  - Painless unilateral cervical adenopathy (scrofula).
  - Meningitis of insidious onset.
  - Bone or joint disease.
  - When any of the above are unresponsive to antibiotics.
- PPD test (Mantoux test).
- Interferon-Gamma Release Assays (IGRAs)
  - QuantiFERON®-TB Gold test (QFT-GIT).
  - T-SPOT®.*TB* test (T-Spot).
- Culture (gastric aspirates, sputum, pleural fluid, cerebrospinal fluid, urine, or other body fluids).
- Look for the adult source.
- Acid-fast stain or PCR.

TREATMENT

- Prompt treatment is necessary as TB can disseminate quickly in the very young.
- Two to four or more drugs (isoniazid, rifampin, pyrazinamide, ethambutol, streptomycin) are used for a minimum of 6 months for active disease.
- Isoniazid for is used for 6–9 months for infection without active disease (rifampin if isoniazid resistant).

Cystic Fibrosis (CF)

 A 3-year-old child presents with constant cough with sputum. He has had six episodes of pneumonia, with *Pseudomonas* being isolated from sputum; loose stools; and is at the 20th percentile for growth. *Think: Cystic fibrosis.*
CF is an inherited multisystem disorder resulting in chronic lung disease, exocrine pancreatic insufficiency, and failure to thrive.

DEFINITION

This disease of exocrine glands causes viscous secretions and:
- Chronic respiratory infection.
- Pancreatic insufficiency.
- Increased electrolytes in sweat.

EXAM TIP

The gene affected in cystic fibrosis codes for the cystic fibrosis transmembrane conductance regulator (CFTR) protein; the most common mutation is deletion of delta F508 on chromosome 7. Defects interfere with chloride movement out of the cell.

EXAM TIP

Fat-soluble vitamin deficiencies include:
A—night blindness.
D—decreased bone density.
E—neurologic dysfunction.
K—bleeding.

WARD TIP

Pseudomonas aeruginosa is the most common bacteria to cause chronic infection in CF lungs.

WARD TIP

False-positive sweat test (not CF) shows:
- Nephrogenic diabetes insipidus
- Myxedema/hypothyroidism
- Mucopolysaccharidosis
- Adrenal insufficiency
- Ectodermal dysplasia

WARD TIP

Features of CF: CF PANCREAS
Chronic cough
Failure to thrive
Pancreatic insufficiency
Alkalosis
Nasal polyps
Clubbing
Rectal prolapse
Electrolytes increased in sweat
Absence of vas deferens
Sputum mucoid

ETIOLOGY

- Defect of cyclic adenosine monophosphate (cAMP)–activated chloride ion channel of exocrine epithelial cells in pancreas, sweat glands, salivary glands, intestines, respiratory tract, and reproductive system.
- Autosomal recessive.

PATHOPHYSIOLOGY

- Decreased chloride secretion from cells in lungs and GI tract.
- Dysfunction of salt and water balance, causing thickened secretions and increased loss of salt in sweat (see Diagnosis below).

EPIDEMIOLOGY

- Cystic fibrosis is the most common cause of severe, chronic lung disease in children.
- It occurs in one in 2000–3000 live births in whites of European descent.

SIGNS AND SYMPTOMS

- Respiratory symptoms include:
  - Cough (persistent and productive, most common symptom).
  - Wheezing, dyspnea, exercise intolerance.
  - Bronchiectasis, recurrent pneumonia.
  - Sinusitis, nasal polyps.
  - Reactive airway disease or hemoptysis that results in anemia.
  - Increased AP chest diameter.
  - Hyperresonant lungs.
  - Clubbing of nails.
- Gastrointestinal (GI) symptoms include:
  - Failure to thrive.
  - Meconium ileus (10%).
  - Constipation, rectal prolapse.
  - Intestinal obstruction.
  - Pancreatic insufficiency, including:
    - Malabsorption with steatorrhea.
    - Fat-soluble vitamin deficiencies.
    - Glucose intolerance.
  - Biliary cirrhosis (uncommon): jaundice, ascites, hematemesis from esophageal varices.
- Reproductive tract symptoms include decreased or absent fertility with thick cervical secretions or azoospermia.
- Sweat glands contribute to:
  - Salty skin.
  - Hypochloremic alkalosis in severe cases.
- Complications may include pneumothorax, chronic pulmonary hypertension, cor pulmonale, atelectasis, allergic bronchopulmonary aspergillosis, respiratory failure, and gastroesophageal reflux.

DIAGNOSIS

- Sweat test—chloride concentration >60 mEq/L (gold standard).
- Routine newborn screening done in all 50 states by IRT (immunoreactive trypsinogen) assay (increased in CF) and reflex DNA analysis (CFTR mutations). A sweat test is performed after 2 weeks of age.
- Genetic studies identify most, but not all, mutations.
- *In utero* screening is available.
- Pulmonary function tests (PFTs) include obstructive and restrictive abnormalities.
- Prenatal diagnosis via gene proves CF mutations or linkage analysis.

TREATMENT

- A multidisciplinary team approach includes the pediatrician, physiotherapist, dietitian, nursing staff, teacher, child, and parents.
- Respiratory treatment includes:
  - Chest physical therapy to promote mucociliary clearance.
  - Exercise.
  - Coughing to move secretions and mucous plugs.
  - Bronchodilators.
  - Normal saline aerosol.
  - Anti-inflammatory medications.
  - Dornase-alfa nebulizer (breaks down mucus).
- Pancreatic/digestive treatment includes:
  - Enteric coated pancreatic enzyme supplements (add to all meals).
  - Fat-soluble vitamin supplements.
  - High-calorie, high-protein diet.
- Antibiotics: sputum cultures guide antibiotic choice. Pseudomonal infections are common. Macrolide antibiotics are most commonly used.
- CFTR modulators (only work with specific CFTR mutations).
- Lung transplant.
- Gene therapy is being aggressively studied.

PROGNOSIS

Therapy advances have increased life expectancy into adulthood.

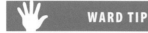

WARD TIP

Ninety-nine percent of cases of meconium ileus are due to CF.

Tonsils/Adenoids

ENLARGED TONSILS AND ADENOIDS

ANATOMY

- Tonsils—two faucial/palatine tonsils.
- Adenoids—nasopharyngeal tonsils.

CAUSES

- Acute infection (frequently with pharyngitis).
- Persistent infection.
- Allergens.
- Irritants.
- Enlarged tonsils, which may be normal in some children.

SIGNS AND SYMPTOMS—ENLARGED TONSILS

- Sore throat.
- Pain with swallowing.
- May have whitish exudate on tonsils.
- Chronic tonsillitis, defined as:
  - Seven in past year.
  - Five in each of the past 2 years.
  - Three in each of the past 3 years.

SIGNS AND SYMPTOMS—ENLARGED ADENOIDS

- Mouth breathing.
- Persistent rhinitis.
- Snoring.
- Mucopurulent nasal discharge.
- Hyponasal speech.

WARD TIP

Palatine tonsils and adenoids are part of Waldeyer's ring that circles the pharynx; the two other components are the lingual tonsils (at the back of the tongue) and the tubal tonsils (at the exit of the Eustachian tubes).

WARD TIP

It can be normal for tonsils to be relatively large during childhood.

WARD TIP

Enlarged adenoids are the most common cause of nasal obstruction in children.

WARD TIP

Trismus is the limited ability to open the mouth and distinguishes peritonsillar abscess from severe pharyngitis or tonsillitis.

EXAM TIP

Always look for the presence of an upper-airway obstruction in peritonsillar abscess.

WARD TIP

Lymph nodes in the retropharyngeal space usually disappear by the third to fourth year of life.

WARD TIP

The retropharyngeal space is widened if >7mm at C2 level or >14mm at C6 level of a soft-tissue lateral neck x-ray.

- Adenoid facies—open mouth, flattened/elongated midface, retracted upper lip, narrowed hard palate with crowded maxillary teeth.
- Recurrent otitis media or nasopharyngitis.

DIAGNOSIS

- Digital palpation and direct visualization.
- Indirect laryngoscopy.

TREATMENT

- A tonsillectomy and/or an adenoidectomy is used for chronic inflammation, OSA, and recurrent or chronic otitis media.
- Large size alone is not an indication to remove tonsils.
- A tonsillectomy should not be performed routinely with an adenoidectomy unless a separate indication exists.

PERITONSILLAR ABSCESS

DEFINITION

This walled-off infection occurs in the space between the superior-pharyngeal constrictor muscle and the capsule of the palatine tonsils. It is the most common deep-neck infection.

ETIOLOGY

- GABHS.
- Anaerobes.

EPIDEMIOLOGY

Usually preadolescent

SIGNS AND SYMPTOMS

- Preceded by acute tonsillopharyngitis.
- Severe throat pain, usually unilateral.
- Trismus.
- Refusal to swallow or speak.
- "Hot potato voice."
- Markedly swollen and inflamed tonsil.
- Uvula displaced to opposite side.

TREATMENT

- Antibiotics covering staph and strep, typically, IV ampicillin—sulbactam or clindamycin. If no response, add vancomycin or linezolid.
- Supportive care follows needle aspiration or incision and drainage.

Retropharyngeal Abscess

DEFINITION

This is an infection of the potential space between the posterior pharyngeal wall and the prevertebral fascia. It commonly occurs in children <5 years old.

ETIOLOGY

It is usually a complication of pharyngitis caused by:

- GABHS.
- Oral anaerobes.
- S. *aureus*.

SIGNS AND SYMPTOMS

- Associated with recent URI.
- Sudden onset of high fever with difficulty in swallowing.
- Refusal of feeding due to dysphagia and odynophagia.
- Throat pain.
- Toxicity (common).
- May cause meningismus with the extension of the neck causing pain.

DIAGNOSIS

- A lateral neck x-ray shows a widened pre-vertebral/retropharyngeal space (see Figure 12–4).
- Reversal of lordosis and the normal cervical spine curvature may also be seen.

TREATMENT

- IV clindamycin or ampicillin—sulbactam.
- If the airway is compromised, perform an immediate surgical drainage.

Asthma

 A 5-year-old boy with a history of sleeping problems presents with a non-productive nocturnal cough and shortness of breath and cough during exercise. *Think: Asthma.*

Start a bronchodilator trial, which is helpful in the demonstration of reversible-airway obstruction (increase in forced expiratory volume in 1 second [FEV_1]). Asthma is an inflammatory disease. A diagnosis of asthma should be considered in the presence of recurrent wheezing in a child with a family history of asthma.

DEFINITION

This chronic inflammatory and hypersensitivity airway disorder causes recurrent cough, wheezing, and difficulty breathing. The hallmark is reversible-airway obstruction.

ETIOLOGY

Airway hyper-responsiveness to a variety of stimuli, including:
- Respiratory infection.
- Air pollutants.
- Allergens: seasonal, dust, mold, animal dander.
- Foods.
- Exercise.
- Emotions.

PATHOPHYSIOLOGY

- Bronchospasm (acute).
- Mucus production (acute).
- Inflammation and edema of the airway mucosa (chronic).
- Underlying abnormalities in asthma include increased pulmonary vascular pressure, diffuse airway narrowing, increased residual volume and functional residual capacity, and increased total ventilation maintaining normal or reduced PCO_2 despite increased dead space.

SIGNS AND SYMPTOMS

- Cough, wheezing, dyspnea, and tachypnea.
- Increased work of breathing (retractions, accessory muscle use, nasal flaring, abdominal breathing).

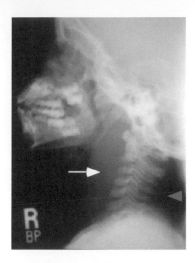

FIGURE 12-4. Lateral radiograph of the soft tissue of the neck. Note the large amount of prevertebral edema (solid arrow). Findings are consistent with retropharyngeal abscess. (Reproduced, with permission, from Dr. Gregory J. Schears.)

 WARD TIP

Asthma is the most common chronic lung disease in children.

 EXAM TIP

It is important to ask for allergy history and family history of asthma.

 WARD TIP

Lack of wheezing does not exclude asthma.

 WARD TIP

In asthma, the cellular infiltration of mucosa by eosinophils, activated helper T cells, and mast cells are seen.

 WARD TIP

Asthma is the most common cause of cough in school-age children.

TABLE 12-4. **Asthma Severity Classification**

CLASSIFYING SEVERITY OF ASTHMA EXACERBATIONS IN THE URGENT OR EMERGENCY CARE SETTING	
Mild	Dyspnea only with activity PEFR >70% predicted personal best
Moderate	Dyspnea interferes with or limits usual activity PEFR 40–69% predicted personal best
Severe	Dyspnea at rest, interferes with conversation PEFR <40% predicted personal best
Life threatening	Too dyspneic to speak PEFR <25% predicted personal best

PEFR, peak expiratory flow rate.

(Adapted from National Asthma Education & Prevention Program Expert Panel Report 3: Guidelines for the Diagnosis & Management of Asthma NHLBI guidelines, *Summary Report 2007:* 54. National Heart, Lung, and Blood Institute; National Institutes of Health; U.S. Department of Health and Human Services.)

EXAM TIP

Before puberty, boys have a higher prevalence of asthma.

WARD TIP

URI is the most important triggering factor for patients with asthma of all ages.

WARD TIP

The classic trilogy of asthma includes:
- Bronchospasm
- Mucus production
- Inflammation and edema of the airway mucosa

EXAM TIP

Respiratory drive is not inhibited in asthma.

WARD TIP

All wheezing is not caused by asthma; all asthmatics do not wheeze.

- Decreased air movement on auscultation.
- Prolongation of expiratory phase.
- Acidosis and hypoxia may result from airway obstruction.
- See Table 12-4 for classification of severity.

DIAGNOSIS

- Asthma is primarily a clinical diagnosis.
- A peak expiratory flow rate (PEFR) assesses the severity of an acute exacerbation.
  - Note a maximal airflow rate during forced exhalation after a maximal inhalation.
- Normal values depend on age and height:
  - Mild (80% of predicted).
  - Moderate (50–80% of predicted).
  - Severe (<50% of predicted).
- Spirometry is the preferred method of diagnosis of airflow obstruction
  - Recommended >5 years old if asthma is suspected.
  - Measure forced vital capacity (FVC) and forced expiratory volume in 1 second (FEV_1).
  - Airway obstruction is present if $FEV_1 < 80\%$; $FEV_1/FVC < 85\%$.
- A chest x-ray may show hyperinflation and can diagnose pneumonia or foreign body for first-time wheezing.
- Pulse oximetry may demonstrate hypoxia.
- Arterial blood gas (ABG) shows hypoxia in severe exacerbations; hypercapnia is suggestive of impending respiratory failure.
- Bloodwork should not be routinely ordered in the evaluation of asthma.

TREATMENT

The treatment goals are to improve bronchodilation, avoid allergens, decrease inflammation, and educate the patient.

FIRST-LINE AGENTS FOR ACUTE EXACERBATIONS

- Oxygen if O_2 saturation <92% on room air.
- Inhaled short-acting β_2 agonist (SABA):
  - Targets bronchospasm.
  - Albuterol (metered dose inhaler or nebulized).

- SABA is a short-acting/rescue medication that treats only symptoms, not the underlying process.
- This bronchial smooth-muscle relaxant increases airflow.
- Side effects include tachycardia, tremors, and hypokalemia.
- Systemic corticosteroids (sooner is better):
  - Target inflammation.
  - Oral prednisone, IV methylprednisolone, or IV or PO dexamethasone.
  - Precaution: active varicella or herpes infection.
- Anticholinergic agents:
  - Ipratropium bromide (nebulized).
  - Acts synergistically with albuterol and is not for monotherapy in exacerbation.
  - Bind to cholinergic receptors in the medium and large airways.
  - Improved clinical outcome in children when used for acute exacerbation in ED.

SECOND-LINE TREATMENT

- Magnesium sulfate—bronchodilation via direct effect on smooth muscle.
- Heliox—mixture of 60–70% helium and 30–40% oxygen:
  - Decreases the work of breathing by improving laminar-gas flow (nonintubated patients).
  - Improves oxygenation and decreased peak airway pressure (intubated patients).
- Mechanical ventilation indications include:
  - Failure of maximal pharmacologic therapy.
  - Hypoxemia.
  - Hypercarbia.
  - Change in mental status.
  - Respiratory fatigue or impending failure.
- Generally speaking, there is no role in acute asthma exacerbation for theophylline or aminophylline.

ASTHMA CONTROL AND LONG-TERM CARE

- Classification of severity using the NHLBI asthma management guideline directs therapy:
  - Short acting β_2 agonist, as needed.
  - Inhaled corticosteroids:
    - Daily controller.
    - Use lowest dose to control symptoms.
    - Slows growth rate slightly, with the final height unaffected.
  - Leukotriene modifiers:
    - Inflammatory mediators.
    - Improve lung function.
  - Cromolyn and nedocromil:
    - Mast cell stabilizers.
    - Can be used in maintenance therapy.
    - Used in exercise-induced asthma.
    - May reduce dosage requirements of inhaled steroid.

STATUS ASTHMATICUS

DEFINITION

- Life-threatening form of asthma.
- Progressively worsening episode unresponsive to usual therapy.

 WARD TIP
An asthmatic patient in severe respiratory distress may not wheeze due to poor air movement.

 WARD TIP
O_2 is indicated for all asthmatics to keep O_2 saturation >95%.

 WARD TIP
Low-dose daily inhaled corticosteroids are the first-line controller therapy for mild, persistent asthma.

 WARD TIP
Spirometry is the most important study in asthma.

 WARD TIP
A long-acting β_2 agonist (salmeterol) should not be used for acute asthma exacerbation.

 WARD TIP
Dehydration may be present in status asthmaticus, but overhydration should be avoided (risk for syndrome of inappropriate antidiuretic hormone secretion [SIADH]).

 WARD TIP
An asthmatic child's ability to use an inhaler correctly should be regularly assessed and should be used with a spacer to ensure the most effective administration of dose.

EXAM TIP

The most important risk factor for morbidity is failure to diagnose asthma from recurrent wheezing.

WARD TIP

Leukocytosis does not always signify infection in status asthmaticus.

WARD TIP

Ketamine is used for sedation/analgesia before intubating a child with asthma in respiratory failure due to its bronchodilatory properties.

WARD TIP

Prevention is key! Keep small food and objects away from young children.

WARD TIP

Caution! Do not try to remove foreign bodies causing partial upper-airway obstruction because these attempts may result in complete glottic obstruction.

WARD TIP

Most foreign body aspirations in children end up on the right, and most of these lodge in the right main-stem bronchus.

SIGNS AND SYMPTOMS

Look for:

- Pulsus paradoxus >20 mm Hg.
- Hypotension, tachycardia.
- Cyanosis.
- One- to two-word dyspnea.
- Lethargy.
- Agitation.
- Retractions.
- Silent chest (no wheezes—poor air exchange).

Foreign Body Aspiration

 A 2-year-old boy is brought to the ED with a history of choking or gagging episodes followed by coughing spells. In the ED, he was noted to have wheezing. His respiratory rate is 24, and he has mild intercostal retractions. His babysitter found him playing in his room. *Think: Foreign body aspiration.*

A previously healthy 12-year-old boy presented with a cough for almost a year. He had a persistent dry cough during the day and night that was occasionally productive. His parents reported a history of pneumonia with consolidation of the right lower lobe on three different occasions in 6 months. On physical examination, no nasal congestion is noted. Decreased air entry and wheezing is noted on the right side of his chest. *Think: Foreign body aspiration.*

Note that this classic triad (sudden onset of paroxysmal coughing, wheezing, and diminished breath sounds on the ipsilateral side) may not be present in all children with foreign-body aspiration.

PATHOPHYSIOLOGY

The cough reflex usually protects against aspiration.

EPIDEMIOLOGY

- Twice as likely to occur in males, particularly 6-month-olds to 3-year-olds.
- Peak incidence: 1–2 years of age.

SIGNS AND SYMPTOMS

- Symptoms are determined by the nature of the object, location, and degree of obstruction.
- The narrowest portion of the pediatric airway is at the cricoid ring.
- An upper-airway foreign body may cause respiratory distress with severe retractions and stridor.
- With lower-airway foreign bodies (most common [80%]), symptoms may be subtle.
- Initial respiratory symptoms may disappear for hours to weeks after the incident.
- The most common aspirated foreign body is a peanut.
- The most common foreign body aspirations resulting in death are caused by balloons.
- Potential complications if the object is not removed include pneumonitis/pneumonia, abscess, bronchiectasis, pulmonary hemorrhage, erosion, and perforation.

DIAGNOSIS/TREATMENT

Larynx

- Croupy cough; may have stridor, aphonia, hemoptysis, cyanosis.
- Lateral x-ray.
- Direct laryngoscopy—confirm diagnosis and remove object.

TRACHEA

- Stridor, audible slap, and palpable thud due to expiratory impaction.
- Inspiratory and expiratory chest x-rays, bronchoscopy.

BRONCHI

- Initial choking, gagging, wheezing, coughing.
- Latent period with some coughing, wheezing, possible hemoptysis, recurrent lobar pneumonia, or intractable asthma.
- Tracheal shift, decreased breath sounds.
- Midline obstruction can cause severe dyspnea or asphyxia.
- Can lead to chronic bronchopulmonary disease if not treated.
- Direct bronchoscopic visualization (Figure 12-5).
- An expiratory chest x-ray can show air trapping as result of ball-valve effect from foreign body.
- Antibiotics for secondary infection, if prolonged exposure.
- Emergency treatment of local upper airway obstruction, if necessary.
- If the child can cough and verbalize:
  - Provide supplemental oxygen.
  - Maintain position of comfort.
  - Immediate consult with ENT and anesthesiologist.
- If the child cannot cough or verbalize, initiate basic life support.

Laryngomalacia

DEFINITION

- Collapse of supraglottic structures during inspiration.
- Caused by a disproportionately small and soft larynx.

SIGNS AND SYMPTOMS

- Usually begins within first month of life.
- Noisy breathing, snoring.
- A "wet" inspiratory stridor is the most frequent cause of stridor in children.
- Symptoms can be intermittent.
- Hoarseness or aphonia (laryngeal crow).
- Feeding difficulty occurs, as well as gastroesophageal reflux and laryngopharyngeal reflux.
- Symptoms worsen when crying or lying on back.

DIAGNOSIS

- Flexible fiberoptic laryngoscopy.
- The laryngeal structure collapses during inspiration, especially the arytenoid cartilages.

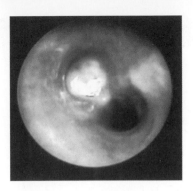

FIGURE 12-5. **Foreign body (peanut) in the right mainstem bronchus visualized by bronchoscopy.** Foreign bodies tend to lodge most commonly in the right mainstem bronchus due to the larger anatomic angle that makes traveling down right mainstem easier. (Reproduced, with permission, from Dr. Gregory J. Schears.)

 WARD TIP

Percussion of Lung Fields
- Hyperresonant = overinflation
- Dull = atelectasis

 WARD TIP

Rigid bronchoscopy is the procedure of choice to identify and remove an object.

 WARD TIP

Tracheomalacia is the collapse of the trachea during *expiration* causing airway obstruction; the presentation and management are similar to laryngomalacia.

TREATMENT

- Provide reassurance.
- No specific therapy is required.
- Usually resolves spontaneously by 18 months.
- Surgery is rare and only performed if severe.

Congenital Lobar Emphysema

DEFINITION

Developmental anomaly of the lower respiratory tract characterized by hyper-inflation of one or more of the pulmonary lobes

EPIDEMIOLOGY

- Most common congenital lung lesion.
- More common in males (3:1).

PATHOPHYSIOLOGY

No significant parenchymal destruction

SIGNS AND SYMPTOMS

- Affected infants appear normal at birth.
- Cough, wheezing, dyspnea, and cyanosis occur within a few days.
- Decreased breath sounds and hyper-resonance to percussion occur over involved lobe.

DIAGNOSIS

- Chest x-ray shows:
  - Distention of the affected lobe.
  - Can see compressive atelectasis of contralateral lung.
  - Radiolucency.
  - Mediastinal shift to opposite side.
  - Flattened diaphragm.

TREATMENT

Lobectomy

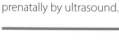

Both congenital lobar emphysema and congenital pulmonary airway malformation (CPAM) can be diagnosed prenatally by ultrasound.

Congenital Pulmonary Airway Malformation (CPAM)

DEFINITION

- Formerly called congenital cystic adenomatoid malformation (CCAM).
- Developmental anomaly of the lower respiratory tract.
- Excessive overgrowth of bronchioles.
- Increase in terminal respiratory structure.
- Hamartomatous lesions in tracheal, bronchial, bronchiolar, and alveolar tissues.

EPIDEMIOLOGY

Second-most common congenital lung lesion

Increased expression of HOXB5 gene has been noted in patients with CPAM.

In patients with CPAM, avoid attempted aspiration or chest-tube placement because a risk of spreading infection exists.

SIGNS AND SYMPTOMS

- Neonatal respiratory distress.
- Recurrent pneumonia in same location.
- Pneumothorax.
- May be confused with diaphragmatic hernia in neonatal period.
- Can be asymptomatic.

DIAGNOSIS

- Chest x-ray (posteroanterior, lateral, and decubitus).
- Cystic mass (multiple grapelike sacs) and mediastinal shift.
- Air-fluid level.
- CT scan shows small and large air- or fluid-filled cysts.

TREATMENT

- Of newborns with prenatal CPAM diagnosis, 75% will be asymptomatic at birth.
  - Close followup is required; some infants develop symptoms as cystic lesions expand with air.
- Surgical excision of affected lobe is typically reserved for symptomatic infants.

EXAM TIP

Congenital pulmonary airway malformation increases the risk for pulmonary neoplasia, specifically pleuropulmonary blastoma and bronchoalveolar carcinoma.

NOTES

Cardiovascular Disease

Murmurs

NORMAL HEART SOUNDS

- S1, produced by tricuspid and mitral valve closure, may split with respirations.
- S2, produced by aortic (A2) and pulmonic (P2) valve closure, normally splits.
  - P2 should be soft after infancy.
- S3 can represent normal, rapid ventricular refilling; early diastolic gallop rhythm
- S4 can represent high output state or poor compliance of ventricular walls; late diastolic gallop

EPIDEMIOLOGY

- Up to 90% of children have a murmur at some point in their lives.
- 2–7% of murmurs in children represent pathology.

DESCRIPTION AND GRADING

Murmurs are graded for intensity on a six-point system:
- **Grade I:** Very soft, detected after careful auscultation in a quiet environment.
- **Grade II:** Soft, readily heard but faint, roughly equal to S1/S2.
- **Grade III:** Moderately intense, louder than S1/S2, without a palpable precordial thrill.
- **Grade IV:** Loud with a palpable precordial thrill present.
- **Grade V:** Loud, heard with only the stethoscope edge touching the chest.
- **Grade VI:** Loud, heard without the stethoscope touching the chest.

SITES OF AUSCULTATION

See Figure 13-1 to correlate the following points:

1. **Carotid arteries.** Common murmurs heard here: carotid bruit, aortic stenosis (AS).
2. **Aortic valve.** Right upper-sternal border. Common murmur: AS. Valvular stenosis will often have an ejection click.
3. **Pulmonic valve.** Left upper-sternal border. Common murmurs: pulmonary valve stenosis, atrial septal defect (ASD), pulmonary flow murmur, pulmonary artery stenosis, patent ductus arteriosus (PDA).

WARD TIP

Murmur grading is usually written as "Grade [#]/6." Any murmur > Grade III is likely pathologic.

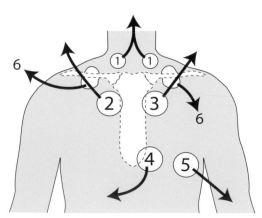

FIGURE 13-1. Sites of auscultation.

4. **Tricuspid valve.** Left lower-sternal border. Common murmurs: ventricular septal defect (VSD), Still's murmur, hypertrophic obstructive cardiomyopathy (HOCM), tricuspid regurgitation, endocardial cushion defect.
5. **Mitral valve.** Apex. Common murmurs: mitral regurgitation, mitral valve prolapse, Still's murmur.
6. This site correlates with areas of **venous confluence.** Common murmurs: venous hum or subclavian bruit.

INNOCENT MURMURS

- Typically from turbulent blood flow rather than structural disease, and lacking hemodynamic significance.
- Common to all innocent murmurs are:
  - Absence of structural heart defects.
  - Normal heart sounds (S1, S2) with normal peripheral pulses.
  - Normal chest radiographs and electrocardiogram (ECG).
  - Asymptomatic.
  - Usually systolic and graded less than III.
  - No association with cardiovascular disease.
  - Accentuated in high-output states (fever and anemia).
- Pulmonary flow murmurs and Still's murmurs are heard best in supine patients.
- A Still's murmur may disappear with the Valsalva maneuver.
- Pulmonary flow murmurs are augmented by exhalation and diminished by inhalation.
- A venous hum is continuous, disappears in the supine position, and can be eliminated with digital compression of the jugular vein.
- See Table 13-1.

Interpretation of Pediatric ECGs

- Always approach an ECG systematically:
  1. Rate: measure atrial and ventricular rates.
  2. Rhythm: define the rhythm (sinus, or other).
  3. Axis: measure the axis of the P waves, QRS complexes, and T waves.
  4. Intervals: measure the P-R interval, QRS duration, and Q-T interval.
  5. Morphology: look for abnormalities of wave patterns and voltages.
- Pediatric considerations:
  - The interpretation is age dependent.
  - Heart rate is age dependent, and is higher in young children (Table 13-2).
- The PR interval and QRS duration are shorter in children.
- QTc is longer in infants (QT interval varies with heart rate).

ECG PAPER

- Speed = 25 mm/s
- Small box = 0.04 second = 1 mm
- Large box = 0.20 second = 5 mm

ATRIAL RATE

- If the number of P waves is greater than the number of QRS complexes, an atrial dysrhythmia may be present.
- Premature atrial contractions (PACs) are common in infancy.

TABLE 13-1. Innocent Murmurs

Murmur	Cause	Epidemiology	Location	Sound	Characteristics
Pulmonary flow murmur	Turbulent flow through a normal pulmonary valve	Most common between 8 and 14 years	Mid to upper left sternal border	Midfrequency, crescendo–decrescendo, systolic	Louder when patient is supine than upright
Still's (vibratory) murmur	Possibly turbulent flow in the left ventricular outflow tract region	Most common between 3 and 6 years; uncommon < 2 years	Lower left sternal border	Musical or vibratory with mid-systolic accentuation	Louder supine, may disappear with Valsalva, softer during inspiration
Venous hum	Turbulent flow of systemic venous return in the jugular veins and superior vena cava	Most common between 3 and 6 years	Infra- and supraclavicular, base of neck	High frequency, best heard with diaphragm, during systole and diastole	More prominent on right than left, can be accentuated or eliminated with head position, disappears supine or digital compression of jugular vein
Carotid bruit or subclavian bruit	Turbulent flow from abrupt transition from large-bore aorta to smaller carotid and brachiocephalic arteries	Any age	Over carotid arteries with radiation to head	Systolic	Rarely, a faint thrill is palpable over the artery
Physiologic pulmonary branch stenosis (PPS)	Turbulent flow as blood enters right and left pulmonary arteries that are relatively hypoplastic at birth due to patent ductus arteriosus predominance	Newborns, especially low birth weight (usually disappears by 3–6 months)	Upper left sternal border, axillae, and back	Crescendo-decrescendo, systolic	Louder supine
Patent ductus arteriosus	Turbulent flow as blood is shunted left to right from the aorta to the pulmonary artery	Can be innocent in newborns, abnormal if persists	Upper left sternal border	Continuous, machinery-like, louder in systole	

VENTRICULAR RATE

- Count the number of QRS complexes in typical 6-second ECG and multiply by 10.
- If the rate is irregular or fast, count R-R cycles in six large boxes, and then multiply by 50.

BRADYCARDIA

- Hypoxemia is a common cause of bradycardia in children.

TABLE 13-2.   Heart Rate by Age

AGE	NORMAL RANGE
0–1 month	95–180
1–6 months	110–180
6–12 months	110–170
1–3 years	90–150
4–5 years	65–135
6–8 years	60–130
8–16 years	60–110
Adult	60–100

- Many other causes: sleep, sedation, vagal stimulation (stooling, cough, or gag), hypothyroid, hyperkalemia, hypothermia, hypoglycemia, hypoxia, athletic heart, second- or third-degree atrioventricular (AV) block, junctional rhythm, increased intracranial pressure, medicine (i.e., digitalis, β blockers)

TACHYCARDIA

Found in fever, anxiety, pain, hypovolemia, sepsis, congestive heart failure (CHF), hyperthyroidism, supraventricular tachycardia (SVT), ventricular tachycardia, atrial flutter and fibrillation, medications (i.e., theophylline, stimulants)

RHYTHM

Check for sinus rhythm (depolarization originating from the sinus node):
- Verify a P wave is present before each QRS complex, and a QRS complex occurs after each P wave.
- Examine morphology: all P waves in a given lead should look the same.
- Normal P wave axis (0° to +90°) with upright P waves in leads I and aVF.
- Normal P wave:
  - <0.10 second in children (1/2 big box).
  - <0.08 second in infant (2 small boxes).

SINUS ARRHYTHMIA

This is a common, normal variation in heart rate due to inspiration and expiration.

ABNORMAL RHYTHMS

Premature Atrial Contraction (PAC)

- A premature P wave can be followed by a normal QRS and a compensatory pause, or it can be non-conducted.
- It has no hemodynamic significance.
- This is the most common arrhythmia in newborn infants; most cases self-resolve.

Premature Ventricular Contraction (PVC)

- Premature and wide QRS, no P wave, T wave opposite to QRS.
- May be benign if they are uniform and decrease with exercise.
- Must evaluate further for runs of multiple PVCs or if they occur regularly.

Atrial Flutter

- A rapid atrial rate (~300 bpm) in a sawtooth pattern, with a varying ventricular rate depending on degree of block (i.e., 2:1, 3:1).
- Normal QRS.
- Can suggest significant pathology (atrial enlargement).

Atrial Fibrillation

- Rapid atrial rate (350–600 bpm) with an irregularly irregular ventricular response.
- No P waves; normal QRS.
- Very rare in children and adolescents.
- Usually suggests significant pathology.

Supraventricular Tachycardia (SVT)

- Narrow QRS complex, no R-R interval variability, without discernible P waves.
- Sudden onset and resolution either spontaneously or with Valsalva maneuvers.
- Most often due to a reentrant tachycardia that uses the AV node or an accessory pathway in the reentrant circuit.
- Usually associated with structurally normal hearts.
- Most common tachyarrhythmia in infants and children.
- SVT with aberrant conduction producing wide QRS may look like V-tach.

Ventricular Tachycardia

- Series of 3 or more PVCs with a heart rate between 120 and 200 bpm.
- Wide, unusually shaped QRS complexes, indicating depolarization traveling outside of the His-Purkinje system.
- T waves in the opposite direction of the QRS complex.
- Usually suggests significant pathology and should be terminated electrically (if unstable) or medically (if stable).

Ventricular Fibrillation

- Very irregular QRS complexes without P waves.
- The rate is rapid and irregular.
- This is a terminal arrhythmia. The heart cannot fill and maintain effective circulation; the rhythm should be terminated with an AED.

AXIS

QRS Axis

- Examine leads I and aVF.
    - If net positive deflection in lead I, the axis range is between +90° and −90°.
    - If net positive deflection in lead aVF, the QRS is also between 0° and +180°.
- Superimpose the ranges. The region of overlap is the quadrant where the QRS lies.
- If positive (upward) in I and aVF, the axis is normal.

EXAM TIP

Axis Summary

Normal = [+] in lead I, [+] in aVF

I[+], aVF[−] = Left-axis deviation

I[−], aVF[+] = Right-axis deviation

I[−], aVF[−] = Extreme-axis deviation (direction based on Q wave).

Abnormal Axis

- Right-axis deviation (RAD): severe pulmonary stenosis with right ventricular hypertrophy (RVH), pulmonary hypertension (HTN), conduction disturbances (RBBB).
- Left-axis deviation (LAD) with RVH is highly suggestive of AV canal; consider especially with Down syndrome.
- Mild LAD with left-ventricular hypertrophy (LVH) in a cyanotic infant suggests tricuspid atresia.

P Axis

- Normal is [+] deflection in II, [−] in aVR. This defines sinus rhythm and normally related atria (atrial situs solitus).
- P axis > +90° suggests atrial inversion, an ectopic atrial rhythm, or misplaced leads.

ABNORMAL WAVE PATTERNS AND VOLTAGES

Abnormal Q Waves

- New onset Q waves or waves of increased duration may represent myocardial infarction (MI).
- Causes of ischemia and infarction: anomalous origin of left coronary artery from pulmonary artery, coronary artery aneurysm and thrombosis in Kawasaki disease, asphyxia, cardiomyopathy, severe aortic stenosis, myocarditis, cocaine use.
- A deep, wide Q wave in aVL is a marker for LV infarction. Suspect anomalous origin of left coronary artery, particularly in a child <2 months old.

ST Segment

- End of S to beginning of T.
- Causes of ST displacement: pericarditis, myocarditis, cor pulmonale, pneumopericardium, head injury, pneumothorax.
- Elevation may result from ischemia or pericarditis.

T Wave

- Peaked, pointed T waves occur with **hyperkalemia**, LVH, and head injury.
- Flattened T waves are seen in **hypokalemia** and hypothyroidism.

Right Atrial Enlargement

- Peaked P waves (leads II and V1).
- Causes include cor pulmonale (pulmonary HTN, RVH), anomalous pulmonary venous connection, large ASD, or Ebstein's anomaly.

Left Atrial Enlargement

- Wide P wave (notched in II, deep terminal inversion in V1).
- Causes include VSD, PDA, mitral stenosis, or regurgitation.
- Wider and deeper terminal components suggest more severe enlargement.

Right Ventricular Hypertrophy (RVH)

- RAD alone is not enough as a criterion for RVH; other criteria exist.
- Causes include ASD, TAPVR, pulmonary stenosis, tetralogy of Fallot (TOF), large VSD with pulmonary HTN, and coarctation in the newborn.

Left Ventricular Hypertrophy (LVH)

- Excessive LAD supports LVH but is insufficient to make the diagnosis.
- Causes include VSD, PDA, anemia, complete AV block, aortic stenosis, systemic HTN, obstructive, and nonobstructive hypertrophic cardiomyopathies.

Combined Ventricular Hypertrophy (CVH)

- If criteria for RVH exist and left-ventricular forces exceed normal mean values for age, the patient has CVH. If LVH is present, similar reasoning may apply to the diagnosis of RVH.
- Causes include left-to-right shunts with pulmonary HTN (large VSD) and complex structural heart disease.
- Cannot diagnose ventricular hypertrophy in the absence of normal conduction (RBBB).

Decreased QRS Voltage

- <5 mm in limb leads.
- Causes include pericardial effusion, pericarditis, and hypothyroidism.
- Some normal newborns have reduced voltages.

Wolff-Parkinson-White Syndrome

- Ventricular preexcitation via accessory (Bundle of Kent) conduction pathway.
- Accessory pathway conducts more rapidly but takes longer to recover.
- Shortened PR interval, widened QRS caused by slurred upstroke (**delta wave**).
- Associated with Ebstein's anomaly.
- Increased risk of SVT and sudden death.
- Treatment: antiarrhythmic medications; definitive therapy is surgical ablation of accessory pathway.

> **EXAM TIP**
>
> Causes of Sudden Cardiac Deaths in Young Athlete:
> - Hypertrophic cardiomyopathy (HOCM)
> - Arrhythmogenic right ventricular cardiomyopathy
> - Congenital coronary artery anomalies
> - Aortic rupture with Marfan syndrome
> - Wolff-Parkinson-White syndrome
> - Congenital long QT syndrome

Basics of Echocardiography

- Trans-thoracic echocardiography (TTE): this is the most commonly used method to delineate cardiac anatomy.
- Transesophageal echocardiography: a transducer is introduced into the esophagus to enhance imaging during cardiac surgery or catheterization.
- Fetal Echocardiography: for the prenatal diagnosis and counseling of congenital heart diseases (CHD)
  - Indications: abnormal obstetric ultrasound, extracardiac anomalies, chromosomal abnormalities, increased first-trimester nuchal translucency measurement (trisomy 21 and Turner syndrome), family history of CHD, maternal disease (lupus, diabetes, phenylketonuria).

Interpretation of Pediatric Chest X-Rays

HEART SIZE

Cardiothoracic Ratio

- Measure largest heart width and divide by the largest chest diameter. A normal ratio is <0.6.
- The CXR requires a good inspiratory effort, which is difficult to accomplish in newborns and infants.
- Cardiomegaly on CXR is most suggestive of volume overload.

> **EXAM TIP**
>
> In newborns and small infants, the upper aspects of the heart are obscured by a large "boat sail–shaped" opacity—the thymus. This organ will involute after puberty. It is often not seen in premature newborns.

PULMONARY VASCULAR MARKINGS

Increased Pulmonary Vascular Markings

- Visualization of pulmonary vasculature in the lateral third of the lung field; this represents increased pulmonary vascular blood flow.
- In an **acyanotic** child, causes include ASD, VSD, PDA, or endocardial cushion defect (**left to right shunting**).
- In a **cyanotic** child, causes include transposition of the great vessels, TAPVR, hypoplastic left heart syndrome, persistent truncus arteriosus, or single ventricle (**right to left shunting**).

Decreased Pulmonary Vascular Markings

- The lung fields are dark, with small vessels.
- Seen in conditions limiting pulmonary vascular blood flow, such as pulmonary stenosis and atresia, tricuspid stenosis and atresia, and tetralogy of Fallot with severe pulmonary stenosis or atresia, and some conditions causing pulmonary HTN.

Pulmonary Venous Congestion

- Manifested as hazy lung fields.
- Kerley B lines may be present (short horizontal lines in the periphery representing intralobular septae).
- Caused by LV failure or pulmonary vein obstruction, causing pulmonary venous HTN.
- Seen in mitral stenosis, TAPVR, hypoplastic left-heart syndrome, or any left-sided obstructive lesion with heart failure.

> **WARD TIP**
>
> Conditions that cause right-to-left shunts lead to cyanosis. Conditions that cause left-to-right shunting lead to CHF and pulmonary vascular congestion.

ABNORMAL CARDIAC SILHOUETTES

Tetralogy of Fallot

- A "boot-shaped" heart with decreased pulmonary vascular markings is sometimes seen. The shape is due to the hypoplastic main pulmonary artery and RVH.

Transposition of the Great Vessels

- An "egg-shaped" heart is sometimes seen.
- The narrow superior aspect of the cardiac silhouette is due to the absence of the thymus and the irregular relationship of the great arteries.

Total Anomalous Pulmonary Venous Return with Supracardiac Venous Drainage.

- A "snowman" shape is sometimes seen.
- The left vertical vein, left innominate (brachiocephalic) vein, and dilated superior vena cava create the "snowman's" head.

Rheumatic Fever (RF)

DEFINITION

- RF is a delayed immunologic sequela of a group A streptococcal pharyngeal infection.
- Cutaneous streptococcal infection causes glomerulonephritis, not RF.
- RF affects the brain, heart, joints, and skin.

EXAM TIP

Rheumatic fever can cause long-term valvular disease, both stenosis and insufficiency.

WARD TIP

Carditis (inflammation of the heart) is a manifestation of rheumatic fever that can cause permanent cardiac damage. Therefore, once rheumatic fever is definitively diagnosed, anti-inflammatory therapy (with NSAIDS [e.g., naproxen] or prednisone in extreme cases) should be started.

WARD TIP

If a patient's arthritis does not improve within 48 hours of therapeutic aspirin therapy, the patient probably does not have rheumatic fever.

EXAM TIP

The chorea of rheumatic fever is known as Sydenham chorea, or St. Vitus' dance.

EPIDEMIOLOGY

- Incidence: common worldwide. It is uncommon in the U.S., but small outbreaks occur.
- Peak age range: 5–15 years.
- Increased risk with a positive family history of RF.
- RF risk after untreated strep pharyngitis is 1–3%.
- Follows pharyngitis by 1–5 weeks (average: 3 weeks).
- Rate of recurrent RF with subsequent strep infection approaches 60%.

CLINICAL FEATURES

Carditis

- Incidence: 30–70% of patients.
- Tachycardia is common.
- Heart murmur, most commonly valvulitis, in order of decreasing frequency:
  - Mitral valve regurgitation.
  - Aortic valve regurgitation.
  - Tricuspid valve regurgitation.
  - Pericarditis (may hear a friction rub).
  - Cardiomegaly.
  - CHF (may hear a gallop).

Arthritis

- It affects 40–70% of patients and is usually the first symptom of RF.
- Usually affects the large joints, but can affect the spine, temporomandibular and sternoclavicular joints.
- Migratory, affecting new joints as other affected joints resolve.
- Joints are red, warm, swollen, and very tender, particularly if moved.
- Responds well to aspirin therapy.
- Duration is usually <1 month, even without treatment.

Chorea

- Incidence: 10–30% of patients.
- Initial emotional lability: behaviors characteristic of attention deficit/hyperactivity and obsessive-compulsive disorders may precede the movement disorder.
- Loss of motor coordination.
- Spontaneous, purposeless movement.
- Motor weakness.
- Has a longer latent period than other symptoms, presenting 1–8 months after strep infection, lasts for months, and then slowly diminishes.

Erythema Marginatum

- Incidence: <15% of patients.
- Evanescent, migratory, pink, erythematous, nonpruritic macular rash.
- Often has a clear center and serpiginous outline.
- Disappears when cold, reappears when warm.
- Found primarily on the trunk and proximal extremities, but not on the face.

Subcutaneous Nodules

- Incidence: 0–10% of patients.
- Hard, painless, 0.5–1 cm swellings over bony prominences, primarily the extensor tendons of the hand, but also on the scalp and along the spine.
- Not transient, lasting for weeks.

DIAGNOSIS

- Acute rheumatic fever (ARF) is confirmed by fulfilling the modified Jones criteria.
- In addition to evidence of a preceding GAS infection, the initial diagnosis of ARF requires two "major" manifestations OR one "major" and two "minor" manifestations.
- Criteria vary between Low Risk groups and Moderate to High Risk groups.
  - Low Risk groups are defined as ARF incidence in the population ≤1/1000.
  - Moderate to High Risk groups are defined as ARF incidence in the population >1/1000.
- Major criteria include:
  - Carditis
  - Arthritis (Low Risk: polyarthritis; High Risk: mono OR polyarthritis, or polyarthralgia)
  - Chorea
  - Erythema marginatum
  - Subcutaneous nodules
- Minor criteria:
  - Arthralgia (Low Risk: polyarthralgia; High Risk: monoarthralgia)
  - Fever (Low Risk: ≥ 38.5°C; High Risk: ≥ 38°C)
  - Elevated ESR (Low Risk: ESR ≥ 60mm/hr; High Risk: ESR ≥ 30mm/hr) and/or CRP ≥ 3.0 mg/dL
  - Pronounced PR interval (unless carditis is a major criterion)
- Aschoff bodies (found in atrial myocardium) are diagnostic.
- Antistreptolysin O (ASO) antibody titer is the most common test. It is elevated in 80% of ARF patients and 20% of normal individuals.
- Other antibody tests exist (antihyaluronidase, antistreptokinase, antideoxyribonuclease B) wherein at least one will be positive in 85% of ARF patients.
- Positive throat cultures and "rapid strep tests" are less reliable; they do not differentiate acute infection versus chronic carrier state.

TREATMENT

- ARF patients should receive NSAIDS (e.g., naproxen) to reduce fever and alleviate arthritis symptoms, and penicillin (eradicate the streptococci). Although historically a first line anti-inflammatory agent, aspirin is used less commonly in pediatric ARF patients now.
- Patients allergic to penicillin can receive five days of azithromycin.
- Prophylaxis should be initiated:
  - Benzathine penicillin G IM every 3–4 weeks *or*
  - Penicillin PO three times per day *or*
  - Sulfadiazine PO once per day.
- The prophylaxis duration is often advocated at least throughout adolescence, if not indefinitely. Compliance becomes an issue.
- Most patients recover within six weeks, but the recurrence risk is 40–60%.

WARD TIP

Subcutaneous nodules in rheumatic fever have a significant association with carditis. They are painless and palpable nodules, usually found on extensor surfaces and over bony prominences. Subcutaneous nodules are also found in connective tissue diseases, such as systemic lupus erythematosus (SLE) and rheumatoid arthritis

WARD TIP

A history of sore throat or scarlet fever is insufficient evidence for rheumatic fever without a positive strep test.

WARD TIP

To diagnose rheumatic fever, patients must have laboratory evidence of preceding group A strep infection, **in addition to** a combination of "major" and "minor" symptoms collectively known as the "Jones criteria." These criteria were most recently updated in 2015 by the American Heart Association.

Endocarditis

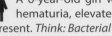

A 6-year-old girl with PDA develops fever and anorexia. Her Hgb is 9; she has hematuria, elevated ESR, positive rheumatoid factor, and immune complexes are present. *Think: Bacterial endocarditis.*
Predisposition: congenital heart disease
Greatest risk factor: systemic-pulmonary arterial communications such as PDA
Possible additional findings: chronic anemia, microscopic hematuria, elevated ESR, positive rheumatoid factor, circulating immune complexes, and low complement levels.

EXAM TIP

If a child has a cyanotic congenital heart disease with a positive blood culture, suspect endocarditis.

ETIOLOGY

- α-Hemolytic streptococci are most common (70%): *Streptococcus pneumoniae* and *Streptococcus viridans.*
- *Staphylococcus aureus* accounts for 20% of cases.
- If related to cardiac surgery complications, *Staphylococcus epidermidis,* gram-negative bacilli, and fungi should be considered.
- In culture-negative endocarditis, consider *Coxiella burnetii* or *Bartonella.*
- Most endocarditis in children is left-sided.

PATHOPHYSIOLOGY

- Turbulent blood flow across an abnormal valve: congenitally abnormal (bicuspid or atretic), damaged by RF or other mechanism, or a prosthetic replacement.
- Turbulent blood flow from another cardiac defect across a normal valve.

SIGNS AND SYMPTOMS

- Fever is the most common symptom.
- New or changing heart murmur.
- Chest pain, dyspnea, arthralgia, myalgia, headache.
- Embolic phenomena:
  - Hematuria with red cell casts.
  - Acute brain ischemia (embolic stroke caused by septic emboli).
  - Roth spots, splinter hemorrhages, Osler nodes, Janeway lesions (less common in children).

WARD TIP

Janeway lesions—
Small, painless, erythematous, on palms and soles
Caused by septic embolic that create micro-abscesses and necrosis of the dermis.
Osler nodes—
Red, painful, on the hands and feet
Caused by immune complex deposition

PREDISPOSING CONDITIONS

- High risk:
  - Prosthetic cardiac valves.
  - Previous bacterial endocarditis (due to scar formation on valve).
  - Congenital heart disease: complex cyanotic types.
  - Surgical pulmonary-systemic shunts to correct cyanotic heart disease.
- Moderate risk:
  - Acquired valvular dysfunction (i.e., radiation therapy or lupus).
  - Rheumatic heart disease, Libman-Sacks valve (lupus associated nonbacterial endocarditis), antiphospholipid syndrome–associated valve disease.
- Hypertrophic cardiomyopathy.
- Complicated mitral-valve prolapse (valvular regurgitation, thickened valve leaflets).

DIAGNOSIS

- A least three sets of blood cultures over 48 hours from different sites.
- Most common findings:
  - Positive blood cultures.
  - Elevated ESR.

- Hematuria.
- Anemia.
- Echocardiographic evidence of vegetations or thrombi is diagnostic.

TREATMENT

- Four to eight weeks of organism-specific IV antibiotic therapy.
- Surgery is necessary for medically refractory endocarditis, and it is considered for prosthetic valves, fungal endocarditis, and hemodynamic compromise.

PROPHYLAXIS RECOMMENDATIONS FOR PATIENTS WITH STRUCTURAL HEART DISEASE

- American Heart Association guidelines from 2007, re-affirmed in 2021, have significantly narrowed the patient population who is to receive pre-procedure prophylaxis for infective endocarditis. This change is based on evidence that the majority of infective endocarditis episodes were from an oral source during routine daily activity. There is now a larger focus on daily oral care.
- Prophylaxis with oral amoxicillin (cephalexin, azithromycin, or clarithromycin if allergic) prior to a serious dental procedure that involves manipulation of the gingival tissue or periapical region of the teeth or disruption of the oral mucosa is now recommended only for patients with:
  - Prosthetic cardiac valves or prosthetic material used as part of a cardiac repair.
  - A previous history of infective endocarditis.
  - Unrepaired cyanotic congenital heart defect (CHD), or a repaired CHD with residual shunts, patches, or prosthetic devices.
  - A cardiac transplant with subsequent cardiac valvulopathy.
- Prophylaxis is *not* usually recommended with:
  - Shedding of primary teeth.
  - Dental x-rays.
  - Placement or adjustment of orthodontic appliances (braces, etc.).
  - Oral trauma with bleeding.

EXAM TIP

Risk Factors for Endocarditis:
- Previous endocarditis
- Dental procedures
- Indwelling central venous catheters
- IV drug use (usually affects the tricuspid valve)
- Cardiac transplant patients with valvulopathy
- Prior cardiac surgery with prosthetic material

Myocarditis

ETIOLOGY

- Viruses: Coxsackievirus, echovirus, COVID and adenovirus are most common causes.
- Immune-mediated diseases (e.g., ARF, Kawasaki disease).
- Toxic ingestions: alcohol, amphetamines, anthracyclines, clozapine.

EPIDEMIOLOGY

Clinically recognizable myocarditis is rare in the United States. Chagas disease is a common cause in developing countries.

PATHOPHYSIOLOGY

Heart-muscle inflammation, caused by an insult such as a viral infection, can cause dilated cardiomyopathy and heart failure.

SIGNS AND SYMPTOMS

- Depending on the injury, findings range from asymptomatic to fulminant CHF.
- Common symptoms are fever, dyspnea, GI/upper respiratory symptoms, and lethargy.
- Consider CHF in patients with tachycardia, tachypnea, and a gallop.

DIAGNOSIS

- ECG findings: sinus tachycardia, low voltages, nonspecific S-T changes, prolonged QT interval, premature beats.
- Radiology: chest radiographs will show cardiomegaly.
- Echocardiography: chamber enlargement is present with impaired ventricular function.
- Lab findings: elevated inflammatory markers, elevated troponin.
- Definitive diagnosis is made by myocardial biopsy or cardiac MRI.

TREATMENT

- Treat the underlying cause (i.e., antibiotics if bacterial, but most are viral).
- Treatment is largely supportive. Rest and activity limitation is important.
- CHF treatment may be needed (i.e., diuretics, inotropic agents). Consider gamma globulin.

Pericarditis

ETIOLOGY

- Viral (most common).
- Other causes: *S. aureus, Haemophilus influenzae, Neisseria meningitidis,* streptococci, tuberculosis.
- Acute rheumatic fever.
- Heart surgery complications.
- Collagen vascular diseases.
- Uremia.
- Medications (i.e., dantrolene, oncology agents).

PATHOPHYSIOLOGY

- Inflammation of the pericardium.
- Pericardial effusion; tamponade can result if significant fluid accumulates.

SIGNS AND SYMPTOMS

- Precordial pain with shoulder and neck radiation (often relieved by standing or leaning forward).
- Pericardial friction rub on auscultation.
- Signs of cardiac tamponade:
  - Distant heart sounds.
  - Tachycardia.
  - Pulsus paradoxus.
  - Hepatomegaly and venous distention.

DIAGNOSIS

- CXR: a pear- or water bottle–shaped heart indicates a large effusion.
- Echocardiography is diagnostic (can also detect tamponade).

TREATMENT

- Treat the underlying disease process, likely supportive (often viral).
- NSAIDS or steroids to decrease inflammation.
- Pericardiocentesis for hemodynamically significant effusions.
- Urgent drainage is indicated for tamponade symptoms.

Congestive Heart Failure (CHF)

ETIOLOGY

- Caused from either CHD or acquired heart disease.
- CHD: most common cause is from volume or pressure overload.
- VSD, PDA, and endocardial cushion defects are the most common causes of CHF in the first six months of life.
- ASD can cause CHF in adulthood with cor pulmonale, if unrepaired.
- Acquired heart disease:
    - Metabolic abnormalities (i.e., hypoxia, acidosis, hypoglycemia, hypocalcemia).
    - Myocarditis.
    - Rheumatic fever with carditis.
    - Cardiomyopathy.
    - Drug toxicity.

SIGNS AND SYMPTOMS

- Symptoms similar to those seen in respiratory illnesses: tachycardia, tachypnea, shortness of breath, rales and rhonchi, intercostal retractions.
- Poor weight gain/poor feeding.
- Cold sweat on forehead.
- Peripheral edema in older children.
- Gallop on auscultation.
- Hepatomegaly, jugular venous distention (JVD).

DIAGNOSIS

- CXR: cardiomegaly, evidence of pulmonary edema.
- Echo: enlarged ventricular chamber, impaired ventricular function.

TREATMENT

- Treat the underlying cause (i.e., surgical correction of CHD, correction of metabolic defects).
- Oxygen for patients with hypoxic or in respiratory distress.
- Medication:
    - Digitalis is used to improve ventricular function. It is contraindicated in complete heart block and hypertrophic cardiomyopathy.
    - Diuretics are used to decrease volume overload and pulmonary edema. The most common are the "loop diuretics" (i.e., furosemide).
    - Afterload-reducing agents (i.e., angiotensin-converting enzyme [ACE] inhibitors, calcium channel blockers, nitroglycerin) are used to dilate peripheral vasculature and thus decrease the work on the heart.

WARD TIP

Bedside ultrasonography is useful in the aiding diagnosis of pericarditis with effusion and in cases of tamponade.

WARD TIP

The onset of CHF is dependent on the fall of pulmonary vascular resistance and the subsequent increased left-to-right shunting.

WARD TIP

A left-to-right shunt usually takes about six weeks to become significant enough to stress the left ventricle.

WARD TIP

Use of diuretics in CHF is preferred to salt and fluid restriction. Watch out for hypokalemia since some diuretics, loop diuretics specifically, cause significant potassium loss. Hypokalemia can also precipitate digitalis toxicity.

Vasculitides

HENOCH-SCHÖNLEIN PURPURA (HSP) (SEE CHAPTER 21)

KAWASAKI DISEASE

> A 2-year-old boy has seven days of fever reaching 104°F (40°C), develops nonexudative conjunctival injection bilaterally; intensely erythematous lips, palms, and soles; generalized rash, and an enlarged, tender anterior-cervical lymph node. Blood cultures are sterile, and platelets are elevated. *Think: Kawasaki disease.*
>
> The fever lasts five or more days and at least four of the following features make the diagnosis: conjunctival injection, oropharyngeal mucous membrane changes, extremity swelling, polymorphous rash, and cervical lymphadenopathy. Coronary aneurysms and MI are the most serious consequences.

DEFINITION

- Also known as mucocutaneous lymph-node syndrome
- Most common acquired heart disease in children

ETIOLOGY

Acute vasculitis of mostly medium-sized arteries of unknown etiology

EPIDEMIOLOGY

- Affects infants and young children (>80% under age 4 years).
- More common in Asians than other racial groups.
- More common in males.
- Most common in winter/spring months.

SIGNS AND SYMPTOMS

Kawasaki disease is a clinical diagnosis; helpful findings include:
- Sterile pyuria.
- Aseptic meningitis.
- Thrombocytosis (usually after 7 days of fever).
- Desquamation of fingers and toes.
- Elevated ESR or CRP.
- Elevated transaminases.
- Most significant sequelae:
  - Coronary aneurysms (resolves within 12 months with therapy).
  - Pericardial effusion.
  - CHF

DIAGNOSIS

- Diagnostic criteria: fever for more than five days plus at least four of the following:
  1. Bilateral conjunctivitis (without exudate)
  2. Mucocutaneous lesions ("strawberry" tongue; dry, red, cracked lips; diffuse erythema of oral cavity)
  3. Erythema and/or edema of hands and/or feet
  4. Polymorphic rash (usually truncal)
  5. Cervical lymphadenopathy (>1.5 cm), usually unilateral
- Echocardiogram: conduct baseline study at diagnosis to evaluate for early coronary aneurysms; conduct a follow-up echo to establish presence or absence.

TREATMENT

- Used to prevent cardiac sequelae; the actual vasculitis self-resolves.
- Intravenous immune globulin (IVIG): usually, one dose reduces coronary-artery dilation incidence from 25% incidence to <4%.
- High-dose aspirin until 48–72 hours after fever defervescence.
- If no coronary artery abnormalities are present, administer low-dose aspirin for 6–8 weeks, or until normal platelet count and ESR.
- If coronary arteries are abnormal, continue anticoagulation indefinitely in consultation with a pediatric cardiologist.
- Steroid use is typically reserved for cases refractory to repeat doses of IVIG.

POLYARTERITIS NODOSA

DEFINITION

- A necrotizing inflammation of the small- and medium-sized muscular arteries.
- Involves renal and visceral vessels, spares pulmonary circulation.

SIGNS AND SYMPTOMS

- Prolonged fever, weight loss, malaise, subcutaneous nodules on extremities.
- Various rashes can be seen such as livedo reticularis.
- Often waxes and wanes.
- Distal extremity gangrene due to deep skin infarctions seen in severe disease.

DIAGNOSIS

- No diagnostic tests.
- Associated with thrombocytosis and leukocytosis; proteinuria, hematuria, and red cell casts; elevated acute-phase reactants, and perinuclear anti-neutrophil cytoplasmic antibody (p-ANCA).
- Conclusive with findings of medium-sized artery aneurysms.
- Coronary-artery aneurysms on echocardiogram are diagnostic if other clinical evidence is present.

TREATMENT

- Corticosteroids suppress the clinical manifestations.
- Cyclophosphamide or azathioprine may be required to induce remission.

TAKAYASU ARTERITIS (AORTOARTERITIS)

DEFINITION

- A large vessel vasculitis of unknown cause.
- Chronic inflammatory disease involving:
  - Aorta.
  - Arterial branches from the aorta.
  - Pulmonary vasculature.

PATHOPHYSIOLOGY

- Lesions are segmental and often obliterative.
- Aneurysmal and saccular dilation also occur.
- Thoracoabdominal aorta is the predominantly affected site in pediatrics.

EPIDEMIOLOGY

Most patients are female, aged 4–45 years.

EXAM TIP

Reye syndrome is associated with aspirin therapy during an infection with any viral etiology, commonly influenza or varicella. It presents as a progressive encephalopathy with liver dysfunction. Therefore, the use of aspirin in children for Kawasaki disease is an exception to its general avoidance in pediatrics.

WARD TIP

Hypertension and abdominal pain can be important diagnostic clues in the diagnosis of polyarteritis nodosa.

WARD TIP

Infantile polyarteritis nodosa occurs before the age of 2 years and most commonly causes coronary-artery aneurysms. Diagnosis is made postmortem because it clinically mimics Kawasaki disease.

EXAM TIP

Takayasu arteritis is also known as "pulseless disease" because peripheral artery pulses can be absent, decreased, or unequal.

EXAM TIP

Essentially, Takayasu arteritis is giant cell arteritis of the aorta (and large branches).

EXAM TIP

In central cyanosis, systemic arterial desaturation is found. In peripheral cyanosis, systemic arterial oxygenation is normal, but increased oxygen extraction by the tissues is noted.

EXAM TIP

Cyanotic Heart Defects
Five T's and a P:
Truncus arteriosus
Transposition of the great vessels
Tricuspid atresia
Tetralogy of Fallot
Total anomalous pulmonary venous return (obstructive)
Pulmonic atresia

WARD TIP

Children with congenital heart disease are at increased risk for ischemic stroke.

WARD TIP

Key features of TOF:
- **VSD** (typically large enough to equalize pressures in right and left ventricles)
- **RVOTO** (e.g., pulmonary stenosis)
- **Aortic override** is variable.
- **RVH** is secondary to the RVOTO.

WARD TIP

Conotruncal facies is also described in DiGeorge syndrome. Children have hypertelorism, lateral displacement of the inner canthi, a flat nasal bridge, narrow palpebral fissures, and ear anomalies.

SIGNS AND SYMPTOMS

- Many patients have LV dysfunction and CHF (even without coronary-artery involvement, HTN, or valvular abnormalities).
- A lymphocytic infiltration consistent with myocarditis is present in about 50% of patients.
- Other symptoms include fever, polyarthralgia, polyarthritis, and loss of radial pulsations.

TREATMENT

Corticosteroids may induce remission.

Cyanotic Heart Defects

CENTRAL CYANOSIS VS. ACROCYANOSIS

Central cyanosis:
- Involves mucous membrane, often evident as blue-tinged lips.
- Is always pathologic in a newborn.
- In neonates is usually due to either pulmonary or cardiac disease.
- Has >5 mg/dL of deoxyhemoglobin.

Acrocyanosis:
- Involves distal extremities.
- Is normal in newborns.
- Related to peripheral cyanosis due to cold exposure and reduced peripheral perfusion.

TETRALOGY OF FALLOT (TOF)

The most common form of cyanotic CHD in the post-infancy period.

DEFINITION

Four anomalies constitute the tetralogy (Figure 13-2A)

1. Right ventricular outflow tract obstruction (RVOTO)
2. VSD
3. Overriding aorta
4. RVH

ETIOLOGY

Associated prenatal factors include maternal rubella or viral illness.

PATHOPHYSIOLOGY

The severity of the RVOT obstruction dictates the degree of shunting:
- Minimal obstruction: pulmonary blood flow will increase across the VSD as the PVR decreases, eventually causing CHF.
- Mild obstruction: hemodynamic balance pressure between right and left ventricles is equal, thus no net shunting ("pink tet").
- Severe obstruction: blood cannot exit through the RVOT; pulmonary blood flow decreases causing cyanosis.

EPIDEMIOLOGY

This is the most common cyanotic heart defect in children who survive infancy.

SIGNS AND SYMPTOMS

- Failure to thrive (FTT), if diagnosed late.
- "Conotruncal facies."
- Variable cyanosis (clubbing later if unrepaired).
- RV impulse; single S2, systolic ejection murmur at the upper-left sternal border with or without ejection click.
- Squatting is a common posture in older children with uncorrected TOF.
  - This often occurs after exercise.
  - Desaturated blood is trapped in the lower extremities and SVR is increased, but the RVOT is fixed. Squatting causes a decrease in the R to L shunt, increased pulmonary blood flow, and increased arterial saturation.

"TET SPELLS"

- Most common: 2–6 months of age.
- Occur in the morning or after a nap when SVR is low.
- Precipitating factors:
  - Stress
  - Drugs that decrease SVR.
  - Hot baths.
  - Fever.
  - Exercise.
- Mechanism: unknown, but it is likely due to increased cardiac output with fixed RVOT, causing increased right-to-left shunting and cyanosis.
- If prolonged or severe: syncope, seizures, cardiac arrest.

DIAGNOSIS

- CXR (Figure 13-2).
- "Boot-shaped heart."
- Decreased pulmonary vascular markings.
- Right aortic arch (25%).

WARD TIP

During a "Tet spell" (a paroxysmal cyanotic event), the object is to increase systemic vascular resistance (SVR) or reduce pulmonary hypertension to reduce the right-to-left shunting. Strategies include lifting legs to chest, squatting, giving oxygen, or giving morphine (which reduces infundibular spasm resulting in increased pulmonary blood flow).

WARD TIP

CXR with the boot shape, decreased pulmonary vascular markings, and a right aortic arch. *Think: tetralogy of Fallot.*

WARD TIP

The Blalock-Thomas-Taussig shunt increases pulmonary blood flow by grafting the subclavian or carotid artery to the pulmonary artery.

Tetralogy of Fallot

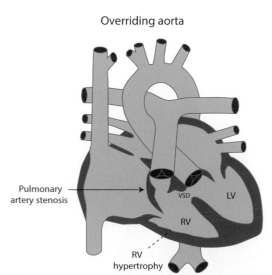

Overriding aorta

Pulmonary artery stenosis

VSD

LV

RV

RV hypertrophy

Figure 13-2A

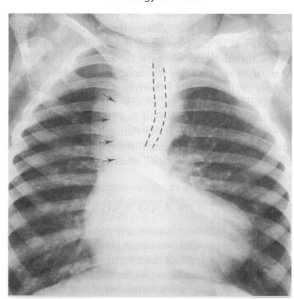

Figure 13-2B

FIGURE 13-2. **Figure 13-2A. Diagram of tetralogy of Fallot. Figure 13-2B. Chest x-ray in tetralogy of Fallot.** Arrows indicate right-sided aortic arch and upper thoracic aorta. Dashed lines indicate right-sided aortic indentation on the air bronchogram. (X-ray reproduced, with permission, from Rudolph CD, et al (eds). *Rudolph's Pediatrics*, 21st ed. New York: McGraw-Hill, 2002: 1821.)

TREATMENT

- The patient's clinical status may prevent definitive repair initially.
- Shunting (i.e., Blalock-Thomas-Taussig [BTT] shunt) is often used when pulmonary stenosis is severe, requiring an alternative route for blood to reach the lungs.
- Complete repair entails:
  - VSD closure.
  - Relief of RVOTO.
  - Ligation of shunts.
  - ASD/patent foramen ovale (PFO) closure.

TRANSPOSITION OF THE GREAT VESSELS

This is the most common cyanotic heart lesion in the newborn period.

PATHOPHYSIOLOGY

This lesion occurs when, in the development of the heart, the primitive heart loops to the left instead of the right and the following result (see Figure 13-3):
- Aorta originates from the RV.
- Pulmonary artery (PA) originates from LV.
- **A**orta is **a**nterior; **p**ulmonary trunk is **p**osterior.
- Right and left hearts are in parallel:
  - Pulmonary venous return goes to the pulmonary artery via the left ventricle.
  - Systemic venous return goes to the aorta via the right ventricle.
- Requires a mixing lesion for survival, i.e., VSD, ASD, or PDA (Table 13-3).
- A PDA alone is often insufficient in the extrauterine environment.
- Cyanosis becomes more prevalent with the closure of the PDA.
- Presentation: CHF in the first week of life.
- CXR: egg-shaped heart with a narrow mediastinum. Cardiomegaly with increased pulmonary vascular marking.

TRUNCUS ARTERIOSUS

DEFINITION

- A single arterial trunk that emerges from the ventricles, supplying the coronary, pulmonary, and systemic circulations (see Figure 13-4).
- Association: DiGeorge syndrome.

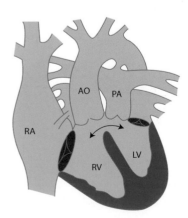

FIGURE 13-3. **Transposition of the great vessels.**

TABLE 13-3. **Characteristics of Transposition of Great Vessels**

INTACT VENTRICULAR SEPTUM (WITH NO VALVE ABNORMALITY)	WITH VSD (A LARGE VSD ALLOWS ADEQUATE MIXING)
SIGNS AND SYMPTOMS	
▪ Early cyanosis, a single S2, and no murmur	▪ Symptoms are related to ↑ pulmonary blood flow, with CHF sometimes occurring early.
▪ An intact atrial septum or very restrictive PFO is a medical emergency.	▪ May have little cyanosis
DIAGNOSIS	
▪ ECG will be normal initially but will demonstrate right-ventricular hypertrophy by 1 month.	▪ ECG: right or biventricular hypertrophy
▪ CXR: "Egg on a string"	
TREATMENT	
▪ Patient is "ductal dependent" and will require prostaglandin E1 (PGE1) to keep the PDA patent.	▪ PA band to control ↑ pulmonary blood flow
▪ Early balloon atrial septostomy (BAS) is necessary to allow mixing of oxygenated and deoxygenated blood.	▪ Arterial switch with VSD closure is definitive.
▪ Arterial switch procedure is definitive.	

TYPES

- **I**: Short common pulmonary trunk arising from right side of the common trunk, just above truncal valve.
- **II**: Pulmonary arteries (PAs) arise directly from the ascending aorta, from the posterior surface.
- **III**: This type is similar to type II, with PAs arising more laterally and more distant from truncal valves.

PATHOPHYSIOLOGY

- The truncal valve has 1–6 leaflets and is often poorly functioning.
- The truncus overrides a VSD.

SIGNS AND SYMPTOMS

- Presentation: CHF and cyanosis in the first week.
- Initial left-to-right shunt symptoms include:
  - Dyspnea.
  - Frequent respiratory infections.
  - FTT

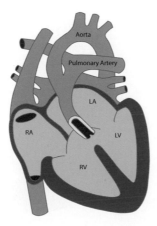

FIGURE 13-4. **Truncus arteriosus.**

- If the pulmonary vascular resistance increases, so will the cyanosis.
- The second heart sound is prominent and single due to the single semilunar valve.
- Peripheral pulses are strong, often bounding.
- Often, a systolic ejection click can be appreciated.

DIAGNOSIS

CXR shows cardiomegaly and increased pulmonary vascular markings.

TREATMENT

- Conduct surgery (Rastelli procedure) by 3–4 months of age to preclude pulmonary vascular disease.
- VSD is surgically closed, leaving the valve on the LV side.
- The PAs are freed from the truncus and connected to a valved conduit, which serves as the new pulmonary trunk.

HYPOPLASTIC LEFT HEART SYNDROME (HLHS)

DEFINITION

The syndrome consists of the following (see Figure 13-5):
- Aortic valve stenosis or atresia, with or without mitral valve stenosis or atresia.
- Hypoplasia of the ascending aorta.
- LV hypoplasia or agenesis.
- The result is a single (right) ventricle providing blood to the pulmonary system, the systemic circulation via the PDA, and coronary system via retrograde flow after crossing the PDA.
- In utero:
  - All systemic blood flow is ductus dependent.
  - Pulmonary resistance > systemic vascular resistance.
  - Normal perfusion pressure is maintained with right-to-left PDA shunt.
- At birth:
  - PDA closes.
  - Systemic vascular resistance > pulmonary resistance.
  - PDA closure → decreased cardiac output and decreased systemic perfusion → metabolic acidosis.
  - Thus, the lesion is PDA dependent until definitive intervention.

EPIDEMIOLOGY

- This is the second-most common CHD, presenting in the first week of life.
- This is the most common cause of death from CHD in the first month of life.

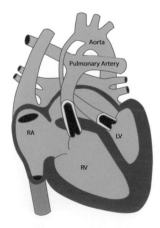

FIGURE 13-5. **Hypoplastic left heart syndrome.** Note small size of left ventricle.

SIGNS AND SYMPTOMS

- Pulses range from normal to absent (depending on ductal patency).
- Hyperdynamic RV impulse.
- Single S2 of increased intensity.
- Nonspecific systolic murmur at left-sternal border.
- Skin may have a characteristic grayish pallor.

DIAGNOSIS

- CXR: cardiomegaly with globular-shaped heart; increased pulmonary vascular markings, pulmonary edema.
- Echocardiogram is diagnostic, and HLHS is often detected in utero.

TREATMENT

- Although treatment and outcomes have improved, high mortality and a complicated surgical course result in ethical dilemmas in some cases.
- Three-stage surgery:
  1. Norwood procedure: the pulmonary trunk is used to reconstruct the hypoplastic aorta; the right ventricle now becomes the functional left ventricle. The pulmonary blood flow is then reestablished via systemic to pulmonary conduits either from the subclavian artery (BTT shunt) or from the right ventricle (Sano shunt).
  2. Bidirectional Glenn procedure: the superior vena cava (SVC) is connected to the right PA, restoring partial venous return to the lungs. The systemic-to-pulmonary shunt placed during the Norwood procedure is removed.
  3. Fontan procedure: the inferior vena cava is anastomosed to the PAs, resulting in venous diversion from the systemic circulation to the lungs.
- Heart transplant: a primary alternative if an organ is available or if palliative surgeries are insufficient.

Acyanotic Heart Defects

Left-to-right shunt (see Figure 13-6).

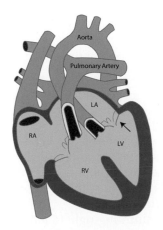
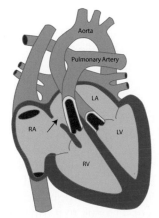
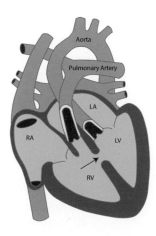
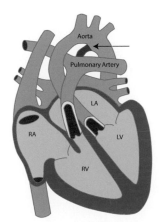

| Subendocardial cushion defect | Atrial septal defect | Ventricular septal defect | Patent ductus arteriosus |

FIGURE 13-6.   Acyanotic heart defects.

SUBENDOCARDIAL CUSHION DEFECT

PATHOPHYSIOLOGY

An abnormal AV canal (endocardial cushions) development resulting in:
- VSD.
- An ostium primum ASD.
- Clefts in the mitral and tricuspid valves or a common AV valve.

EPIDEMIOLOGY

- Association: Down syndrome.
- Also frequently found with asplenia and polysplenia syndromes.

SIGNS AND SYMPTOMS

- Often the result of the specific components of the accumulated defects:
  - Holosystolic murmur from the VSD, if restrictive.
  - Systolic murmur from mitral and tricuspid valve insufficiency.
- High risk of developing Eisenmenger syndrome.
- ECG: superior QRS axis, RVH, RBBB, LVH, and a prolonged PR interval.

TREATMENT

Surgical correction is sometimes the only option (despite high risk) when patient has an unbalanced AV canal.

ATRIAL SEPTAL DEFECT (ASD)

This defect represents 10% of all congenital heart disease.

DEFINITION

Three types:
- Secundum defect (50–70%): located in the central portion of the atrial septum.
- Primum defect (30%):
  - Located at the atrial lower margin.
  - Associated with mitral and tricuspid valve abnormalities.
- Sinus venosus defect (about 10%): located at the upper portion of the atrial septum and often extends into the SVC; results in anomalous return of the right upper-pulmonary vein to the right atrium.

EPIDEMIOLOGY

- A common "co-conspirator" in CHD.
- As many as 50% of CHD patients have an ASD as one of the defects.
- More common in females.

SIGNS AND SYMPTOMS

- Children with ASDs are typically asymptomatic.
- Widely split and fixed S2 because right-sided volume overload causes delayed pulmonic value closing. Murmurs are uncommon, but they may occur as patient gets older. Murmur is a secondary pulmonary flow murmur.
- Symptoms of CHF and pulmonary HTN occur in adults (second and third decades) due to persistent right-side overload.
- Can lead to strokes or TIA due to a thrombus shunting right to left.

DIAGNOSIS

- ECG: the left-to-right shunt may produce right-atrial enlargement and RVH.
- CXR: cardiomegaly with increased pulmonary vascular markings occurs.

TREATMENT

- Nearly 90% will close spontaneously.
- One hundred percent close if <3 mm.
- ASDs >8 mm are unlikely to close spontaneously.
- Surgical or catheter closure ("clamshell" or "umbrella" device) if needed.

PATENT FORAMEN OVALE (PFO)

- Prenatally, the PFO delivers oxygenated blood from the placenta to the left atrium.
- It functionally closes when increased left-atrial pressure causes the septa to press against each other, although some remain "probe-patent" into adulthood.
- Occasionally, the atrial septum tissue insufficiently covers the foramen (insufficient growth or it is stretched from increased pressure or volume).
- Some CHDs require a PFO for survival (tricuspid and mitral atresia, TAPVR).

VENTRICULAR SEPTAL DEFECT (VSD)

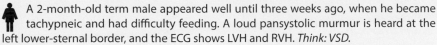 A 2-month-old term male appeared well until three weeks ago, when he became tachypneic and had difficulty feeding. A loud pansystolic murmur is heard at the left lower-sternal border, and the ECG shows LVH and RVH. *Think: VSD.*

Small VSD causes no symptoms. Large VSD may result in left-to-right shunt and pulmonary HTN. Left-sided volume overload and RVH are suggestive of a large VSD.

> **EXAM TIP**
>
> VSD is the most common congenital heart disorder requiring intervention in children.

EPIDEMIOLOGY

- The most common form of recognized CHD (30–60% of all CHDs).
- Usually membranous, as opposed to in the muscular septum.
- Occurs in 2 per 1000 live births.

SIGNS AND SYMPTOMS

Dependent on defect size:
- Small VSDs:
    - Usually asymptomatic.
    - Normal growth and development.
    - High-pitched, holosystolic murmur (more turbulent flow).
    - No ECG or CXR changes.
- Large VSDs:
    - Can cause CHF and pulmonary HTN.
    - May have FTT.
    - Lower-pitched murmur (less turbulent flow); intensity dependent on the degree of shunting.

> **EXAM TIP**
>
> Spontaneous closure occurs in 30–50% of VSDs.

DIAGNOSIS

- ECG: LVH.
- CXR: cardiomegaly with increased pulmonary vascular markings.

TREATMENT

- With a spontaneous closure:
    - Muscular defects often close in the first year of life (up to 50%).
    - Inlet and infundibular defects do not reduce in size or close.
- Intervention required for CHF, pulmonary HTN, and growth failure.
- Initial management with diuretics and digitalis.
- Surgical closure is indicated when medical therapy fails.
- Catheter-induced closure less commonly used than with ASDs.

Patent Ductus Arteriosus (PDA)

PATHOPHYSIOLOGY

- This is most often a problem in premature neonates.
  - Left-to-right shunts are poorly handled by premature infants.
  - Many develop idiopathic respiratory distress syndrome
  - Some progress to develop left-ventricular failure
- Failure of spontaneous closure:
  - Premature infants: failure is due to ineffective response to oxygen tension.
  - Mature infants: failure is due to structural abnormality of ductal smooth muscle.

EPIDEMIOLOGY

- PDA is more common in females.
- An increased incidence is noted at higher altitudes (lower atmospheric oxygen tension).
- First trimester maternal rubella is a cause of PDA.

SIGNS AND SYMPTOMS

- Small PDAs usually are asymptomatic.
- Large PDAs have higher incidence of lower-respiratory tract infections and CHF.
- The machinery-like murmur is louder with supination.
- Bounding peripheral pulses and wide pulse pressure
- If Eisenmenger syndrome results, lower-extremity cyanosis occurs (oxygen poor blood mixes into the aorta distal to the subclavian arteries).

TREATMENT

- Indomethacin is used in premature infants. It inhibits prostaglandin synthesis, resulting in closure.
- Catheter closure via devices such as double-umbrella devices and coils.
- Surgical ligation and division via a left-lateral thoracotomy
  - An occasional complication is recurrent laryngeal nerve injury (hoarseness).
- Eisenmenger syndrome is a contraindication to closure.

PDA-Dependent Congenital Heart Abnormalities

- PDA-dependent congenital heart abnormalities include:
  - Tetralogy of Fallot, with severe pulmonary stenosis.
  - Tricuspid atresia.
  - Aortic coarctation (severe).
  - Pulmonic atresia.
  - Hypoplastic left heart.
- Using prostaglandin E_1 (PGE_1) to keep the ductus open can be lifesaving in a cyanotic newborn with PDA-dependent CHD.
- CHD presenting in first two to three weeks of life are usually ductal-dependent lesions.

INDICATIONS FOR PGE₁ ADMINISTRATION

- Critically ill newborn with:
  - Suspected LV outflow tract obstruction.

- Side effects:
  - Apnea: endotracheal intubation prior to transport.
  - Fever, hypotension, and seizures.
- Do not delay PGE_1 administration in critically ill neonates with suspected ductal-dependent CHDs pending definitive diagnosis.

Eisenmenger Syndrome

- This syndrome can occur in unrepaired left-to-right shunts (i.e., VSD) that cause an increased pressure load on the pulmonary vasculature.
- Pulmonary vasculature pressure overload can result in irreversible arteriole changes.
- Pulmonary vascular obstructive disease may develop over several years.
- The pulmonary HTN reverses the left-to-right shunt.
- Persistent HTN maintains an enlarged right ventricle and can dilate the main pulmonary segment (evident on CXR).
- Avoidance via surgical correction of CHD is essential.

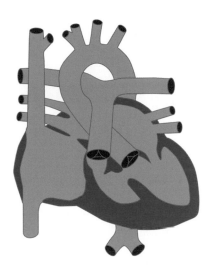

Tricuspid atresia

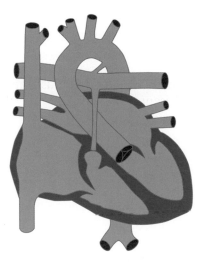

Pulmonary atresia

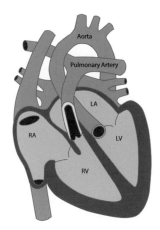

Aortic insufficiency

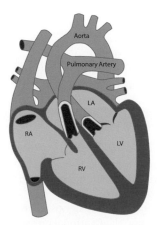

Mitral stenosis

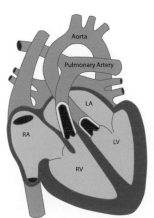

Mitral valve prolapse

FIGURE 13-7.   Congenital valvular defects.

Congenital Valvular Defects

TRICUSPID ATRESIA

DEFINITION

RV inlet is absent or nearly absent:

- Eighty-nine percent have no evidence of tricuspid valve tissue, only dimple.

EPIDEMIOLOGY

- ASD and/or VSD is usually present.
- Seventy-five percent have cyanosis within the first week.

SIGNS AND SYMPTOMS

LV impulse displaced laterally

DIAGNOSIS

ECG: LVH, prominent LV forces (due to decreased RV voltages)

TREATMENT

- PGE_1 to maintain ductal patency.
- Surgical intervention.
- Modified Blalock-Taussig shunt.
- Glenn procedure, followed by Fontan procedure.

PULMONARY ATRESIA (WITH INTACT VENTRICULAR SEPTUM)

SIGNS AND SYMPTOMS

- Cyanosis within hours of birth (PDA closing).
- Hypotension, tachypnea, acidosis.
- Often form fistulae between the RV and coronary arteries (high ischemia risk).
- Single S2, with a holosystolic murmur (tricuspid regurgitation).

DIAGNOSIS

- ECG: reduced RV forces and occasionally RVH.
- CXR: normal to enlarged RV with decreased pulmonary vascular markings.

TREATMENT

- PGE_1 to maintain ductal patency.
- Balloon atrial septostomy (less common).
- RVOT reconstruction with transannular patch or pulmonary valvotomy.
- ASD left open to prevent systemic venous HTN.

AORTIC STENOSIS

 A 4-year-old boy with recurrent episodes of syncope while playing has a harsh systolic murmur radiating to the carotids, diminished cardiac pulses, and severe LVH. *Think: Congenital aortic stenosis.*

Angina, syncope, and CHF are signs of aortic stenosis. Syncope during exertion occurs due to the reduced cerebral perfusion when arterial pressure declines. However, many patients are diagnosed prior to these symptoms based on the systolic murmur and echocardiography.

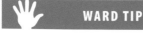
WARD TIP

Bicuspid aortic valve is the most common congenital heart defect, occurring in 1–2% of the population. This defect goes largely unrecognized. Bicuspid aortic valve predisposes to premature aortic valve calcification and stenosis.

EPIDEMIOLOGY

Eighty-five percent of congenitally stenotic aortic valves are bicuspid.

SIGNS AND SYMPTOMS

- Severe stenosis generally presents shortly after birth.
- Older children may complain of chest or stomach pain (epigastric).
- Untreated severe aortic stenosis is a risk factor for syncope and sudden death.
- The characteristic murmur is a crescendo-decrescendo systolic murmur.
- A systolic ejection click is also common (particularly if bicuspid aortic valve).
- In severe disease, paradoxical S2 splitting seen (split narrows with inspiration).

DIAGNOSIS

- Clinical findings, including ECG findings, and symptoms can be deceiving.
- Echo or catheterization to evaluate pressure differences between the aorta and left ventricle is essential.

TREATMENT

- Surgical valvotomy or interventional balloon valvuloplasty.
- Valvuloplasty is the most common intervention:
  - The indication is a measured cathetrization gradient >50 mm Hg.
  - There is a high incidence of recurrent stenosis.
- Valve replacement is deferred, when possible, until the patient completes growth.

EXAM TIP

Supravalvular aortic stenosis is associated with idiopathic hypercalcemia and with Williams syndrome.

AORTIC INSUFFICIENCY

EPIDEMIOLOGY

Uncommon and usually associated with mitral valve disease or aortic stenosis as in the case of rheumatic heart disease.

SIGNS AND SYMPTOMS

- A left upper-sternal border diastolic, decrescendo murmur is present.
- Presentation with symptoms indicates advanced disease.
- Chest pain and CHF are ominous signs.

DIAGNOSIS

CXR: LV enlargement, dilated ascending aorta

TREATMENT

- Valvuloplasty to treat aortic stenosis may worsen the insufficiency.
- Aortic valve replacement is the only definitive therapy.

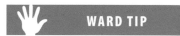

WARD TIP

Patients with Marfan syndrome frequently have aortic insufficiency as well.

MITRAL STENOSIS

 A 16-year-old girl complains of some shortness of breath. She was adopted from the Ukraine as a child, and her vaccination status is unknown. She has a diastolic murmur. *Think: mitral stenosis.*

Mitral stenosis is usually a sequela of untreated ARF, rarely seen in the United States. Diastolic murmurs are *always* pathologic.

EPIDEMIOLOGY

- It is rare in children, usually a sequela of ARF.
- Congenital forms are generally severe.

SIGNS AND SYMPTOMS

- When symptomatic, dyspnea is the most common symptom.
- Weak peripheral pulses with narrow pulse pressure.
- An opening snap is heard as atrial pressures snap open the stiff, calcified valve; a presystolic (late diastolic) murmur may be heard.
- Pulmonary venous congestion occurs, leading to:
    - CXR evidence of interstitial edema.
    - Hemoptysis from small bronchial vessel rupture.

TREATMENT

- Balloon valvuloplasty.
- Surgical:
    - Commissurotomy.
    - Valve replacement.

WARD TIP

Differentiate opening **snap** (mitral stenosis) and mid-systolic **click** (mitral prolapse).

MITRAL VALVE PROLAPSE

PATHOPHYSIOLOGY

Thick and redundant valve leaflets bulge into the mitral annulus.

EPIDEMIOLOGY

- Usually occurs in older children and adolescents.
- Has a familial component (autosomal dominant).
- Present in nearly all patients with Marfan syndrome.

SIGNS AND SYMPTOMS

- Auscultation: mid-systolic click and late systolic murmur.
- Often asymptomatic, but palpitations and chest pain can occur.

TREATMENT

Management is symptomatic (e.g., β-blocker for chest pain).

Other Congenital Cardiovascular Defects

COARCTATION OF THE AORTA

PATHOPHYSIOLOGY

- Most commonly found in the juxtaductal position (where the ductus arteriosus joins the aorta). (See Figure 13.8).
- Symptoms may develop with PDA closure (the PDA provides room for blood to reach the post-ductal aorta).

EPIDEMIOLOGY

- More common in males.
- Association: seen in one-third of patients with Turner syndrome.

WARD TIP

Coarctation of the aorta is associated with Turner syndrome.

WARD TIP

The presence of decreased pulses in the lower extremities is the clue for the diagnosis of coarctation.

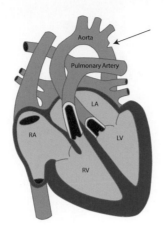

FIGURE 13-8. **Coarctation of the aorta.**

SIGNS AND SYMPTOMS

Clinical Presentation of Symptomatic Infants

- FTT, respiratory distress, and CHF develop in the first two to three months of life.
- Lower extremity changes include decreased lower extremity pulses.
- Acidosis may develop (the lower body receives insufficient blood).
- Usually, a murmur is heard over the left back.

Clinical Presentation of Asymptomatic Infants or Children

- Normal growth and development.
- Occasional complaint of leg weakness or pain after exertion.
- Decreased pulses in the lower extremities.
- Upper-extremity BPs greater than in the lower extremities.

DIAGNOSIS

CXR: "3 sign," dilated ascending aorta that displaces the SVC to the right.

TREATMENT

- Preferred: resection of the coarctation segment with end-to-end anastomosis.
- Allograft patch augmentation can also be used.
- Catheter balloon dilation can be used:
    - Has a higher restenosis rate than surgery.
    - Has an increased risk of producing aortic aneurysms.
    - Balloon dilation is used for stenosis at the surgical site of a primary re-anastomosis, or in older patients where a larger stent can be placed.

EBSTEIN ANOMALY

DEFINITION

Components of the defect (see Figure 13-9):
- The tricuspid valve is displaced apically in the right ventricle.
- The valve leaflets are redundant and plastered against the ventricular wall, often causing functional tricuspid or pulmonary atresia.
- The right atrium is frequently the largest structure.

EPIDEMIOLOGY

Without intervention:
- CHF occurs in first 6 months.
- Nearly 40% mortality.

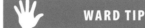
WARD TIP

Comparison of the right upper-extremity blood pressures and pulse oximeter readings with the lower extremity should be performed with a possible diagnosis of coarctation.

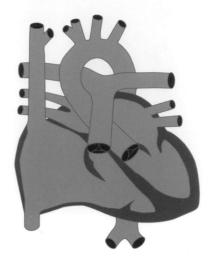

FIGURE 13-9. Ebstein's anomaly.

SIGNS AND SYMPTOMS

- Growth and development can be normal, depending on severity of the lesion.
- Older patients usually complain of dyspnea, cyanosis, and palpitations.
- A widely split S1, fixed split S2, variable S3, and S4 (characteristic triple or quadruple rhythm) can be found.
- A holosystolic murmur occurs at the left lower-sternal border.
- An opening snap occurs.
- Cyanosis from atrial right-to-left shunt is present.

DIAGNOSIS

- ECG: RAD, right atrial enlargement, RBBB. WPW is present in 20% (dilated right atrium predisposes to accessory pathway formation [increased surface area]).
- CXR: cardiomegaly ("balloon-shaped") "wall-to-wall heart" in severely affected infants.
- Enlarged heart on CXR.
- Echocardiogram is diagnostic.

TREATMENT

Intervention:
- Glenn procedure (passive venous blood flow to pulmonary artery).
- Severely affected infants may require an aortopulmonary shunt.
- Tricuspid valve replacement or reconstruction.
- Right-atrial reduction surgery.
- Ablation of accessory conduction pathways.

TOTAL ANOMALOUS PULMONARY VENOUS RETURN (TAPVR)

The pulmonary veins return blood to the right rather than the left atrium.

PATHOPHYSIOLOGY

- See Figure 13-10A and B.
- No communication exists between the pulmonary veins and the left atrium.
- All pulmonary veins drain to a common vein.
- The common vein drains into the:

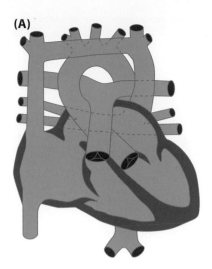
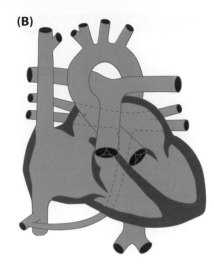

FIGURE 13-10. **Total anomalous pulmonary venous return.** (A) Supracardiac return. (B) Infracardiac return.

- Right SVC (50%)
- Coronary sinus or right atrium (20%)
- Portal vein or inferior vena cava (20%)
- Combination of the above types (10%)
- An ASD is needed for survival.

EPIDEMIOLOGY

Dramatically more common in males

SIGNS AND SYMPTOMS/DIAGNOSIS/TREATMENT

The presence of pulmonary venous obstruction changes the clinical presentation.

TAPVR with Obstruction

- Defined as obstruction of the egress of the pulmonary veins, often at the level of the diaphragm in infradiaphragmatic TAPVR, and results in increased pulmonary-artery pressure (and subsequent pulmonary edema).
- Increased pulmonary pressures result in right-ventricular and ultimately right-atrial pressures. Right-to-left shunt and cyanosis ultimately occur.
- Presents with early, severe respiratory distress and cyanosis, no murmur, and hepatomegaly.
- PGE is contraindicated as it will worsen the pulmonary edema.
- CXR: normal-size heart, pulmonary edema.
- Echocardiogram is diagnostic.
- Management is accomplished by balloon atrial septostomy followed by urgent corrective surgery.

TAPVR Without Obstruction

- Free communication between right atrium and left atrium.
- Large right-to-left shunt ("large ASD").
- Presents later in the first year of life with mild FTT, recurrent pulmonary infections, tachypnea, right heart failure, and rarely cyanosis.
- CXR: cardiomegaly, large PAs; increased pulmonary vascular markings ("snowman" or "figure eight" sign).
- Management is accomplished by surgical movement of pulmonary veins to the left atrium.

HYPERTROPHIC OBSTRUCTIVE CARDIOMYOPATHY

- Autosomal dominant 60%, sporadic 40%.
- Sudden death: 4% to 6% incidence.
- Asymmetrical septal hypertrophy or idiopathic hypertrophic subaortic stenosis is the most common form.
- Systolic ejection murmur heard best with maneuvers that decrease preload (e.g., Valsalva, standing). Decreased preload causes lower ventricular volume, closer proximity of the hypertrophic ventricular septum to the aortic outflow tract, increased turbulence, and a murmur.
- Murmur decreases with increased preload.
- ECG: LVH and left-atrial enlargement, large Q wave (indicates septal hypertrophy).
- Echo: asymmetrical septal hypertrophy, outflow obstruction (which predict the severity of disease).

TREATMENT

- Moderate restriction of physical activity.
- β blocker or calcium channel blocker to improve filling.

Renal, Gynecologic, and Urinary Disease

WARD TIP

Blood gas results, whether arterial or venous, are reported in this order: pH/PCO_2/PO_2/calculated HCO_3^-/calculated base excess or deficit/calculated Sao_2.

WARD TIP

Normal ABG values = $7.36 - 7.44/36 - 44/80 - 100/21 - 27/-4$ to $+2/95\text{-}100\%$

WARD TIP

ABGs show a calculated value of bicarbonate. Electrolyte panels show a measured value of bicarbonate (venous CO_2) and are, therefore, more reliable.

WARD TIP

The observation that hemoglobin's oxygen-binding affinity is inversely related to the acidity and concentration of carbon dioxide is termed the Bohr effect, described by Christian Bohr in 1904.

WARD TIP

Causes of anion gap metabolic acidosis:

MUDPILES

Methanol
Uremia
Diabetic ketoacidosis (DKA)
Propylene glycol/Paraldehyde
Isoniazid
Lactate
Ethylene glycol
Salicylates

Acid-Base Disorders

NORMAL ACID-BASE BALANCE

- pH 7.4
- PCO_2 40
- O_2 sat 98–100%
- Bicarbonate 22–28

DIAGNOSIS

- Diagnose acid-base disorders by obtaining an arterial blood gas (ABG—pH and PCO_2) and an electrolyte panel (HCO_3^-).
- Assess the acid-base disorder step by step:
  - Is the primary disorder an acidosis (pH <7.36) or alkalosis (pH >7.44)?
  - Is the disorder respiratory (pH and PCO_2 move in opposite directions)?
  - Is the disorder metabolic (pH and PCO_2 move in the same direction)?
  - Has there been respiratory/metabolic compensation? Is it a simple or mixed disorder?

ACIDOSIS

- Acidemia is an arterial pH <7.36 caused by metabolic (decreased serum HCO_3^-) or respiratory (increased PCO_2) acidosis.
- An extracellular shift of potassium (exchange of hydrogen for potassium cation), and decreased binding of calcium to albumin, may lead to hyperkalemia and hypercalcemia.
- A lower affinity between O_2 and Hb results in more oxygen release to tissues, shifting the oxygen dissociation curve to the right.

METABOLIC ACIDOSIS

- A drop in pH occurs due to a decreased serum HCO_3^-.
- Decreased serum HCO_3^- may result from (1) increased production of acids, (2) decreased excretion of acids, or (3) loss of alkaline fluids.
- The anion gap (AG) helps identify the cause of metabolic acidosis. It reflects unmeasured serum ions (organic acids, phosphates, etc.).
  - $AG = [Na^+] - ([Cl^-] + [HCO_3^-])$.
  - In children, an AG above 14 is considered elevated.
- Normal AG metabolic acidosis (hyperchloremic metabolic acidosis) results when low serum HCO_3^- is balanced by increased renal Cl^- reabsorption. Etiologies include:
  - Diarrhea (most common), due to gastrointestinal HCO_3^- loss
  - Renal tubular acidosis, caused by ineffective HCO_3^- reabsorption proximally (type 2) or ineffective H^+ excretion distally (type 1)
- AG metabolic acidosis can be caused by exogenous sources (drugs), endogenous acid production (lactic acidosis, ketoacidosis, etc.), or acid retention due to renal failure (uremia). See MUDPILES Ward Tip.
- Respiratory compensation (tachypnea) begins within 30 minutes. Severe metabolic acidosis (pH <7.2) results in compensatory hyperventilation (Kussmaul's breathing).
  - Appropriate change in PCO_2 can be predicted with the Winter's formula, i.e. expected $PCO_2 = (1.5 \times \text{serum } HCO_3^-) + 8 \pm 2$.
- Treat by correcting the underlying disorder. Oral bicarbonate may be used for chronic metabolic acidosis. For acute metabolic acidosis, use IV bicarbonate only in severe cases (pH <7.1).

RESPIRATORY ACIDOSIS

- A drop in pH may occur due to pulmonary retention of CO_2 ($PaCO_2$ >40 mm Hg).
- It may be acute or chronic. Causes include respiratory suppression due to the loss of CNS control, muscular dysfunction, acute lung injury, chronic lung disease, and chest-wall restriction.
- Renal compensation consists of increased H^+ excretion and HCO_3^- reabsorption.
- Children with acute respiratory acidosis due to hypoventilation require close monitoring and may need ventilator support. Correct electrolyte abnormalities, ensure adequate O_2, and correct reversible causes.

ALKALOSIS

- Alkalemia is an arterial pH >7.44 caused by metabolic (increased HCO_3^-) or respiratory (decreased PCO_2) alkalosis.
- It may induce hypokalemia (intracellular exchange of potassium for hydrogen ions) and hypocalcemia (increased binding to albumin).
- Increased affinity occurs between O_2 and Hb and decreased oxygen delivery results; it moves curve to the left.

METABOLIC ALKALOSIS

 A 6-week-old child has a 2-day history of projectile vomiting that is not bile-stained. He is dehydrated and slightly jaundiced. *Think: Pyloric stenosis.*
The classic symptom of pyloric stenosis is nonbilious, projectile vomiting. Progressive vomiting results in hypochloremic hypokalemic metabolic alkalosis from loss of gastric HCl. A classic but infrequent physical exam finding is an olive-shaped mass in the right upper quadrant. Treatment includes IV fluids to normalize acid-base status and correct electrolyte abnormalities and a surgical consult for pyloromyotomy.

- Increase in pH due to increased serum HCO_3^-
- In children, metabolic alkalosis is most commonly caused by gastric (acidic) fluid loss (vomiting). Other causes include volume contraction due to diuretics, cystic fibrosis, primary hyperaldosteronism, Bartter syndrome, Liddle syndrome, and milk-alkali syndrome.
  - Urinalysis (UA) is the best initial step to determine if the extracellular fluid (ECF) volume is contracted or expanded.
- Respiratory compensation is expected to cause 0.7 mm Hg increase in $PaCO_2$ for every 1 mEq/L increase in serum HCO_3^-.
- Treatment includes volume repletion for ECF contraction, correction of electrolyte abnormalities, potassium-sparing diuretics or acetazolamide for patients with high-volume states, dialysis in renal failure patients, and reversal of the underlying cause.

RESPIRATORY ALKALOSIS

- An increase in serum pH occurs due to **hyperventilation**, leading to loss of CO_2 ($PaCO_2$ <40 mm Hg).
- Causes include anxiety, asthma, pulmonary embolism, and pneumonia.
- Renal compensation occurs via excretion of HCO_3^-.
- Correct the underlying disorder. Breathing into a paper bag helps with psychogenic hyperventilation.

 WARD TIP

Expected PCO_2 in metabolic acidosis should be calculated with Winter's formula and compared with measured PCO_2 to see if the compensation is appropriate.

$$Expected\ PCO_2 = (Measured\ HCO_3^- \times 1.5) + 8 \pm 2$$

Failure of compensation is indicative of a mixed acid-base disorder.

 WARD TIP

Vomiting causes dehydration with a metabolic alkalosis and low urine chloride (loss of hydrogen and chloride with emesis).

 WARD TIP

Hypokalemia is a common electrolyte abnormality seen in metabolic alkalosis. Treat with KCl.

 WARD TIP

In metabolic disorders, respiratory compensation occurs immediately. In respiratory disorders, metabolic compensation takes longer to occur.

 WARD TIP

What do you do with an asthmatic in respiratory distress who has a normal pH and normal PCO_2? Get ready for intubation—they are tiring out. An asthmatic in only mild distress is expected to have respiratory alkalosis from tachypnea.

MIXED ACID-BASE DISORDER

- Simultaneous presence of more than one acid-base disorder.
- Suspect mixed acid-base disorder when the compensation is less than or greater than expected.
- Compensation rarely corrects to a normal pH, so suspect a mixed disorder with a normal pH and abnormal PCO_2 or HCO_3^-.

Renal Tubular Acidosis (RTA)

 A 1-year-old child is brought into the ED with vomiting, constipation, and decreased urine production. The child is found to have normal anion gap metabolic acidosis. A renal ultrasound reveals nephrocalcinosis. *Think: Renal tubular acidosis.*

Renal tubular acidosis is characterized by normal anion gap metabolic acidosis. A urine pH <5.5 suggests proximal RTA, whereas urine pH >5.5 suggests distal RTA. The presence of nephrocalcinosis and hypercalciuria is also suggestive of distal RTA.

DEFINITION

- A disorder of the renal tubules with preservation of glomerular function.
- Normal anion gap (hyperchloremic) metabolic acidosis due to:
    - Impaired distal acidification (retention of H^+, type 1).
    - Reduced proximal bicarbonate resorption (type 2).
    - Aldosterone deficiency or resistance (type 4).
    - Type 3, or mixed RTA, a rare autosomal recessive deficiency of carbonic anhydrase, a classification that is infrequently used.

TYPE 1—DISTAL RTA

PATHOPHYSIOLOGY

- Hyperchloremic metabolic acidosis with an abnormally high urinary pH (>5.5) due to impaired acid secretion by the distal tubule and collecting duct.
- Compensatory excretion of other cations causes hypokalemia and elevated calcium in urine.
- Serum bicarbonate is much lower in RTA type 1 than in other types ($HCO_3^- <10$ mEq/L) because of impaired distal H^+ secretion.

ETIOLOGY

May be due to genetic causes or acquired causes (obstructive uropathy, autoimmune disorders, amphotericin B).

SIGNS AND SYMPTOMS

- Clinical manifestation and severity depend on etiology.
- Presentation may include vomiting, dehydration, poor growth, nephrocalcinosis, and hypokalemia.

TREATMENT

Correct acidosis with bicarbonate therapy; a chronic cause of metabolic acidosis

TYPE 2—PROXIMAL RTA

PATHOPHYSIOLOGY

- Hyperchloremic metabolic acidosis usually *without* a high urinary pH (<5.5) due to decreased proximal tubular reabsorption of bicarbonate.
- Normal distal tubules function allows urine acidification. In severe cases, this mechanism is overwhelmed and urine pH increases to >5.5.
- Increased sodium delivery to the distal tubule increases aldosterone secretion, leading to hypokalemia.

ETIOLOGY

- May occur as an isolated disorder or as a generalized defect in proximal tubular transport (Fanconi syndrome)
  - Isolated proximal RTA is rare in children.

SIGNS AND SYMPTOMS

Clinical presentation depends on the underlying etiology (see section on Fanconi syndrome).

TREATMENT

Correct acidosis with alkali replacement. Larger alkali doses are needed for type 2 RTA due to bicarbonate loss via urine. Bicarbonate diuresis may cause hypokalemia, which can be treated with potassium citrate.

TYPE 4—MINERALOCORTICOID DEFICIENCY RTA

PATHOPHYSIOLOGY AND ETIOLOGY

- Caused by aldosterone deficiency (congenital adrenal insufficiency, aldosterone synthase deficiency, medication, HIV) or aldosterone resistance (mineralocorticoid deficiency)
  - The most common cause of hypoaldosteronism in children is medication—NSAIDs, trimethoprim, heparin, and potassium-sparing diuretics.
  - Characterized by hyperkalemia, acidic urine—urinary pH <5.5 (distal tubule H^+ pump functions normally).

SIGNS AND SYMPTOMS

- Failure to thrive.
- Persistent hyperkalemia.
- Mild metabolic acidosis and hyponatremia.

TREATMENT

- Correct acidosis and any electrolyte imbalance.
- Replace any deficient hormones.

PROGNOSIS OF RTA TYPE 1, 2, AND 4

- Distal RTA can be a lifelong disease and may lead to renal failure.
- Proximal RTA and mineralocorticoid RTA usually resolve within 12 months.

EXAM TIP

Type 1 and type 2 RTA are associated with **hypokalemia** due to aldosterone activation. Type 4 RTA is associated with **hyperkalemia** due to aldosterone deficiency or resistance.

Fanconi Syndrome

DEFINITION

- This rare disorder is characterized by generalized proximal tubular dysfunction with hypophosphatemia.
  - Loss of phosphate, glucose, amino acids, protein in urine, as well as proximal RTA (as above).

ETIOLOGY

- Can be inherited or acquired.
- Inherited causes include:
  - Cystinosis, galactosemia, hereditary fructose intolerance, tyrosinemia type I, and Wilson disease.
- Acquired secondary to exposure to:
  - Drugs (ifosfamide, cisplatin, aminoglycosides, and valproic acid).
  - Heavy metals (lead, mercury, cadmium).

SIGNS AND SYMPTOMS

- Hypophosphatemia and low vitamin D commonly cause bony abnormalities (rickets/osteomalacia) and growth failure.
- Loss of ions causes polyuria and hypovolemia.
- Hypokalemia causes constipation and muscle weakness.

DIAGNOSIS

Look for metabolic abnormalities, including hypophosphatemia, hypokalemia, proteinuria, and hyperchloremic metabolic acidosis.

TREATMENT

See above section on proximal RTA.

Acute Kidney Injury (AKI)

A 2-year-old boy develops bloody diarrhea a few days after eating in a fast-food restaurant. About 48 hours later, he develops facial edema, pallor, lethargy, and decreased urine output. Blood work shows a low hematocrit and platelet count. A UA reveals blood and protein. *Think: Hemolytic uremic syndrome (HUS) secondary to Escherichia coli O157:H7 infection.*

HUS is usually preceded by either gastroenteritis (usually diarrheal) or an upper respiratory tract infection. *E. coli* can be acquired by eating undercooked red meat or, in some cases, unwashed vegetables. The sudden onset of pallor, lethargy, and oliguria following an infection suggests HUS. Hemolytic uremic syndrome is characterized by hemolytic anemia, thrombocytopenia, and uremia from endothelial damage in small vessels like the kidney. The peripheral smear may show schistocytes and burr cells.

DEFINITION

- Formerly known as acute renal failure (ARF).
- Abrupt decline in renal function, reflected by acute rise in BUN (azotemia), serum creatinine, or both; often transient, but always <3 months
  - AKI is defined as a serum creatinine increase by 50% within 7 days or by 0.3 mg/dL within 2 days, or the presence of oliguria.
  - Acute kidney disease (AKD) is defined as AKI or a decreased GFR <60 mL/1.73 m^2 (or by >35%) for <3 months. AKI is a subset of AKD.

WARD TIP

Fanconi syndrome is one of the causes of proximal RTA.

WARD TIP

It is important to distinguish Fanconi syndrome from Fanconi anemia. Fanconi anemia is an inherited disorder of bone marrow failure, whereas Fanconi syndrome is a disorder of renal tubules.

WARD TIP

AKI: <3 months duration
CKD: >3 months duration

- There are three main types: prerenal, renal (intrinsic), and postrenal.
- Prerenal is the most common cause of AKI.

> A 4-year-old boy develops oliguria 12 hours after surgery for a ruptured appendix. Creatinine (Cr) is 0.5 mg/dL, blood urea nitrogen (BUN) is 23 mg/dL, urine sodium is 12 mEq/L. *Think: Prerenal AKI (or prerenal azotemia).*
>
> Oliguria is most often due to dehydration. Historical features include vomiting, diarrhea, and poor oral intake. A BUN-to-serum creatinine ratio of >20:1 is suggestive of prerenal AKI. Other features are decreased concentration of urinary sodium, increased urinary excretion of creatinine, and a high urine osmolality. Note that a normal or slightly elevated creatinine level does not exclude prerenal AKI. The precipitating event for prerenal AKI is renal hypoperfusion. Give normal saline for blood volume expansion. Reversibility with treatment of the underlying cause is the hallmark.

PATHOPHYSIOLOGY

- **Prerenal:**
    - Kidney hypoperfusion occurs due to blood loss, intestinal fluid loss, sepsis, heart failure.
    - Gastroenteritis is the most common cause of hypovolemia.
    - Oliguria is always present.
    - Prolonged renal hypoperfusion can cause acute tubular necrosis (ATN), which is an intrinsic renal disease; it is potentially reversible if the blood flow is restored quickly.
- **Renal (Intrinsic):**
    - Renal parenchymal damage is caused by:
        - Glomerular disease (e.g., poststreptococcal glomerulonephritis).
        - Vascular disease (e.g., hemolytic uremic syndrome).
        - Tubulointerstitial disease (secondary to drugs, UTIs, myoglobinuria from rhabdomyolysis).
    - The kidneys are unable to concentrate urine effectively.
- **Postrenal:**
    - Postrenal is caused by any significant physical or functional urinary-tract obstruction (posterior urethral valves, bilateral ureteropelvic or uretero-vesical obstruction, renal stones, neurogenic bladder, medications).
    - Often associated with infection.
    - Prolonged obstruction can lead to intrinsic renal disease.

SIGNS AND SYMPTOMS

- Signs and symptoms vary by etiology but commonly include:
    - Oliguria or anuria, dysuria.
    - Edema.
    - Gross or microscopic hematuria.
    - Hypertension (HTN).

DIAGNOSIS

- Obtain a careful history to determine the cause of AKI.
- Catheterize the patient to monitor output and obtain urine studies.
- Check serum and urine chemistry to help identify the cause.
    - Prerenal: BUN:Cr >20:1 with FENa <1%.
    - Renal: BUN:Cr <20:1 and FENa >1%.
- In intrinsic AKI, urinalysis may reveal proteinuria or hematuria. UA in pre-renal AKI is normal. UA in postrenal AKI can be normal or have varying degrees of hematuria.
- In children with postrenal AKI, a renal ultrasound will show dilation of the renal pelvis and collecting system.

EXAM TIP

A common cause of AKI in toddlers is hemolytic-uremic syndrome (HUS).

WARD TIP

AKI may be due to pre-renal, renal (intrinsic), or post-renal causes.

WARD TIP

Normal urinary output is 1–4 mL/kg/hr.

WARD TIP

The *fractional excretion of sodium*, or FENa, is the percentage of sodium filtered by the kidney that is excreted in the urine. It is useful to assess patients with AKI who are not on diuretics. Values for both plasma and urine sodium and creatinine are needed:
FENa = (PCr * UNa)/(PNa * UCr)
<1%—prerenal
1-4%—intrinsic
>4%—post-renal

WARD TIP

Oliguria
Infants: <1 mL/kg/hr for more than 6 hours
Older children: <0.5 mL/kg/hr for more than 6 hours

TREATMENT

- Treat patients with hypovolemia (as in prerenal AKI) with volume replacement and monitor I/Os to prevent worsening AKI.
- For oliguric patients leading to hypervolemia, treat with fluid restriction and/or furosemide. In critically ill patients with intrinsic AKI, consider dialysis.
- Monitor and treat electrolyte imbalances (hyperkalemia, metabolic acidosis).
- Avoid drugs that can precipitate or worsen AKI (NSAIDs, contrast dyes). Adjust the dosing of any renally excreted medications.

COMPLICATIONS OF AKI

AKI can lead to chronic kidney disease (CKD; >3 month) and can have profound electrolyte abnormalities. See CKD section for more information.

Chronic Kidney Disease (CKD)

On a routine exam, a 10-year-old girl has HTN of 160/90 in all extremities. *Think: Renal disease.*
BP should be measured at least twice with the appropriate cuff size. A short or narrow cuff may artificially raise BP measurement. Renal parenchymal disease and coarctation of the aorta are common causes of hypertension in children 1–10 years of age. Coarctation of the aorta would present with a higher BP in the upper extremities, while renal disease presents with consistent BP readings throughout. The most appropriate next test is UA.

DEFINITION

- CKD is a result of irreversible kidney damage, which may lead to end-stage renal failure.
- GFR <60 mL/min/1.73m² for >3 months
  OR
- GFR >60 mL/min/1.73m² with evidence of structural damage or functional kidney abnormalities (pathologic abnormalities on histology, proteinuria, casts, renal tubular disorders, imaging abnormalities).

ETIOLOGY

- Most commonly due to congenital abnormalities—obstructive uropathy, hypoplastic or dysplastic kidneys, reflux nephropathy, polycystic kidney disease.
- Focal segmental glomerulosclerosis is the most common glomerular disease seen in patients with CKD.
- Diverse etiologies can cause initial kidney damage. The kidney then compensates by adaptive hyperfiltration. Adaptive hyperfiltration and/or repeated insults due to the primary disease causes further glomerular damage. The cycle repeats, causing progressive renal insufficiency.

SIGNS AND SYMPTOMS

- Asymptomatic in the early stages with gradual symptom onset; may have polyuria or nocturia.
- Patients may develop headache, fatigue, lethargy, anorexia, nausea, vomiting, polyuria, and growth failure. In cases of glomerular disorders, proteinuria, discolored urine, and edema may accompany other findings.

COMPLICATIONS

- HTN: the renin-angiotensin-aldosterone system is stimulated by diminished GFR.
- Anemia: anemia occurs due to decreased kidney erythropoietin production.
- Electrolyte imbalances include:
    - Hyperkalemia due to impaired renal tubule function and renal tubular acidosis (ion shifts due to acidosis)
        - A serum potassium >6.5 mEq/L, which can lead to arrhythmias and must be treated emergently. Give calcium gluconate to stabilize the myocardium, sodium bicarbonate, glucose and insulin, Kayexalate (sodium polystyrene), and albuterol.
- Metabolic acidosis occurs due to hyperuricemia.
    - **Hypocalcemia** may result from the kidney's inability to hydroxylate vitamin D into an active form responsible for calcium GI absorption.
        - To compensate for low calcium, hyperparathyroidism may occur, which can cause bone loss and lead to growth impairment.
    - **Hyperphosphatemia** occurs due to the kidney's inability to excrete phosphate and causes itching.
    - **Hyponatremia** may result from excessive hypotonic fluids administration to oliguric patients. Patients with a serum sodium <120 are at risk for cerebral edema and CNS hemorrhage. Partial correction is undertaken to raise the sodium level to at least 120 mEq.
- In dyslipidemia, lipid metabolism is abnormal in patients with CKD; an increased risk for cardiovascular disease is seen.
- See Table 14-1 for a listing of symptoms of uremia.

TREATMENT

- Address the underlying etiology, treat any reversible kidney damage to slow CKD progression, and treat symptoms and complications.
    - Growth failure is common; ensure adequate caloric intake. Recombinant human growth hormone therapy can improve linear growth.
    - HTN: use strict BP control with ACE inhibitors or ARBs.
    - Anemia: treat with iron supplementation and erythropoietin.
    - Bone disorders: treat secondary hyperparathyroidism by normalizing the serum calcium and phosphorus levels with calcium supplements and phosphate binders, and vitamin D replacement.
    - Address any other fluid and electrolyte imbalances.
- Renal replacement therapy (e.g., transplant, dialysis) is necessary for patients with GFR <15. In children, it may be considered earlier (GFR <30).

WARD TIP

Cardiac arrest from hyperkalemia is a life-threatening complication of both AKI and CKD.

WARD TIP

Correcting hyponatremia too rapidly (>8 mEq/L in 24 hours) can lead to central pontine myelinolysis due to severe damage neurons in the pons. This can cause paralysis, difficulty speaking and swallowing, and other neurologic symptoms. A more recent term, osmotic demyelination syndrome (ODS) reflects recent observations that rapid osmotic changes can also cause demyelination outside the pons.

WARD TIP

Indications for emergent dialysis: **AEIOU**
Acidosis: (intractable to meds)
Electrolyte abnormalities (high K or Ca, low Na)
Toxic **I**ngestion (lithium, ASA, etc.)
Fluid **O**verload: (intractable to meds)
Uremia (symptomatic, i.e., pericarditis, seizures, nausea, bleeding) (keep BUN <100.)

TABLE 14-1.   Symptoms of Uremia

Azotemia (accumulation of nitrogen products)	Bleeding tendency
Acidosis	Infection
Sodium wasting	Neurologic (headache, drowsiness, muscle weakness, seizures)
Sodium retention	
Urinary concentrating defect	Gastrointestinal ulceration
Hyperkalemia	Hypertension
Renal osteodystrophy	Hypertriglyceridemia
Growth retardation	Pericarditis and cardiomyopathy
Anemia	Glucose intolerance

End-Stage Renal Disease (ESRD)

 An 8-year-old patient receiving peritoneal dialysis for ESRD develops abdominal pain and fever. *Think: Peritonitis.*

The most serious complication of peritoneal dialysis is peritonitis. It should be suspected in dialysis patients with abdominal pain and fever. Common causative organisms are coagulase-negative staphylococci, *S. aureus*, streptococci, *Escherichia coli*, *Pseudomonas*, and other gram-negative organisms.

DEFINITION

The last stage of CKD, when the kidney function becomes irreversibly compromised and the GFR falls below 15 mL/min/1.73m^2

TREATMENT

- Renal replacement therapy is necessary at GFR <15. It may be initiated earlier to allow adequate nutrition and normal growth.
- **Dialysis:** no significant difference in outcomes has been shown between hemodialysis (HD) and peritoneal dialysis (PD). The mode should be chosen based on contraindications and the patient/family's preference.
  - Infants and younger children may prefer PD due to certain advantages (less restrictive diet, therapy performed at home, no repeated venipuncture).
  - Hemodialysis is performed in children with contraindications to PD (intra-abdominal pathology).
- **Renal transplant:** renal transplantation is the preferred treatment mode for most children with ESRD.
  - Transplant contraindications include metastatic malignancy, systemic sepsis, elevated anti-GBM antibodies, severe multi-organ failure, extra-renal disorder not correctable by renal transplant, and other surgical contraindications. HIV infection is not an absolute transplant contraindication.

Hypertension

DEFINITION

Hypertension in children is defined as systolic and/or diastolic BP above the 95th percentile, measured on ≥3 separate occasions. The normal range for BP depends on age, gender, and height.

ETIOLOGY

- In older children (>age 15), primary HTN is the most common cause.
  - Risk factors include obesity, male gender, African American ethnicity, family history.
- In younger children (<age 15), HTN is most likely from a secondary cause, including:
  - Renal parenchymal disease (glomerulonephritis, polycystic kidney disease, CKD).
  - Endocrine disease (thyroid disease, corticosteroid excess, catecholamine-producing tumors).

- Renovascular disease (fibromuscular dysplasia, renal artery hypoplasia)
- Cardiac disease (coarctation of aorta).
- Drugs.

DIAGNOSIS

- Initially, BP should be obtained from all four extremities.
- Conduct a careful history and physical to determine primary versus secondary etiology.
- Initial testing should include BMP, CBC, UA, renal ultrasound (US), and echocardiogram.
- For mild HTN and no comorbidities, recommend lifestyle changes.
- For more severe HTN or comorbidities (renal disease, end-organ damage, diabetes), initiate pharmacologic treatment. Thiazide diuretics, angiotensin converting enzyme (ACE) inhibitors, calcium channel blockers (CCBs), and beta-blockers are most often used in children.
- For secondary HTN, address the underlying etiology.

EXAM TIP

The most common causes of HTN in children younger than 15 years are secondary causes, and ~80% of these are due to kidney or vascular abnormalities. Primary HTN is more common in children >15 years and adults.

Proteinuria

APPROACH

- Proteinuria up to 150 mg/day may be normal (can be higher in neonates).
- Transient proteinuria is the most common cause and can be induced by many factors including fever, exercise, dehydration, and seizures.
- Orthostatic/postural proteinuria: increased protein excretion occurs in the upright position, which returns to normal when the patient is lying down. It is especially common in adolescent males. The first morning void should be negative for protein.
- Persistent proteinuria should be evaluated for a glomerular lesion.

WARD TIP

Nephrotic range (or "heavy") proteinuria = Protein excretion of >40 mg/m^2/hr. Random urine protein/creatinine ratio >3.0.

Glomerular Diseases (Nephrotic and Nephritic Syndromes)

- Glomerular disorders are often classified as causes of nephrotic syndrome, nephritic syndrome, or both (Table 14-2).

WARD TIP

Nephritic syndrome: hematuria, edema, and hypertension
Nephrotic syndrome: pronounced edema, proteinuria, hyperlipidemia, and hypoalbuminemia

NEPHROTIC SYNDROME

A 2-year-old boy has a 1-week history of edema. On examination, he is normotensive with generalized edema and ascites. Lab values show Cr 0.4 (normal), albumin 1.4 g/dL (low), and cholesterol 569 mg/dL (high). A UA shows 4+ protein and no blood. *Think: Nephrotic syndrome.*

The common age of presentation is 2–6 years. Minimal change disease (MCD) is the most common nephrotic syndrome in children. Periorbital and peripheral edema is typically present. Histopathologic examination shows no glomerular abnormalities on light microscopy in minimal change disease.

TABLE 14-2. Contrast of Nephrotic and Nephritic Syndrome

NEPHROTIC SYNDROME	OVERLAP	NEPHRITIC SYNDROME
Minimal Change Disease	Membranoproliferative Glomerulonephritis	Poststreptococcal Glomerulonephritis
Focal segmental Glomerulosclerosis		Rapidly progressive Glomerulonephritis
Membranous Nephropathy		IgA nephropathy (Berger's)
		Alport syndrome

WARD TIP

Patients can develop a hypercoagulable state due to nephrotic loss of antithrombin III.

DEFINITION

- Nephrotic syndrome is caused by renal diseases that increase the permeability across the glomerulus. It is characterized by:
    - Nephrotic range proteinuria (>40 mg/m^2/hr).
    - Hypoalbuminemia (serum level <3g/dL).
    - Edema.
    - Hyperlipidemia.

ETIOLOGIES

- Minimal change disease (MCD, the most common nephrotic syndrome in children).
- Focal segmental glomerular sclerosis (FSGS).
- Membranous nephropathy.
- Nephrotic syndrome can also be secondary to systemic illnesses such as lupus and Henoch-Schönlein purpura.

PATHOPHYSIOLOGY

- Glomerular capillary wall permeability is normally regulated by charge selectivity (negatively charged to prevent passage of anions) and size selectivity. In nephrotic syndrome, this barrier is disrupted.
- In minimal change disease, a loss of anionic charge in the glomerular capillary wall with no structural damage on light microscopy is found.

EPIDEMIOLOGY

Primary nephrotic syndrome is most common in children between 2 and 6 years of age, and it commonly follows a viral upper respiratory infection.

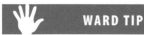

WARD TIP

Minimal change disease is the most common cause of nephrotic syndrome in children.

SIGNS AND SYMPTOMS

- Edema is the most common presenting symptom for all nephrotic syndromes.
    - It often presents initially as periorbital edema, usually pitting, and can become as severe as anasarca (generalized massive total-body edema).
- Nonspecific complaints (malaise, headache, fatigue, irritability) are common.
- Hematuria may be present, depending on nephrotic-syndrome etiology (more likely if secondary to glomerulonephritis).
- Labs show nephrotic-range proteinuria (>40 mg/m^2/hr), hypoalbuminemia (serum level <3 g/dL), and hyperlipidemia.

DIAGNOSIS

- The diagnosis is usually made clinically, with supportive lab values.
- Patients are empirically treated with steroids; a majority respond since most have MCD. A renal biopsy is needed for patients who do not respond.

TREATMENT

- Over 90 percent of children with MCD will respond to steroids (4–6 weeks of prednisone).
- For relapse, steroids remain the first-line agent.
- In patients with significant steroid side effects (growth impairment, weight gain) or relapsing nephrotic syndrome, other available agents include cyclophosphamide, cyclosporine, mycophenolate mofetil, tacrolimus, and rituximab.
- For other etiologies of nephrotic syndrome (FSGS, membranous nephropathy), steroids remain the first-line treatment, although the response is usually poor with progression to CKD.

COMPLICATIONS

- Infection is common (urinary loss of immunoglobulins). URI, UTI, and spontaneous bacterial peritonitis are the three most frequent infections.
    - In spontaneous bacterial peritonitis, the two most common organisms are *Streptococcus pneumoniae* and *Escherichia coli*.
- Thromboembolism: hypercoagulability results due to thrombocytosis and decreased levels of antithrombin III, plasminogen, and protein S (urinary loss).
    - Renal-vein thrombosis, deep-vein thrombosis, and pulmonary embolism occur.
- Renal insufficiency: can progress to end-stage renal disease, especially in those who are steroid-resistant.
- Anasarca.
- Hypovolemia: despite markedly increased extracellular fluid volume, children can present with third spacing of fluid and signs of decreased effective circulating volume (tachycardia, oliguria, peripheral vasoconstriction).

GLOMERULONEPHRITIS (GN)

DEFINITION

- Group of diseases that can cause glomerular injury via inflammation.
- May also cause nephritic syndrome.

CLINICAL SYMPTOMS

- Edema.
- Gross hematuria.
- Hypertension.
- Proteinuria may be present (less than nephrotic-range proteinuria).

DISEASE COURSE

- Acute glomerulonephritis—sudden onset hematuria, possible mild proteinuria, decreased GFR, and sodium and water retention leading to hypertension and edema
    - Most commonly caused by poststreptococcal glomerulonephritis (PSGN).

WARD TIP

Begin steroid therapy for MCD without renal biopsy in patients who:
- Are >1 year old and <12 years old
- Have symptoms of nephrotic syndrome
- None of the following are present:
    - Hypertension
    - Gross hematuria
    - Marked serum-creatinine elevation
    - Abnormal serum-complement levels
- If any of the above findings are present, this suggests an alternative etiology than minimal change disease

EXAM TIP

A urine dipstick is not the most accurate measure of protein excretion; a urine protein/creatinine ratio is more sensitive.

WARD TIP

In membranous nephropathy, immune complexes deposit in the glomeruli and cause nephrotic syndrome. Although it is the most common cause of nephrotic syndrome in adults, it is uncommon in children. Microscopy can show deposits of IgG and C3. It is associated with lupus, hepatitis B, and hepatitis C.

WARD TIP

Causes of gross hematuria include:
- Urinary tract infections
- Trauma
- Irritation of urethral meatus
- Nephrolithiasis
- Sickle cell disease/trait
- Coagulopathy
- Glomerular disease
- Malignancies
- Drug-induced hemorrhagic cystitis (cyclophosphamide)

- Rapidly progressive glomerulonephritis (RPGN) features acute GN and progressive loss of renal function over a relatively short period.
  - Rare in children and can be from any cause of glomerulonephritis.
  - Crescent-shaped scars are present in most glomeruli.
  - Treatment involves the use of steroids, cyclophosphamide or rituximab, and sometimes plasmapheresis. The prognosis is typically poor; most patients require dialysis.
- Chronic glomerulonephritis: patients often have asymptomatic hematuria or proteinuria but can also have acute glomerulonephritis and progress to CKD.

POSTSTREPTOCOCCAL GLOMERULONEPHRITIS (PSGN)

A 4-year-old girl presents with malaise, generalized edema, and red-brown colored urine. She had a strep throat infection 2 weeks prior. C3 level is decreased, and an antistreptolysin O (ASO) titer is positive. *Think: PSGN.*

PSGN occurs after an infection of the throat or skin by a nephritic strain of group A beta-hemolytic streptococci. It is manifested as an acute nephritic syndrome or as isolated hematuria. It is mediated by immune complexes, which is suggested by the low complement level.

DEFINITION

- Acute glomerulonephritis mediated by immune complex deposition is induced by group A beta-hemolytic streptococcus.
- It typically occurs following GAS pharyngitis or skin infection (impetigo).

EPIDEMIOLOGY

- This is the most common cause of acute glomerulonephritis globally, but it primarily occurs in developing countries.
- 2:1 male-to-female ratio, increased risk in ages 5–12.
- PSGN is the classic pediatric example of postinfectious glomerulonephritis (PIGN).
- In adults, most common cause of PIGN is staphylococcus.

SIGNS/SYMPTOMS

Most common presenting symptoms are edema, gross hematuria, hypertension, and possibly proteinuria.

DIAGNOSIS

- Based on clinical findings and evidence of recent Group A strep infection:
  - Renal function: variable decline in GFR, can see rise in serum Cr.
  - Positive throat cultures or antibody titers to streptococcal antigen.
  - UA: RBC casts, RBCs, varying amounts of protein, and sometimes pyuria.
  - Serum complement: low C3 in first 2 weeks of illness; resolves within 4–8 weeks.
  - Renal biopsy: typically not needed as PSGN tends to resolve within 1 week of presentation.

TREATMENT AND PROGNOSIS

- Treatment is primarily supportive.
- Monitor for hypertension and pulmonary edema. Treat with sodium and water restriction and loop diuretics, if needed.
- Treatment with penicillin will not prevent PSGN, but it can help prevent development of rheumatic fever.
- Treat renal failure or life-threatening fluid overload with peritoneal dialysis.
- Microscopic hematuria usually will resolve within 3–6 months.
- Proteinuria clears more slowly; a mild increase in protein excretion can still be present up to 10 years later.

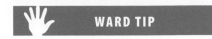

WARD TIP

Treatment with penicillin does not prevent the development of PSGN, although it does prevent development of rheumatic fever.

> A patient presents with hemoptysis, sinusitis, and glomerulonephritis. *Think: Granulomatosis with polyangiitis* (formerly called Wegener's granulomatosis).
> Granulomatosis with polyangiitis is a systemic vasculitis involving the upper and lower airways and kidneys. It is rare before adolescence. Features include necrotizing granulomatous lesions in the upper and lower respiratory tracts, necrotizing vasculitis, and focal glomerulonephritis. Most patients present with respiratory symptoms. Patients are typically c-ANCA positive. The radiographic findings may include nodular infiltrates, pulmonary nodule, cavitation, and diffuse alveolar hemorrhage.

MEMBRANOPROLIFERATIVE GLOMERULONEPHRITIS

DEFINITION

- Renal biopsy glomerular injury is characterized by mesangial hypercellularity and basement membrane thickening, often described as a "tram-track" pattern.
- May present with nephrotic and/or nephritic syndrome.
- Two primary mechanisms include:
  - Immune complex deposition leading to complement activation.
  - Dysregulation and persistent activation of complement pathway.

ETIOLOGIES

Associated with infections (HBV/HCV, chronic bacterial/fungal infections), autoimmune diseases (Sjögren's, SLE), monoclonal gammopathies, etc.

SIGNS AND SYMPTOMS

Varied presentation including nephrotic syndrome, nephritic syndrome, microscopic hematuria, and possibly proteinuria

DIAGNOSIS

- Renal biopsy.
- Serum complement levels often low.

TREATMENT AND PROGNOSIS

- Treat any underlying cause if present.
- Poor prognosis, especially with nephrotic syndrome, elevated serum creatinine, hypertension, or RPGN; often progresses to CKD.
- No definitive therapy is recommended; some patients respond to steroids.

A patient presents with dyspnea, hemoptysis, and AKI. *Think: Goodpasture syndrome.*
Goodpasture syndrome is an antiglomerular-basement membrane disease.

- Triad: glomerulonephritis, pulmonary hemorrhage, and antibody to basement membrane antigens
- Respiratory manifestations: cough, dyspnea, and hemoptysis associated with pulmonary hemorrhage
- Renal manifestations: acute-nephritic syndrome with hematuria, proteinuria, and HTN. UA may show active sediment with RBCs and RBC casts.

IGA NEPHROPATHY (BERGER DISEASE)

DEFINITION

Glomerulonephritis is thought to be caused by deposition of IgA (often complexed with C3 and IgG) in the mesangium and along the glomerular capillary wall.

EPIDEMIOLOGY

- Most common cause of acute glomerulonephritis in the developed world.
- Most common in the second and third decades of life, but it can present at any age.

SIGNS AND SYMPTOMS

- Typically follows an upper respiratory tract infection.
- 40–50% present with one or recurrent episodes of gross hematuria.
- 30–40% have microscopic hematuria and mild proteinuria; these are detected incidentally.
- Less than 10% present with nephrotic syndrome or acute RPGN with edema, hypertension, and renal insufficiency.

DIAGNOSIS

- Suspicion is generally based on clinical history and lab data.
- Diagnosis is confirmed with renal biopsy with immunofluorescence studies for IgA deposits.
  - Identical to renal biopsy findings seen in Henoch-Schönlein purpura since both are caused by IgA deposition.
- A biopsy is performed only if signs of more severe or progressive disease (excessive proteinuria, elevated creatinine).

TREATMENT

- Can be benign, but slow progression to ESRD occurs in up to 50% of affected patients over 20–50 years.
- ACE inhibitors or angiotensin receptor blockers (ARBs) are used for blood pressure control and to slow renal disease progression.
- Use steroid therapy only for patients with declining GFR or persistent proteinuria despite ACE inhibitor/ARB therapy or evidence of active disease on renal biopsy.
- Use renal-replacement therapy if progression to CKD or ESRD.

WARD TIP

IgA vasculitis (Henoch-Schönlein purpura) is a systemic disease that typically affects children and is often preceded by a throat infection. It is a small-vessel vasculitis that can cause purpuric rash on the lower extremities and other symptoms. In the kidneys, deposition of IgA and C3 can cause hematuria and proteinuria. Although renal biopsy results are the same as IgA nephropathy, HSP is a systemic disease and IgA nephropathy only affects the kidneys.

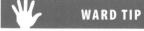
WARD TIP

IgA nephropathy is a common cause of recurrent gross hematuria, seen most often in young adults.

ALPORT SYNDROME

DEFINITION

Also called hereditary nephritis; inherited glomerular disease associated with sensorineural hearing loss and ocular abnormalities

SIGNS AND SYMPTOMS

- Initial renal manifestation is asymptomatic, persistent microscopic hematuria.
- Over time, proteinuria, hypertension, and renal insufficiency develop.

DIAGNOSIS

- Generally suspected from family history of deafness and renal failure.
- Can be confirmed by skin or renal biopsy or molecular genetic testing.

TREATMENT

No specific treatment is currently available; use renal transplant for renal failure (disease does not occur in transplanted kidney).

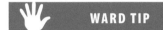

WARD TIP

Suspect Alport syndrome in patients with deafness and a family history of renal failure.

SYSTEMIC LUPUS ERYTHEMATOSUS (SLE) NEPHRITIS

DEFINITION

- SLE is a systemic autoimmune disease that can affect skin, joints, kidneys, lungs, the nervous system, and other organ systems.
  - The most common initial symptoms are fever, weight loss, and malaise over several months.

PATHOPHYSIOLOGY

- Clinical manifestations are mediated by autoantibody formation and immune complex deposition.
- Immune complexes deposit in the glomeruli, which activates complement, causing renal dysfunction.

EPIDEMIOLOGY

- Most common in adolescent females.
- Can occur at any age, but incidence increases after 5 years of age and even further after the first decade.

SIGNS AND SYMPTOMS

- Hematuria.
- Proteinuria.
- Reduced renal function.
- Nephrotic syndrome.
- Renal disease is more frequent early in the disease course in children and is often more severe.

DIAGNOSIS

- Specific American College of Rheumatology classification criteria are widely available.

- Antinuclear antibodies (ANA) are highly sensitive, whereas anti-Smith antibodies and anti-double-stranded DNA antibodies (anti-dsDNA) are highly specific for SLE.
- Markers of disease activity include:
  - Anti-double-stranded DNA.
  - Low complement levels C3 and C4 during active disease.

TREATMENT

- Immunosuppressive therapy (e.g., prednisone, azathioprine, hydroxychloroquine) to help reduce/prevent flare-ups, but cannot cure the disease.
- Mycophenolate mofetil, cyclophosphamide, voclosporin, belimumab, and rituximab are used in more severe/refractory cases of lupus nephritis.

ACUTE INTERSTITIAL NEPHRITIS (AIN)

DEFINITION

Inflammation in the interstitium between the glomeruli in the areas surrounding the tubules

RISK FACTORS

- Reaction to medications (NSAIDs, penicillin, cephalosporins, sulfonamides, ciprofloxacin, cimetidine, PPIs, rifampin, thiazides, furosemide, allopurinol) is the most common cause.
- Infections (especially in children).
- Systemic diseases (SLE, Sjögren's, and sarcoidosis).

SIGNS AND SYMPTOMS

- Nonspecific signs/symptoms of acute renal dysfunction including nausea, vomiting, and malaise; may be asymptomatic.
  - Oliguria can be seen. Gross hematuria and proteinuria are very rare.
- In drug-induced AIN, one or more of the classical triad of rash, fever, and eosinophilia may also be present, although not necessary for diagnosis.

DIAGNOSIS

- Suspect if elevated serum creatinine, or urinalysis shows WBCs, WBC casts, and possibly eosinophiluria.
- Renal biopsy demonstrates interstitial edema and marked interstitial infiltrate of inflammatory cells.

TREATMENT

- Remove offending agent if drug induced.
- Immunosuppressive therapy with steroids is sometimes used.
- Prognosis is variable.

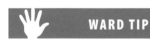

WARD TIP

Classic triad in acute interstitial nephritis is rash, fever, and eosinophilia.

Renal Parenchymal Malformations

- **Renal dysplasia:** abnormal embryonic cell differentiation resulting in atypical structure and decreased number of nephrons and presence of nonrenal tissues (cartilage and bone); can affect all or part of the kidney.
- **Renal hypoplasia:** nondysplastic small kidney that has decreased number but structurally normal calyces and nephrons.
- **Renal hypodysplasia:** congenitally small kidney with dysplastic features.

A 1-week-old male newborn has a wrinkled abdomen that lacks anterior abdominal musculature. He also has clubbed feet and is in respiratory distress. His bladder is distended and easily palpable, and neither testis is in his scrotum. Lab findings include BUN 30, Cr 2, and HCO3 15. *Think: Prune belly syndrome.*

Triad: **absent abdominal wall muscles, undescended testes,** and **renal dysplasia**. The renal collecting system is dilated and nephrons are incompletely differentiated. Abnormalities of bladder, testicles, prostate, and/or ureter are common. Respiratory distress may be present due to pulmonary hypoplasia secondary to severe oligohydramnios.

Renal Agenesis

DEFINITION

- Uni- or bilateral congenital absence of renal parenchymal tissue
  - Bilateral renal agenesis is incompatible with life.
  - Children with a solitary kidney are at increased risk for long-term CKD, thought to be due to glomerular hyperfiltration.
  - Diagnosis should prompt evaluation for associated abnormalities such as chromosomal anomalies and VACTERL association (vertebral anomalies, anal atresia, cardiac defects, TE fistula, renal defects, limb defects).

WARD TIP

VACTERL Association should be suspected with congenital renal abnormalities, including:
  Vertebral anomalies
  Anal atresia
  Cardiac defects
  TE fistula
  Renal defects
  Limb defects

Polycystic Kidney Disease (PKD)

An 8-month-old girl has an easily palpable kidney. Ultrasound (US) shows cystic kidneys, hepatic fibrosis, and portal HTN. *Think: Autosomal-recessive polycystic kidney disease.*

The classic presentation includes bilateral flank masses during the neonatal period or early infancy. US may show uniformly hyperechogenic kidneys. Presence of hepatic fibrosis supports this diagnosis.

DEFINITION

- An inherited disorder that causes bilateral renal cysts without dysplasia.
- Two types: Autosomal-Recessive PKD (ARPKD) and Autosomal-Dominant PKD (ADPKD).

AUTOSOMAL-RECESSIVE PKD (ARPKD)

PATHOPHYSIOLOGY

- Previously known as infantile polycystic kidney disease.
- Most commonly caused by PKHD1 gene mutations, which encodes for fibrocystin.
- Primarily affects the kidney and the hepatobiliary tract
  - Enlarged kidneys are present with numerous microcysts (cystic-collecting duct dilations) that radiate from the medulla to the cortex. No urinary flow obstruction is present, but it is a progressive disease; larger cysts and interstitial fibrosis develop and can cause renal dysfunction.
  - Biliary dysgenesis leads to congenital hepatic fibrosis and intrahepatic bile duct dilation. Hepatomegaly and portal HTN result over time.

SIGNS AND SYMPTOMS

- May be detected prenatally by ultrasound; a normal finding does not rule out ARPKD.
- In severe cases, neonates will present with respiratory distress and/or other features of the Potter syndrome (flat nose, recessed chin, low-set ears, limb abnormalities, pulmonary hypoplasia).
- In less severe cases, infants or older children will present with progressively deteriorating renal function, portal HTN, and increased risk of cholangitis.

DIAGNOSIS

Diagnosed with abdominal ultrasound, showing enlarged hyperechogenic kidneys with poor corticomedullary differentiation and hepatobiliary disease

TREATMENT

- Supportive.
- Renal replacement therapy for children who progress to ESRD.

WARD TIP

ARPKD—innumerable tiny cysts
ADPKD—large cysts

AUTOSOMAL-DOMINANT PKD (ADPKD)

PATHOPHYSIOLOGY

- Previously known as adult polycystic kidney disease.
- Caused by mutations in PKD1 or PKD2 gene, which encodes for polycystin 1 and polycystin 2, respectively.
- Characterized by macrocysts (large cystic dilatations in all parts of the nephron, including all tubular segments and the Bowman's capsule).
- Complications commonly seen in adults, such as cysts in the liver/pancreas or cerebral AV malformations, are rare in children.

SIGNS AND SYMPTOMS

- Commonly presents in adulthood but may present in childhood.
- Even if cysts develop early, most patients remain asymptomatic until adulthood.
- May present with gross or microscopic hematuria, proteinuria, infection of the cyst, HTN, and abdominal, flank, or back pain.
- Renal insufficiency can occur during childhood but is rare.

DIAGNOSIS

- Family history is helpful, but 10% present without a family history.
- Diagnosed with renal ultrasound, which reveals cysts.

TREATMENT

- Supportive (BP control, pain management, treatment for UTI).
- Renal-replacement therapy is used for patients who develop ESRD.

WARD TIP

The most common cause of end-stage renal disease in children is congenital renal anomalies.

Horseshoe Kidney

DEFINITION

- Midline fusion of the lower kidney poles.
- Kidney does not ascend fully due to tethering by the inferior mesenteric artery; kidney is found in the pelvis or lower-lumbar vertebral levels.
- Majority of patients are asymptomatic.

ASSOCIATED CONDITIONS

- Urologic and genital anomalies are commonly found (e.g., vesicoureteral reflux, ureteropelvic junction obstruction, bicornuate uterus, hypospadias, and undescended testis).
- Horseshoe kidney can be a feature of many syndromes, including Turner syndrome and is common in Trisomy syndromes (13, 18, and 21).
- An increased risk for developing Wilms tumor is found.

Wilms Tumor (See Oncologic Disease Chapter)

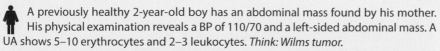 A previously healthy 2-year-old boy has an abdominal mass found by his mother. His physical examination reveals a BP of 110/70 and a left-sided abdominal mass. A UA shows 5–10 erythrocytes and 2–3 leukocytes. *Think: Wilms tumor.*

The usual presentation of Wilms tumor is an abdominal mass, and it is not uncommon for the parent to discover this asymptomatic mass. The most appropriate next diagnostic test is an ultrasound of the abdomen and urinary tract. Because Wilms tumor metastasizes to the lungs, a chest radiograph should be obtained.

 WARD TIP

The characteristic features of Beckwith-Wiedemann syndrome include omphalocele, macroglossia, and macrosomia. Also notable are the presence of hemihypertrophy (asymmetric growth), neonatal hypoglycemia, and increased risk for embryonal tumors, including Wilms tumor (5–10% chance).

Renal Vein Thrombosis (RVT) in Infancy

DEFINITION

- Thrombus formation in the renal vein.
- A common cause of venous thromboembolism during the neonatal period.
- Risk factors include:
    - Prematurity (especially with history of umbilical vein catheter), perinatal asphyxia, shock, dehydration, sepsis, polycythemia, cyanotic heart disease, maternal diabetes, and inherited prothrombotic conditions.
    - In older children, RVT is associated with nephrotic syndrome, burns, systemic lupus erythematosus, or renal transplant.

SIGNS AND SYMPTOMS

- Most often, an insidious onset occurs with no symptoms referable to the kidney.
- Gross hematuria, proteinuria, anuria, thrombocytopenia, vomiting, and hypovolemia are found.

DIAGNOSIS

- US shows swollen and echogenic kidneys.
- Doppler flow studies may show absent intrarenal and renal venous flow.
- Coagulation and prothrombotic disorder studies are considered on a case-by-case basis.

TREATMENT

- Correction of fluid and electrolyte abnormalities.
- Unilateral renal vein thrombosis without compromised renal function or extension into the inferior vena cava (IVC) can be managed with supportive care.
- For extension into the IVC, compromised renal function or bilateral thrombosis, anticoagulate with unfractionated heparin.

Nephrolithiasis

 An 8-year-old boy presents with left-flank pain radiating to his left testicle. The colicky pain does not change with movement or positioning. Urine dip is positive for blood. *Think: Nephrolithiasis.*

The pain begins in the flank, extends around the abdomen, and may radiate into the groin. Ipsilateral costovertebral tenderness may be present. Children with a history of multiple UTIs may be at risk of renal stones. UA typically shows hematuria, but the absence of hematuria does not exclude the diagnosis of nephrolithiasis.

WARD TIP

Urinary metabolic abnormalities are often the cause of pediatric stones. They include:
- Hypercalciuria (most common)
- Hyperoxaluria
- Hypocitraturia

WARD TIP

Uric acid stones are radiolucent and thus cannot be seen on x-ray.

EPIDEMIOLOGY

- Lower incidence in children, with increased occurrence after 12 years.
- In most children, it is associated with metabolic abnormalities, urinary tract abnormalities, or urinary tract infection.

ETIOLOGY

- Made of calcium oxalate (most common), calcium phosphate, struvite, uric acid, or cystine that accumulates in the calyx or bladder.
- Calcium stones are:
  - Radiopaque, envelope-shaped stones.
  - Secondary to hypercalciuria due to increased intestinal absorption, decreased renal reabsorption, or increased bone resorption.
- Struvite stones are:
  - Radiopaque, coffin-lid shaped stones composed of magnesium ammonia phosphate.
  - Most commonly secondary to UTIs by urease-producing bacteria such as *Proteus* and *Klebsiella*.
- Uric acid stones are:
  - Rare in children.
  - Radiolucent, rhomboid-shaped stones associated with high serum uric-acid levels (idiopathic hyperuricosuria, Lesch-Nyhan syndrome, chemotherapy [tumor lysis syndrome], and myeloproliferative disorders.
- Cystine stones are:
  - Radiopaque, hexagonal-shaped stones associated with cystinuria, an autosomal-recessive disorder causing excessive excretion of dibasic amino acids (cystine, lysine, arginine, and ornithine) by the renal epithelial cells.

SIGNS AND SYMPTOMS

- Most common presenting symptom is abdominal/flank pain radiating to the genitalia (renal colic).
- Microscopic or gross hematuria.
- Dysuria and urgency, sometimes with concurrent UTI.
- Particularly in younger children, can be asymptomatic and diagnosed incidentally on abdominal imaging.

DIAGNOSIS

- Three imaging modalities are used for diagnosis—noncontrast helical ("spiral") abdominal CT, ultrasound, and plain abdominal radiography.
  - A plain abdominal x-ray will show radiopaque stones (calcium, struvite, and cystine) but could miss small ones or those overlying bones.
  - Abdominal CT is the most sensitive modality and can help detect ureteral stones, radiolucent stones, and small stones that may be missed on x-ray. It will also show structural anomalies or hydronephrosis.

- Ultrasound is effective and avoids radiation; it should be used in pregnancy. It is limited in ability to detect small, papillary, or ureteral stones. It can, however, identify hydronephrosis that may help guide next steps.

TREATMENT

- Acute treatment:
  - Pain management: NSAIDs are mainstay; opiates may be needed.
  - Aggressive IV hydration.
  - Should obtain urine culture given high rate of concurrent UTI.
  - Majority of stones <5 mm will pass spontaneously.
  - Should undergo intervention to remove calculi if they are >5 mm, if signs of infection, obstruction, or renal insufficiency are present, or if the stone does not pass.
  - Options for intervention include extracorporeal shock wave lithotripsy, percutaneous nephrostolithotomy, and ureteroscopy.
- Prevention of recurrence depends on metabolic abnormality.

WARD TIP

The most sensitive test for identifying stones in the urinary system is a noncontrast helical (spiral) abdominal CT scan.

Urinary Tract Infection (UTI)

 A 3-week-old infant presents with fever, vomiting, and decreased fluid intake. A UA reveals 100 WBC/HPF. *Think: E. coli UTI. Next step: Urine culture.*

Infants have nonspecific UTI symptoms, such as irritability, fever, and vomiting. *E. coli* is the most common organism in children of all ages. UA may show positive urinary leukocyte esterase, positive urinary nitrite, pyuria (>5 WBC/HPF), and bacteriuria.

 A 7-year-old girl presents with urinary urgency, frequency, suprapubic pain, and no flank pain or mass. UA shows many leukocytes, 2–5 RBC/HPF, and no protein or casts. *Next step: Urine culture.*

Older children have more localized UTI symptoms, such as frequency, dysuria, and abdominal pain. The definitive diagnosis requires a positive urine culture from a specimen obtained with sterile techniques.

DEFINITION

- Infection of the urinary tract by bacterial pathogens.
- UTIs are typically caused by fecal or genital bacteria. The most common is *E. coli* (85%), followed by *Klebsiella*, *Proteus*, and enterococci. *Staphylococcus saprophyticus* is seen among female adolescents.
- UTIs are more common in males in the first year of life and in females afterward.
- UTI occurs in 3–8% of girls and 1–2% of boys.

PREDISPOSING FACTORS

- Female sex.
- Uncircumcised male.
- Vesicoureteral reflux.
- Anatomic abnormalities.
- Bowel and bladder dysfunction (incontinence, holding urine, and eliminating with abnormal frequency or urgency).
- Sexual activity.
- Neurogenic bladder.

WARD TIP

The differential for dysuria includes:

- Infections (UTIs, reproductive tract infections)
- Trauma (stones, urethral stricture, labial adhesions, sexual activity)
- Systemic illness (Stevens-Johnson, Behçet, reactive arthritis)
- Other (elimination dysfunction, virginal ulcers, psychogenic)

CLASSIFICATION OF UTIs

- **Pyelonephritis** is an infection of the kidney characterized by abdominal or flank pain, fever, malaise, nausea, vomiting, and diarrhea (systemic symptoms).
- **Cystitis** is an infection of the bladder whose common symptoms include dysuria, urgency, frequency, suprapubic pain, incontinence, and malodorous urine (localized symptoms). Cystitis does not typically cause fever.
- **Asymptomatic bacteriuria** is the presence of >50,000/mL of a single bacterial organism on two successive urine cultures in a patient without any UTI-like symptoms or pyuria. No treatment is needed unless pregnant.

SIGNS AND SYMPTOMS

Symptoms vary with age:

- Neonates exhibit fever, failure to thrive, vomiting, and jaundice. All febrile neonates should be evaluated for UTI.
- Infants 2 months–2 years exhibit fever, poor feeding, vomiting, strong smelling urine, abdominal pain, and irritability. Fever without a source may be evaluated for UTI based on clinical judgment.
- Infants >2 years exhibit urinary urgency and frequency, bed-wetting, dysuria, strong smelling urine, and abdominal or flank pain.
- Complications include renal scarring (loss of renal parenchyma), hypertension, and end-stage renal disease. Complications are more common with pyelonephritis, recurrent UTIs, and vesicoureteral reflux.

DIAGNOSIS

- Gold standard: urine culture PLUS urinalysis. If child is not toilet trained, cultures must be obtained via suprapubic tap or catheterization.
- Diagnostic criteria: pyuria (WBC >5/HPF) and/or positive Gram stain on UA and presence of >50,000 colonies in the urine culture. In asymptomatic children, pyuria must be present for diagnosis.
  - Urine nitrite is not sensitive in children because they empty their bladders frequently. The conversion of nitrates to nitrites by bacteria requires approximately 4 hours in the bladder. It is highly specific when present.
  - Leukocyte esterase is positive.
  - +/− Hematuria, white cell casts.

TREATMENT

Treatment varies depending on the age of the child:

- It is difficult to differentiate cystitis from pyelonephritis in children <2 years old, so treat the same initially.
- For infants <2 months: administer 10–14 days of IV antibiotics. Start broad and narrow based on cultures. The usual choice is cephalosporin (cefotaxime). Gentamycin is added if <7 days old.
- Infants >2 months: administer 7–14 days of oral or IV antibiotics based on local sensitivities. Usual choices include cephalosporins, amoxicillin-clavulanate, or trimethoprim-sulfamethoxazole.
- Bladder and renal ultrasounds can identify factors predisposing to UTIs, including hydronephrosis, dilation or duplication of distal ureters, solitary kidney, echogenic stones, and perinephric abscess. Indications for ultrasound include:
  - Children with two or more febrile UTIs.
  - Children <2 years old with one febrile UTI.
  - Children with nonfebrile UTI and risk factors (poor growth, hypertension, or a family history of urologic/renal disease).
  - Children who do not respond to antibiotics.

- A voiding cystourethrogram (VCUG) is used to diagnose vesicoureteral reflux, in which urine flows backward from the bladder toward the kidneys during urination. To perform a VCUG, the bladder is filled with contrast via a catheter and images are taken during urination. Perform VCUG in:
  - Children with two or more febrile UTIs.
  - Children with one febrile UTI and an abnormal ultrasound or clinical risk factors.
- Renal cortical scintigraphy with DMSA determines acute functioning of the renal cortex and chronic renal scarring. It is done following an ultrasound that suggests renal damage. Radiotracer is injected into a vein and excreted by the kidneys.

INDICATIONS FOR INPATIENT TREATMENT

- Child cannot tolerate oral antibiotics.
- Toxic appearing.
- Pyelonephritis.

Vesicoureteral Reflux (VUR)

DEFINITION

- Retrograde flow of urine from the bladder to the ureter and renal pelvis
- Reflux predisposes to pyelonephritis by facilitating the transport of bacteria from the bladder to the upper urinary tract.
- The most common cause of VUR is inadequate closure at the uretero-vesicular junction, which commonly resolves spontaneously with growth.
- VUR may also be caused by abnormally high bladder pressures seen with posterior urethral valves and neurogenic bladder.

EPIDEMIOLOGY

- 30–45% of children with UTIs have reflux.
- More common in females.
- More common in children <2 years old.

DIAGNOSIS

- Often diagnosed by voiding cystourethrogram (VCUG) during a UTI workup.
- Patients with prenatal ultrasonography showing hydronephrosis should receive a postnatal ultrasound; a VCUG will help determine if VUR is present.

GRADING

Reflux is graded on a scale of 1 (most mild) to 5 (most severe), depending on the extent of dilation of the ureter and kidney findings on VCUG.

TREATMENT

- The goal of treatment is to prevent pyelonephritis and renal injury.
- Treatment options include watchful waiting, antibiotic prophylaxis (sterile urine does not damage the kidney), and surgical correction.
- Dimercaptosuccinic acid (DMSA) scans help determine renal function.
- Surgical management is more appropriate with higher grade reflux and reflux beyond age 2–3.

WARD TIP

VCUG must be done in all children with two or more febrile UTIs, even if they have a normal ultrasound, to assess for vesicoureteral reflux.

WARD TIP

Perform urinalysis immediately after obtaining a clean-catch specimen. A delay of 1–2 hours may cause bacterial multiplication and false positives.

Outflow Tract Obstruction

DEFINITION

- Anomalies resulting in a physical barrier between the uterus and vaginal introitus include:
  - Imperforate hymen and incomplete hymenal fenestration.
  - Transverse or longitudinal vaginal septum.
  - Vaginal agenesis ("Müllerian aplasia," Mayer-Rokitansky-Kuster-Hauser syndrome) is upper vaginal, and possibly uterus, absence due to the underdevelopment of the Müllerian system. It is associated with congenital anomalies (i.e., renal agenesis, horseshoe kidneys). The external exam is normal due to separate development of urogenital sinus.

SIGNS AND SYMPTOMS

- Imperforate hymen and transverse vaginal membrane are total obstructions that can present in infancy as bulging (maternal estrogen withdrawal secretions). If not identified, mucus is reabsorbed; the anomaly presents in adolescence with cyclical abdominal pain, primary amenorrhea, introitus bulging, potentially with a bluish membrane.
- Incomplete hymenal fenestration and longitudinal vaginal septa are incomplete obstructions that can be asymptomatic, cause dyspareunia or pain with tampon insertion, or cause retained blood leading to spotting, malodorous discharge, or infection.
- Vaginal agenesis is the most common obstructive cause of primary amenorrhea, often detected in adolescence.

DIAGNOSIS

Diagnosis is clinical or made via ultrasound.

TREATMENT

Surgery is the treatment. If asymptomatic, longitudinal septa do not require intervention. Dilators may be used for vaginal agenesis.

Polycystic Ovarian Syndrome (PCOS)

DEFINITION

- PCOS is the most commonly diagnosed ovarian cause of infertility and anovulation.
- Consider PCOS in female adolescents who present with:
  - Hirsutism (excessive male-pattern hair growth on face, back, or chest).
  - Treatment-resistant inflammatory acne.
  - Menstrual irregularities.
  - Obesity accompanied by menstrual irregularities.

PATHOPHYSIOLOGY

- Excess androgen production by the ovaries.
- Linked to insulin resistance and obesity, but about 1/2 are not obese.

SIGNS AND SYMPTOMS

- Hirsutism, acne, alopecia, menstrual abnormalities, infertility, and obesity.
- Insulin resistance, as evidenced by acanthosis nigricans, metabolic syndrome (increased risk for type 2 diabetes and cardiovascular disease), fatty liver disease.
- PCOS is a risk factor for endometrial hyperplasia and carcinoma.

DIAGNOSIS

- Clinical diagnosis for 1–2 years of abnormal uterine bleeding and evidence of hyperandrogenism.
- Abnormal uterine bleeding includes:
  - Primary amenorrhea: no menarche by age 15 or by 3 years after breast development.
  - Secondary amenorrhea: no menses for over 90 days after menarche.
  - Oligomenorrhea: <4 periods in the first year, <6 in year 2, <8 in year 3–5, <9 in year 6+.
  - Excessive uterine bleeding: more often than every 21 days (or 19 days in year 1), lasting over 7 days, or soaking through a pad or tampon every 1–2 hours.
- Evidence of hyperandrogenism includes high testosterone (best test) or moderate to severe hirsutism (clinically).
- Ultrasound is **not recommended** for diagnosis due to poor specificity, but it can be used to rule out adrenal and ovarian tumors.
- Adolescent females often have irregular menses during the first few years after menarche. Make sure they actually fit the criteria for abnormal uterine bleeding!
- Other causes of hyperandrogenism to consider include congenital adrenal hyperplasia, adrenal tumors, cortisone reductase deficiency, Cushing syndrome, and thyroid dysfunction.

TREATMENT

- Combined estrogen/progestin oral contraceptive pills regulate menses, decrease androgen production, and reduce endometrial hyperplasia.
- Alternatives: progestin-only contraception, gonadotropin-releasing hormone agonists.
- For hirsutism: hair reduction (creams, laser therapy), antiandrogens (spironolactone).
- Lifestyle modification, glucose monitoring, possible metformin for insulin resistance.

Ovarian Torsion

DEFINITION

Twisting of the ovary on its vascular pedicle; an **obstetrical emergency**

EPIDEMIOLOGY

- Most common in women of reproductive age, but can occur in all ages.
- The biggest risk factors are large (>5 cm) ovarian masses, including cysts and neoplasms.
- Risk factors include pregnancy and ovulation induction.

SIGNS AND SYMPTOMS

- Acute sharp lower abdominal pain with nausea and vomiting.
- Pain may be unilateral or diffuse. In children pre-menses, pain is often diffuse, leading to delays in diagnosis.
- An adnexal mass may be palpated.

DIAGNOSIS

- A definitive diagnosis is made intraoperatively by direct visualization.
- A presumptive diagnosis is made clinically and on Doppler ultrasound showing decreased or absent blood flow, fluid around the ovary, and a change in gonadal location or size.

TREATMENT

- Surgical detorsion with ovary salvage, if possible, and cystectomy, if found.
- If ovary is not viable, an oophorectomy is performed.
- Torsion is a surgical emergency. Prolonged torsion reduces ovary viability.

Testicular Torsion

 A 15-year-old boy presents with sudden onset of severe pain in his right testicle. A physical exam reveals a tender, swollen, firm testicle with a transverse lie. No cremasteric reflex on the right is found. *Think: Testicular torsion.*

Testicular torsion presents with nausea, vomiting, and severe and acute testicular pain. The diagnosis is made clinically, and surgical exploration should occur immediately in cases of high clinical suspicion.

DEFINITION

- Twisting of the testicle on its vascular pedicle.
- Most often due to poor testis fixation to the intra-scrotal tunica vaginalis.

EPIDEMIOLOGY

- Most common in boys 12–18 years; also occurs in utero and in neonates.
- Undescended testes are a significant risk factor.
- A bell-clapper deformity increases risk due to increased testicular mobility.

SIGNS AND SYMPTOMS

- Acute pain, erythema, and swelling of the scrotum.
- Nausea and vomiting.
- Absent cremasteric reflex (testicular elevation provoked by stroking the inner thigh).

DIAGNOSIS

- A definitive diagnosis is made by direct visualization in surgery.
- A presumptive diagnosis is made clinically, and Doppler ultrasound shows decreased or absent blood flow, perigonadal fluid, and a change in gonadal location or size.

TREATMENT

- Torsion is a surgical emergency: "Time is testes."
- Surgical detorsion is followed by fixation in scrotum (orchiopexy) or removal of the testicle (orchiectomy) if the tissue is already dead.
- The contralateral testis is also explored, and orchiopexy may be performed.

Phimosis/Paraphimosis

DEFINITION

- Phimosis is the inability to retract the prepuce (foreskin) over the glans penis. In newborns and younger children, phimosis is normal. In older males, it is pathologic (from scarring).

WARD TIP

Testicular torsion would cause decreased flow on ultrasound, while epididymitis causes increased flow with ultrasound. Epididymitis also presents with fever and presents with more gradual pain localized to the epididymis (see also Adolescent chapter).

WARD TIP

Do not force retraction of the foreskin in phimosis. This may lead to paraphimosis. Return the foreskin over the glans after cleaning and sex.

- Paraphimosis is the inability to return the prepuce over the glans from a retracted position. Leaving the prepuce retracted may cause venous and lymphatic congestion, followed by arterial compromise and penile infarction, which is a urologic emergency.
- Risk factors for paraphimosis include:
  - Phimosis.
  - Recurrent infections.
  - Failure to return the foreskin over the glans after manipulation.
  - Forceful retraction of the foreskin resulting in scarring.
  - Penile piercing.

SIGNS AND SYMPTOMS

- Phimosis predisposes to urinary retention, UTIs, and inflammation of glans and prepuce.
- Epithelial cells may get trapped under phimotic foreskin and form benign cysts. Cysts help the phimotic foreskin to retract and resolve.
- Phimotic foreskin may balloon out with urination, which is benign unless urine is retained.
- Paraphimosis may present with swelling and tenderness of the penis and a band of circumferential tissue.

TREATMENT

- Phimosis: reassurance and hygiene education. Most resolve spontaneously. Topical steroids and gentle manual stretching loosen the phimotic ring. Circumcision may be offered.
- Paraphimosis: pain control, reduce local swelling, and manually return the foreskin over the glans. In few cases where color change is present, urology consult may be needed.

Balanitis and Balanoposthitis

DEFINITION

- Balanitis: inflammation of the glans penis.
- Balanoposthitis: inflammation of the glans penis and prepuce (foreskin); can only occur in uncircumcised males.
- Multiple possible causes, including:
  - Infections: fungal (candida); bacterial (*E. coli*, enterococcus, staphylococcus); viral (HPV, HSV 1 & 2); protozoal (*Trichomonas vaginalis*, *Entamoeba histolytica*).
  - Irritants: poor hygiene; irritant dermatitis.
  - Trauma.

SIGNS AND SYMPTOMS

- Pain or itching.
- Urinary outflow obstruction due to inflammation.
- Erythema.
- Irritation or erosions.
- Dysuria.
- Penile discharge (must be distinguished from STI urethral discharge).

TREATMENT

- Local hygiene, proper foreskin hygiene.
- Avoid irritants.

- Topical antifungals and antibiotics (avoid neomycin, can cause dermatitis).
- Oral antibiotics if suspected group A strep or staph.
- Consider sexual abuse if STIs suspected in children.

Hypospadias

DEFINITION

- Congenital anomaly resulting in ventral displacement of the male urethra.
- Urethra located between the glans and perineum.
- If hypospadias occurs with undescended testes, consider disorders of sexual development.
- If hypospadias occurs with other congenital anomalies, perform an ultrasound of the upper urinary tract for anomalies.

SIGNS AND SYMPTOMS

- "Two urethral openings," with the second blind ending crevice at normal urethral position.
- "Dorsal hooded prepuce" (foreskin remains open ventrally, looks partially circumcised).
- Abnormal penile curvature (chordee).
- Difficulty controlling urine direction.
- Severe hypospadias may cause erectile dysfunction and infertility.

TREATMENT

- No intervention or surgical repair until 6–18 months, depending on severity.
- Avoid circumcision. It is not safe with a dorsal, hooded prepuce, and the foreskin is used for the future hypospadias surgery.

WARD TIP

It is important to not circumcise newborns with hypospadias because the foreskin may be used in the repair.

Epispadias

- Dorsal opening of the urethra on the penile shaft.
- Associated with more serious congenital abnormalities, such as bladder exstrophy (inside-out bladder that is exposed to the environment due to abnormal abdominal wall development), and/or cloacal exstrophy (exstrophy of bladder and large intestine).

Cryptorchidism (Undescended Testes)

 A 16-year-old healthy boy has sudden onset of abdominal and scrotal pain. A physical examination shows severe tenderness in the right inguinal canal, and the right scrotum is empty. *Think: Testicular torsion of an undescended testicle.*

Most undescended testes are in or distal to the inguinal canal. Torsion should be considered with inguinal pain or swelling in a boy with an undescended testis. Fixation of undescended testes may help prevent torsion.

DEFINITION

- Absent or undescended testicle not in the scrotum by 4 months of age
  - Testes may be absent (agenesis or intrauterine testicular torsion and necrosis ["vanishing testes syndrome"]).

- True undescended testes are in the abdomen (least common), inguinal canal, or at the external ring (most common).
- Retractile undescended testes are elevated and can be manually brought into correct position.
- Acquired undescended testes start descending and then ascend.
- Ectopic testes descend, and then move to perineal, femoral, suprapubic, or contralateral scrotal areas (rare).
- Prematurity is a risk factor (not completely descended in 30% of premature males).

SIGNS AND SYMPTOMS

- Empty, under-formed, or poorly rugated scrotal sac or hemiscrotum.
- May cause inguinal fullness, palpable testes at the external ring or in the inguinal canal.
- Absence of testes on the left more common; may also be bilateral.
- Increased risk for subfertility, malignancy, hernias, torsion, testicular cancer, and trauma.

TREATMENT

- Most descend spontaneously by 3–4 months.
- If born with testes nonpalpable bilaterally or unilaterally with hypospadias, consider sexual development disorders.
- If testes are not palpated or appear atrophic, do exploratory surgery at 6–12 months.
- Orchiopexy at 6–12 months reduces torsion and subfertility risks. Malignancy risk remains increased, but the testes can be examined more easily.
- If retractile, watch and wait until non-descent or descent is confirmed at puberty.

WARD TIP

Orchiopexy does not reduce the risk of testicular malignancy in cryptorchidism, but the testes can be examined more easily.

NOTES

Hematologic Disease

TABLE 15-1. Normal Hemoglobin (Hgb) and Mean Corpuscular Volume (MCV) by Age

AGE	HGB (G/DL)	MCV (FL)
Birth	14–20	100–120
2 month	10–13	78–94
6 month	10.5–13	69–82
1 year	10.5–13.5	70–86
2–12 years	11.5–15.5	70–90
12–18 years	12–16	78–102

Normal Hemoglobin (Hgb) and Mean Corpuscular Volume (MCV) by Age

- Red blood cell (RBC) parameters vary with age, race, and gender (Table 15-1).
- Lower limit of normal (3rd percentile) Hgb from age 1–10 years = 11 + (0.1xAge).
- Lower limit of normal (3rd percentile) MCV from age 1–10 years = 70 + Age.

Anemia

DEFINITION

- Physiological: Hgb level too low to meet cellular oxygen demands.
- Practical: Hgb level 2 SD below mean for age, gender, and race.

CLASSIFICATION

- Based on red blood cell (RBC) size, also known as MCV (see Table 15-2).
- Classification is based on mechanism:
  - Blood loss or RBC sequestration (e.g., trauma).
  - RBC destruction (high reticulocyte count) (e.g., ABO incompatibility in newborn).
  - Decreased RBC production (low reticulocyte count) (e.g., aplastic anemia).
- Hemolytic anemia is mediated by either intrinsic RBC defects or disorders extrinsic to the red cell (see Figure 15-1).

PATHOPHYSIOLOGY

- Less oxygen transport and decreased blood volume lead to clinical consequences.
- Physiological adaptations include:
  - Increased heart rate and stroke volume (increases cardiac output).
  - Increased 2,3 diphosphoglycerate (DPG) levels (leads to decreased O_2 affinity of Hgb and better O_2 delivery).
  - Vasodilatation (expands blood volume).

TABLE 15-2.   Anemias

MCV	ANEMIA	LABS
Microcytic	Iron deficiency	Low ferritin, high TIBC, high platelet count
	Thalassemia	Normal to high RBC count, microcytosis disproportionate to anemia, normal iron studies
	Anemia of chronic disease	High ferritin and low TIBC
	Sideroblastic anemia	Normal or high ferritin
	Some hemoglobinopathies (HbC, HbE, unstable Hbs)	Abnormal hemoglobin electrophoresis
Normocytic	Acute blood loss	
	Hemolytic anemia	High bilirubin/LDH
	Anemia of chronic disease	Very low reticulocyte count
	Hemoglobinopathy	
	Transient erythroblastopenia of childhood	
Macrocytic	Hemolytic	High bilirubin/LDH
	Liver disease, hypothyroidism	
	Drug effect (e.g. hydroxyurea)	Abnormal T_4/TSH
	Diamond Blackfan anemia	Very low reticulocyte count
	Aplastic anemia and myelodysplastic syndromes	Very low reticulocyte count and other cell lines down
Macrocytic with megaloblastic bone marrow	Folate deficiency	Low serum/RBC folate, high homocysteine
	B_{12} deficiency	High serum cobalamin, methylmalonic acid and homocysteine

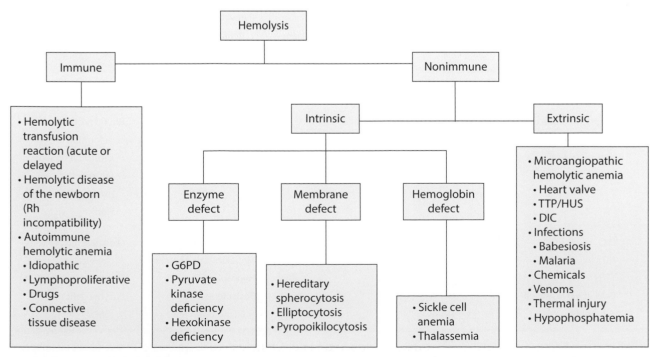

FIGURE 15-1.   Hemolytic anemias.

SIGNS AND SYMPTOMS

- Somnolence, light-headedness, headache, and easy fatiguability.
- Exertional dyspnea, palpitations, sinus tachycardia, and flow murmur.
- Pallor: palpebral conjunctiva, oral mucosa, nail beds; in severe cases, palmar creases.
- Hepatosplenomegaly and/or jaundice in some instances, such as hemolysis.

DIAGNOSIS

- Family history of anemia, gallstones or splenectomy, and ethnic origin.
- Birth history of phototherapy and anemia.
- Dietary history including milk intake.
- Past medical history, including underlying chronic disease, transfusions, and bleeding.
- Physical exam: signs of congestive heart failure, jaundice, hepatosplenomegaly, associated physical anomalies.
- Complete blood count (CBC) with differential and blood smear (Tables 15-2 and 15-3).
- Elevated reticulocyte count response expected in normal marrow in anemia.

TABLE 15-3. Some Erythrocyte Morphology and Inclusion Bodies

CELL	SPHEROCYTE	TARGET CELL	ECHINOCYTE (BURR)	ACANTHOCYTE	DACROCYTE
Description	Round, no central clearing	Central red area within zone of central pallor	Evenly spaced rounded projections off the surface	Irregularly spaced pointy projections off the surface	Teardrop shape
Etiologies	Hereditary spherocytosis Autoimmune and alloimmune hemolytic anemia	Liver disease Hemoglobinopathies (e.g., Hgb C, S) Postsplenectomy Thalassemia	Liver/renal disease Posttransfusion Burns Phosphate deficiency	Liver/renal disease Hyposplenism Pyruvate kinase deficiency	Myelofibrosis Iron deficiency

CELL	SCHISTOCYTE	SICKLE CELLS	BASOPHILIC STIPPLING	HOWELL-JOLLY BODY	HEINZ BODIES
Description	Fragmented due to mechanical damage	Pointed ends with crescentic or boat shape	Round, dark-blue granules in the cell representing aggregated ribosomes	Densely blue cytoplasmic inclusions representing nuclear fragments	Round protuberances deforming the cell on supravital staining, representing oxidized/denatured Hgb
Etiologies	DIC HUS TTP Cardiac valve related hemolysis	Sickle cell disease	Lead poisoning	Hemolytic anemia Megaloblastic anemia Hyposplenism Postsplenectomy	Oxidative medications, chemicals Abnormal Hgb (H, Köln) Enzyme deficiencies (G6PD)

DIC, disseminated intravascular coagulation; G6PD, glucose-6-phosphate dehydrogenase; HUS, hemolytic-uremic syndrome; TTP: thrombotic thrombocytopenic purpura; RBC, red blood cell.

TABLE 15-4. **Hemolytic anemia classification**

CONGENITAL	ACQUIRED
Hemoglobinopathies	Immune mediated
Thalassemia	Warm autoimmune hemolytic anemia
Sickle cell disease	Cold agglutinin
HbC, HbE, other mutations	Paroxysmal cold hemoglobinuria
Unstable hemoglobins	Hemolytic disease of newborn
	Transfusion reaction
Hereditary membrane syndromes	Non immune
such as spherocytosis, elliptocytosis,	Thrombotic microangiopathy such as HUS, TTP and DIC
stomatocytosis and xerocytosis	Mechanical hemolysis due to heart disease
	PNH
Enzymopathies such as G6PD deficiency,	Toxins/drugs
pyruvate kinase deficiency, hexokinase	Thermal burns
deficiency and aldolase deficiency	Wilson Disease

DIC, disseminated intravascular coagulation; HUS, hemolytic uremic syndrome; TTP, thrombotic thrombocytopenic purpura.

- Possible bone marrow aspirate/biopsy—cellularity, morphology, stroma, and flow cytometry.
- Chemistry—liver function tests (LFTs), lactic dehydrogenase (LDH), creatinine (Cr), uric acid.
- Other special tests—ferritin and other iron studies, B_{12}/folate levels, direct Coombs test, haptoglobin, Hgb quantitative methods such as electrophoresis, and lead level.
- In hemolytic anemia, blood tests show reticulocytosis, high LDH and indirect bilirubin, low haptoglobin; polychromasia seen on blood smear.

TREATMENT

- Treat underlying cause.
- RBC transfusion if hemodynamically unstable or severely symptomatic.

WARD TIP

Coombs test: *Direct*—detects IgG bound RBCs (autoimmune hemolysis, hemolytic disease of newborn); *Indirect*—detects unbound autoantibodies to RBCs (antenatal, pretransfusion testing).

PHYSIOLOGIC ANEMIA OF INFANCY

- Normal newborns have a high initial Hgb (14–20 g/dL).
- Decreases to 9–11 g/dL by 8–12 weeks.
- Decline in Hgb is more extreme and more rapid in premature infants: 7–9 g/dL by 3–6 weeks.

ETIOLOGY

- Abrupt cessation of erythropoiesis occurs with the onset of respiration.
- Decreased survival of fetal RBCs compared to adults (60 days versus 120 days).
- Expansion of blood volume in the first 3 months.

TREATMENT

Not normally required: as Hgb approaches its nadir, erythropoietin is produced, with subsequent resumption of erythropoiesis.

TRANSIENT ERYTHROBLASTOPENIA OF CHILDHOOD

> A previously healthy 1-year-old male infant had a cold 8 weeks ago. He now is pale and irritable and refuses to eat. A CBC shows Hgb 5.0, Hct 10%, MCV 80, reticulocyte count 0.1%, WBC 9K, platelets 400K. *Think: Transient erythroblastopenia of childhood (TEC).*

ETIOLOGY

- Transient failure of bone marrow to produce RBCs in a healthy child
- The etiology is unclear, but likely an IgG antibody inhibits erythropoiesis.

CLINICAL FEATURES

- Gradual onset of pallor in a child between the ages of 6 to 60 months (usually >12 months) with clinically appearance better than expected for Hgb level
- Normocytic anemia (Hgb 5–7 g/dL) with reticulocytopenia (<1%); normal or slightly reduced neutrophils

TREATMENT

- Supportive, including transfusion as needed, until spontaneous recovery occurs (typically in 2–3 months)
- If spontaneous resolution does not occur, further investigation is indicated.

DIAMOND BLACKFAN ANEMIA (DBA)

ETIOLOGY

Congenital, genetic failure of bone marrow to produce RBCs

CLINICAL FEATURES

- Presents with pallor in first year of life (usually <3 months).
- DBA should be differentiated from TEC based on MCV and other parameters:

	DBA	TEC
Reticulocytes	low	low
Hemoglobin	low	low
Erythrocyte adenosine deaminase level	elevated	normal
HbF	elevated	normal
MCV	elevated	normal
Congenital anomalies	present in 50%	absent

- DBA is associated with long-term risk of malignancy.
- Draw blood for diagnostic studies before transfusing the patient; post-transfusion values are difficult to interpret.

TREATMENT

RBC transfusion and steroids.

IRON DEFICIENCY ANEMIA

A 15-month-old child drinking 40 ounces of milk a day presents with the following lab values: Hgb 7.5 g/dL, MCV 62, RBC 3.2. *Think: Iron deficiency anemia or IDA.* Consumption of large amounts of cow's milk is the most common dietary pattern in toddlers with IDA. Cow's milk has poor iron bioavailability, reduces iron absorption from other foods, and damages gut mucosa, resulting in small amounts of bleeding.

ETIOLOGY

- Inadequate intake of iron rich foods.
- Loss of iron due to bleeding: heavy menses, inflammatory bowel disease, *H. pylori* gastritis.
- Malabsorption (rare): celiac disease, genetic defects of iron absorption.
- Prematurity (low iron stores).

CLINICAL FEATURES

- Usual symptoms of anemia.
- Pica (desire to eat unusual things such as clay, paper, mud), ice craving.
- Koilonychia (spoon-shaped nails) in chronic cases.

DIAGNOSIS

- Low serum ferritin (earliest finding), low fasting serum iron, low transferrin saturation, and high iron-binding capacity.
- Low MCV and mean corpuscular hemoglobin (MCH), high red cell distribution width (RDW), and low mean reticulocyte hemoglobin content (CHR) or reticulocyte hemoglobin equivalent (Ret-He).
- High platelet count.
- Bone marrow studies: hypercellular marrow with erythroid hyperplasia and reduction of stainable iron.

TREATMENT

- Administer ferrous sulfate (or other iron formulations) 3–6 mg/kg/day of elemental iron for at least 3 months to replenish iron stores.
- Intravenous iron preparations are available for malabsorption or poor oral tolerance.

FOLATE DEFICIENCY

ETIOLOGY

- Deficient intake (e.g., fed with goat's milk) or absorption.
- Pregnancy (increases requirement).
- Very-low-birth-weight (VLBW) infants.
- Drugs (phenytoin, methotrexate).

CLINICAL FEATURES

- Features of anemia.
- Chronic diarrhea and failure to gain weight.
- Angular stomatitis, glossitis, and loss of taste.

DIAGNOSIS

- Macrocytic anemia, mild thrombocytopenia and neutropenia, with hypersegmented neutrophils.
- Low reticulocyte count.

WARD TIP

Mentzer Index
MCV/RBC
≥ 13.5 Iron deficiency (also will see an increased RDW)
≤ 11.5 Thalassemia trait

WARD TIP

Ferritin is an acute-phase reactant. A normal or high ferritin does not exclude iron deficiency during an acute infection.

WARD TIP

Chronic lead poisoning interferes with iron utilization and hemoglobin synthesis, thus leading to anemia. Risk assessment for lead poisoning is recommended between 6 months and 6 years of age, with blood lead testing if the risk assessment is positive. A characteristic feature is basophilic stippling of RBCs.

WARD TIP

Goat's milk is folate deficient, and it is not an acceptable alternative source of infant nutrition to breast milk or formula. Unpasteurized goat's milk can also contain *Brucella.*

WARD TIP

Green vegetables, fruits, liver, and legumes contain folate.

- High LDH.
- Bone marrow: hypercellular with megaloblastic changes.
- Low serum and RBC folate levels, high homocysteine level.

TREATMENT

- Folic acid supplementation
- A high folic acid intake in patients with vitamin B$_{12}$ deficiency will mask anemia, yet B$_{12}$ deficiency neurologic symptoms will progress.

VITAMIN B$_{12}$ DEFICIENCY

ETIOLOGY

- Inadequate intake (exclusively breastfed baby of a vegan mom).
- Pernicious anemia (autoimmune intrinsic factor deficiency prevents adequate B$_{12}$ absorption).
- Malabsorption: stomach (e.g., gastric bypass) or terminal ileum surgery.

CLINICAL FEATURES

- Features of anemia.
- Red, beefy tongue and glossitis.
- Weakness, irritability, and anorexia.
- Neurologic (ataxia, paresthesias, hyporeflexia, Babinski response, and clonus).

DIAGNOSIS

- Macrocytic anemia, mild thrombocytopenia and neutropenia, with hypersegmented neutrophils.
- High LDH.
- Bone marrow: hypercellular with megaloblastic changes.
- Low serum B$_{12}$ and high homocysteine and methionine levels with methylmalonic aciduria.
- Anti-intrinsic factor antibody and Schilling test to determine cause.

TREATMENT

Vitamin B$_{12}$ supplementation, typically IM.

ANEMIA OF CHRONIC DISEASE

ETIOLOGY

- Juvenile idiopathic arthritis (JIA), systemic lupus erythematosus (SLE), and ulcerative colitis.
- Malignancies.
- Renal disease.

CLINICAL FEATURES

Signs and symptoms of underlying disease.

DIAGNOSIS

- Can be normochromic and normocytic or hypochromic and microcytic.
- Low serum iron with normal or low total iron-binding capacity (TIBC).
- Elevated serum ferritin.

TREATMENT

- Treat underlying disease.
- Iron, if concomitant iron deficiency is present.

HEMOLYTIC DISEASE OF THE NEWBORN

ETIOLOGY

- Neonatal or fetal RBC destruction caused by maternal IgG antibodies to Rh, ABO, or other blood system antigens (e.g., Kell, Duffy).
- When an Rh-positive (or other alloantibody) infant is carried by an Rh-negative mother:
  - Maternal blood comes into contact with fetal blood cells presenting the D antigen (Rh$^+$), a different blood group, or other blood system antigens.
  - Maternal antibodies are produced against the "foreign" antigen.
  - Maternal IgG antibodies may cross the placenta and bind to fetal RBC, causing hemolysis.
- Fetal RBC destruction causes increased unconjugated bilirubin, becoming clinically apparent only after delivery (as the placenta effectively clears bilirubin).
- Severe cases may lead to extramedullary erythropoiesis, with potential replacement of hepatic parenchyma.

CLINICAL FEATURES

- These range from mild, self-limited, hemolytic disease to severe life-threatening anemia (hydrops fetalis).
- Hemolytic anemia.
- Fetal hydrops, including:
  - Large placenta.
  - Rapidly progressive jaundice after birth, kernicterus.
  - Abdominal distention: hepatosplenomegaly, ascites, and hepatic dysfunction.
  - Scalp or skin edema.
  - Pleural or pericardial effusion.
  - Cyanosis.

DIAGNOSIS

Features of hemolysis and positive direct Coombs test (also known as direct antiglobulin test [DAT]).

PREVENTION

RhoGAM (pooled anti-D antibodies) is given to Rh$^-$ mothers during pregnancy, and immediately after delivery of Rh$^+$ infants, decreasing their risk of developing anti-D antibodies and Rh sensitization.

TREATMENT

- RBC transfusion may be performed in utero for severely affected fetuses.
- Supportive care with intensive phototherapy is provided after delivery.
- IVIG may be used to decrease the need for exchange transfusion in Rh and ABO hemolytic disease, but data are mixed and further research is required.
- Exchange transfusion may be required with severe hemolysis.

SICKLE CELL DISEASE (SCD)

A 16-month-old African-American boy is brought to the ED because of crying and refusal to stand. He has no fever, vomiting, or diarrhea. His parents denied trauma or fall. On examination, he is afebrile. He cries when his right leg is touched. An X-ray of his right leg showed no fracture. *Think: Sickle cell disease.*

Acute sickle cell painful episode (pain crisis) is the most common presentation in children with SCD. Newborn screening has resulted in detection in early infancy. Labs show chronic hemolytic anemia. Peripheral smear may show sickled forms, target cells, and polychromasia suggestive of reticulocytosis.

ETIOLOGY

- Autosomal recessive disorder due to mutation in β-globin of Hgb with substitution of glutamic acid at sixth position of β-chain by valine.
- HbS molecules aggregate in a deoxygenated state to form polymers, especially in states of low O_2 saturation→polymers bend to make rigid sickle RBCs→block capillaries→vaso-occlusion and hemolysis.
- Pathophysiology is multifactorial, including: oxidative stress, inflammation and hypercoagulability.

CLINICAL FEATURES

- One in 365 U.S. African-Americans are born with SCD; 1 in 13 have the sickle cell trait.
- Signs and symptoms appear after 6 months of age as the protective HbF levels decline.
    - Anemia (due to hemolysis): reduced exercise tolerance, cardiomegaly, poor growth.
    - Vaso-occlusive crises: recurrent painful events, dactylitis (swollen hands and feet), acute chest syndrome (ACS; pulmonary infiltrate with respiratory signs and symptoms), acute splenic sequestration (ASSC; sudden splenic enlargement with drop in Hgb), stroke, priapism.
    - Infection with encapsulated organisms (*Pneumococcus*, *Meningococcus*, *Haemophilus influenzae*, *Salmonella*) due to functional hyposplenism leading to overwhelming sepsis.
    - Splenomegaly initially, followed by splenic infarction that leads to functional asplenia.
    - Aplastic crisis: severe anemia due to bone marrow suppression by parvovirus.
    - Hemolytic crises: acute on chronic hemolysis due to trigger such as infection or medication.
    - Sleep disordered breathing, pulmonary hypertension, and cardiomyopathy.
    - Delayed sexual maturation, fertility issues and vitamin D deficiency.
    - Nocturnal enuresis, hyposthenuria, and renal failure.
    - Sickle cell retinopathy.
    - Venous stasis ulcers and avascular osteonecrosis (femoral and/or humeral head).
    - Neurocognitive deficits and academic underachievement (cerebral infarction).

DIAGNOSIS

- Newborn screening in all states leads to early diagnosis in the U.S.
- Hgb electrophoresis: HbS 90%, HbF 2-10% and HbA 0%.

TREATMENT

- Clinical surveillance for complications.

- Infection prevention: additional pneumococcus and meningococcus vaccines, penicillin prophylaxis until 5 years of age, immediate medical attention for fever with empirical antibiotics.
- Supportive care: hydration, analgesics, transfusion for severe complications.
- Acute exchange transfusion for stroke, multi-organ dysfunction, or other situations needing rapid HbS reduction without causing hyperviscosity associated with increase in Hgb.
- Hydroxyurea reduces the incidence of acute painful episodes and hospitalizations through multiple mechanisms, mainly increasing HbF.
- L-glutamine, crizanlizumab (P-selectin inhibitor), and voxelotor (HbS polymerization inhibitor) are other agents for long-term use.
- Stem cell transplant is curative, and gene therapy is undergoing clinical trials.

THALASSEMIA

 A 2-year-old boy has required transfusion since early infancy. *Think:* β-*thalassemia major.*
Children with β-thalassemia usually become symptomatic in early infancy because of progressive hemolytic anemia and cardiac decompensation. Severe hypochromia and microcytosis are the characteristics of β-thalassemia. The hemoglobin level declines progressively in the first year and may be as low as 3–4 g/dL, requiring transfusion.

ETIOLOGY

- Defective synthesis of alpha or beta globins due to gene mutations.
- **α-Thalassemia** (based on mutation inheritance pattern in 4 alpha genes αα/αα):
    - Hb Bart's (four-gene deletion or --/--).
    - HbH (three-gene deletion or --/-α).
    - **α**-Thalassemia minor (two-gene deletion, either -α /-α or --/αα).
    - Silent carrier (one-gene deletion, –α/αα).
- **β-Thalassemia** (based on mutation inheritance pattern in 2 beta genes β/β):
    - Classification into thalassemia major, intermedia, and minor based on clinical phenotype.

CLINICAL FEATURES

Anemia signs and symptoms, hepatosplenomegaly, and bony overgrowth due to extramedullary hematopoiesis (classic facies: maxillary overgrowth and skull bossing).

DIAGNOSIS

- Hypochromic, microcytic anemia with reticulocytopenia and high LDH due to ineffective erythropoiesis.
- Hgb electrophoresis: HbA2 and HbF high in β thalassemia, HbH or Barts Hgb may be present in α thalassemia.

TREATMENT

- β-Thalassemia major: monthly RBC transfusions to prevent extramedullary hematopoiesis, iron chelation therapy, and stem cell transplant, if possible.
- Splenectomy if requiring >240 mL/kg of packed RBCs/year.
- Transfusions as needed for moderate phenotypes.
- Thalassemia trait requires no management other than genetic counseling and avoidance of unnecessary iron therapy.

WARD TIP

β-Thalassemia major is fatal without regular transfusion.

WARD TIP

Hemosiderosis is an iron-overload disorder that can lead to cardiomyopathy, cirrhosis, and diabetes due to deposition of hemosiderin.

GLUCOSE-6-PHOSPHATE DEHYDROGENASE (G6PD) DEFICIENCY

A previously well 2-year-old African-American male is treated with trimethoprim/sulfamethoxazole. Two days into treatment he develops fever, back pain, dark urine, and anemia. Blood smear shows fragmented erythrocytes. *Think: G6PD deficiency.*

G6PD deficiency is a recessive X-linked trait; therefore, males are at higher risk. It is caused by exposures that cause oxidant stress, such as infection or drugs. Sulfonamides and antimalarial drugs (primaquine and chloroquine) are the common agents. Most patients are asymptomatic unless exposed to an oxidant stress that results in episodic hemolytic crises. Heinz bodies, indicative of denatured hemoglobin, are typically present and can be detected by a methyl violet stain. G6PD levels can be deceptively normal during an acute crisis because of elevated numbers of reticulocytes and young erythrocytes with near normal enzymatic function.

ETIOLOGY

- This X-linked recessive disorder causes a low G6PD level, an enzyme defect of the hexose monophosphate (HMP) pathway, that results in hemolysis 24 to 48 hours after exposure to stresses such as infection or certain drugs.
- G6PD normally maintains an adequate level of glutathione in a <u>reduced</u> state in RBCs. However, <u>oxidized</u> glutathione complexes with Hgb, forming Heinz bodies→RBCs become less deformable→splenic macrophages "bite out" RBCs leading to blister cells and bite cells seen on peripheral smear.

CLINICAL FEATURES

- Most common hemolytic enzymopathy.
- Higher incidence in African-American, Middle Eastern, and Mediterranean populations.
- Episodic intravascular hemolysis secondary to oxidant stress (drugs, fava beans).
- Chronic nonspherocytic hemolytic anemia in severe cases (Mediterranean variant).
- Jaundice, dark urine.
- Splenomegaly.

DIAGNOSIS

- Reduced G6PD activity in RBCs (<10% in Mediterranean variant and 10–60% in African-American variant).
- Anemia, Heinz bodies, and bite cells on peripheral smear.
- Hemolysis with major intravascular component: reticulocytosis, elevated serum bilirubin and LDH, low serum haptoglobin, and hemoglobinuria.

TREATMENT

- Removal of oxidant stressor.
- Avoidance of known triggers.
- Oxygen.
- Transfusion of packed RBC for Hgb <7, hemodynamic instability, and ongoing hemolysis.

PYRUVATE KINASE (PK) DEFICIENCY

ETIOLOGY

Autosomal recessive defect, resulting in deficiency of RBC PK, an enzyme that catalyzes the final step in the glycolytic pathway.

CLINICAL FEATURES

- Chronic hemolytic anemia.
- Hyperbilirubinemia/failure to thrive (FTT) in newborn.
- Severity of hemolysis is variable, but it may require chronic transfusions.

DIAGNOSIS

Low RBC PK activity.

TREATMENT

- An exchange transfusion may be needed for neonatal hyperbilirubinemia.
- Transfusion of packed RBCs for severe anemia or aplastic crisis.
- Splenectomy (after 5–6 years of age), if persistently severe anemia or frequent transfusion requirement.
- Folate supplementation.

HEREDITARY SPHEROCYTOSIS

 A 4-year-old boy has pallor and a family history of gallstone surgery. His Hgb is 8 g/dL, reticulocyte count 11%, bilirubin 2.0 mg/dL. *Think: Hereditary spherocytosis.*
Hereditary spherocytosis is a common inherited autosomal-dominant hemolytic anemia. The characteristic feature is spherocytic red cells that are intrinsically defective. Splenomegaly and gallstones are common. Spherocytes are present in the peripheral blood smear. Splenectomy is helpful in reducing the rate of hemolysis.

ETIOLOGY

- Autosomal-dominant disorder leading to defect in erythrocyte membrane proteins.
- Abnormal proteins result in a destabilized RBC membrane that leads to spherocytes.
- Abnormal RBCs become sequestered in the spleen and hemolyze.
- 30% of cases are sporadic.

CLINICAL FEATURES

- Commonly asymptomatic.
- Possible neonatal jaundice and anemia needing transfusion.
- Aplastic/hemolytic crisis.
- Splenomegaly.
- Gallstones at a young age.
- Chronic anemia is usually mild and detected on blood tests.

DIAGNOSIS

- A family history of hemolytic anemia and spherocytes on blood smear is diagnostic.
- An osmotic fragility test historically used to confirm diagnosis is not reliable in neonates. The eosin-5-maleimide (EMA) binding assay is more sensitive and specific.

TREATMENT

- Supportive in mild cases with transfusion, as needed.
- Full or partial splenectomy (avoid or at least delay until >5 years old).

EXAM TIP

Spherocytosis is the most common erythrocyte membrane defect.

WARD TIP

Hereditary spherocytosis has the following characteristics: increased osmotic fragility, increased reticulocyte count, positive family history (in 70% of cases), and splenomegaly. Coombs test is negative.

WARD TIP

Splenectomy predisposes patients to overwhelming post-splenectomy infections (OPSIs) caused by encapsulated organisms:
- *Streptococcus pneumoniae*
- *Neisseria meningitidis*
- *Haemophilus influenzae*

WARD TIP

The onset of paroxysmal nocturnal hemoglobinuria is in late childhood.

EXAM TIP

Causes of aplastic anemia include drug exposure (e.g., chloramphenicol) and chemical exposure (e.g., benzene).

PAROXYSMAL NOCTURNAL HEMOGLOBINURIA (PNH)

ETIOLOGY

- Complement-induced hemolytic anemia is caused by acquired defect in RBC membrane.
- PIG-A gene mutation leads to a lack of membrane proteins CD55 and CD59, making RBC sensitive to complement-mediated destruction.

CLINICAL FEATURES

- Red urine: intravascular hemolysis is worse with relative nocturnal hypoxia and/or more concentrated urine.
- Thrombosis, particularly in intra-abdominal and cerebral veins.
- Possible marrow failure leading to pancytopenia.
- Intermittent or chronic hemolytic anemia.
- Increased risk of leukemia.

DIAGNOSIS

- Features of hemolysis, especially low haptoglobin and macrocytosis.
- Sucrose lysis test, Ham's acid hemolysis test historically used.
- Flow cytometry detects diagnostic clones with absent CD55 and CD59.

TREATMENT

- Bone marrow transplantation for severe disease, especially with aplasia.
- Splenectomy not indicated.
- Eculizumab: humanized monoclonal antibody that inhibits the activation of terminal complement components (blocks the split of C5 into C5a and C5b).
- Iron supplementation (urinary iron loss).
- Folic acid supplementation.

Aplastic Anemia

- Rare group of closely related disorders with reduced numbers in 2 or more cell lines (pancytopenia).
- Bone marrow is replaced with fat and shows reduced cellularity (<25% on bone marrow biopsy: severe aplastic anemia).

ETIOLOGY

- Idiopathic: aberrant immune response causes T cell mediated stem cell destruction.
- Other causes (rare) include: drugs/chemicals, radiation, viruses (hepatitis, EBV), secondary to other diseases such as autoimmune disease, PNH, and myelodysplastic syndrome.
- Genetic causes of marrow failure syndromes (e.g., Fanconi anemia).

CLINICAL FEATURES

- Fatigue (fewer RBCs).
- Infections (fewer WBCs).
- Bleeding (fewer platelets).
- Increased risk of leukemia.

DIAGNOSIS

- CBC is suspicious if at least two cell lines are down.
- Bone marrow biopsy is definitive.
- Decreased reticulocyte count.

TREATMENT

- Supportive care: platelet and RBC transfusions, granulocyte colony-stimulating factor (G-CSF) or granulocyte-macrophage colony-stimulating factor (GM-CSF), as needed.
- Immunosuppressive therapy—antithymocyte globulin (ATG) and cyclosporine.
- Eltrombopag is a newer agent sometimes added to the therapy above.
- Stem cell transplantation is curative: it is the first-line treatment if a matched sibling donor is available.

Thrombotic Thrombocytopenic Purpura (TTP)

ETIOLOGY

Hereditary (rare) or acquired von Willebrand factor (vWF) cleaving protease deficiency (ADAMTS13) leads to hemolytic anemia from vWF multimer deposition into microvasculature.

CLINICAL FEATURES

- Fever may be present.
- Microangiopathic hemolytic anemia.
- Thrombocytopenia.
- Abnormal renal function.
- Neurologic signs.
- Risk of stroke, cardiac ischemia, and mesenteric ischemia.

DIAGNOSIS

- Normal prothrombin time (PT) and activated partial thromboplastin time (aPTT).
- Microangiopathic hemolytic anemia with schistocytes, spherocytes, and helmet cells.
- High reticulocyte count with negative direct antiglobulin test (DAT / direct Coombs test).
- Thrombocytopenia.

TREATMENT

- Plasmapheresis and steroids are the main therapy.
- Splenectomy, rituximab, and caplacizumab are used in severe or refractory cases.

WARD TIP

Diagnostic pentad for TTP:
FATRN
- **F**ever
- **A**nemia
- **T**hrombocytopenia
- **R**enal dysfunction
- **N**eurologic abnormality

Hemolytic Uremic Syndrome (HUS)

 Ten days after an episode of diarrhea, a 2-year-old boy has pallor and icterus and petechiae of the skin and mucous membranes. His mother reports that he has not urinated for 24 hours. Characteristic lab findings include fragmented erythrocytes on smear, high blood urea nitrogen (BUN), high reticulocyte count, indirect hyperbilirubinemia, and normal platelet count. *Think: HUS.*

HUS is a common cause of renal failure in children. Triad: microangiopathic hemolytic anemia, thrombocytopenia, and uremia. The onset is usually preceded by gastroenteritis. The platelet count is usually low, but it may be normal early in the course of illness.

ETIOLOGY

- Acquired HUS: acute gastroenteritis caused by *Escherichia coli* O157:H7 (produces a Shiga-like toxin); responsible for 90% of HUS cases.

- Hereditary HUS: complement gene-mutation errors (most common hereditary cause), cobalamin C metabolism, and diacylglycerol kinase epsilon (DGKE) gene mutations (rare).

CLINICAL FEATURES

- Hemolytic anemia.
- Thrombocytopenia.
- Acute renal failure (ARF).

DIAGNOSIS

- History of bloody diarrhea.
- Abnormal red cell morphology (schistocytes).
- Thrombocytopenia with normal marrow megakaryocytes.
- Urine: protein, RBCs, and casts.

TREATMENT

- Fluid management and dialysis, if needed.
- Eculizumab for atypical HUS.
- Plasmapheresis (for neurologic complications).
- Antibiotics not indicated.

Infections Causing Hemolytic Anemia

- Sepsis and productions of hemolysins: clostridium, staphylococcus, and streptococcus.
- Warm autoimmune hemolytic anemia triggered by viral infections.
- Cold agglutinin hemolytic anemia: listeria, mycoplasma, and EBV.
- Congenital infections causing hemolysis: CMV, toxoplasma, syphilis, rubella, and HSV.
- Malarial anemia: mechanical hemolysis with splenomegaly, possible immune-mediated destruction (DAT+), defective marrow response (non-hemolytic component).

Bleeding Disorders

- Bleeding due to platelet problems usually occurs immediately and is mucocutaneous.
- Bleeding due to clotting-factor deficiencies is often "deeper" bleeding (intra-articular, intramuscular) and can be delayed.
- See Table 15-5 for diagnostic tests.

IMMUNE THROMBOCYTOPENIC PURPURA (ITP)

EXAM TIP

ITP is the most common thrombocytopenia of childhood.

WARD TIP

Purpuric lesions do not blanch.

A 4-year-old previously healthy girl with purple skin lesions had a visit to the ED with an upper respiratory infection (URI) a month ago. CBC is normal except for low platelets. *Think: ITP.*

Typical presentation: A sudden onset of generalized petechiae and purpura occurs in a previously healthy child. Often, there is a history of a viral infection weeks before the onset. Physical examination is usually normal except for the petechiae and purpura. Complete remission occurs in most children.

TABLE 15-5. **Coagulation Tests**

Test	Purpose	
PT (INR)	Extrinsic system	Elevated in DIC, warfarin use, liver failure, myelofibrosis, vitamin K deficiency, fat malabsorption, circulating anticoagulants, factor deficiencies
aPTT	Intrinsic	Elevated in factor deficiencies, circulating anticoagulants, heparin use, higher doses of warfarin
Bleeding time	Surgical	Related to platelet count If lengthened and platelet count is normal, consider qualitative platelet defect
Platelet count	Related to bleeding time	<100,000/mm³—mild prolongation of bleeding time <50,000/mm³—easy bruising <20,000/mm³—↑ incidence of spontaneous bleeding
Platelet aggregation	Qualitative	May be abnormal even with normal platelet count—qualitative platelet disorders (Glanzmann's thrombasthenia and Bernard Soulier syndrome), von Willebrand factor deficiency
D-dimer	Intravascular fibrinolysis	Elevated in DIC, trauma, inflammatory disease Sensitive for active clotting, but not specific
Assays for specific factors	Quantitative	Hemophilia A (VIII), hemophilia B (IX), von Willebrand factor deficiency (VIII, vWF antigen and activity)

aPTT, activated partial thromboplastin time; DIC, disseminated intravascular coagulation; INR, International Normalized Ratio; PT, prothrombin time.

ETIOLOGY

- Immune platelet destruction by autoantibodies after an infection or unknown trigger.
- Antibody binds to the platelet membrane and results in accelerated destruction by macrophages, predominantly in the spleen.
- Associated with antecedent viral illnesses in 50–65% of cases.

CLINICAL FEATURES

- Abrupt onset of petechial, purpura, and epistaxis.
- Usually 1–4 weeks after a viral infection.
- <1% of patients with acute ITP will have intracranial bleed.

DIAGNOSIS

- Diagnosis of exclusion.
- WBC and Hgb levels normal.
- Normal peripheral smear except thrombocytopenia.
- Bone marrow (not always indicated): normal to increased megakaryocytes.

TREATMENT

- Observation in the absence of active bleeding (>80% recover within several months without treatment); educate on avoiding injury and medications affecting platelets
- Admit if platelet count is <20,000/mm³.

Primary ITP is a diagnosis of exclusion.

WARD TIP

Historically, prednisone was not given in ITP without a marrow examination. It is now acceptable to give steroids after a careful peripheral smear evaluation (large platelets and absence of blasts on smear point toward ITP) if a low suspicion for a malignant process exists.

WARD TIP

Anti-Rho antibodies can only be used if patient is Rh⁺.

- For active or prolonged bleeding: intravenous immune globulin (IVIG) or anti-Rho antibodies.
- Oral or intravenous steroids may also be given for active bleeding.
- Other therapies in refractory or chronic cases include: rituximab, thrombopoietin mimetics (romiplostim and eltrombopag), and splenectomy.
- Splenectomy is indicated urgently for intracranial hemorrhage.
- Platelet transfusion is generally not helpful.

DISSEMINATED INTRAVASCULAR COAGULATION (DIC)

ETIOLOGY

- Sepsis.
- Incompatible transfusion.
- Rickettsial infection.
- Snake bite.
- Acute promyelocytic leukemia.

CLINICAL FEATURES

- Early stage of hypercoagulation followed by bleeding symptoms.
- Petechiae and ecchymoses.
- Hemolysis.

DIAGNOSIS

- Prolonged PT and aPTT.
- Low fibrinogen and platelets.
- High d-dimer.

TREATMENT

- Treat underlying cause.
- Replacement therapy includes:
  - Platelets (thrombocytopenia).
  - Cryoprecipitate (hypofibrinogenemia).
  - Fresh-frozen plasma (FFP) (replacement of coagulation factors).
- Cautiously administered heparin prevents the consumption of coagulation factors.

VON WILLEBRAND DISEASE

 A child presents with epistaxis, prolonged bleeding time, and a normal platelet count. *Think: von Willebrand disease.*

von Willebrand disease is the most common inherited bleeding disorder. A family history of an established bleeding disorder should be sought. Typical presentation is mucocutaneous bleeding (excessive bruising, epistaxis, and menorrhagia). The evaluation involves qualitative and quantitative measurements of von Willebrand factor (vWF).

ETIOLOGY

- Autosomal dominant (type 1, most common) or recessive (type 3, rare) gene mutations leading to qualitative (type 2) or quantitative (type 1 and type 3) vWF deficiency.

- Defective platelet function and reduced half-life of factor VIII (both due to defective vWF) contribute to bleeding symptoms.

CLINICAL FEATURES

- Easy bruising.
- Heavy or prolonged menstruation.
- Frequent or prolonged epistaxis.
- Prolonged bleeding after injury, surgery (circumcision), or invasive dental procedures.

DIAGNOSIS

- Family or personal history of bleeding episodes.
- aPTT normal or prolonged.
- Normal PT and platelet count.
- Abnormal vWF panel: low vWF antigen and activity and normal or low factor VIII activity.

TREATMENT

- Supportive care: avoid trauma and medications that can cause bleeding.
- Desmopressin (DDAVP) for surgery, if needed.
- Antifibrinolytics as needed: tranexamic acid and aminocaproic acid.
- Recombinant vWF before major surgery or bleeding.

HEMOPHILIA

ETIOLOGY

- X-linked recessive coagulation defect.
- Hemophilia A: Factor VIII deficiency.
- Hemophilia B: Factor IX deficiency.

CLINICAL FEATURES

- Hemophilia A is more common than hemophilia B.
- Hemophilia A is more likely to be severe.
- Easy bruising occurs.
- Intramuscular hematomas occur.
- Hemarthroses, especially into a large joint, leads to joint destruction if untreated.
- Spontaneous hemorrhaging if levels <5%, i.e., severe disease.

DIAGNOSIS

- Family history.
- aPTT 2–3 times upper limit of normal.
- Normal PT and platelet count.
- Specific factor assays.

TREATMENT

- Early diagnosis.
- Prevent trauma.
- Prompt management of bleeding.
- Recombinant factors (prophylactic versus on-demand).
- Avoid certain medications (anticoagulants, aspirin, NSAIDs).
- Amount and frequency of factor replacement depends on clinical need (see Table 15-6).

WARD TIP

Patient should have therapeutic trial of DDAVP to measure response before use.

EXAM TIP

Side effects of DDAVP include: tachyphylaxis, redness/flushing, and hyponatremia.

EXAM TIP

Hemophilia A and hemophilia B are X-linked recessive diseases that present in male children of carrier females.

WARD TIP

Patients with hemophilia may lose large amounts of blood into an iliopsoas hematoma.

WARD TIP

Severe hemophilia <1% of factor activity.

EXAM TIP

Only 30% of male infants with hemophilia bleed at circumcision.

EXAM TIP

In hemophilia, aPTT corrects in mixing studies.

WARD TIP

- 1 unit of VIII/kg raises FVIII level by 2%
- 1 unit of IX/kg raises FIX level by 1%

TABLE 15-6. Factor VIII Replacement

TYPE OF HEMORRHAGE	DESIRED LEVEL (%) VIII
Joint or superficial muscle (except iliopsoas)	40–60% for 2–3 days
Iliopsoas or deep muscle with neurovascular injury	100% for 1–2 days, 50% for 3–5 days
Dental extraction	50–80% pre-operative
Head injury	100% for 1–7 days, 50% for 8–21 days
Major surgery	100% pre-operative, gradual taper over 7–14 days

Hypercoagulable States

- Thrombosis can be due to hereditary or acquired risk factors that lead to disturbances in the three areas of Virchow's triad:
  - Endothelial damage (e.g., inflammation, trauma, burns, infection, surgery, central lines, artificial heart valves).
  - Change in blood flow (e.g., immobilization, local pressure, congestive heart failure, dehydration, hyperviscosity, and pregnancy).
  - Hypercoagulability (e.g., factor release secondary to surgery, trauma, malignancy); antiphospholipid antibodies, lupus, oral contraceptive use; genetic predispositions such as deficiencies of protein S, protein C, antithrombin III, or mutations such as factor V Leiden and prothrombin G20210A; nephrotic syndrome, polycythemia vera, sickle cell anemia, homocystinemia, dysfibrinogenemia, TTP.

SIGNS AND SYMPTOMS

- Deep-vein thrombosis.
- Pulmonary embolism.
- Myocardial infarction.
- Stroke.

DIAGNOSIS

- Family history of thrombosis at an early age or recurrent pregnancy loss.
- Patient history of recurrent, early, unusual, or idiopathic thromboses.
- Appropriate screening.
- Risk factor assessment.

TREATMENT

- Reduce risk factors: mobilize patients, stop smoking and using alcohol, and hydrate.
- Aspirin, unfractionated heparin intravenous drip or subcutaneous low molecular weight heparin, warfarin, direct oral anticoagulants, as appropriate.

Transfusion Medicine

GENERAL INDICATIONS FOR TRANSFUSION OF BLOOD PRODUCTS

- Packed RBCs: Hgb <7g/dl or 7–10g/dl if symptomatic (higher Hgb cut-off for certain situations, such as thalassemia, neonates, and severe heart disease).

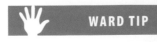

WARD TIP

Children rarely have febrile reactions to initial transfusion unless they are immunoglobulin A (IgA) deficient.

- Platelets: platelet count <10,000/μL; 10,000−50,000/μL if bleeding; <50,000/μL in preparation for most surgeries (<100,000/μL for eye or central nervous system), platelet function disorders with bleeding.
- FFP: bleeding from vitamin K deficiency or warfarin overdose, liver disease, plasma exchange for TTP, DIC, factor deficiencies (e.g., fibrinogen, factor V, severe protein C or S).
- Cryoprecipitate: hypofibrinogenemia, hemophilia A, vWF deficiency, and factor XIII deficiency.

COMPLICATIONS

- Transfusion reactions: most are febrile non-hemolytic or urticarial (see Table 15-7).
- Disease transmission (e.g., HIV, hepatitis B virus [HBV], hepatitis C virus [HCV], human T-lymphotropic virus [HTLV], cytomegalovirus [CMV], parvovirus).
- Iron overload, electrolyte disturbances.
- Fluid overload, hypothermia.

WARD TIP

Life-threatening transfusion reactions are nearly always due to clerical errors (wrong ABO blood type).

Methemoglobinemia

ETIOLOGY

- Congenital
  - Deficiency of cytochrome b5 reductase.
  - Hemoglobin M disease (inability to convert methemoglobin back to hemoglobin).
- Acquired
  - Increased production of methemoglobin typically results from specific drugs or agents that cause an increase in methemoglobin production (nitrites [contaminated water], xylocaine/benzocaine [teething gel], sulfonamides, benzene, aniline dyes, and potassium chlorate).
- Altered state of hemoglobin (ferrous irons of heme [Fe^{++}] are oxidized to ferric [Fe^{+++}]), and ferric form is unable to transport oxygen.

CLINICAL FEATURES

Depends on the concentration:

- 10−30%: cyanosis.
- 30−50%: dyspnea, tachycardia, dizziness.
- 50−70%: lethargy, stupor.
- >70%: death.

DIAGNOSIS

Methemoglobin level, co-oximetry studies.

TREATMENT

- <30%: treatment not needed; 30−70%: IV methylene blue.
- Hyperbaric O_2.
- Oral ascorbic acid (200−500 mg).

WARD TIP

Suspect methemoglobinemia if:
- oxygen-unresponsive cyanosis.
- chocolate-brown blood.

Porphyria

ETIOLOGY

A group of inherited and acquired disorders due to inherited heme biosynthetic pathway deficiency.

EXAM TIP

Porphyria cutanea tarda is the most common of the porphyrias.

TABLE 15-7. **Transfusion Reactions**

Type	Etiology	Signs and Symptoms	Treatment	Prevention
Acute hemolytic	RBC blood group incompatibility	Fever, chills, nausea, dyspnea, flank pain, abdominal pain, infusion site pain, tachycardia, hypotension, hemoglobinuria	Stop transfusion and send DAT Manage blood pressure and renal perfusion Control DIC	Pretransfusion testing Accurate labeling, unit inspection Proper patient identification
Delayed hemolytic	Antibodies to minor blood group antigens during prior transfusion (Kidd, Duffy, Rh, Kell)	Hemolytic symptoms as above, usually mild, 3–10 days post-transfusion; can cause profound anemia	Send DAT; supportive	
Allergic	Antibodies to plasma proteins	Hives, itching, local erythema	Antihistamines	Pretransfusion antihistamines Washed blood products
Anaphylactic	Antibodies to IgA in IgA deficient individuals	Cough, respiratory distress, bronchospasm Nausea, vomiting, abdominal cramps, diarrhea Shock, vascular instability, loss of consciousness	Stop transfusion Epinephrine Supportive care	IgA-deficient plasma products Washed blood products
Febrile nonhemolytic	Antibodies to granulocytes Cytokines and other pyrogens released from leukocytes/platelets	Fever, chills, diaphoresis	Stop transfusion while investigating cause Antipyretics	Pretransfusion antipyretics Leukocyte-reduced blood products
Transfusion-related acute lung injury (TRALI)	Antigranulocyte or anti HLA antibodies in donor product	Bilateral pulmonary infiltrates with fever, chills Cyanosis, hypoxemia Respiratory distress, cough Hypotension, normal central venous pressure ARDS-like picture	Supportive, including O_2 and mechanical ventilation	Do not use plasma products from implicated donor
Transfusion associated circulatory overload (TACO)	Hypervolemia Rapid infusion CHF	Dyspnea, cyanosis, hypoxemia Tachycardia Pulmonary edema, cough	Diuretics Oxygen Phlebotomy	Pretransfusion diuretics Slow infusion Limit volume

ARDS, adult respiratory distress syndrome; CHF, congestive heart failure; DIC, disseminated intravascular coagulation; IgA, immunoglobulin A; RBC, red blood cell.

CLINICAL FEATURES

- Acute (hepatic) porphyria: abdominal pain, vomiting, neuropathy, mental disturbances, seizures, autonomic nervous system dysfunction, arrythmias, tachycardia; risk of hepatocellular carcinoma over lifetime.
- Cutaneous (erythropoietic) porphyria: edema, blister formation, increased hair growth, photosensitivity, and red urine.
- Precipitated by drugs, infection.

DIAGNOSIS

- Spectroscopy: blood, urine, and stool.
- Serum/urine porphyrin levels.
- Measurement of porphyrin precursors ALA and PBG.

TREATMENT

- Acute attacks: analgesia, hydration, maintain electrolytes, IV hematin especially if low serum sodium or status epilepticus, high-carbohydrate diet, glucose 10% infusion.
- For long-term management:
  - Avoid alcohol and drugs that can precipitate an attack.
  - Sunscreen.

Disorders of White Blood Cells

NEUTROPENIA

DEFINITION

Absolute neutrophil count (ANC) <1500/μL:

- Mild: 1000−1500/μL.
- Moderate: 500−1000/μL.
- Severe: <500/μL.

ETIOLOGY

- Congenital: severe congenital neutropenia (most common is Kostmann syndrome), cyclic neutropenia, Shwachman-Diamond syndrome, bone marrow failure syndromes, neutropenia associated with immunodeficiencies or metabolic disorders, and familial benign neutropenia.
- Acquired: infection, drugs, autoimmune, nutritional deficiencies (B_{12}, folate, copper), bone marrow infiltration, hypersplenism.

CLINICAL FEATURES

- High susceptibility to bacterial and fungal infections (especially Pseudomonas) when ANC <500/μL.
- Stomatitis, gingivitis, recurrent otitis media, cellulitis, pneumonia, and septicemia.

TRANSIENT LEUKEMOID REACTION

- Leukocyte counts more than 50,000/μL.
- Peripheral smear with immature myeloid cells.
- Caused by infections or inflammatory syndromes; resolves upon addressing underlying etiology.
- May resemble acute leukemia.
- May be seen in infants with trisomy 21.

WARD TIP

ANC = Total WBC × (Segs% + Bands%).

NOTES

Oncology

Leukemia

 A 3-year-old girl has had fever, anorexia, and fatigue for the past month. She has lost 5 kg. She has pallor, cervical adenopathy, splenomegaly, skin ecchymoses, and petechiae. *Think: Acute leukemia.*

The typical presentation is pancytopenia—anemia (pallor and fatigue) and thrombocytopenia (epistaxis, ecchymoses, and petechiae); white cells may be low or high. The initial presentation may be nonspecific and subtle and develop over weeks to months. The final diagnosis depends on the results of bone marrow aspirate and biopsy.

EPIDEMIOLOGY

- Leukemia is the most common childhood malignancy (brain tumors are number two).
- Leukemia represents 30% of all childhood malignancies.
- Acute lymphocytic leukemia (ALL) is five times more common than acute myelogenous leukemia (AML).

RISK FACTORS

- Trisomy 21.
- Fanconi anemia and other inherited marrow failure syndromes.
- Bloom syndrome.
- Immune deficiency syndromes, including ataxia-telangiectasia

CLINICAL FEATURES

- Fever.
- Pallor.
- Bleeding.
- Bone pain.
- Lymphadenopathy.
- Hepatosplenomegaly.

TREATMENT

- Chemotherapy specific to type of leukemia.
- Infection prevention: empiric antibiotics for febrile neutropenia and isolation, if necessary.
- Monitoring for occurrence of tumor lysis, hydration, allopurinol, or rasburicase.
- Transfusions, as needed.
- Hyperleukocytosis: leukapheresis and hydroxyurea.

ACUTE LYMPHOBLASTIC LEUKEMIA (ALL)

- Most common malignancy in children.
- Eighty percent of leukemia in children.

CLINICAL FEATURES

- Fatigue, anorexia, lethargy, pallor.
- Bone pain.
- Fever.
- Bleeding, bruising, petechiae.
- Lymphadenopathy.
- Hepatosplenomegaly.

WARD TIP

Between 70 and 80% of childhood cases of ALL are of the precursor B cell lineage.

- Testicular swelling.
- Septicemia.

DIAGNOSIS

- CBC: anemia, abnormal white count, low platelet count.
- Abnormal electrolytes: low calcium, high phosphorus, high uric acid, high LDH.
- Chest x-ray (mediastinal mass).
- Bone marrow: hypercellular, increased lymphoblasts.
- Cerebrospinal fluid (CSF): blasts.
- Cytogenetics and flow cytometry for risk stratification and classification.

TREATMENT

- Remission induction: vincristine, prednisone, asparaginase, doxorubicin.
- Consolidation and delayed intensification: 6-mercaptopurine (6MP), etoposide, cytarabine, cyclophosphamide, high dose methotrexate.
- Maintenance therapy: 2 years—methotrexate, 6MP, vincristine, and prednisone.
- CNS prophylaxis/treatment: intrathecal methotrexate, possibly cytarabine and/or irradiation.
- Targeted therapy in individual cases.
- Allogeneic stem cell transplant in high-risk/refractory cases.
- Chimeric antigen receptor or CAR T-cell therapy in high-risk/refractory cases.

ACUTE MYELOGENOUS LEUKEMIA (AML)

- Fifteen to twenty percent of leukemia cases.
- Predisposing factors, including toxins (benzene) and medications (etoposide, cyclophosphamide).

CLINICAL FEATURES

- Manifestations of anemia, thrombocytopenia, or neutropenia, including fatigue, bleeding, and infection.
- Chloroma: localized mass of leukemic cells.
- Bone/joint pain.
- Hepatosplenomcgaly.
- Lymphadenopathy.

DIAGNOSIS

- More than 20% myeloblasts in the bone marrow, hypercellular.
- Similar to ALL.

TREATMENT

- Remission induction: etoposide, daunorubicin (anthracycline) and cytarabine.
- Intensification: high-dose cytarabine, mitoxantrone (anthracycline), etoposide.
- CNS prophylaxis/treatment: intrathecal cytarabine, irradiation.
- Possible addition of targeted therapy in individual cases.
- Allogeneic stem cell transplant in high-risk/refractory cases (needed more often than ALL).

CHRONIC MYELOGENOUS LEUKEMIA (CML)

- Clonal hematopoietic stem cell disorder with Philadelphia translocation—t(9;22)(q34;q11).

WARD TIP

A marrow exam is essential to confirm the diagnosis of ALL.

WARD TIP

Tumor lysis syndrome—rapid leukemic cell lysis at presentation or after initiating chemotherapy
- Acute renal failure
- Hyperphosphatemia
- Hyperuricemia
- Hyperkalemia
- Hypocalcemia

EXAM TIP

Philadelphia chromosome t(9:22) BCR/ABLI translocation = poor prognosis.

- Uncontrolled production of mature and maturing granulocytes, predominantly neutrophils.
- Less common in children.

CLINICAL FEATURES

- Usually insidious onset, but can present as acute blast crisis.
- Splenomegaly (massive).
- Fever, bone pain, anemia.

TREATMENT

- Tyrosine kinase inhibitors (imatinib, dasatinib) are therapy mainstays.
- Stem cell transplant may be required in some cases.

JUVENILE MYELOMONOCYTIC LEUKEMIA (JMML)

- Clonal condition involving pluripotent stem cell.
- <4 years.

CLINICAL FEATURES

- Pallor, fatigue, weakness, and dry cough.
- Skin lesions (maculopapular rash, xanthoma, café au lait spots, chloroma).
- Lymphadenopathy.
- Hepatosplenomegaly.

DIAGNOSIS

- Absolute monocyte count >1000/μL.
- Increased marrow monocyte precursors with <20% blasts (>20% is AML).
- Philadelphia chromosome absent.
- Specific genetic mutations of the RAS pathway.

TREATMENT

- Complete remissions occur in up to 50% with stem cell transplant.
- Some (35–40%) experience relapse.

Lymphoma

- This is the most common childhood cancer in the 15- to 19-year-old age group.
- Lymphoid malignancy arising in a single lymph node or lymphoid region (liver, spleen, bone marrow).
- Broadly categorized as Hodgkin and non-Hodgkin (50% each).
- Hodgkin lymphoma (HL) can be classical HL or nodular-lymphocyte predominant (NLPHL).
- Four subtypes of classical HL are treated similarly:
  - Nodular sclerosing (most common)
  - Mixed cellularity
  - Lymphocyte predominance
  - Lymphocyte depletion
- Non-Hodgkin includes:
  - Lymphoblastic (treated similar to ALL)
  - Burkitt
  - Diffuse large B cell (DLBCL)
  - Anaplastic large cell (ALCL)

WARD TIP

CML often gets diagnosed when CBC shows elevated WBCs.

EXAM TIP

Neurofibromatosis is associated with an increased incidence of JMML.

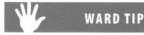

WARD TIP

Reed-Sternberg cells are characteristic of Hodgkin lymphoma.

WARD TIP

The four histological classifications of classical Hodgkin lymphoma include:
- Nodular sclerosis.
- Mixed cellularity.
- Lymphocyte depleted.
- Lymphocyte rich.

CLINICAL FEATURES

- "B symptoms:" fever for 3 days, drenching night sweats, weight loss >10% in 6 months.
- Loss of appetite.
- Cough, dysphagia, dyspnea.
- Lymphadenopathy persistent for weeks—lower cervical, supraclavicular.
- Hepatosplenomegaly.
- Mediastinal mass.

DIAGNOSIS

- CBC normal in early stages, high erythrocyte sedimentation rate (ESR).
- High uric acid and LDH.
- Chest x-ray (mediastinal mass).
- Computed tomography (CT) and positron-emission tomography (PET) scans of chest, abdomen, and pelvis.
- Lymph node or bone marrow (rare) biopsy.

TREATMENT

- Chemotherapy is the mainstay of therapy.
- Radiation and stem cell transplants are used in high-risk cases.
- Surgery is used for NLPHL.

Malignant Bone Tumors

OSTEOSARCOMA

 A patient has had dull, aching pain in the left leg for several months that has suddenly become more severe. *Think: Osteosarcoma.*

Osteosarcoma is a common cancer in adolescence. Symptoms may be present for a significant period before it is diagnosed. Pain, particularly with activity, is a common symptom. Distal femur and proximal tibia are commonly involved bones. On examination, a palpable mass may be present. Since osteosarcoma is not radiosensitive, surgery may be needed.

- The most frequent sites of origin are the metaphyseal regions.
- Most osteosarcomas develop in patients 10–20 years of age.
- Osteosarcomas most frequently occur during maximal growth periods.

CLINICAL FEATURES

- Bone pain.
- Typically in long bones (distal femur and proximal tibia) and flat bones (pelvis 10%).

DIAGNOSIS

- Radiographs show mixed sclerotic and lytic lesions arising in the metaphyseal region, often described as a *sunburst pattern* with periosteal elevation. (Figure 16-1).
- MRI of the lesion and joints on either side, CT chest, bone scan.
- Biopsy of lesion for definitive diagnosis.

TREATMENT AND PROGNOSIS

- Chemotherapy: **m**ethotrexate, **A**driamycin (doxorubicin), cis**p**latin (called MAP).
- Amputation and limb salvage are effective in achieving local control.

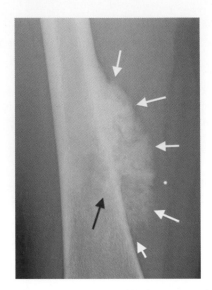

FIGURE 16-1. Osteosarcoma. Shows osteoid matrix (black arrow) and soft tissue ossifications (white arrows) in a patient with known osteosarcoma. (Reproduced, with permission, from Wilson FC, Lin PP. General Orthopedics. New York: McGraw Hill, 1997.)

- The survival rate is 75% in nonmetastatic disease.
- Death is usually due to pulmonary metastasis.
- Metastatic disease carries a poor prognosis.

EWING SARCOMA

A 10-year-old boy complains of pain in his left leg. On examination, he has localized swelling and pain in the middle of his left femur. His temperature is 100.8°F (38.2°C), and ESR is elevated. Further questioning reveals a 2-month history of increasing fatigue and weight loss. *Think: Ewing sarcoma.*

Ewing sarcoma is a common malignant bone tumor in young patients. Most patients present with either pain or a mass. The most common site for metastases is the lung. Periosteal reaction and new bone formation with an onion-skin appearance are suggestive of Ewing sarcoma. Most tumors are considered radiosensitive.

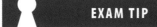
EXAM TIP

Primary site is split almost evenly between the extremities and the central axis.

- Malignant tumor of bone arising in medullary tissue.
- Most common bone tumor in first decade; second to osteosarcoma in second decade.
- Very strong Caucasian and male predilection.

CLINICAL FEATURES

- Bone pain.
- Systemic signs: fever, weight loss, fatigue.

EXAM TIP

Bone pain is a presenting symptom of Ewing sarcoma in 80–90% of cases.

DIAGNOSIS

- Radiographs show calcified periosteal elevation, termed *onion skin*, and radiolucent lytic bone lesions in the diaphyseal region.
- MRI of involved site, CT of the chest, bone scan/PET scan, and biopsy of lesions are used for staging purposes.

TREATMENT AND PROGNOSIS

- Radiotherapy.
- Chemotherapy: vincristine, doxorubicin, cyclophosphamide, etoposide, ifosfamide (VDC/IE).
- Surgical resection.
- Autologous bone marrow transplant for high-risk/relapsed patients.
- Patients with a small, localized tumor have a 50–70% long-term disease-free survival rate.
- Patients with metastatic disease have a poor prognosis.

Malignant Soft Tissue Tumors

- Broadly categorized as rhabdomyosarcoma (RMS) and non-RMS soft tissue tumors (NRSTS).
- RMS is the most common soft-tissue sarcoma in children.
- Treatment includes a combination of chemotherapy, surgery, radiation, and especially proton therapy.

Brain Tumors

- Most common solid tumor of childhood.
- Third-most common pediatric tumor (#1 leukemia, #2 lymphoma).
- Arise from glial cells, neurons or choroid plexus in 90% and extracranial sources in 10% (germ cell tumor and craniopharyngioma).
- Low-grade gliomas (LGGs) are most common: astrocytomas, ependymomas, oligodendroglioma.
- Primitive neuroectodermal tumor (PNET): medulloblastoma (a common PNET only in childhood), pineoblastoma.

CLINICAL FEATURES

- Signs and symptoms of raised ICP (infants) or focal neurologic signs (adolescents).
- Personality alterations are often the first brain tumor symptoms.
- Nystagmus and ataxia occur in posterior fossa tumors.
- Hydrocephalus is secondary to CSF flow obstruction.

CEREBELLAR PILOCYTIC ASTROCYTOMA

- Most common posterior fossa tumor of childhood.
- Slow-growing and more benign than the adult-onset astrocytomas.
- Histologically shows fibrillary astrocytes with dense cytoplasmic inclusions (Rosenthal fibers).
- Associated with neurofibromatosis type 1 (NF1).
- Good prognosis: 5-year survival >90% after gross total resection, achieved in 70% of the cases.

MEDULLOBLASTOMA

- Second-most common posterior fossa tumor and most prevalent brain tumor in children <7y.
- Arises from the undifferentiated neural cells in the region of cerebellar vermis.
- Rapidly growing and tends to spread along CSF pathways and the spine.

CLINICAL FEATURES

- Histologically shows deeply staining nuclei with scant cytoplasm arranged in pseudorosettes.
- Presents with intracranial hypertension and ataxia; papilledema is absent.
- MRI: brightly enhancing mass with cystic lesion.
- Classified as standard versus high risk based on size, dissemination, histology, and genetics.

TREATMENT AND PROGNOSIS

- Surgical resection followed by craniospinal irradiation and chemotherapy.
- Five-year survival rate is >75% for standard risk and 40–60% for high risk.

CRANIOPHARYNGIOMA

- A supratentorial brain tumor arising from cells in the Rathke's pouch.
- Pituitary dysfunction and progressive visual loss are common initial signs.
- Typically slow growing and benign but locally aggressive; may be confined to the sella turcica or extend through the diaphragma sellae and compress the optic nerve or, rarely, obstruct CSF flow.
- Due to location, surgical resection is often subtotal and risk of recurrence is high.
- Ninety percent show calcification on CT scan; an MRI is more effective for surrounding structures.
- Baseline endocrine studies and visual fields should be done prior to surgery.

Other Common Tumors of Childhood

NEUROBLASTOMA

- Small, round blue-cell tumor that arises during neural-crest cell development.
- Most commonly diagnosed cancer of infancy; 90% diagnosed before age 5.
- N-myc amplification associated with poor prognosis.

CLINICAL FEATURES

- Forty percent present with localized disease in the abdomen, pelvis, thorax, cervix, and/or paraspinal ganglia.
- Abdominal pain, hypertension, superior vena cava syndrome, Horner's syndrome, spinal cord compression occur.
- More than 50% are metastatic at presentation, including bone, bone marrow, and liver.
- Proptosis and periorbital ecchymoses (raccoon eyes) occur due to periorbital bone infiltration, fever, failure to thrive, pallor, and bruising.
- Opsoclonus-myoclonus: "dancing eyes, dancing feet" is the telltale symptom of this disease (secondary to paraneoplastic antibodies).

DIAGNOSIS

- Ultrasound of primary site and CT or MRI scans.
- MIBG (metaiodobenzylguanidine) scintigraphy (accumulates in adrenal medullary chromaffin cells and in pre-synaptic granules of adrenergic neurons).
- Bone marrow aspirates and biopsies from both iliac crests for staging.
- Urinary vanillylmandelic acid (VMA) and homovanillic acid (HVA) are high in 95% of cases.

TREATMENT AND PROGNOSIS

- Surgical resection for early stages.
- Intermediate-risk disease: chemotherapy and surgery lead to >90% overall survival rate.
- High-risk disease: overall survival 30–40% despite combination of chemotherapy, myeloablative therapy supported by autologous stem cell transplant, radiotherapy, and immunotherapy.

GERM CELL TUMORS (GCT)

- Gonadal tumors are more common after puberty.
    - Testicular GCT: painless scrotal swelling; abdominal pain and dyspnea due to metastases.
    - Ovarian GCT: pelvic mass; acute pain due to rupture/hemorrhage/torsion.
- Sacrococcygeal tumors present in first 5 years of life (often at birth), predominantly in females.
- Mediastinal GCT during infancy are usually teratomas; post infancy they are yolk sac tumors or embryonal carcinomas; after puberty, seminoma/dysgerminoma are common.
- Perinatal GCTs are mostly benign with survival rates of 85%.
- USG (testes), CT, or MRI of abdomen and pelvis are used to determine extent.
- Tumor markers are tested prior to surgery: AFP (yolk sac component), beta-HCG (choriocarcinoma), and LDH.
- Treatment is primarily surgical resection with cisplatin-based chemotherapy for advanced stages.

HISTIOCYTOSIS

- This group of disorders is characterized by histiocytic infiltration.
- The exact cause is unclear: histiocytosis has both reactive and neoplastic features, likely due to environmental and genetic factors.
- Langerhans cell histiocytosis (LCH) most commonly involves bone (punched-out lytic lesions) and skin (nonspecific rash); it can also present as diabetes insipidus, lymphadenopathy, and hepatosplenomegaly.
    - The mean age of diagnosis is 2 years.
    - The expression of CD1a marker and the presence of Birbeck granules are characteristic.
- Hemophagocytic lymphohistiocytosis (HLH) is more rapidly progressive with persistent high-grade fever, cytopenias, splenomegaly, and highly elevated ferritin level.
    - Fatal if left untreated.
    - Can be primary (familial) or secondary to infections like EBV, JRA, or malignancy.
    - Treated with steroids and etoposide; stem cell transplant may be used for primary HLH.

HEPATOBLASTOMA

- Usually affects children <5 years of age.
- Associated with Beckwith-Wiedemann syndrome (BWS) and hemihyperplasia.

CLINICAL FEATURES

- Large, asymptomatic abdominal mass.
- Abdominal distention and increased liver size.
- Weight loss, anorexia, vomiting, and abdominal pain (as disease progresses).
- May spread to regional lymph nodes.

DIAGNOSIS

- The α-fetoprotein (AFP) level may be helpful as a marker.
- An ultrasound may be used to detect a mass; a CT of the chest/abdomen/ pelvis or an MRI may be useful.

TREATMENT AND PROGNOSIS

- Complete surgical resection is key and may necessitate liver transplantation.
- Chemotherapy: cisplatin, doxorubicin, 5-fluoruracil (5-FU).
- More than 90% survival with multimodal treatment (surgery with chemotherapy).

WILMS TUMOR (NEPHROBLASTOMA)

 A previously healthy 2-year-old boy has a left-sided abdominal mass discovered by his mother. His physical examination reveals a BP of 110/70 and a large mass arising in his left abdomen. A UA shows 5–10 erythrocytes and 2–3 leukocytes. *Think: Wilms tumor.*
The usual presentation of Wilms tumor is an abdominal mass, and it is not uncommon for the parent to discover this mass. It is often asymptomatic at presentation.

WARD TIP

The characteristic features of Beckwith-Wiedemann syndrome include omphalocele, macroglossia, and macrosomia. Also notable are the presence of hemihypertrophy (asymmetric growth), neonatal hypoglycemia, and increased risk for embryonal tumors, including Wilms tumor.

- This is the most common renal malignancy in children.
- The median age of diagnosis is 3.5 years.
  - Derived from the embryonic renal precursor cells (mesenchymal cells)
- Certain gene mutations are associated with syndromes that predispose to Wilms tumor.
  - WT1 deletion (11p13): WAGR syndrome (Wilms tumor, Aniridia, GU anomalies, mental Retardation).
  - WT2 mutation (11p15): Beckwith-Wiedemann syndrome (macrosomia, macroglossia, hemihypertrophy, umbilical hernia).

CLINICAL FEATURES

- This condition most commonly presents with an isolated abdominal/flank mass that rarely crosses the midline (as opposed to neuroblastoma).
- If present, symptoms include abdominal pain, hematuria, fever, and hypertension.
- Mostly solitary, but can be bilateral (5–7%) or multifocal within a single kidney (10%).
- May metastasize to the lung, liver, bone, and brain.

DIAGNOSIS

- Renal ultrasound: hydronephrosis and echogenic masses may contain cystic areas.
- CT or MRI will determine tumor origin and extent of spread.
- Chest imaging is used for lung metastases.
- A definitive diagnosis is made after surgical excision or surgical biopsy. Transcutaneous biopsy is not recommended because it can spill tumor cells into the abdomen.

TREATMENT

- In general, low-stage tumors are treated with nephrectomy and chemotherapy. High-stage or high-risk tumors require radiation therapy.
- Chemotherapy: vincristine, dactinomycin, doxorubicin, cyclophosphamide, etoposide, carboplatin.
- Stage 5 (bilateral) tumors: preoperative chemotherapy followed by renal parenchymal-sparing surgical tumor resection.

DISORDERS OF GLUCOSE HOMEOSTASIS

Diabetes Mellitus

 A 10-year-old girl has blood glucose of 300 mg/dL and a large amount of glucose with trace ketones in her urine. She has lost 1 kg of weight and has had polyuria and polydipsia for the past few weeks. *Think: Type 1 diabetes.*

A 16-year-old obese male with blood sugar of 300 mg/dL has a thickened rash on the back of his neck. *Think: Type 2 diabetes.*

Typical history: For type I diabetes, polyuria, polydipsia, polyphagia, and weight loss are often found. The initial hyperglycemia symptoms may be nonspecific. Exogenous insulin is required to correct the metabolic derangement due to insulin deficiency. Children with type 2 diabetes mellitus are usually overweight, often showing signs of insulin resistance, such as acanthosis nigricans. A family history of type 2 diabetes is often noted.

WARD TIP

Consider testing urine glucose with the onset of enuresis in a previously toilet-trained child.

DEFINITION

Diabetes mellitus is a group of metabolic diseases characterized by hyperglycemia resulting from defects in insulin secretion, insulin action, or both (Table 17-1). Diabetes is associated with long-term damage, dysfunction, and failure of various organs, especially the eyes, kidneys, nerves, heart, and blood vessels.

TABLE 17-1. Diabetes

TYPE I (INSULIN DEPENDENT)	TYPE II (NON-INSULIN DEPENDENT)
Absolute insulin deficiency (require insulin for survival)	Insulin is ↑, normal, or ↓ (insulin is not required for survival)
Immune mediated	Insulin resistance
Juvenile onset	Usually adult onset but incidence is rising in children
Shorter duration of symptoms with history of weight loss at diagnosis	Mild symptoms, 85% overweight at diagnosis
Ketosis common	Ketosis infrequent but occurs under stressful conditions
DKA is a complication of uncontrolled diabetes	Hyperglycemic hyperosmolar state is a rare complication
HLA-DR3 and HLA-DR4 (chromosome 6)	Not HLA associated
5% have diabetic relative	74–100% have a diabetic relative

DKA, diabetic ketoacidosis; HLA, human leukocyte antigen.

EPIDEMIOLOGY

- Diabetes is one of the most common endocrine disorders of pediatrics.
- Classification:
    - **Type 1 diabetes** is caused by *absolute* insulin deficiency.
        - The classic presentation is polyuria, polydipsia, polyphagia, and weight loss.
        - Positive urine ketones at onset is commonly seen.
        - It may present as diabetic ketoacidosis or may be an incidental discovery.
        - Most children are positive for beta-cell destruction immune markers (islet cell antibodies, antiglutamic acid decarboxylase antibodies, and insulin autoantibody).
    - **Type 2 diabetes** is a heterogeneous disorder characterized by insulin resistance, hyperglycemia, and *relative* insulin deficiency (impaired secretion).
        - It is insidious in onset; diagnosis is often delayed due to a lack of symptoms early in the disease course.
        - The incidence is increasing due to the rise in childhood obesity.
        - Many patients have acanthosis nigricans (velvety hyperpigmented skin thickening in intertriginous sites, such as the neck and axillae).

PATHOPHYSIOLOGY

It revolves around relative insulin deficiency or insulin resistance leading to:
- decreased glucose utilization.
- increased hepatic glucose production causing hyperglycemia.

SIGNS AND SYMPTOMS

- Triad of polyuria, polydipsia, and polyphagia (more abrupt in type 1 diabetes).
- Weight loss and enuresis are common in type 1 diabetes.
- Vomiting, dehydration, and abdominal pain are often seen with diabetic ketoacidosis.

DIAGNOSIS

- Fasting blood glucose ≥126 mg/dL.
- Random blood glucose ≥200 mg/dL along with symptoms of diabetes.
- Two-hour glucose >200 mg/dL during an oral glucose tolerance test.
- Hemoglobin A1C ≥6.5%.
- Screening for type 2 diabetes begins at 10 years of age or puberty (whichever comes first) and is repeated every 3 years. Testing is done sooner for overweight or obese children who have two or more risk factors such as:
    - family history of type 2 diabetes (first- and second-degree relatives).
    - race (Native American, Black, Hispanic, and Asian-American or Pacific Islander).
    - signs and symptoms of insulin resistance (acanthosis nigricans, dyslipidemia, hypertension [HTN], polycystic ovarian syndrome, or small-for–gestational-age birth weight).
    - maternal history of diabetes or gestational diabetes.

TREATMENT

- Treatment includes patient education and counseling, especially about nutrition for all.
- Insulin is the mainstay of treatment in type 1 diabetes.
- Oral hypoglycemics are used in type 2 diabetes (such as metformin, sulfonylureas, thiazolidinediones), along with diet and exercise.

EXAM TIP

The prevalence of type 1 diabetes is rising, particularly in those under the age of 5 years, for unclear reasons. The prevalence of type 2 diabetes is increasing in children, secondary to the increasing prevalence of childhood obesity.

EXAM TIP

Insulin-dependent diabetes mellitus in children is associated with islet cell antibodies and ↑ prevalence of human leukocyte antigen (HLA)-DR3 and HLA-DR4 or both.

Diabetic Ketoacidosis (DKA)

A 3½-year-old boy is found unconscious and is difficult to rouse. He has a flushed face, pulse of 160/min, respiratory rate of 30/min with shallow breaths, blood pressure 40/20 mm Hg, and an unusual odor on his breath. His mucous membranes are dry. His parents report a weight loss of 5 pounds in the past month and noted increased drinking. *Think: DKA,* and check serum glucose.

Diabetic ketoacidosis (DKA) is an acute, life-threatening complication of mainly type 1 diabetes. A complex disordered metabolic state of hyperglycemia, ketoacidosis, and ketonuria occurs. Weight loss is due to hyperglycemia and glucosuria causing lipolysis. Ketosis also leads to anorexia and nausea contributing to weight loss. Shallow breathing is a respiratory compensation for metabolic acidosis secondary to ketoacid accumulation. Severe dehydration is due to glucosuria, resulting in osmotic diuresis and volume depletion.

DEFINITION

- Hyperglycemia >200 mg/dL.
- Acidosis pH < 7.30.
- Bicarbonate <15 mmol/L.
- Ketonemia (Beta hydroxybutyrate >3 mmol/L) and ketonuria >2+.

ETIOLOGY/PATHOPHYSIOLOGY

- An insulin deficiency causes accelerated hepatic and renal glucose production and impaired glucose utilization, lipolysis (release of free fatty acids into serum), and increased fatty acid oxidation to ketone bodies. The result is ketosis and hyperglycemia.
- Precipitating factors include: stress, infection, and trauma.

SIGNS AND SYMPTOMS

Polyuria, polydipsia, dehydration, weight loss, fatigue, headache, nausea, vomiting, abdominal pain, tachycardia, tachypnea (Kussmaul breathing)

OTHER LABORATORY FINDINGS

- Elevated anion gap (>12–16 mEq).
- Increased hemoglobin and hematocrit due to hemoconcentration.
- High white blood cell count.
- Low serum sodium (pseudohyponatremia from hyperglycemia and/or hypertriglyceridemia).
- Normal or high potassium (K+) (shift from intra- to extracellular K+ from acidosis).
- Normal or high phosphate (osmotic diuresis).
- Urinalysis revealing glucose and ketones.

TREATMENT

- Careful fluid and electrolyte replacement is used to avoid cerebral edema.
- The initial bolus should be 10 mL/kg normal saline. Repeat the bolus, if needed.
- Potassium should be given as potassium chloride *and* potassium phosphate.
- Regular insulin (0.1 U/kg/hr).
- Glucose is used: add glucose to IV fluids when blood glucose is <250–300 mg/dL.

COMPLICATIONS

- Hypoglycemia.
- Hypokalemia.

WARD TIP

Dehydration in DKA is primarily intracellular and is often underestimated.

WARD TIP

Serum Na ↓ 1.6 mEq/L for every 100 mg/dL rise in glucose through osmotic dilution; sodium corrects as glucose is corrected. You may also see calculators use a factor of 2.4 mEq/L for glucoses >400 mg/dL, reflecting more recent research.

EXAM TIP

Total body potassium and phosphate may be considerably depleted, even when serum levels are normal or ↑.

- Cerebral edema can cause death in DKA patients (symptoms such as headache/mental status changes indicate acute intracranial pressure elevation); treatment includes 3% saline administration and/or mannitol.

Hypoglycemia

A 14-year-old boy with an 8-year history of diabetes mellitus has had frequent admissions for DKA in the past 18 months. His school performance has been deteriorating. Recently, he has had frequent episodes of hypoglycemia. He is Tanner stage 2 in pubertal development and has mild hepatomegaly. *Think: Poorly controlled diabetes mellitus due to noncompliance.*

Adolescence is a difficult age for management of any chronic disease. Treatment regimen nonadherence is common in teenagers. Often, blood sugar levels are high because of missing insulin doses. Inappropriate insulin administration may result in secondary hypoglycemia. Recurrent hospitalization is the hallmark of noncompliance. Hepatomegaly is most likely due to poorly controlled diabetes mellitus

ETIOLOGY

- Hyperinsulinism.
- Hormone deficiencies (glucocorticoid, growth hormone).
- Glycogen storage disease.
- Defect in gluconeogenesis.
- Fatty acid oxidation defects.
- Organic acidemias.
- Ketotic hypoglycemia.
- Malnutrition, prematurity, SGA.
- Liver failure.
- Congenital heart diseases.
- Tumors.
- Poisons/drugs (salicylates, alcohol).
- Systemic disease: sepsis, burns, cardiogenic shock.

TREATMENT

- Acute symptomatic hypoglycemia: if the patient is conscious and able to drink, rapidly absorbed carbohydrates (e.g., fruit juice) should be given by mouth. In children with altered level of consciousness, IV $D_{10}W$ dextrose should be administered.
- In hyperinsulinemia patients, subcutaneous glucagon can reverse the hypoglycemia.

Hyperinsulinism

A 2-hour-old newborn has plasma glucose of 20 mg/dL. Physical examination shows a large plethoric newborn. Birth weight is >90th percentile. *Think: Hyperinsulinism.*

Hyperinsulinism is a common cause of hypoglycemia in early infancy. These infants may have macrosomia. Hypoglycemia may develop on the first day of life. The diagnostic criterion is the presence of signs and symptoms of hypoglycemia with low plasma glucose level and an inappropriately elevated insulin level. Macrosomia is due to hyperinsulinemia (insulin is an intrauterine growth factor). Transient hyperinsulinism may occur due to maternal diabetes. Persistent hyperinsulinism can be a genetically inherited disorder.

EPIDEMIOLOGY

Hyperinsulinemia is the most common cause of recurrent hypoglycemia in early infancy. Clinical manifestations may include jitteriness/tremors, sweating, irritability, pallor, tachypnea, and poor suck or feeding. In severe hypoglycemia, changes in level of consciousness and seizures may be seen.

TRANSIENT HYPERINSULINEMIA

- Excessive insulin secretion in infants from transient islet cell dysfunction.
- Inadequate glucose supply (low glycogen stores, impaired glucose production).
- Risk factors include:
  - small for gestational age, large for gestational age, or premature infants.
  - perinatal hypoxia/asphyxia.
  - infant of diabetic mother.
  - erythroblastosis fetalis (alloimmune hemolytic disease of the newborn due to Rh or ABO incompatibility).
  - polycythemia.
  - sepsis.
  - surreptitious insulin administration.

CONGENITAL HYPERINSULINEMIA

- It is caused by a mutation in the genes coding a component of K_{ATP} (adenosine triphosphate-sensitive potassium) channel involved in glucose-regulated insulin release.
- Autosomal-dominant forms of hyperinsulinism are usually responsive to diazoxide.

TREATMENT

- Feed every 3 to 4 hours to reduce the frequency and severity of hypoglycemic events.
- Administer IV glucose, if necessary.
- In severe cases, treatment with diazoxide, octreotide, and/or pancreatectomy may be necessary.

DISORDERS OF THYROID/ADRENALS

Hyperthyroidism

DEFINITION

Increased synthesis and secretion of thyroid hormone

GRAVES DISEASE

- This disease is a common cause of hyperthyroidism in children and adolescents.
- It occurs about five times more frequently in females.
- It is a triad of:
  - hyperthyroidism, often with diffuse goiter.
  - ophthalmopathy with proptosis.
  - dermopathy: pretibial myxedema is less common in children than adults.

ETIOLOGY

- This autoimmune disorder has antibodies against the thyroid-stimulating hormone (TSH) receptor, causing chronic stimulation which leads to inappropriate thyroid stimulation, gland enlargement, and increased thyroid hormone production.

SIGNS AND SYMPTOMS

- Gradual onset (6–12 months).
- Emotional disturbance, change in academic performance.
- Insomnia.
- Palpitations.
- Fatigue, muscle weakness, increased sweating.
- Increased appetite, usually without weight gain.
- Goiter.
- Heat intolerance.
- Fine tremors.
- Exophthalmos.
- Menstrual irregularities
- Thyroid storm is a life-threatening condition characterized by:
    - hyperpyrexia.
    - tachycardia out of proportion to fever, leading to high-output heart failure.
    - central nervous system manifestations (agitation, delirium, psychosis, confusion, obtundation, coma, and convulsions).
    - severe vomiting, diarrhea, abdominal pain.

LABORATORY FINDINGS

- Elevated total and free thyroxine (T_4) and free triiodothyronine (T_3) levels.
- Low TSH.
- Elevated TSH receptor antibody.

TREATMENT OF HYPERTHYROIDISM

- Treatment depends on the patient's age and disease severity, and it may include anti-thyroid medications, radioiodine ablation, or surgical thyroidectomy.
    - Anti-thyroid medication therapy (methimazole) is often the first-line treatment.
    - Radioactive iodine ablation may be indicated for patients without adequate response (or side effects) with anti-thyroid medication or in those >10 years of age, often requiring lifelong thyroid hormone replacement.
    - Thyroidectomy is immediately effective and requires lifelong thyroid hormone replacement.
- For thyroid storm, in addition to methimazole and beta-blockers to decreased adrenergic effects, bile acid sequestrants, saturated solution of potassium iodide (SSKI), and glucocorticoids may also be given. Propylthiouracil (PTU) and glucocorticoids inhibit the peripheral conversion of T_4 to T_3.

> **WARD TIP**
>
> Goiter is usually present in hyperthyroidism and typically is symmetrical, smooth, soft, and nontender.

Hypothyroidism

DEFINITION

- Decreased thyroid hormone production from a primary defect at the thyroid level or secondary to hypothalamic pituitary disorder.

CONGENITAL HYPOTHYROIDISM

Incidence is 1 in 2000 to 4000 worldwide. It is a preventable cause of intellectual disability.

ETIOLOGY

- Sporadic: most common and due to thyroid dysgenesis (absent, hypoplastic, or ectopic thyroid).
- Iodine deficiency remains a cause of transient congenital hypothyroidism worldwide.
- Prenatal radioiodine or antithyroid medication exposure can cause transient congenital hypothyroidism.
- It is rarely hereditary, caused by thyroid dyshormonogenesis (defect in thyroid hormone synthesis) and generalized thyroid hormone resistance.

SIGNS AND SYMPTOMS

- Most cases are asymptomatic at birth, as there is some passage of maternal T4 through the placenta.
- Initial physical findings may include:
    - wide fontanelle, particularly the posterior fontanelle.
    - umbilical hernia.
- Signs and symptoms that develop include:
    - prolonged jaundice.
    - macroglossia and feeding problems.
    - hoarse cry.
    - abdominal distention, constipation.
    - hypotonia or lethargy.
    - goiter (in some dyshormonogenesis).
- If left untreated:
    - slowed development, late teeth, late milestones, and short stature may result.
    - eventual intellectual disability will occur.

DIAGNOSIS

Newborn screening: measurement on filter paper blood spots T4 and/or TSH based on region-specific protocols

TREATMENT

- Oral levothyroxine is initiated as early as possible.

ACQUIRED HYPOTHYROIDISM

 A 10-year-old girl has a 3-year history of growth failure. A moderate-sized goiter is palpated. T_4 is low, and TSH is high. *Think: Acquired hypothyroidism.*
Congenital hypothyroidism is generally diagnosed early via newborn screening. Childhood hypothyroidism is usually Hashimoto disease. Initial signs and symptoms may be subtle. Growth retardation is usually not severe. If it remains unrecognized, linear growth is retarded, and sexual maturation is delayed. Goiter is the hallmark of classic Hashimoto disease. The thyroid function test results depend on the stage of the disease. TSH is elevated. Antithyroglobulin and anti–thyroid peroxidase (anti-TPO antibody) may be present.

- Lymphocytic thyroiditis (Hashimoto) is the most common cause. It is an autoimmune disorder with thyroid lymphocytic infiltration and the presence of:
    - antithyroglobulin antibodies.
    - anti-thyroid peroxidase (anti-TPO) antibodies.
- Hashimoto thyroiditis is about four to six times more common in girls.
- Other causes include thyroid surgery and irradiation, medications (iodine, lithium, amiodarone), and pituitary or hypothalamic dysfunction (secondary or tertiary acquired hypothyroidism).

SIGNS AND SYMPTOMS

- Goiter.
- Growth deceleration.
- Delayed skeletal maturation.
- Fatigue, lethargy.
- Constipation.
- Cold intolerance.
- Bradycardia.
- Dry skin.
- Weight gain.
- Delayed deep tendon reflexes.

TREATMENT

Levothyroxine

Thyroid Neoplasm

EPIDEMIOLOGY

- Up to 2% of children have palpable thyroid nodules. Most are benign.
- Family history (medullary thyroid cancer seen with multiple endocrine neoplasia [MEN2]).
- Prior irradiation (papillary thyroid cancer).

TYPES

- Benign thyroid adenomas: follicular adenomas are the most common, with a small number causing hyperthyroidism.
- Thyroid carcinoma, which arises from:
  - Follicular epithelium
    - Papillary carcinoma (most common; focal calcification)
    - Follicular carcinoma (especially with iodine deficiency)
    - Insular carcinoma (poorly differentiated)
  - Parafollicular (C) cells (produce calcitonin): medullary carcinoma is associated with type 2 multiple endocrine neoplasia (MEN)

SIGNS AND SYMPTOMS

Solitary or multiple thyroid nodules (malignancy risk in solitary nodules in children is 10–50%).

DIAGNOSIS

- Thyroid profile (thyroid functions are usually normal).
- Calcitonin (for medullary cancer).
- Thyroid ultrasound.
- Fine-needle aspiration.
- Definite diagnosis by surgical excision.

TREATMENT

- Papillary and follicular cancer:
  - Total thyroidectomy, occasionally with modified neck dissection, if needed.
  - Postoperative ^{131}I ablation.
  - Replacement thyroxine.
- Medullary thyroid cancer:
  - Total thyroidectomy.
  - Prophylactic thyroidectomy if positive for MEN mutation, before age 5 years in MEN 2A and in the first year of life with MEN 2B.

WARD TIP

Cervical lymphadenopathy: rapid and painless enlargement of a thyroid growth may suggest neoplasia.

EXAM TIP

The incidence of malignancy of a thyroid nodule is higher in children than in adults.

WARD TIP

A newborn with ambiguous genitalia is a medical and social emergency.

Congenital Adrenal Hyperplasia (CAH)

DEFINITION

- Genetic defect of adrenal corticosteroid and/or mineralocorticoid synthesis.

ETIOLOGY

- 21-hydroxylase deficiency (95% of all CAH):
  - A defect occurs in conversion of progesterone and 17-hydroxyprogesterone to 11-deoxyycorticosterone and 11-deoxycortisol.
  - About three-quarters of cases are salt wasters.
  - Ambiguous genitalia are present in females (clitoral enlargement and a common urethral-vaginal orifice, normal uterus, and ovaries); normal genitalia are present in males.
  - Nonclassical variant has normal female genitalia, but it presents with premature pubarche in both genders.
- 11β-hydroxylase deficiency: HTN with low K is frequently present due to excessive deoxycorticosterone (DOC).
- Ambiguous genitalia are present in females and precocious puberty in males.
- 3β-hydroxysteroid dehydrogenase:
  - Ambiguous genitalia are present in both sexes.
  - Salt wasting is present.
- 17-hydroxylase deficiency:
  - Normal genitalia are present in females; undervirilized or ambiguous genitalia are present in males.
  - Females have delayed puberty, primary amenorrhea, and lack of secondary sexual characteristics.
  - HTN with low K is frequently present.
- Lipoid adrenal hyperplasia:
  - It is a rare but severe form of CAH.
  - All adrenal hormones and their precursors are low.
  - Normal genitalia are present in females; undervirilized or ambiguous genitalia are present in males.
  - Salt wasting is present and severe.

PATHOPHYSIOLOGY

- Decrease in cortisol secretion results in absent hypothalamic and pituitary gland feedback.
- Increased ACTH secretion results in elevated production of the precursors before the block.

EPIDEMIOLOGY

- CAH is the most common cause of ambiguous genitalia.

SIGNS AND SYMPTOMS

- Clinical features result from the hormonal deficiencies (cortisol, aldosterone) and excessive precursor production (17-hydroxyprogesterone, androstenedione, DOC).
- Female pseudohermaphroditism: ambiguous female genitalia are present with normal 46,XX chromosome (21-hydroxylase, 11β-hydroxylase, 3β-hydroxysteroid dehydrogenase deficiency).
- Male pseudohermaphroditism: ambiguous male genitalia are present with 46,XY chromosome (3β-hydroxysteroid dehydrogenase, 17-hydroxylase deficiency, lipoid adrenal hyperplasia).

- Hypoglycemia (cortisol deficiency).
- Salt wasting (21-hydroxylase, 3β-hydroxysteroid dehydrogenase, lipoid adrenal hyperplasia).
- HTN with hypokalemia (11β-hydroxylase, 17 hydroxylase deficiency).
- Vomiting, dehydration, and shock at 2–4 weeks of age.

DIAGNOSIS

- Newborn screening (elevated 17-hydroxyprogesterone level for 21-hydroxylase).
- Karyotype.
- Hyponatremia, hyperkalemia, hypochloremia, hypoglycemia.
- For 21-hydroxylase: markedly increased 17-hydroxyprogesteronenal level.
- Low baseline and low cortisol level after 1–24 ACTH stimulation.
- Elevated plasma renin activity.
- Genetic testing (DNA analysis for genetic mutations in the affected gene).
- Prenatal diagnosis in pregnancy with increased risk.

TREATMENT

- Fluid and electrolyte replacement.
- Normal saline (NS) bolus, then maintenance plus ongoing fluid losses with D₅NS.
- Management of hypoglycemia.
- Stress dose of hydrocortisone (mineralocorticoid and glucocorticoid activity).
- Fludrocortisone (mineralocorticoid).
- Salt replacement (formula and breast milk sodium content is low).
- Treat with dexamethasone any pregnant mothers at risk for 21-hydroxylase deficiency.

Cushing Syndrome

DEFINITION

Cushing syndrome is a characteristic pattern of obesity with or without HTN due to excessive endogenous glucocorticoid production or exogenous exposure.

ETIOLOGY

- Most common etiology of Cushing syndrome: exogenous corticosteroid.
- Cushing disease is bilateral adrenal hyperplasia due to excessive ACTH secretion, usually due to a pituitary microadenoma. It is the most common cause of endogenous Cushing syndrome in children.
- Other causes of endogenous Cushing syndrome include:
    - excess cortisol secretion: unilateral adrenocortical tumors (adenoma, carcinoma) or bilateral adrenal hyperplasia (primary pigmented micronodular adrenal hyperplasia).
    - ectopic ACTH syndrome: malignant nonendocrine tumor, e.g., small cell lung carcinoma produces an excessive amount of ACTH. It is extremely rare in children.

SIGNS AND SYMPTOMS

Truncal obesity, rounded moon facies, buffalo hump, purple striae, easy bruising, muscle weakness, osteopenia, delayed growth, acne, hirsutism, hyperpigmentation, HTN, hyperglycemia, depression, cognitive impairment

The combination of hyperkalemia and hyponatremia is a clue to the diagnosis of classical salt-wasting CAH.

WARD TIP

Most urgent tests for congenital adrenal hyperplasia:
1. Serum glucose
2. Serum electrolytes
Other tests: cortisol, testosterone, 17-OH progesterone

In CAH, blood should be drawn for steroid profile before the administration of hydrocortisone.

Cushing disease is a state of hypercortisolism secondary to adrenocorticotropic hormone (ACTH)-producing pituitary adenoma.

Endogenous Cushing syndrome occurs when the body produces excess cortisol. Cushing disease occurs when a tumor on the pituitary produces excess ACTH.

DIAGNOSIS

- Screening:
  - Elevated 24-hour urine test for free cortisol (UFC).
  - Elevated 8 AM serum ACTH and UFC levels suggest Cushing disease or ectopic ACTH production.
  - Elevated midnight serum cortisol and ACTH levels suggestive of Cushing syndrome or disease.
- Confirmation/localization when screening tests suggest Cushing syndrome or disease:
  - Low-dose dexamethasone suppression test
    - Cushing syndrome refuted if cortisol, ACTH, and UFC levels suppressed.
    - Elevated UFC or cortisol, suggesting Cushing syndrome or disease.
  - High-dose dexamethasone suppression test:
    - Low cortisol, ACTH, and UFC levels suggest Cushing disease, while high levels suggest Cushing syndrome.
    - 24 UFC paradoxically rises in primary pigmented nodular adrenal disease after a high-dose dexamethasone suppression test.
- An elevated ACTH level from petrosal sinus sample after IV corticotropin-releasing hormone suggests Cushing disease.
- Polycythemia, lymphopenia, and eosinopenia can be associated findings.
- Abdominal computed tomography (CT) (adrenal tumors).
- Pituitary magnetic resonance imaging (MRI) (pituitary adenoma).

DIFFERENTIAL DIAGNOSIS

- Exogenous obesity (pseudo-Cushing state).

TREATMENT

- Pediatric endocrine, surgical, and neurosurgical consultation.
- Adrenalectomy (unilateral or bilateral for adrenal tumors or bilateral nodular hyperplasia, respectively).
- Chemotherapy for adrenal cancer with metastasis (after surgery).
- Transsphenoidal resection of pituitary adenoma.
- Fractionated radiotherapy for recurrent pituitary adenoma.

WARD TIP

Growth retardation may be the early manifestation of Cushing syndrome. Virilization may indicate adrenal carcinoma.

Adrenal Insufficiency

DEFINITION

- The adrenal cortex fails to produce glucocorticoid in response to stress.
- It may be primary adrenal disorder or secondary to ACTH deficiency/resistance.
- Mineralocorticoid deficiency is found in primary adrenal disorder but not secondary adrenal insufficiency since aldosterone secretion depends on renin/angiotensin system.

ETIOLOGY

Primary Adrenal Insufficiency (Low Cortisol/Elevated ACTH)
- Congenital:
  - CAH.
  - Congenital adrenal hypoplasia (X-linked).
  - ACTH resistance.
  - Adrenal leukodystrophy (X-linked-recessive disorder of metabolism of very long chain fatty acids).

- Acquired (Addison disease):
    - Autoimmune destruction (most common).
    - Tuberculosis.
    - Bilateral adrenal hemorrhages (meningococcal septicemia).
    - AIDS (opportunistic infections).
    - Drugs (ketoconazole, mitotane, etomidate).

Secondary Adrenal Insufficiency (Low Cortisol/Low ACTH)
- Congenital:
    - Congenital hypopituitarism.
    - Septo-optic dysplasia.
- Acquired:
    - Iatrogenic: abrupt glucocorticoid discontinuation after prolonged use.
    - Pituitary or hypothalamic tumors.

SIGNS AND SYMPTOMS

- Weakness, fatigue, anorexia, nausea, vomiting, weight loss.
- Postural hypotension (more marked in primary adrenal insufficiency).
- Hyperpigmentation of skin and mucosal surfaces (in primary adrenal insufficiency due to elevated ACTH/melanocyte-stimulating hormone [MSH]).
- Salt craving (in primary adrenal insufficiency).
- Adrenal crisis (fever, vomiting, dehydration, and shock precipitated by infection, trauma, or surgery in susceptible patient).

DIAGNOSIS

- Hyponatremia, hyperkalemia, acidosis, hypoglycemia.
- Obtain morning plasma cortisol and ACTH level:
    - Low morning plasma cortisol suggests adrenal insufficiency.
    - Basal plasma ACTH level is high in primary adrenal insufficiency, while a normal level does not rule out secondary causes.
- Anti-adrenal antibodies (in autoimmune destruction of adrenal glands).
- ACTH stimulation test.
- CT scan of adrenal glands (primary adrenal insufficiency).
- Pituitary gland and hypothalamus MRI (secondary adrenal insufficiency).

TREATMENT

- Oral hydrocortisone, increased for febrile illness or injury.
- Fludrocortisone.
- In acute adrenal insufficiency (adrenal crisis):
    - volume replacement.
    - high-dose intravenous hydrocortisone.
    - switch to oral therapy in 2–3 days.

Pheochromocytoma

DEFINITION

- Catecholamine-producing tumor of chromaffin tissue of adrenal medulla (80–85% of cases) or extra-adrenal origin (paraganglioma) (15–20% of cases).
- Usually benign, well encapsulated (<10% malignant).
- In children: frequently familial, bilateral, and multifocal.
- Recurrent tumor may appear years after initial diagnosis.

WARD TIP

Failure of a suntan to disappear may be an early manifestation of adrenal insufficiency; however, the absence of hyperpigmentation does not exclude the diagnosis.

EXAM TIP

Tumors arising in the adrenal medulla produce both epinephrine and norepinephrine. Extra-adrenal tumors produce only norepinephrine.

ETIOLOGY

- It may occur in isolation.
- It is also seen in the multiple endocrine neoplasia (MEN) syndromes, von Hippel–Lindau, neurofibromatosis type 1, and tuberous sclerosis.

SIGNS AND SYMPTOMS

- Nonspecific symptoms.
- Headache, palpitations, increased sweating, anxiety.
- Nausea, vomiting, weight loss, tremor, fatigue, chest or abdominal pain, and flushing.
- Sustained HTN (in children).
- Hyperglycemia.

DIAGNOSIS

- Elevated plasma metanephrines and normetanephrines.
- Increased urinary catecholamines (or metabolites) and vanillylmandelic acid.
- Serum chromogranin A.
- Abdominal ultrasound (US).
- Abdominal CT and MRI.
- ^{123}I MIBG (metaiodobenzylguanidine) scan.

TREATMENT

- Surgical excision.
- Preoperative α_1 and α_2 adrenoreceptor and β adrenoreceptor blockade is required to prevent hypertensive crisis and arrhythmias, respectively.
- Evaluate yearly for recurrence, especially for those with familial disease.

DISORDERS OF CALCIUM AND BONE METABOLISM

Hyperparathyroidism

 A 10-year-old girl has severe abdominal pain and gross hematuria. She passes a calculus in her urine. She had received no medication and has no family history of renal stones. *Think: Primary hyperparathyroidism.*

Symptoms of primary hyperparathyroidism include painful *bones*, renal *stones*, abdominal pain (*groans*), and psychiatric *moans* (poor concentration, depression, fatigue). It is a common cause of hypercalcemia. Hypercalcemia in the presence of an elevated serum parathyroid hormone level confirms the diagnosis of primary hyperparathyroidism. Other biochemical findings include hypercalciuria and hypophosphatemia.

DEFINITION

Hypercalcemia with increased parathyroid hormone (PTH) level

EPIDEMIOLOGY

Uncommon in children

ETIOLOGY

- Primary (defect of parathyroid gland):
  - Parathyroid adenoma is the most common cause.
  - Familial is isolated or as part of MEN 1 and MEN 2A.
- Secondary (in response to hypocalcemia):
  - Chronic renal failure (CRF).
  - Renal tubular acidosis.
  - Vitamin D–deficiency rickets.
  - Treatment (with phosphorus) for hypophosphatemic rickets.
  - Liver failure.
- Tertiary hyperparathyroidism: adenomatous change in parathyroid in the setting of CRF leading to overexcretion of PTH and subsequent hypercalcemia.

SIGNS AND SYMPTOMS

- Clinical manifestation of hypercalcemia.
- Muscle weakness, anorexia, nausea, vomiting, constipation, polyuria, dehydration, failure to thrive, coma, seizures, fever, renal stones.

DIAGNOSIS

- Elevated serum and urinary Ca.
- Decreased serum phosphorus.
- Increased PTH level.
- Subperiosteal resorption of the hand on a plain radiographs.
- CT, USG, or ^{99m}Tc-sestamibi scanning for parathyroid adenoma.

TREATMENT

- For significant hypercalcemia:
  - Hydration.
  - Furosemide (increase Na and Ca excretion).
  - Glucocorticoids (decreases intestinal Ca absorption).
  - Calcitonin.
  - Bisphosphonates (inhibit osteoclast-mediated bone resorption).
  - Calcimimetics, to suppress PTH.
  - Dialysis as a last resort.
- Primary hyperparathyroidism:
  - Resection of isolated adenoma.
  - For generalized hyperplasia, subtotal resection.
  - Vitamin D and calcium for post-op hypocalcemia, which can be severe and prolonged due to "hungry bone syndrome" (hypocalcemia, hypophosphatemia, hypomagnesemia, and hyperkalemia).
- Secondary hyperparathyroidism: treatment of the underlying cause.

WARD TIP

Patients with hyperparathyroidism can develop nephrocalcinosis.

Hypoparathyroidism

DEFINITION

- Decreased PTH or abnormal tissue responsiveness to PTH.
- Can lead to hypocalcemia and increased serum phosphate levels.

ETIOLOGY

- Autoimmune.
- Post-surgical after thyroid, parathyroid, or radical neck surgery.
- Familial: autosomal dominant or recessive and X-linked recessive forms.
- DiGeorge syndrome (deletion of chromosome 22q.11.2).
- Acute illness (PTH secretion is impaired in critical illness.)
- Severe hypomagnesemia (usually <1 mg/dL).

WARD TIP

Hypoparathyroidism can be seen with polyglandular autoimmune endocrinopathy: thyroiditis, diabetes, adrenal insufficiency, mucocutaneous candidiasis.

SIGNS AND SYMPTOMS

- The presentation is related to hypocalcemia: numbness, tingling, paresthesia, and muscle cramps.
- In severe cases: seizure, tetany, and mental status changes.
- In older asymptomatic patients, hyperreflexia, Chvostek's (facial twitching), and Trousseau's (carpopedal spasm) signs can be elicited.
- EKG may reveal prolongation of the QTc interval leading to arrhythmias.

DIAGNOSIS

- Decreased serum total and ionized Ca.
- Increased serum phosphate.
- Markedly decreased PTH.
- Prolonged QTc interval.

DIFFERENTIAL DIAGNOSIS

Pseudohypoparathyroidism (PTH unresponsiveness; markedly high PTH level)

TREATMENT

- Correct hypocalcemia:
  - Intravenous route for acute symptomatic hypocalcemia.
  - Transition to PO calcium as soon as possible.
- Correct hypomagnesemia.
- Vitamin D (calcitriol).

WARD TIP

Pay attention to the heart rate with treatment for hypoparathyroidism; bradycardia is an indication to stop calcium infusion.

Metabolic Bone Disease

- Osteopenia: bone mass deficiency relative to age, sex, and race norms.
- Osteoporosis: loss of bone mineral and bone matrix.
- Osteomalacia: defective mineralization of the bone matrix.
- Rickets: defective mineralization before growth plate fusion.

CLASSIFICATION OF RICKETS

Calcipenic

ETIOLOGY

- Nutritional:
  - Vitamin D deficiency.
  - Calcium deficiency.
- Genetic:
  - Vitamin D–dependent rickets type 1 (1α-hydroxylase deficiency causing defect in the conversion of 25(OH) vitamin D to 1,25(OH)$_2$ vitamin D).
  - Vitamin D–dependent rickets type 2 (mutation in the gene coding the vitamin D receptor causing hereditary vitamin D resistance).
- Drugs:
  - Corticosteroids.
  - Anticonvulsants.
- Prematurity.

Phosphopenic (hypophosphatemic)

- Genetic:
  - autosomal-dominant, recessive, and X-linked hypophosphatemic rickets forms identified.

- tumor-induced hypophosphatemia (small, typically benign tumor mostly of mesenchymal origin).
- Dietary:
    - Intestinal malabsorption.
    - Breast-fed very premature infants.
- Fanconi syndrome (renal loss of glucose, phosphate, amino acids, and bicarbonate).

CLINICAL FEATURES

- Genu varum (bow-legged deformity) during early childhood.
- Genu valgum (knocked-knee deformity) in older children.
- Enlargement of wrists and knees.
- Rachitic rosary (enlargement of costochondral junctions).
- Harrison grooves (groove extending laterally from xiphoid process, corresponds to the diaphragmatic attachment).
- Frontal bossing.
- Craniotabes (generalized softening of calvaria).
- Bone pain.
- Proximal muscle weakness.

RADIOLOGICAL FEATURES

- Widening of epiphyseal plates.
- Cupping, splaying, and formation of cortical spurs.
- Deformities in shaft of long bones.

DIAGNOSIS

- Serum calcium, phosphorous, alkaline phosphatase level:
    - Alkaline phosphatase is markedly elevated in calcium and vitamin D deficiency and mildly elevated in hypophosphatemic rickets.
    - Serum calcium and phosphorus tend to be low or low normal in calcipenic rickets. Serum PTH is elevated.
    - Low serum phosphate with normal calcium level suggests hypophosphatemic rickets.
- 25(OH) vitamin D and 1,25(OH)$_2$ vitamin D level:
    - Low 25(OH) vitamin D is seen in all forms of vitamin D deficiency.
    - Normal 25(OH) vitamin D level with low 1,25(OH)$_2$ vitamin D level point to 1α-hydroxylase deficiency.
    - 1,25(OH)$_2$ vitamin D level is elevated in hereditary vitamin D resistance.
    - 1,25(OH)$_2$ vitamin D level is inappropriately normal in the setting of hypophosphatemia in X-linked and autosomal-dominant hypophosphatemic rickets.
- PTH level:
    - Moderate to severe hyperparathyroidism is seen with calcipenic rickets.
    - In hypophosphatemic rickets, PTH level may be normal or modestly elevated.
- Low tubular reabsorption of phosphorous (usually >95%) with low serum phosphate confirms inappropriate renal loses, characteristic of hypophosphatemic rickets.

TREATMENT

- Nutritional rickets:
    - Oral vitamin D supplementation for several weeks.
    - For noncompliance: single large oral or IM vitamin D dose.
    - Ensure adequate calcium intake.

EXAM TIP

Excluding those with chronic malabsorption syndromes or end-stage renal disease, most cases of rickets occur in dark-skinned breast-fed infants who have received inadequate vitamin D supplementation.

- 1α-hydroxylase deficiency rickets:
    - 1,25(OH)$_2$ vitamin D (calcitriol) orally.
    - Adequate dietary calcium intake.
- Hereditary vitamin D resistance:
    - High doses of 1,25(OH)$_2$ vitamin D.
    - IV calcium in patients who do not respond to vitamin D.
- Hypophosphatemic rickets:
    - Oral phosphate.
    - 1,25(OH)$_2$ vitamin D, which enhances calcium and phosphate absorption and dampens phosphate stimulated PTH secretion.

NEUROENDOCRINE DISORDERS

Diabetes Insipidus (DI)

DEFINITION

Inability of kidneys to concentrate urine

ETIOLOGY

- Central (decreased ADH production):
    - Congenital hypothalamic/pituitary defects (septo-optic dysplasia, holoprosencephaly).
    - Idiopathic, accidental, or surgical trauma, infections (meningitis).
    - Neoplasms (suprasellar tumors).
    - Infiltrative and autoimmune diseases (histiocytosis X).
    - Drugs (ethanol, phenytoin).
- Nephrogenic (renal unresponsiveness to ADH):
    - X-linked recessive: males present in early infancy. Carrier females are asymptomatic.
    - Autosomal recessive or autosomal dominant forms.
    - Idiopathic.
    - Renal diseases.
    - Hypercalcemia.
    - Hypokalemia.
    - Drugs (lithium, demeclocycline).

SIGNS AND SYMPTOMS

- Central:
    - Polyuria (>1.5 L/m^2/day).
    - Polydipsia (excessive thirst).
    - Enuresis.
    - Hypernatremic dehydration.
- Nephrogenic:
    - Polyuria, nocturia, failure to thrive (FTT), fever, vomiting.
    - Hypernatremic dehydration.

DIAGNOSIS

- Increased serum osmolality (normal: <290 mOsm/kg).
- Increased serum Na.
- Decreased urine osmolality.
- Water deprivation test differentiates DI from primary polydipsia.
- Withhold fluids for 8–10 hours. Serum osmolality >300 mOsm/kg with urine osmolality <600 mOsm/kg or plasma sodium >145 mEq/L establishes the diagnosis.

WARD TIP

In diabetes insipidus, there is high urine output despite significant dehydration.

- Once DI is established, give desmopressin (DDAVP).
    - Urine volume falls and osmolality doubles, suggesting central DI.
    - Less than twofold rise in urine osmolality suggests nephrogenic DI.
- Plasma vasopressin (low in central DI and high in nephrogenic DI).
- MRI: posterior pituitary bright spot is diminished or absent in both forms of DI.

TREATMENT

- Central:
    - Fluids (3–4 L/m^2/day without desmopressin, 1 L/m^2/day with desmopressin).
    - Desmopressin orally, intranasally, or subcutaneously.
- Nephrogenic:
    - Fluids.
    - Thiazide diuretic (promotes distal tube Na excretion, a decrease in glomerular filtration rate, and increased proximal tubular reabsorption of Na and water).
    - Indomethacin further enhances proximal tubular sodium and water reabsorption.

Syndrome of Inappropriate Secretion of Antidiuretic Hormone (SIADH)

DEFINITION

Hyponatremia with increased ADH and impaired water excretion

ETIOLOGY

- Can be hereditary.
- CNS disorders: meningoencephalitis, brain tumor, trauma, intracranial bleeding.
- Psychiatric diseases.
- Postictal period after prolonged seizures.
- Rocky Mountain spotted fever.
- Pneumonia.
- AIDS.
- Drugs (carbamazepine, chlorpropamide, vincristine, tricyclic antidepressant).

SIGNS AND SYMPTOMS

- Asymptomatic until Na < 120 mEq/L.
- Headache, nausea, vomiting, irritability, seizure.
- Decrease urine output.

DIAGNOSIS

- Hyponatremia (Na < 135 mEq/L).
- Low serum osmolality (<275 mOsm/kg).
- High urine osmolality (>100 mOsm/kg).
- Increased urine Na (usually >80 mEq/L).
- Low serum uric acid level.
- Normal renal, adrenal, and thyroid function.

TREATMENT

- Treat the underlying disease.
- Symptomatic with hyponatremia: hypertonic (3%) saline.

In SIADH, there is an absence of edema and dehydration.

Urine osmolality <100 mOsm/kg excludes diagnosis of SIADH.

- Asymptomatic:
  - Fluid restriction (1000 mL/m^2/day).
  - Demeclocycline and lithium (diminish collecting tubule responsiveness to ADH, thus increasing water excretion).
  - Selective V2 receptor antagonist (tolvaptan): selective water diuresis without affecting sodium and potassium excretion.
  - Oral urea at low doses reduces natriuresis and at higher doses causes osmotic diuresis.

Cerebral Salt Wasting (CSW)

DEFINITION

Renal Na loss during intracranial disease, causing hyponatremia and extracellular fluid depletion due to inappropriate sodium wasting in the urine

ETIOLOGY

High atrial natriuretic peptide causes natriuresis and diuresis (decreased sodium reabsorption and inhibition of renin release).

SIGNS AND SYMPTOMS

- Acute, intermittent excessive fluid and salt loss.
- Elevated urine output.
- Onset within first week of CNS insult.
- Duration variable usually lasts 2–4 weeks.
- Dehydration.

DIAGNOSIS

- Hyponatremia and low plasma osmolality.
- Inappropriately elevated urine osmolality that is isotonic with plasma.
- Increased urine Na excretion.
- See Table 17-2 for comparison between SIADH and CSW.

TREATMENT

- Water and salt replacement (in contrast to SIADH where water restriction without salt supplementation is indicated).

Prolactin Excess

ETIOLOGY

- Prolactin-secreting adenoma: micro- (<1 cm) or macroadenoma (>1 cm).
- Tumors that disrupt pituitary stalk, preventing inhibitory control.
- Drugs (phenothiazines, risperidone, metoclopramide, estrogen, cocaine).
- Hypothyroidism.
- Physical stress.

CLINICAL FEATURES

- Headache.
- Galactorrhea.
- Gynecomastia.

TABLE 17-2. **Comparison Between SIADH and CSW**

	SIADH	CSW
Body weight and Plasma volume	↑	↓
Serum Na and osmolality	↓	↓
Urine osmolality	Higher than plasma	Isotonic with plasma
Urine flow rate	↓	↑
Plasma renin	↓	↓
Plasma aldosterone and ADH	↑	↓
Plasma ANP	↑	↑
Serum uric acid	↓	Normal

ADH, antidiuretic hormone; ANP, atrial natriuretic peptide; CSW, cerebral salt wasting; SIADH, syndrome of inappropriate secretion of antidiuretic hormone.

DIAGNOSIS

- Elevated prolactin level.
- MRI (hypothalamic-pituitary region).

TREATMENT

- Treatment of the underlying cause, such as hypothyroidism.
- Dopamine agonists (bromocriptine, cabergoline) are the first line of treatment for adenoma.
- Transsphenoidal surgery is warranted if medical treatment is unsuccessful.

GROWTH DISORDERS

Short Stature

DEFINITION

Height >2 standard deviations below the mean for age and gender

Normal Growth
- Chronological age (CA) = Bone age (BA) = Height age (HA).
- Normal growth velocity depends on age and pubertal stage:
  - First 2 years of life: about 30–35 cm.
  - Age 2–4 years: 5.5 to 9 cm/yr.
  - Age 4–6 years: 5 to 8.5 cm/yr.
  - Age 6 years to puberty: 4–6 cm/yr.
  - During puberty (girls Tanner II–III): 8 to 14 cm/yr.
  - During puberty (boys Tanner IV): 8 to 14 cm/yr.

Genetic Potential/Mid-parental Height
- For males: add 13 cm to mother's height and average it with father's height.
- For females: subtract 13 cm from father's height and average it with mother's height.

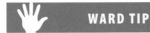

WARD TIP

Prolactin secretion is inhibited by dopamine in pituitary prolactinomas. Therefore, treatment includes dopamine agonists such as bromocriptine.

EXAM TIP

The most common causes of short stature are normal variants including familial short stature and constitutional delay.

Familial (Genetic Short Stature)

- Common cause of short stature.
- Height is within family norm (usually at least one parent is short).
- Normal rate of growth (follow steady channel after 2–3 years of age).
- Normal bone age.
- Puberty at average age.

Constitutional Delay

- Most common cause of short stature.
- Normal variant of growth.
- Normal at birth, then growth decelerates during first 2 years of life.
- Both length and weight gain decelerate until age 2–3 years.
- Resume growth rate by 3–4 years, paralleling a lower percentile curve.
- Delayed puberty (second growth deceleration at age 12–14 years).
- Described as "late bloomers," i.e., catch-up growth upon entering puberty.
- Delayed bone age (bone age = height age but ≠ to chronological age).

EXAM TIP

Children with constitutional delay are the so-called "late bloomers."

Nutritional

- Inflammatory bowel disease.
- Celiac disease.
- HIV infection.
- Other conditions causing malnutrition.

Psychosocial Deprivation

- Resemble children with GH deficiency (bone-age retardation and similar GH findings upon stimulation testing).
- Testing and growth revert to normal upon removal from deprived environment.

Small for Gestational Age (SGA)

- Birth weight and length <10th percentile for gestational age.
- The effects of SGA may persist into adulthood.

Glucocorticoid Therapy

- Effects are dose related.

Intrauterine Growth Retardation

- Pathologically growth-restricted infants.
- Maternal (toxemia, chronic illness), fetal (congenital infection, chromosomal disorders), or placental problems (infarction, separation) are among the causes.
- Prolonged growth and developmental challenges may result.

GROWTH HORMONE DEFICIENCY (GHD)

WARD TIP

Regardless of etiology, the following questions can help guide the evaluation and treatment of children with short stature: (1) How short is the child? (2) Is the child's growth velocity abnormal? (3) What is the child's genetic potential for growth based on predicted adult height?

- Hypoglycemia and micropenis (especially if associated with hypopituitarism).
- Height below genetic potential.
- Decreased growth velocity (<25th percentile for age).
- Downward crossing of percentiles on growth chart after age 2–3 years.
- Decreased muscle mass, increased fat mass.
- Pubertal delay.
- Causes—idiopathic, hereditary, hypothalamic/pituitary malformation, hypothalamic/pituitary tumor, head trauma, CNS surgery or radiation, meningitis/encephalitis, autoimmune hypophysitis, histiocytosis X, sarcoidosis, and hemochromatosis.

DIAGNOSIS

- Delayed bone age.
- Low IGF-1, low IGFBP-3 (insulin-like growth factor-binding protein 3), inadequate response to GH stimulation.

TREATMENT

Biosynthetic human GH.

GROWTH HORMONE INSENSITIVITY (LARON SYNDROME)

- Features similar to GHD.
- GH receptor defect.
- Normal or elevated GH level.
- Low IGF-1, IGF-2, and IGFBP-3.
- Absent or low growth hormone binding protein (GHBP).

TREATMENT

Biosynthetic IGF-1

HYPOTHYROIDISM

- Delayed bone age.
- See discussion above.

CUSHING SYNDROME

- Delayed bone age.
- See discussion above.

CHROMOSOMAL DISORDERS (SEE DISCUSSION IN SPECIFIC CHAPTERS)

- Turner syndrome (45X).
- Down syndrome (trisomy 21).
- Russell-Silver syndrome.
- Prader-Willi syndrome.

Tall Stature

DEFINITION

Height >2 standard deviations above the mean for age and gender.

FAMILIAL OR CONSTITUTIONAL TALL STATURE

- Most common.
- Family history of tall stature.
- Lack of any dysmorphic features.
- Normal bone age.

HORMONAL

- Early/Precocious puberty: increased sex steroids (patient is tall as a child, but short as an adult [early epiphyseal closure]).
- CAH: increased adrenal androgens (tall as child, short as adult).
- Hyperinsulinism/obesity.
- Hypogonadotropic hypogonadism (Kallmann syndrome).

SYNDROMES

- Marfan syndrome (autosomal dominant connective tissue disorder).
- Homocystinuria (inherited inborn error of metabolism).

WARD TIP

Children with poor growth due to nutritional deficiencies are generally short and have low birth weight, whereas children with endocrinologic causes for poor (linear) growth are usually disproportionately heavy.

EXAM TIP

Thyroid hormone is the most important hormone for linear growth in the first 2 years of life.

- Klinefelter syndrome (47XXY).
- Sotos syndrome genetic defect with macrocephaly, large hands and feet, antimongoloid palpebral fissure slant, developmental disability, seizures, and increased risk of neoplasms.
- Beckwith-Wiedemann syndrome: see genetics chapter.

GIGANTISM/ACROMEGALY

- Increased growth hormone (GH).
- If occurs it before epiphyses close, gigantism results.
- If it occurs after epiphyses close, acromegaly results.

ETIOLOGY

- Pituitary gigantism is rare.
- It is most commonly caused by growth hormone (GH)–secreting adenoma.
- It is also seen with McCune Albright syndrome, MEN1, and Carney complex.

CLINICAL FEATURES

- Accelerated rate of linear growth and rapid weight gain.
- Coarsening of facial features (macrocephaly, frontal bossing) and mandibular prominence.
- Enlargement of hands and feet.
- Excessive sweating.
- GH-secreting adenomas associated with amenorrhea, often with galactorrhea in girls and symptoms of tumor compression in boys.

DIAGNOSIS

- Elevated insulin-like growth factor 1 and IGF-binding protein 3.
- GH may be normal or elevated.
- The GH suppression test is the gold standard for diagnosis. The failure of GH concentration to drop to low levels within 2 hours of glucose load suggests GH excess.
- MRI of the pituitary.

TREATMENT

- Transsphenoidal resection of adenoma.
- Somatostatin and dopamine agonist (bromocriptine) for incomplete resection.

Sexual Development

- Pubertal events are classified by Sexual Maturity Rating (SMR, also known as Tanner staging). Puberty progresses with an average duration of 3–4 years, spending about 1 year in each stage.
- See Table 17-3 and Figure 17-1.

NORMAL FEMALE PROGRESSION

Thelarche → pubic hair → height growth spurt → menarche (12.5–13 years). In 20% of girls, pubarche may precede thelarche.

NORMAL MALE PROGRESSION

Testicular enlargement → pubic hair → penile enlargement → height growth spurt (14–15 years) → axillary hair.

TABLE 17-3. Tanner Stages

STAGE	BREAST DEVELOPMENT (FEMALE)	GENITAL DEVELOPMENT (MALE)	PUBIC HAIR (FEMALE AND MALE)
I	Preadolescent	Preadolescent	Preadolescent
II	Breast bud (11 years)	Enlargement of scrotum and testes, darkening of scrotum and texture change (12 years)	Sparse, long, slightly pigmented downy hair (female 12, male 13.5)
III	Continued enlargement, no contour separation (12 years)	Enlargement of penis (13 years)	Darker, coarser, and more curled (female 12.5, male 14)
IV	Secondary mound, projection of areola and papilla (13 years)	Increase in penis breadth and development of glans (14 years)	Hair resembles adult, distributed less than adult and not to medial thighs (female 13, male 14.5)
V	Mature stage (15 years)	Mature stage (15 years)	Mature stage (female 14.5, male 15)

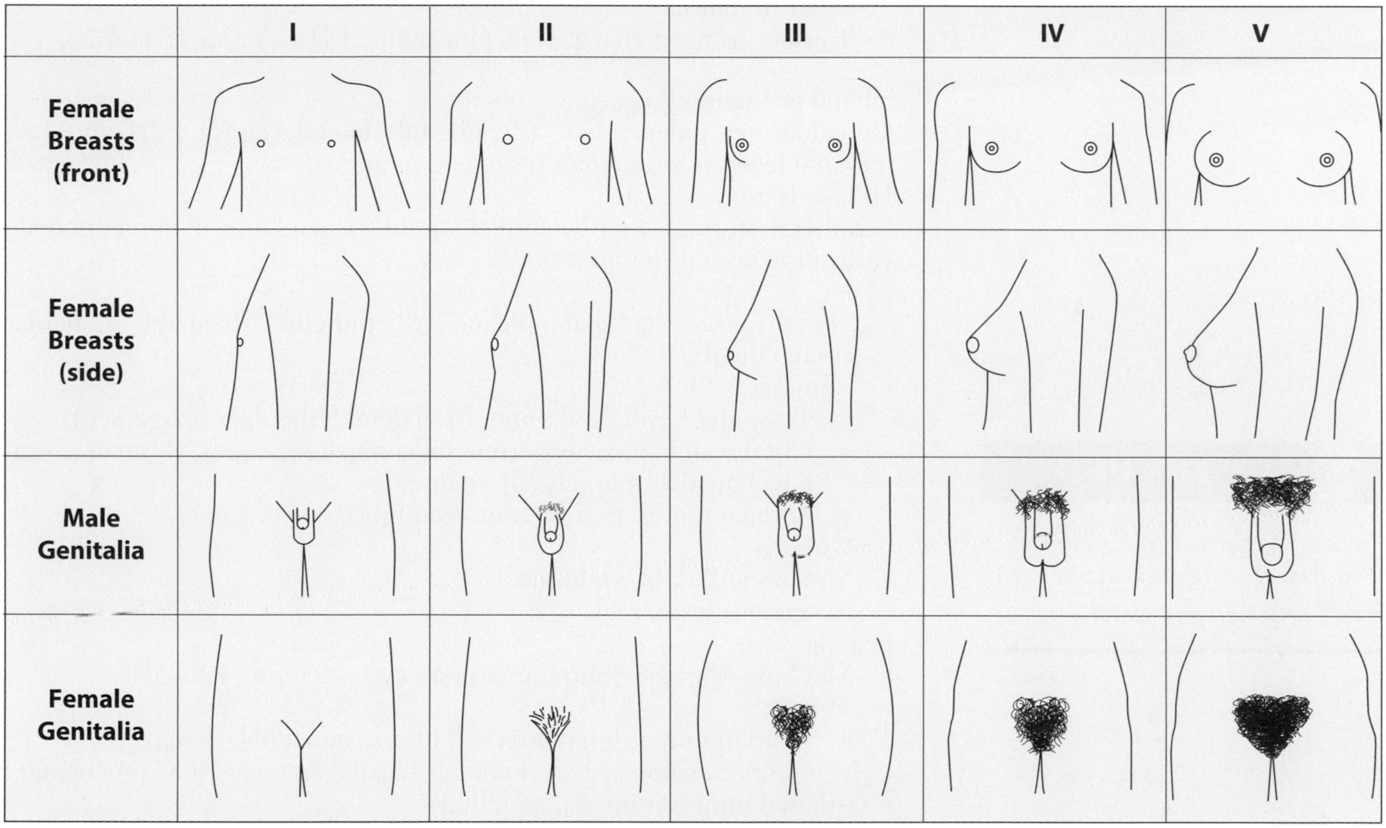

FIGURE 17-1. Tanner stages.

PRECOCIOUS PUBERTY

A 6½-year-old girl develops enlarged breasts. Six months later, she begins to develop pubic and axillary hair. Her menses began at age 9. *Think: Idiopathic precocious puberty.*

Puberty in girls is occurring at an earlier age. The cause of this change in most cases is unknown. Evaluation should include serum FSH, LH, estradiol, and bone age. A brain MRI is considered to rule out a possible underlying intracranial cause.

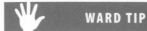

WARD TIP

Most normal 11-year-old girls have pubic hair.

DEFINITION

- Onset of secondary sexual characteristics.
- Girls (<8 years for white, <7 for Black and Hispanics).
- Boys (<9 years).
- Premature breast development (thelarche).
- Premature pubic hair development (pubarche/adrenarche).

ETIOLOGY

Central or True Precocious Puberty

- Premature activation of the hypothalamic-pituitary-gonadal (HPG) axis.
- Gonadotropin dependent: pubertal (high) FSH, LH and sex steroids (testosterone or estradiol).
- Usually idiopathic in girls, but due to organic lesion in boys.
- CNS abnormalities:
    - Hypothalamic hamartoma.
    - Head injury.
    - Hydrocephalus.
    - Radiation.
    - Surgical trauma.
    - Tumors (astrocytoma, glioma, pinealoma, LH-secreting adenoma).

Peripheral or Pseudo Precocious Puberty

- Gonadotropin independent: prepubertal (low) levels of FSH and LH, pubertal levels of sex steroids (estrogens or androgens).
- HPG axis is not activated.
- Peripheral precocity may be correct for child's gender or incorrect (female virilization or male feminization).
- Male:
    - Testotoxicosis: familial precocious puberty (bilateral testicular enlargement).
    - Tumors:
        - Testicular Leydig cell tumor (unilateral testicular enlargement).
        - Choriocarcinoma, dysgerminoma, hepatoblastoma (human chorionic gonadotropin [HCG] producing).
        - Adrenal tumors (testosterone secreting).
    - CAH.
    - McCune-Albright syndrome.
    - Exogenous sex steroid.
- Female:
    - McCune-Albright syndrome: ovarian cysts secreting estrogen.
    - Tumors:
        - Ovarian tumors (granulosa cell tumor, gonadoblastoma).
        - Choriocarcinoma, dysgerminoma, hepatoblastoma (HCG producing).
    - Adrenal tumors (estrogen secreting).
    - Exogenous sex steroids.

EXAM TIP

Precocious puberty in girls is usually idiopathic, while in boys, it usually has an organic cause.

SIGNS AND SYMPTOMS

- Growth acceleration.
- Significantly advanced bone age.
- Progressive sexual development.

DIAGNOSIS

- Prepubertal gonadotropins (FSH, LH) and pubertal levels of estrogen or testosterone suggest gonadotropin-independent process.
- Gonadotropins may be pubertal or prepubertal at baseline, while testosterone or estrogen is usually pubertal in gonadotropin-dependent precocious puberty.

- Gonadotropin-independent precocious puberty: a gonadotropin-releasing hormone (GnRH) agonist stimulation test results in no increase in gonadotropin levels.
- Gonadotropin-dependent precocious puberty: a GnRH agonist stimulation test results in pubertal LH-dominant response.
- Pelvic ultrasound to evaluate ovarian and uterine size and rule out pathology (ovarian cyst, tumor).
- Head MRI to rule out CNS abnormality in central precocious puberty
- CT the abdomen and pelvis; if a tumor is found, peripheral precocious puberty is likely.

TREATMENT

- Treatment of underlying cause for central or peripheral puberty.
- GnRH analogues (in central precocious puberty).
- Androgen antagonist (flutamide) and aromatase inhibitor (blocks conversion of androgen to estrogen) in peripheral precocious puberty.

PREMATURE THELARCHE

DEFINITION

- Isolated breast development.
- Most commonly noted during the first 2 years of life.
- Breast development is usually limited and often regresses.

SIGNS AND SYMPTOMS

- Normal growth rate and bone age.
- Prepubertal level of gonadotropins and estrogen.

TREATMENT

Nonprogressive and self-limiting

PREMATURE ADRENARCHE

DEFINITION

Early sexual hair appearance (premature pubarche) without other sexual development signs

- <8 years in White girls (<7 years in Black and Hispanic).
- < 9 years in boys.
- Adult body odor is another associated feature.

ETIOLOGY

- Increased adrenal androgen production (premature adrenarche).
- Increased risk for later development of polycystic ovarian syndrome.
- Nonclassical CAH may present similarly and can lead to early puberty.

DIAGNOSIS

- Adrenal androgen (dehydroepiandrosterone sulfate [DHEA-S]): normal for pubertal stage but high for chronologic age.
- If androgens are significantly high, CAH and adrenal tumor need to be excluded.

TREATMENT

Self-limiting

DELAYED PUBERTY

DEFINITION

Absence of any pubertal development by 13 years in girls and 14 years in boys

EPIDEMIOLOGY

It is more common in boys.

ETIOLOGY

- Female:
  - Constitutional.
  - Primary ovarian failure (idiopathic, autoimmune, chemotherapy, radiation, galactosemia, fragile X syndrome, gonadotropin receptor mutation).
  - Turner syndrome.
  - Hypogonadotropic hypogonadism (Kallmann syndrome).
  - 17-hydroxylase deficiency CAH.
  - Hypopituitarism (congenital or acquired).
  - HPG axis dysfunction (systemic illness, undernutrition, or strenuous physical activity).
  - Prader-Willi syndrome.
- Male:
  - Constitutional.
  - Primary testicular failure (vanishing testis syndrome, bilateral cryptorchidism/torsion, infection, chemotherapy, radiation, surgical trauma, hemochromatosis, fragile X syndrome, gonadotropin receptor mutation).
  - Klinefelter syndrome.
  - Hypogonadotropic hypogonadism (Kallmann syndrome).
  - Dysfunction of HPG axis secondary to systemic illness or undernutrition.
  - Hypopituitarism (congenital or acquired).
  - Prader-Willi syndrome.

DIAGNOSIS

- FSH, LH, estradiol, testosterone
  - High gonadotropin levels: primary gonadal failure (hypergonadotropic hypogonadism).
  - Low gonadotropin levels: hypogonadotropic hypogonadism or constitutional delay; differentiation of these two conditions difficult until well into adolescence.
- Chromosome analysis for primary gonadal failure.
- Head MRI for hypogonadotropic hypogonadism or hypopituitarism.

EXAM TIP

Kallmann syndrome is usually sporadic; 5% X-linked hypogonadotropic hypogonadism affecting males and rarely females, associated with anosmia, cleft lip/palate, and other midline defects.

TREATMENT

- Treatment of the cause.
- Females: estrogen initially; later, cyclic estrogen–progestin.
- Males: testosterone.

Menstruation

- The mean age for menarche is about 12 years.
- Menarche occurs about 2.5 years after thelarche, typically at Tanner stage IV.
- Many cycles in the first 2 years after menarche are anovulatory.

- The length of a cycle is between 21 and 45 days (average is 28 days).
- The length of flow is 2–7 days.
- Blood loss is 20 to 60 mL.

AMENORRHEA

Primary Amenorrhea

Lack of spontaneous uterine bleeding within 4 years of pubertal development

ETIOLOGY

- Primary ovarian failure (elevated FSH and LH)
- Chromosomal:
  - Turner syndrome (gonadal dysgenesis).
  - Triple X syndrome.
  - Pure gonadal dysgenesis (46,XX or 46,XY).
  - Fragile X.
- Classical galactosemia.
- Constitutional delay of puberty.
- Polycystic ovary syndrome.
- Autoimmune oophoritis.
- Radiation.
- Chemotherapy.
- Gonadal trauma.
- 17-hydroxylase deficiency (CAH).
- Congenital lipid hyperplasia.
- FSH/LH receptor mutation.
- Idiopathic.
- Hypogonadotropic hypogonadism (low FSH and LH): isolated or with hypopituitarism.
- Prader-Willi syndrome.
- Anorexia nervosa.
- Strenuous exercise.
- Structural anomalies:
  - Imperforate hymen.
  - Agenesis of Müllerian structure (Mayer-Rokitansky-Hauser syndrome).
- Other:
  - Complete androgen insensitivity (testicular feminization syndrome).
  - True hermaphroditism.

Secondary Amenorrhea

Menstruation absence for 3 months with prior regular menses or 6 months with irregular menses

EXAM TIP

Turner syndrome is the most common cause of primary amenorrhea.

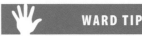

WARD TIP

The initial evaluation of primary amenorrhea can be guided by determining if there is normal breast development and a normal uterus, and by obtaining an FSH level.

A 16-year-old had breast development at age 12 years and menses at age 14. She has not had menses for 2 months. She is active in sports. Physical examination is normal. *Think: Rule out pregnancy, and then consider the sports contribution to her secondary amenorrhea.*

Pregnancy is the most common cause of amenorrhea and is considered in any patient of reproductive age. After pregnancy, thyroid disease and hyperprolactinemia should be considered as potential diagnoses. Amenorrhea can also occur due to exercise. Female athlete triad (disordered eating, amenorrhea, and osteoporosis) is a well-recognized entity. Athletic amenorrhea is due to hypothalamic-pituitary axis suppression, but it is a diagnosis of exclusion. Other testing includes pregnancy, prolactin, FSH, LH, TSH, T_4, DHEA-S, 17 hydroxyprogesterone, and testosterone levels.

ETIOLOGY

- Pregnancy.
- Turner syndrome (mosaicism).
- Hyperandrogenic states (PCOS, CAH).
- Hyperprolactinemia.
- Hypothalamic amenorrhea.
- Causes of primary amenorrhea.

DIFFERENTIAL DIAGNOSIS

- Normal/low FSH:
    - Consider hypothalamic amenorrhea: stress, weight loss, eating disorder, competitive athletics, phenothiazine use, substance abuse.
    - Also consider chronic disease, CNS tumor (i.e., prolactinoma), pituitary infiltration or infarction (postpartum hemorrhage, sickle cell disease), and Asherman syndrome (following endometrial curettage).
- High FSH:
    - Consider gonadal dysgenesis: mosaic Turner syndrome, autoimmune oophoritis, or primary ovarian insufficiency.

DYSMENORRHEA

DEFINITION

Recurrent, crampy lower abdominal pain during menstruation

Primary Dysmenorrhea

Dysmenorrhea, in the absence of any specific, pelvic pathologic condition

ETIOLOGY

- Progesterone during ovulatory cycle increases prostaglandin synthesis.
- Prostaglandins cause uterine contractions, ischemia, and smooth-muscle contraction, explaining the uterine and gastrointestinal pain.

TREATMENT

Prostaglandin inhibitors (NSAIDs) at the onset of flow or pain
Estrogen–progestin oral contraceptives for excessive pain

Secondary Dysmenorrhea

Dysmenorrhea in the presence of a secondary cause

ETIOLOGY

- Underlying vagina, cervix, or uterus abnormality (endometrial polyps, fibroids).
- Pelvic adhesions.
- Endometriosis (endometrial tissue outside the uterus).
- Foreign body such as an intrauterine device.
- Endometritis: infection, especially from sexually transmitted diseases.
- Complications of pregnancy such as ectopic pregnancy.

Testicular Feminization

DEFINITION

- Androgen-insensitivity syndrome (complete and partial form).
- In complete androgen-insensitivity syndrome, XY male appears as a female with a short, blind-ending vaginal pouch and no uterus, but 46 XY

karyotype. Normal breast development is found; testosterone levels are in the normal adult male range. Androgen receptor (AR) is either absent or unable to bind androgen.

■ In partial androgen-insensitivity syndrome, XY cases have either ambiguous or female genitalia with no uterus. Considerable virilization occurs at puberty, but gynecomastia also develops. Androgen receptor binding is low or normal.

SIGNS AND SYMPTOMS

■ Primary amenorrhea.
■ Normal breast development.
■ Pubic hair absent or sparse.
■ Presence of testes in inguinal canal or abdomen.

DIAGNOSIS

■ Testosterone level is elevated.
■ LH is normal or elevated.
■ Sex hormone binding globulin (SHBG) test: unable to suppress SHBG to <80% of the basal value suggests androgen insensitivity.
■ HCG stimulation every other day for 2 days shows normal testosterone response, helping to differentiate partial androgen sensitivity from causes of ambiguous genitalia due to testosterone synthesis defect.
■ Androgen receptor binding studies in cultured genital skin fibroblast.
■ DNA analysis for mutation in AR gene.

True Hermaphroditism

DEFINITION

■ Ovotesticular disorder of sex development (DSD).
■ Gonads comprised of both ovarian and testicular elements (ovotestis).
■ Most are 46,XX.
■ Can be familial.

ETIOLOGY

Abnormal gonadal differentiation

SIGNS AND SYMPTOMS

■ Ambiguous genitalia: significant masculinization (raised as male).
■ Risk of malignant gonadal tissue transformation is lower than XY gonadal dysgenesis.

Pseudohermaphroditism

FEMALE

DEFINITION

Normal ovaries and uterus with external genitalia virilization in a 46, XX patient

ETIOLOGY

■ CAH (21-hydroxylase, 11 β-hydroxylase, or 3 β-hydroxysteroid dehydrogenase deficiency).

- Placental aromatase deficiency (androgens to estrogens conversion is blocked). Estriol level is undetectable. Maternal virilization occurs during pregnancy.
- Luteoma of pregnancy: maternal virilization occurs during pregnancy.

SIGNS AND SYMPTOMS

Virilization of external genitalia (clitoral hypertrophy, labioscrotal fusion)

MALE

DEFINITION

Normal testes with undervirilization or female-appearing genitalia in a 46,XY patient.

ETIOLOGY

- Androgen insensitivity.
- CAH: 3β-hydroxysteroid dehydrogenase deficiency, 17-hydroxylase deficiency, and congenital lipoid adrenal hyperplasia.
- Enzyme defects in testosterone synthesis (17-ketoreductase deficiency).
- 5α-reductase deficiency: conversion of testosterone to dihydrotestosterone is blocked.

SIGNS AND SYMPTOMS

Undervirilization of external genitalia (small phallus, hypospadias, undescended testes) or completely female-appearing genitalia

Gender Dysphoria

- See Psychiatry chapter.

Neurologic Disease

Seizures

DEFINITION

- A paroxysmal electrical discharge of cortical neurons results in an alteration of function or behavior.
- This is the most common pediatric neurologic disorder, affecting 4–10% of children.
- The highest incidence occurs in the first year of life.

ETIOLOGY

Multiple etiologies have been identified for seizures. Provoked causes include:

- Fever.
- Metabolic:
  - Hypoglycemia.
  - Hyponatremia.
  - Hypocalcemia.
  - Inborn errors of metabolism.
- Medications and drugs.
- Trauma (intracranial hemorrhage).
- Infections (encephalitis, meningitis, abscess).
- Vascular events (strokes).
- Hypoxic ischemia encephalopathy.
- Idiopathic.

TYPES OF SEIZURES

See Table 18-1.

Focal (previously known as simple partial) Seizures

These begin in one brain region.

1. Focal seizures without impairment of consciousness (previously simple partial):
   - Brief in duration.
   - Restricted at onset to one focal cortical region.
   - Tend to involve the face, neck, and extremities.
   - Patients may complain of aura, which is a clue for the brain region involved.
   - Seizures can be somatosensory/visual or auditory.

TABLE 18-1. Types of Seizures

Absence	Sudden brief discontinuation of activity and unresponsiveness
Tonic-Clonic	Bilateral symmetrical tonic contraction, then bilateral clonic contractions
Tonic	Sustained muscle contraction for seconds to minutes
Clonic	Repetitive, rhythmic myoclonus at 2–3 Hz
Myoclonic	Sudden, brief (< 50 ms) involuntary contraction of muscles or group of muscles
Atonic	Sudden, brief, 1–2 sec ↓ in tone without preceding myoclonic or tonic event

2. Focal seizures with impairment of consciousness (previously complex partial):
   - Average 1–2 minutes.
   - Commonly include aura.
   - Involve automatisms of the mouth (such as chewing) or extremities (such as manipulation of clothes).
   - Often arise in the temporal lobe.
3. Secondarily generalized seizures:
   - Start as a focal seizure and spread to the entire brain, resulting in generalized seizure.

Generalized Seizures

These begin simultaneously in both cerebral hemispheres. Consciousness is impaired from seizure onset.

1. Typical absence seizures (formerly "petit mal"):
   - Characterized by sudden cessation of motor activity or speech.
   - Involve brief stares (usually a few seconds).
   - Onset typically at 5 to 8 years.
   - Can occur up to hundreds of times a day.
   - Include no aura or postictal state.
   - Can be elicited by hyperventilation.
   - Childhood absence epilepsy is associated with characteristic 3-Hz spike-and-wave pattern.
2. Generalized tonic–clonic (GTC, formerly "grand mal") seizures:
   - Common, may follow a focal seizure.
   - Patients suddenly lose consciousness, their eyes roll back, and their entire musculature undergoes tonic contractions, rarely arresting breathing.
   - Gradually, the hyperextension gives way to a series of rapid clonic jerks.
   - Finally, a period of flaccid relaxation occurs, during which sphincter control is often lost (incontinence).
   - Prodromal symptoms (not aura) often precede the attack by several hours and include mood change, apprehension, insomnia, or loss of appetite.

PEDIATRIC SEIZURE DISORDERS

Febrile Seizure

DEFINITION

- This is a common seizure of childhood.
- Approximately 2–5% of children are affected; peak incidence occurs at about 18 months.
- Defined as a seizure between the ages of 6 months and 5 years associated with temperature of 38°C (100.4°F) or greater and not otherwise explained.
- Risk of recurrence is high, especially if the first episode occurs before the age of 1 year.
- Highest recurrence rate if the episode occurs before 1 year of age (50%).
- Family history is often positive. Autosomal-dominant inheritance pattern is likely.

SIGNS AND SYMPTOMS

- Simple febrile seizure:
  - Generalized, usually tonic–clonic seizure.
  - Duration of 15 minutes or less and not recurrent in 24 hours.
  - No long-term sequelae, and most children will outgrow by age 6.

WARD TIP

The first step in evaluating any seizure disorder is determining the type of seizure.

EXAM TIP

Brief motor activity is the most common symptom of focal seizures without impairment of consciousness (previously called simple partial seizures).

EXAM TIP

The presence of an aura indicates a focal seizure onset. Physiologically, an aura is simply the earliest conscious manifestation of a seizure and corresponds with area of brain involved.

WARD TIP

Automatisms are a common symptom of focal seizures with impairment of consciousness (previously called complex partial seizures).

EXAM TIP

Typical Absence Seizures
- Shorter (seconds)
- Automatism absent
- More frequent (dozens or hundreds per day)
- Quick recovery from seizure
- Hyperventilation induced
- EEG: 3/sec spikes and waves

Focal seizures with impairment of consciousness (previously complex partial)
- Longer (minutes)
- Automatism common
- Less frequent seizures per day
- Gradual recovery post seizure
- Hyperventilation does not induce
- EEG: focal spikes

WARD TIP

Benign neonatal familial convulsions ("fifth-day fits") are a brief self-limited autosomal-dominant condition with generalized seizures beginning in the first week of life and subsiding within 6 weeks. The interictal EEG is normal. The prognosis is excellent; a 10–15% chance of future epilepsy is noted. The family history in neonatal seizures is critical.

EXAM TIP

Immature neonatal brain is more excitable than older children.

WARD TIP

If you are present during a tonic–clonic seizure:

- Keep track of the duration.
- Place the patient between prone and lateral decubitus to allow the tongue and secretions to fall forward.
- Loosen any tight clothing or jewelry around the neck.
- **Do not try to force open the mouth or teeth!**

WARD TIP

If the seizure is brief with fever and immediate complete recovery consistent with febrile seizure, then only good examination and clinically indicated laboratory evaluation to find the cause of fever are indicated. CT and EEG are not routinely indicated. LP is considered for children under one year of age.

- Complex febrile seizure:
  - Seizure longer than 15 minutes.
  - Focal seizure.
  - Recurrent within 24 hours.

DIAGNOSIS

- History and physical examination to identify cause of fever.
- Serum glucose.
- Serum electrolytes typically not needed.
- Lumbar puncture (LP) considered for children under 12 months of age or in complex febrile seizures.
- Neuroimaging reserved for complex febrile seizures or abnormal neurologic exam.

TREATMENT

- Diazepam for ongoing seizures that do not self-resolve.
- Rarely need ongoing anticonvulsant therapy.
- Rectal diazepam PRN for future febrile episodes.
- Antipyretics do not appear to prevent future febrile seizures.

PROGNOSIS

- Risk for development of epilepsy especially if:
  - Complex febrile seizures.
  - Family history of seizures.
  - Neurodevelopmental abnormalities.

Neonatal Seizure

- The most common neurologic manifestation of impaired brain function.
- Higher incidence in low-birth-weight infants.
- Metabolic, toxic, hypoxic, ischemic, and infectious diseases common during the neonatal period place the child at an increased risk for seizures.
- Myelination not complete at birth; GTC seizures uncommon.
- May manifest as spasms, tonic, myoclonic, clonic, or subtle (prolonged nonnutritive sucking, nystagmus, color change, autonomic instability).
- EEG may show burst suppression (alternating high and very low voltages), low-voltage invariance, diffuse or focal background slowing, and focal or multifocal spikes.
- Acute treatment typically with phenobarbital (drug of choice), fosphenytoin, or benzodiazepines.
- Phenytoin intravenous avoided due to myocardial depressive effect and variable metabolism; fosphenytoin preferred.

EPILEPSY

DEFINITION

- A history of at least one unprovoked seizure and either a second seizure or enough ancillary data (EEG or clinical findings) to demonstrate predisposing for recurrence. In clinical practice, the occurrence of two or more unprovoked seizures more than 24 hours apart defines epilepsy.

EPIDEMIOLOGY

Epilepsy occurs in 0.5–1% of the population, usually beginning in childhood.

TABLE 18-2. Characteristic EEG Patterns in Various Seizure Conditions

Seizure Condition	EEG	Drug of Choice
Simple febrile seizure Brief GTC with complete rapid recovery	Not required	Reassurance
Partial seizures with or without impaired consciousness (formerly known as complex and simple partial seizures) Brief (<2 minutes), focal, recurrent	High frequency discharges often in medial temporal lobe	Oxcarbazepine, levetiracetam
West syndrome Hypsarrhythmia, infantile spasms, developmental delay	Hypsarrhythmia	ACTH, vigabatrin
Benign myoclonus of early infancy Imitator of West syndrome but resolves in 3 months, rare after 2 yrs, normal development	Normal	—
Benign myoclonic epilepsy 6 months–3 yrs, brief myoclonic activity or neck and legs flexion with arms extension	Generalized polyspike and slow-wave	Valproate
Benign epilepsy with Centrotemporal Spikes (BECTS) See text	Central-temporal spikes	Carbamazepine, oxcarbazepine, valproic acid
Juvenile myoclonic epilepsy See text	3- to 6-Hz generalized polyspike/wave with photo-paroxysmal response	Valproate Lamotrigine
Childhood absence epilepsy See text	3-Hz spike and wave	Ethosuximide, valproate
Juvenile absence epilepsy See text	4- to 6-Hz spike and wave	Valproate
Lennox-Gastaut syndrome See text	1- to 2-Hz spike and wave in sleep; generalized slowing while awake	Valproate
Landau-Kleffner syndrome See text	Generalized spike and wave	Valproate for seizures; nocturnal diazepam for aphasia
Mesial temporal sclerosis See text	5–7 Hz, rhythmic, sharp theta delta activity	Drug resistance common; surgical remediation can be curative

Signs and Symptoms

- Depends on the seizure pattern, e.g., spasms, tonic, myoclonic, or clonic.
- Electrographically, seizures (ictal activity) are bursts of high-amplitude cortical activity that evolves in both frequency and space. (Table 18-2).
- An aura, a stereotyped symptom such as a buzzing sound or déjà vu that immediately precedes clinical seizure activity, represents the onset of a seizure. Its character can be useful for localizing seizure onset.
- A seizure prodrome, symptoms less stereotyped than an aura, precedes a seizure by hours to days. Symptoms include headache, mood changes, and nausea.

Treatment

- Therapy is directed at preventing the attacks (Table 18-3).

TABLE 18-3. Epilepsy Drugs and Their Use in Different Seizure Types

Drug (U.S. Brand Name)	Seizure Type	Side Effects
Carbamazepine (Tegretol, Carbatrol)	Focal-onset	Aplastic anemia
Ethosuximide (Zarontin)	Absence, some generalized	Drowsiness
Phenytoin (Dilantin)	Generalized or focal	Stevens-Johnson, gingival hyperplasia
Phenobarbital	Focal, generalized	Hyperactivity
Valproate (Depakote, Depacon)	Generalized, focal-onset	Hepatic failure, low platelets, pancreatitis
Topiramate (Topamax)	Partial, generalized	Renal stones, weight loss
Levetiracetam (Keppra)	Partial, generalized, Lennox-Gastaut	Behavior change
Lamotrigine (Lamictal)	Focal, generalized	Stevens-Johnson syndrome
Zonisamide (Zonegran)	Focal, generalized	Don't use if sulfa allergic
Felbamate (Felbatol)	Focal, generalized	Hepatic failure, aplastic anemia

EXAM TIP

Etiologies of neonatal seizure:
- Hypoxic-ischemic encephalopathy
- Intracranial hemorrhage/infarction
- CNS infection
- Metabolic and inborn errors of metabolism
- CNS malformation

EXAM TIP

Unprovoked seizure: unrelated to current acute CNS insult such as infection, increased intracranial pressure (ICP), trauma, toxin, etc.

COMMON EPILEPSY SYNDROMES

Localization-Related Epilepsy

- Seizures secondary to a focal CNS lesion are best candidates for epilepsy surgery.
- Examples include masses (particularly cortical tubers of tuberous sclerosis), cortical dysplasia, postencephalitic gliosis, and arteriovenous malformations.

Benign Epilepsy with Centrotemporal Spikes (BECTS)

A 5-year-old boy has facial twitching and drooling during a nap, followed by generalized body shaking lasting 1–2 minutes. In the ED, he is awake, and his neurological examination is normal. You order an EEG, which shows centrotemporal spikes. *Think: BECTS, formerly known as benign rolandic epilepsy.*

BECTS is a focal epilepsy of childhood. The usual age of presentation is 3–13 years. Typical presentation: seizure with facial involvement during sleep. EEG shows central temporal spikes. Seizures typically resolve spontaneously by early adulthood.

- Common focal epilepsy.
- Onset 3–13 years.
- Particularly nocturnal or early morning before awakening.
- EEG: centrotemporal spikes, especially during sleep or when drowsy.
- Imaging normal.
- Excellent prognosis; most resolve by age 16 years.
- Treatment: carbamazepine, oxcarbazepine, valproic acid.

West Syndrome

- Triad: infantile spasms, developmental regression, and hypsarrhythmia
  - Hypsarrhythmia pattern: large-amplitude chaotic multifocal spikes and slowing.

- Onset is at age 2–12 months.
- Clusters are brief, rapid symmetric flexor/extensor contractions of the neck, trunk, and extremities, up to 100 per day. Clusters can last up to several minutes.
- Symptomatic type is most commonly seen with CNS malformations, brain injury, tuberous sclerosis, or inborn errors of metabolism; they typically have a poor outcome.
- Cryptogenic type has a better prognosis; children typically have an uneventful birth history and reach developmental milestones before seizure onset.
- Treated with adrenocorticotropic hormone (ACTH) or vigabatrin.

Juvenile Myoclonic Epilepsy (JME)

- Onset: 12–16 years.
- Characteristic history: usually early morning on awakening; may be exacerbated by sleep deprivation or photoparoxysmal.
- Seizures: myoclonus, absence (one-fourth of cases), GTC.
- EEG: 3- to 6-Hz polyspike and wave pattern.
- Treatment: valproate, lamotrigine.
- Prognosis: responds well to medications, but generally lifelong.

Childhood Absence Epilepsy (CAE, Pyknolepsy)

- Begin 4 to 8 years of age.
- Up to hundreds of brief absence seizures per day.
- Spontaneous resolution typical, although high lifetime risk of generalized seizures.

Juvenile Absence Epilepsy

- Absence seizures begin in adolescence.
- Seizure frequency is once or twice per week lasting about 20 seconds (longer than CAE).
- Increased incidence of GTC seizures.

Lennox-Gastaut Syndrome (LGS)

- Begin between 2 and 10 years of age.
- Triad of developmental delay, seizures, typical EEG findings
  - Multiple seizure types (tonic, atonic, absence, and myoclonic seizures).
  - EEG: 1- to 2-Hz spike-and-wave pattern in sleep; slow background when awake.
- Cognitive impairment.
- LGS may evolve from West syndrome.
- Seizures are frequent and resistant to treatment.

Landau-Kleffner Syndrome (LKS; Acquired Epileptic Aphasia)

- Language regression in previously normal child.
- Aphasia (primarily receptive or expressive).
- Seizures can be focal or GTC, atypical absence, myoclonic.
- EEG: bitemporal, high-amplitude spike-and-wave discharges, more apparent during non-rapid eye movement sleep.
- Sometimes confused with autism.

Progressive Myoclonic Epilepsies

- This group of diseases includes Unverricht-Lundborg disease, myoclonic epilepsy with ragged-red fibers (MERRF), Lafora disease, neuronal ceroid lipofuscinosis, and sialidosis/mucolipidosis, and Ramsay Hunt syndrome.
- These begin in late childhood to adolescence and entail progressive neurologic deterioration with myoclonic seizures, dementia, and ataxia. Death within 10 years of onset is common, but survival to old age occurs.

WARD TIP

Epilepsy History
- Age, sex, handedness
- Seizure semiology (what the seizures look like, details about right/left); if more than one type, the pattern of progression (if any)
- Seizure duration/history of status epilepticus
- Postictal lethargy or focal neurologic deficits
- Current frequency/tendency to cluster
- Age at onset
- Date of last seizure
- Longest seizure-free interval
- Known precipitants (don't forget to ask if the seizures typically arise out of sleep)
- History of head trauma, difficult birth, intrauterine infection, hypoxic/ischemic insults, meningoencephalitis, or other CNS disease
- Developmental history (delay strongly correlated with poorer prognosis)
- Family history of epilepsy, febrile seizures
- Psychiatric history
- Current AEDs
- AED history (maximum doses, efficacy, reason for stopping)
- Previous EEG, MRI findings

WARD TIP

Loss of language skills in a previously normal child with seizure disorder. *Think: LKS.*

WARD TIP

Evaluate patients following their first seizure (for mass, lesion, etc.) prior to diagnosing and treating epilepsy.

Mesial Temporal Sclerosis

- Gliotic scarring and atrophy of the hippocampal formation occurs, creating a temporal lobe seizure focus. Abnormality is often apparent on high-resolution magnetic resonance imaging (MRI).
- Rhythmic, 5–7 Hz, sharp theta delta activity.
- Phenytoin, phenobarbital, carbamazepine, and valproate are equally effective. Curative resection is often possible if refractory to treatment.

Status Epilepticus (SE)

DEFINITION

Any seizure or recurrent seizures without return to baseline lasting >5 minutes.

ETIOLOGY

- Myriad causes (i.e., metabolic, toxic, infectious, tumor).
- Febrile seizures are a common cause of SE.

PATHOPHYSIOLOGY

Prolonged excitability and reduction of inhibitory neural tissue that can result in neuronal cell death

TREATMENT

- Initial treatment includes assessment of the respiratory and cardiovascular systems (ABCs).
- Management in the ICU with continuous EEG monitoring; anticipate intubation.

MANAGEMENT

- **Stabilization phase** (0–5 minutes of seizure activity): ABCs; give O_2; obtain IV access, monitor vital signs, obtain bedside glucose; obtain additional labs and cultures as indicated.
- **Initial therapy phase** (5–20 minutes of seizure activity): administer IV diazepam, lorazepam, or midazolam. Consider IM midazolam, lorazepam, or diazepam *or* intranasal/buccal midazolam if no IV access.
- **Second therapy phase** (20–40 minutes of seizure activity): consider fosphenytoin, valproic acid, and levetiracetam. IV phenobarbital is an option, but it can worsen respiratory depression.
- **Third therapy phase** (40+ minutes of seizure activity): treatment with repeating second-line therapy or anesthetic doses of thiopental, midazolam, pentobarbital, or propofol.

Rett Syndrome

> A 4-year-old girl with prior history of severe intellectual disability is brought in for evaluation. She had been developing **normally until 18 months of age**, when she began regressing intellectually and her head circumference plateaued. She **wrings her hands, has ataxia, and marked loss of gross motor skills**. *Think: Rett syndrome.*

Rett syndrome is a genetic disorder in which developmental arrest typically occurs between 6 and 18 months of age. Parents may report gross motor

EXAM TIP

In children under age 3, complex febrile seizures are the most likely etiology of status epilepticus.

EXAM TIP

Neonatal status epilepticus that is refractory to the usual measures may respond to pyridoxine. This is seen in pyridoxine dependency (due to diminished glutamate decarboxylase activity, a rare autosomal-recessive condition) or pyridoxine deficiency in children born to mothers on isoniazid.

development delay, disinterest in play, and loss of eye contact. Hand wringing is a hallmark sign. Rett should be considered in a previously healthy child with normal development who develops head growth deceleration.

DEFINITION

A neurodegenerative disorder of early brain growth

EPIDEMIOLOGY

- X-linked recessive with *MECP2* gene mutation occurring almost exclusively in females.
- Prevalence: 1 in 15,000 to 1 in 22,000.

ETIOLOGY

- Most cases result from defect in *MECP2*. Gene testing is available.

SIGNS AND SYMPTOMS

- Normal development until about 12 months.
- The first signs are deceleration of head growth, lack of interest in environment, and hypotonia, followed by a regression of language and motor milestones, including loss of ambulation.
- Ataxia, handwringing by about 6 to 30 months, reduced brain weight, generalized tonic–clinic seizures and episodes of hyperventilation are typical.
- Autistic behavior.

PROGNOSIS

- After the initial period of regression, the disease appears to plateau.
- Death can occur due to cardiac arrhythmias.

EXAM TIP

The hallmark of Rett syndrome is repetitive handwringing and loss of purposeful and spontaneous hand movements.

EXAM TIP

Generally, autistic disorders are more common in boys, except Rett syndrome (more common in girls).

Spinal Muscular Atrophy (SMA)

DEFINITION

An inherited disorder of spinal cord motor neurons that leads to progressive muscle weakness
- Three major phenotypic types in pediatrics:
  - Type 1 (Werdnig-Hoffman) present before 6 months with failing to sit or walk.
  - Type 2 present between 6 and 18 months after failing to walk but achieve sitting.
  - Type 3 present after 18 months of age for those who achieve walking.

ETIOLOGY

- Caused by homozygous deletion in exon 7 of SMN1 gene on chromosome 5q13.

CLINICAL MANIFESTATIONS

- Absence of deep tendon reflexes.
- Peripheral hypotonia for types 1 and 2.
- Bulbar findings for type 1 (loss of gag, sucking and swallowing challenges, weak cry).

DIAGNOSIS

- Thorough history and physical examination suggesting the diagnosis.
- EMG, especially for type 1, where rapid diagnosis may affect interventions.
- Genetic testing, although results may be delayed.

TREATMENT

- Gene therapy: infusion of a working copy of SMN1 gene has resulted in improved outcome, especially in type 1 disease previously universally fatal. Gene therapy in other SMA types is under investigation.
- Supportive care including neurology, orthopedics, and physical therapy.

Neuro-Cutaneous Syndromes

STURGE-WEBER SYNDROME

Dermato-oculo-neural syndrome

EPIDEMIOLOGY

Occurs sporadically in 1 in 50,000

ETIOLOGY

- Abnormal meningeal vasculature development, causing cortical atrophy and calcification.
- Facial capillary hemangioma involving at least trigeminal V1 distribution.

SIGNS AND SYMPTOMS

- A port-wine nevus involves at least trigeminal V1 distribution present at birth (see Figure 18-1).
- Ipsilateral glaucoma may result.
- Ipsilateral brain-surface angiomas cause seizures and intellectual disability.
- CT may reveal intracranial calcifications; a contrast-enhanced MRI may identify leptomeningeal angiomata.
- Seizures are usually refractory, and hemispherectomy improves the prognosis.
- Meningeal involvement without a port-wine stain is unusual, but most children with a port-wine nevus do not have an intracranial angioma.

WARD TIP

If you see "port-wine stain," *think* Sturge-Weber syndrome.

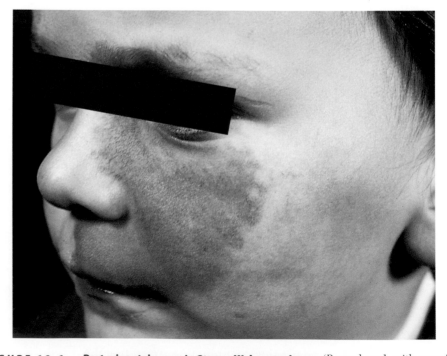

FIGURE 18-1. **Port-wine stain seen in Sturge-Weber syndrome.** (Reproduced, with permission, from Wolff K, Johnson RA, Suurmond D. *Fitzpatrick's Color Atlas & Synopsis of Clinical Dermatology,* 5th ed. New York: McGraw-Hill, 2005:187.)

VON HIPPEL–LINDAU DISEASE

DEFINITION

A neurocutaneous syndrome affecting the cerebellum, spinal cord, medulla, retina, kidneys, pancreas, and epididymis

SIGNS AND SYMPTOMS

The major neurologic findings of this autosomal dominate mutation are:

- Cerebellar/spinal hemangioblastomas, which present in early adult life with increased ICP.
- Retinal angiomata, or small masses of thin-walled capillaries in the peripheral retina.
- Cystic lesions of the pancreas, liver, and kidneys.
- Pheochromocytoma are common.
- Early detection is possible with CT or MRI.
- Photocoagulation for retinal detachment; surgical resection of lesions.

> **EXAM TIP**
>
> Renal carcinoma is the most common cause of death associated with von Hippel–Lindau disease.

NEUROFIBROMATOSIS (NF) (FIGURE 18-2)

EPIDEMIOLOGY

Two different conditions; both display autosomal-recessive inheritance patterns

- Type 1 is common, with an incidence of 1 in 3000 (chromosome 17).
- Type 2 is relatively rare, with an incidence of 1 in 25,000 (chromosome 22).

> **EXAM TIP**
>
> About 50% of NF-1 results from new mutations. Parents should be carefully screened before counseling on the risk to future children.

CLINICAL MANIFESTATIONS

Type 1

- Diagnosis is made by the presence of two or more of the following:
  - Six or more café-au-lait macules (>5 mm prepuberty, >15 mm post puberty), which are almost always present in the first year of life.
  - Axillary or inguinal freckling, typically appearing at 3 to 5 years of age.
  - Two or more iris Lisch nodules, often presenting by 3 to 4 years of age.
  - Two or more cutaneous neurofibromas, usually presenting in adolescence. Can be discrete, or diffuse and disfiguring.

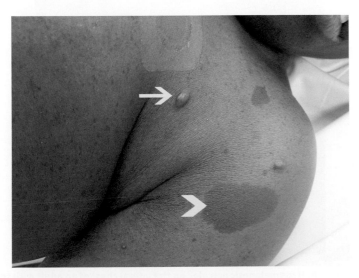

FIGURE 18-2. **This patient has type 1 neurofibromatosis.** Note the cutaneous neurofibromas (arrow) and café-au-lait spots (arrowhead). (Reproduced, with permission, from Kemp WL, Burns DK, Brown TG. *Pathology: The Big Picture.* New York, McGraw Hill, 2008.)

- ■ A characteristic osseous lesion (sphenoid dysplasia, long-bone cortex thinning).
  - ■ Optic glioma.
  - ■ A first-degree relative with confirmed NF-1.
- ■ Learning disabilities, abnormal speech development, and seizures are common.
- ■ CNS lesions such as meningiomas and astrocytomas occur, but they are not as commonly as in NF-2.
- ■ The risk of malignant transformation is about 3%.

Type 2

- ■ Diagnosis is made when one of the following is present:
  - ■ Bilateral CN VIII (vestibular) schwannomas.
  - ■ A parent or sibling with NF-2 or a combination of neurofibroma, meningioma, glioma, or vestibular schwannoma.
- ■ Presenting symptoms include hearing loss, tinnitus, imbalance, and facial weakness.
- ■ Café-au-lait spots and skin neurofibromas are not common findings.
- ■ NF-2 patients are at much higher risk for CNS tumors, often having multiple tumors.

TREATMENT

Treatment is aimed at preventing future complications and early detection of malignancies. Resection of the schwannomas can be performed to preserve hearing.

TUBEROUS SCLEROSIS

EPIDEMIOLOGY

- ■ Inherited as an autosomal-dominant trait, with a frequency of about 1:6,000.
- ■ Two-thirds are new mutations.

FIGURE 18-3. **A. Hypomelanotic macules on the lateral chest of an adult with tuberous sclerosis complex. The macules may be easily overlooked. B. Wood lamp accentuates the macules.** (Reproduced, with permission, from Kang S, Amagai M, Bruckner AL, et al (eds). *Fitzpatrick's Dermatology*, 9th ed. New York, McGraw Hill, 2019.)

PATHOLOGY

- Characteristic brain lesions consist of tubers, located in the convolutions of the cerebrum; they undergo calcification and project into the ventricles.
- There are two recognized genes: TSC1 on chromosome 9, encoding a protein called hamartin, and TSC2 on chromosome 16, encoding a protein called tuberin.
- Tubers may grow into astrocytomas, leading to obstructive hydrocephalus.

CLINICAL MANIFESTATIONS

- Highly variable presentation, even within a family, is common.
- Hypopigmented macules ("Ash leaf" spots) are seen in 90% and are best viewed under a Wood's lamp (violet/ultraviolet light source). (See Figure 18-3).
- Brain imaging shows periventricular calcified hamartomas (tubers).
- Seizures are common. Seizures often present as infantile spasms before age 1, are difficult to control, and are correlated with autism and developmental and learning disabilities.
- Facial angiofibroma (small, raised papules resembling acne on the face in a butterfly pattern) develop between 4 and 6 years of age and are small hamartomas.
- A Shagreen patch (rough, raised, leathery lesion with an orange-peel consistency in the lumbar region), typically does not develop until adolescence.
- Fifty percent of children have heart rhabdomyomas, often diagnosed on prenatal ultrasound, which can cause CHF or arrhythmias but more often regress after birth.
- Ungual or periungual fibroma often develop during adolescence.
- Hamartomas of the kidneys and the lungs are frequently present.

DIAGNOSIS

- A high index of suspicion is required. All children presenting with infantile spasms or cardiac rhabdomyomas should be assessed for skin and retinal lesions.
- Brain CT or MRI will confirm the diagnosis.
- Genetic testing is available.

> **EXAM TIP**
>
> Tuberous sclerosis is the most common cause of infantile spasms, an ominous seizure pattern in infants.

> **EXAM TIP**
>
> **Hamartoma:** a tumor-like overgrowth of tissue normally found in the area surrounding it.

Sleep Disorders

- As a group, these disorders are:
  - Paroxysmal.
  - Predictable in their appearance in the sleep cycle.
  - Nonresponsive to environmental manipulation.
  - Often characterized by retrograde amnesia.
  - Diagnosed by a thorough history; an extensive workup is rarely needed.

NIGHT TERRORS (PAVOR NOCTURNUS)

DEFINITION

- Sudden-onset episodes of terror in which the child cannot be consoled and is unaware of the surroundings, usually lasting several minutes.
- Total amnesia follows the episodes.
- Often prolonged with attempts to awaken the child.
- Sometimes confused with nightmares (Table 18-4).

TABLE 18-4. **Characteristics of Nightmares Versus Night Terrors**

NIGHT TERRORS	NIGHTMARES
■ NREM sleep	■ REM sleep
■ No memory of the event; goes back to sleep	■ Remembers dream and afraid to sleep
■ 2 hours after falling sleep (first third of sleep)	■ Close to morning (last third of sleep)
■ Disappears by age 6	■ Peak 3–6 years; less frequent in adolescent
■ Sleepwalking common	■ No sleepwalking

EXAM TIP

Night terrors, sleepwalking, and nightmares are associated with disturbed sleep, but have no known associated neurologic disorder.

EPIDEMIOLOGY

They occur in 1–6% of the population between ages 2 and 7, and more commonly in boys.

PATHOPHYSIOLOGY

- Sleepwalking is common in the group.
- They occur in stage 3 or 4 (deep) sleep (first third of night sleep).

DIAGNOSIS

- Classic history confirms the diagnosis; further evaluation is usually unnecessary.
- Polysomnography (PSG) is required only in unusual circumstances.

TREATMENT

Reassurance in most cases; usually self-limited and resolves by age 10.

SOMNAMBULANCE (SLEEPWALKING)

- Occurs during deep, non-REM sleep.
- Typically occurs during first third of the night.
- Onset: 10–13 years.
- Awakened only with difficulty and may be confused when awakened.
- Often associated with night terrors.

WARD TIP

Sleep deprivation causes attention deficit, hyperactivity, and behavior disturbances in children—often mistaken for attention deficit/hyperactivity disorder (ADHD).

TREATMENT

Reassurance in most cases; usually resolves by late adolescence.

INSOMNIA

- Affects 10–20% of adolescents.
- Depression is a common cause and should be ruled out.

OBSTRUCTIVE SLEEP APNEA (OSA)

WARD TIP

Obstructive sleep apnea due to adenotonsillar hyperplasia is an indication for tonsillectomy and adenoidectomy.

EPIDEMIOLOGY

- Occurs in about 2–5 % of children, most often between ages 2 and 8.

PATHOPHYSIOLOGY

- Characterized by chronic partial-airway obstruction with intermittent episodes of complete obstruction during sleep, resulting in disturbed sleep.
- Essentially all have snoring, but some pediatric patients snore without OSA.

SIGNS AND SYMPTOMS

- Fatigue/hyperactivity, headache, daytime somnolence, enuresis.
- Narrow airway, tonsillar hypertrophy, obesity.

DIAGNOSIS

- History and physical examination.
- PSG.

TREATMENT

- Variable depending on the cause.
- Possibilities include weight loss, adenotonsillectomy, CPAP, intranasal steroids.

> **EXAM TIP**
>
> Since obstructive sleep apnea causes hypoxia, it may be associated with polycythemia vera, growth failure, and serious cardiorespiratory pathophysiology.

Encephalopathies

MENINGITIS/MENINGOENCEPHALITIS

DEFINITION

- Meningitis: diffuse inflammation involving mostly the meninges.
- Meningoencephalitis: symptoms of both meningitis and encephalitis.
- Viral etiologies are most common, followed by bacteria, fungus, and parasites.

SIGNS AND SYMPTOMS

All are less prominent in immunocompromised patients.
- Fever, headache, and nuchal rigidity.
- Photophobia or myalgia may be present.
- Meningismus (Brudziński and Kernig signs); note these signs are not reliable in children under 1 year of age (see Figures 18-4 and 18-5).
- Altered consciousness, petechial rash, seizures, cranial nerve, or other abnormal neurological findings.

DIAGNOSIS

Due to overlap in findings, CSF analysis is not always predictive of viral or bacterial infection, especially at the onset of the disease (Table 18-5).

> **EXAM TIP**
>
> Take some time to familiarize yourself with Tables 18-6 and 18-7: *You will be asked this!*

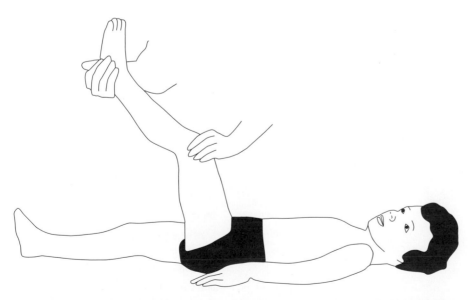

FIGURE 18-4. **Kernig sign.** Flex patient's leg at both hip and knee, and then straighten knee. Pain on extension is a positive sign.

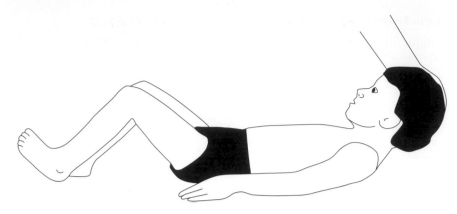

FIGURE 18-5. **Brudzinski sign.** Involuntary flexion of the hips and knees with passive flexion of the neck while supine.

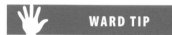

Acute Bacterial Meningitis

- See Table 18-6 for common meningitis-causing bacteria.
- Associated with high rate of complications, chronic morbidity, and death.
- Pathogenesis: 95% bloodborne. Organism enters the CSF, multiplies, and stimulates an inflammatory response. Direct toxin from organism, hypotension, or vasculitis causes a thrombotic event; vasogenic/cytotoxic edema causes increased ICP and decreased blood flow, all of which may contribute to further damage.

Viral Meningoencephalitis

- Enterovirus (85%): echovirus, coxsackievirus, and nonparalytic poliovirus.
- The clinical presentation is similar to bacterial infection but symptoms are usually less severe.
- Children show typical viral-type signs (fever, malaise, myalgia, nausea, and rash), as well as meningeal signs.

TABLE 18-5. **Cerebrospinal Fluid (CSF) Findings in Meningitis**

	NORMAL LEVELS	BACTERIAL	VIRAL	FUNGAL	TB
Appearance		Turbid	Clear	Clear	Fibrinous
Cells	Mononuclear	Polymorphs	Mononuclear	Mononuclear	Mononuclear
Leukocytes (mm³)	< 5	100–1000	50–1000	> 100	100–500
Protein (mg/dL)	20–45	100–500	50–200	25–500	1–5 g/dL
Glucose (mg/dL)	> 50 or 75% serum glucose	↓ < 40 or 66% serum	Generally normal	< 50; continues to decline if untreated	Less than half of the serum
Lab cultures		▪ Gram stain of CSF	▪ Hard to detect ▪ PCR of CSF may show HSV or enteroviruses	▪ Budding yeast may be seen ▪ Cryptococcal antigen may be positive in serum and CSF	Ziehl Neelsen AFB stain PCR

CSF, cerebrospinal fluid; PCR, polymerase chain reaction; HSV, herpes simplex virus.

TABLE 18-6. **Common Causes of Pediatric Bacterial Meningitis**

AGE	BACTERIA	INITIAL TREATMENT
Neonates (< 1 month)	Group B streptococcus Gram-negative enteric bacilli *Listeria monocytogenes* *Escherichia coli*	Ampicillin, and either a third-generation cephalosporin or gentamycin
Infants and children*	*Streptococcus pneumoniae* *Neisseria meningitidis*	Third-generation cephalosporin and vancomycin until susceptibility is known, especially for *S. pneumonia*

*Haemophilus influenzae type B, a leading cause in the past, is now rare in immunocompetent patients owing to widespread vaccine use.

- Children may not be toxic appearing.
- Rarer causes are herpes simplex virus type 1 (HSV-1), Epstein-Barr virus, mumps, influenza, arboviruses, and adenoviruses.

Fungal Meningitis

- Although relatively uncommon, the classic organism is *Cryptococcus*.
- Encountered primarily in the immunocompromised patient (transplants, AIDS, chemotherapy).
- May be rapidly fatal (as quickly as 2 weeks) or evolve over months to years.

TREATMENT

- For suspected neonatal bacterial meningitis:
  - Third-generation cephalosporin (cefotaxime) plus ampicillin for *Listeria*.
  - Alternative treatment: ampicillin plus gentamicin.
- For suspected meningitis outside the newborn period:
  - Third-generation cephalosporin (cefotaxime, ceftriaxone) plus vancomycin (for suspected pneumococci; increased resistance to cephalosporins).
- For the common, enterovirus etiologies, typically supportive care only.
- Consider adding acyclovir for herpes simplex virus infections.
  - HSV-1: most cases occur after the neonatal period.
  - HSV-2: usually bloodborne and results in diffuse meningoencephalitis and other organ involvement. The congenitally acquired form is transmitted to 50% of babies born to a mother with active **primary** vaginal lesions but about 2% for **recurrent** infection.
  - A lack of maternal history does not rule out the potential for HSV infection in a newborn.
- Steroid use is controversial.

Miscellaneous Meningoencephalitides

ETIOLOGY

- *Mycobacterium tuberculosis (common)*, *M. bovis*, and *M. avium-intracellulare*.
  - Nonspecific features develop over days to weeks. Initial complaints include generalized headache, malaise, and weight loss.
  - Later symptoms include confusion, focal neurological signs, cranial nerve palsies, and seizures. In advanced cases, hemiparesis, hemiplegia, or coma are seen.
  - Serious complications include arachnoid fibrosis causing hydrocephalus, arterial occlusion, and infarcts.
  - *M. avium-intracellulare* is common in AIDS patients.
  - Antibiotic regimens are tailored to disease stage and culture results.

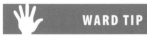

Nuchal rigidity. *Think:* Meningitis.

Undiagnosed congenital syphilis may manifest around age 2 with Hutchinson's triad:

- Interstitial keratitis
- Peg-shaped incisors
- Deafness (cranial nerve VIII)

- Neurosyphilis (tabes dorsalis)
  - Causative organism is *Treponema pallidum*.
  - May present with viral meningoencephalitis pattern.
  - Tertiary syphilis manifests with neurologic, cardiovascular, and granulomatous lesions.
  - Congenital syphilis presents with a maculopapular rash, lymphadenopathy, and mucopurulent rhinitis.
  - Prenatal syphilis screening is mandatory in most states.
- Herpes zoster virus:
  - Can occur after primary or reactivation infection.
  - Usually occurs with a rash, but the outcome is poor in those without a rash.
  - In immunocompetent hosts, 2–6 months after a primary infection, the dormant ganglia virus becomes activated and can cause large-vessel vasculitis and infarcts.
  - In immunocompromised hosts, the dormant virus causes small-vessel vasculitis and gray and white matter hemorrhagic infarcts.
  - EEG will show diffuse slowing and periodic lateralizing epileptiform discharges (PLEDs).
- Rabies:
  - Causes severe encephalitis, coma, and death due to respiratory failure.
  - Transmitted via bite or saliva from an infected animal, commonly dogs, bats, skunks, raccoons, or squirrels.
  - Virus travels from the peripheral nerves from the bite site and enters the brain.
  - Presents with nonspecific symptoms (fever, malaise) and **bite-site paresthesia**. **Hydrophobia**, aerophobia, agitation, **hypersalivation,** and seizures follow. Coma and death are likely.
  - Prophylaxis (rabies immunoglobulin and vaccine) is indicated for potential exposure.

ANTI-NMDA RECEPTOR (AUTOIMMUNE) ENCEPHALITIS

BACKGROUND

- An acute encephalitis, potentially lethal, but high recovery rate with treatment.
- Antibodies against NR1-NR2 NMDA receptors (N-methyl-D-aspartate receptor).
- May be associated with ovarian teratomas in patients older than 12 years.

SIGNS AND SYMPTOMS

- Prodrome of fever, headache, viral-like symptoms possible.
- Abrupt onset of change in consciousness or behavior changes including psychosis with agitation, paranoia, psychosis, violent or bizarre behaviors, and hallucinations.
- Symptoms progress to altered level of consciousness, hypoventilation, seizures, autonomic instability, and dyskinesias.

DIAGNOSIS

- Serum or CSF NMDA-receptor antibodies.
- Pelvic ultrasound to rule out tumor.

TREATMENT

- Early removal of tumor if present.
- IV corticosteroids, IVIG, and plasma-exchange therapy in severe cases.

PROGNOSIS

- The recovery process can take many months or years.
- ~80% will have substantial or full recovery; <10% mortality.

MITOCHONDRIAL ENCEPHALOPATHY

BACKGROUND

A group of disorders caused by mutations in either nuclear or mitochondrial DNA, resulting in a variety of symptoms

Mitochondrial encephalopathy, lactic acidosis, and strokelike episodes (MELAS)

PATHOPHYSIOLOGY/ETIOLOGY

- The most common of mitochondrial encephalopathies.
- Onset between ages 2 and 10 years.

SIGNS AND SYMPTOMS

- Initial development normal, then deterioration.
- Short stature.
- Focal or generalized seizure, recurrent headache, vomiting, cortical blindness, hemianopia.
- Initially neurologic signs are intermittent but progressive, leading to coma and death.

DIAGNOSIS

- MRI shows multiple strokes, not in vascular distribution.
- Lactic acidosis and/or muscle biopsy with ragged-red fibers occurs.

TREATMENT

Steroids, coenzyme Q10, nicotinamide, carnitine

PROGNOSIS

Poor, especially for the full syndrome.

Myoclonic epilepsy with ragged-red fibers (MERRF)

SIGNS AND SYMPTOMS

- Onset may be in childhood or adult life.
- Features include: myoclonus, myoclonic epilepsy, and intermittent muscle weakness.
- Cerebella ataxia (can be confused with Friedreich ataxia), dysarthria, and nystagmus early findings.

DIAGNOSIS

- Lactic acidosis.
- Muscle biopsy with ragged-red fibers.
- Genetic testing.

TREATMENT

- Coenzyme Q10.
- Levetiracetam for seizures.

PROGNOSIS

Slowly progressive condition with poor overall outcome

Reye syndrome

SIGNS AND SYMPTOMS

- Now rare syndrome associated with varicella-zoster or influenza infection and aspirin ingestion.
- Vomiting (early sign of encephalopathy), change in mental status, coma.

DIAGNOSIS

- Hypoglycemia, hyperammonemia, and elevated LFTs without jaundice.
- Liver biopsy with microvesicular steatosis.
- With thorough investigation, most cases of Reye syndrome are due to an identifiable inborn error of metabolism, medium chain acyl Co A dehydrogenase deficiency, urea cycle disorder, or pyruvate metabolism disorder.

TREATMENT

- Supportive care with attention to maintaining glucose control.
- Mannitol and hyperventilation to reduce intracranial pressure.

PROGNOSIS

- Up to 30% mortality previously described.

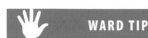

WARD TIP

In general, salicylates should be avoided in children to prevent Reye syndrome.

HEPATIC ENCEPHALOPATHY

SIGNS AND SYMPTOMS

- Acute or chronic symptoms of malaise, lethargy, jaundice, dark urine, and abnormal liver function tests (LFTs).
- Sleep disturbance, change in affect, drowsiness, asterixis (flapping tremor).
- Decerebrate posturing may occur in the terminal stages.

DIAGNOSIS

- Direct and indirect hyperbilirubinemia.
- Elevated LFTs early, possibly returning to normal as liver deteriorates.
- Prolonged PT and INR.

TREATMENT

- Manage cerebral, renal, and cardiovascular function while awaiting liver regeneration or transplant:
    - Control ammonia level (decrease dietary protein, stop gastrointestinal bleed, treat constipation).
    - Avoid cerebral edema (fluid restriction, use of hyperosmolar agents [mannitol]).
- Treat coagulopathy with vitamin K and fresh-frozen plasma.

PROGNOSIS

- Patients who recover or have transplant typically do well.

HIV/AIDS ENCEPHALOPATHY

SIGNS AND SYMPTOMS

- All pregnant mothers should be tested for HIV infection and treated to decrease transmission.
    - Appropriately treated newborns born to treated HIV+ mothers are rarely infected.
- CNS involvement is high in perinatally infected children.

- Many infected infants are symptomatic by 18 months of age.
    - Progressive encephalopathy and hepatosplenomegaly.
    - Failure to meet developmental milestones.
    - Impaired brain growth and symmetrical motor dysfunction.
- Opportunistic infections such as toxoplasmosis typically occur later in adolescence.

DIAGNOSIS

- HIV IgG antibody for patients >18 months PLUS a confirmatory HIV DNA PCR.

TREATMENT

Highly active antiretroviral therapy (HAART)

PROGNOSIS

Good with early diagnosis and treatment compliance

LEAD ENCEPHALOPATHY

SIGNS AND SYMPTOMS

- Acute: vomiting, abdominal pain, seizures, impaired consciousness, respiratory arrest.
- Chronic: gradual confusion, behavior changes, sleep problems, seizures, ataxia. Peripheral neuropathy is common in adults but rare in children.

DIAGNOSIS

- History of pica.
- Microcytic hypochromic anemia and basophilic stippling often described.
- Blood-lead level testing definitive.
    - Blood lead level >5 μg/dL is considered abnormal.

TREATMENT

- Remove the lead source.
- Chelation therapy when blood lead level >45 μg/dL.

PROGNOSIS

- Decreased IQ and neurobehavioral abnormalities, especially for higher lead levels.

EXAM TIP

Old lead paint is the number one cause of lead toxicity.

Transverse Myelitis

DEFINITION

- An acute condition of spinal cord inflammation, likely of viral origin. The most common affected region is the thoracic spinal cord.

SIGNS AND SYMPTOMS

- Nonspecific fever, lethargy, malaise, muscle pains 1 to 3 weeks prior.
- Begins acutely and progresses within 1–2 days.
- Back or neck pain occurs at the level of the involved cord.
- Numbness, anesthesia, ataxia, areflexia, and weakness are distal to the lesion.
- Urinary retention is common.

EXAM TIP

Numerous viruses (HSV, varicella, CMV, EBV), as well as the rabies vaccination and smallpox vaccination, have been implicated without good evidence to transverse myelitis.

DIAGNOSIS

- MRI: enhanced T2 signals.
- CSF: elevated monocyte level.

TREATMENT

IV steroids are the mainstay; trial of intravenous immunoglobulins or plasma exchange may be considered.

PROGNOSIS

Recovery is slow, and about 40% have permanent disability.

Acute Disseminated Encephalomyelitis (ADEM)

DEFINITION

- An immune-mediated demyelinating encephalopathy manifest by widespread inflammation of the brain, spinal cord, and nerves, with white matter destruction.

PATHOPHYSIOLOGY/ETIOLOGY

- Commonly has a history of an antecedent viral infection.
- More common in 5- to 8-year-old population.
- Some features resemble multiple sclerosis.

SIGNS AND SYMPTOMS

- Initial symptoms include fever, headache, lethargy, meningeal signs, and seizures.
- Encephalopathy invariable is present.
- Focal neurologic signs are seen, but are often difficult to identify owing to encephalopathy.

DIAGNOSIS

MRI: ADEM lesions are characteristically multiple, bilateral but asymmetric, and widespread within the CNS.

TREATMENT

First-line high-dose IV steroids, also intravenous immune globulin (IVIG)

PROGNOSIS

Most children recover completely or with mild sequelae.

WARD TIP

ADEM is associated with bilateral optic neuritis and MS is usually unilateral.

Multiple Sclerosis

DEFINITION

- Chronic and relapsing demyelinating disorder of brain, spinal cord, and optic nerves.
- Typically presents in pediatrics after age 10 years.
- Female predominance.

ETIOLOGY

- Demyelination and axonal loss of unknown etiology.
- Helper CD4+ and CD8+ T cells play a central role in pathogenesis.

CLINICAL MANIFESTATIONS

- Acute or subacute neurologic symptoms, depending on CNS site affected.
- Common pediatric findings include hemiparesis or paraparesis, focal sensory loss, ataxia, optic neuritis.
- Encephalopathy less common and suggests ADEM.

DIAGNOSIS

- MRI demonstrates T2 lesions in cerebral white matter, brainstem, cerebellum, and spinal cord.
- CSF findings include increased IgG and/or oligoclonal bands.
- Visual, auditory, and somatosensory evoked potentials may be abnormal.

TREATMENT

- Steroids for acute attack.
- While not approved in children, disease-modulating agents, including interferon α and glatiramer acetate, are often employed. Newer agents are under investigation.

Tetanus

 A 1-week-old child born to an immunocompromised mother presents with difficulty feeding, trismus, and other rigid muscles. *Think: Tetanus.*
Tetanus is a toxin-mediated disease characterized by severe skeletal muscle spasms. Initial symptoms can be nonspecific. Inability to suck and difficulty in swallowing are important clinical features, followed by stiffness and seizures. It can be prevented by immunizing mothers before or during pregnancy.

DEFINITION

- An acute illness of painful muscle spasms and hypertonia caused by the neurotoxin produced by *Clostridium tetani*.
- The symptoms usually start in the jaw/facial muscles and progress to other muscles.

PATHOPHYSIOLOGY/ETIOLOGY

- Incubation period 5 to 14 days after infection.
- In infants, a history of animal excreta applied to the umbilical stump for hemostasis.

SIGNS AND SYMPTOMS

- Trismus (masseter muscle spasm) and Risus sardonicus (a grin caused by facial spasm) are classically described.
- Pharyngeal spasm may cause dysphagia; laryngospasm may result in asphyxia.
- Trunk and thigh involvement results in an arched posture in which only the head and heels touch the bed.
- Sudden, severe tonic contractions of the muscles occur with fist clenching, flexion, and adduction of the upper limb and extension of the lower limb.
- Autonomic dysfunction includes sweating, and fever can occur.

DIAGNOSIS

- Diagnosis is clinical: trismus, dysphagia, rigidity, and muscle spasms.
- Laboratory studies are usually normal; leukocytosis may be present.
- CSF is normal.

 WARD TIP

Tetanic contractions can be triggered by minor stimuli, such as a flashing light. Patients should be sedated, intubated, and, for severe cases, put in a dark room.

TREATMENT

- Maintain airway.
- Rapid administration of human tetanus immune globulin.
- IV penicillin G is the drug of choice.
- Surgical excision and debridement of the wound.
- Muscle relaxants, such as diazepam to promote relaxation and seizure control; neuromuscular blocking agents like vecuronium also used.

PROGNOSIS

- Mortality rate: 5–35%

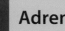

EXAM TIP

Tetanus is an entirely preventable disease via immunization.

Adrenoleukodystrophy

PATHOPHYSIOLOGY/ETIOLOGY

- X-linked recessive peroxisomal disorder causing defect in the ability to catabolize very long-chain fatty acids (VLCFAs), resulting in CNS and peripheral nerve demyelination and adrenal insufficiency.
- Presents in 4- to 8-year-old boy.

SIGNS AND SYMPTOMS

- Symptoms of attention deficit hyperactivity disorder, followed by cognitive delays, visual abnormalities, ataxia, and seizures.
- Adrenal dysfunction essentially universal.

DIAGNOSIS

- White matter abnormality on MRI.
- Increased serum levels of very-long-chain fatty acids.
- Abnormal cortisol response to ACTH stimulation tests.

TREATMENT

- Adrenal hormone supplementation.
- Pharmacologic reduction in VLCFA levels.
- Bone marrow transplantation, especially if no neurologic symptoms.

PROGNOSIS

- Depends on exact phenotype, but prognosis is poor without bone marrow transplant.

Movement Disorders

Can be classified by a paucity of movement (hypokinetic) versus excessive or exaggerated movement (hyperkinetic). Hyperkinetic movement disorders predominate in children.

SYDENHAM CHOREA

PATHOPHYSIOLOGY/ETIOLOGY

- Most frequent cause of new onset chorea in children.
- Autoimmune mediated reaction aimed at basal ganglia.
- Twice as common in females.

- Onset: age 5–15 years.
- Postinfectious chorea appearing 4–8 weeks after a group A streptococcal pharyngitis.
- Cardinal feature of rheumatic fever.

SIGNS AND SYMPTOMS

- Rapid, brief, unsustained, non-stereotypical movements of the body.
- Mood swings, emotional lability.

DIAGNOSIS

- Recent throat infection (anti-streptolysin O, DNase B).

TREATMENT

- Steroids reduce time to remission.
- Treat primary infection.

PROGNOSIS

Most resolve after 8–9 months; relapse is not uncommon.

TOURETTE AND OTHER TIC DISORDERS

 A 13-year-old boy has had **uncontrollable blinking** since he was 9 years old. Recently, he has embarrassing **barking noises**. *Think: Tourette syndrome.*
It is characterized by motor and phonic (or vocal) tics. Tics are defined as involuntary, sudden, intermittent, repetitive movements (motor tics) or sounds (phonic tics). Comorbidities, such as ADHD and obsessive-compulsive disorder, are common. The age of onset is before 18 years, but most children show readily identifiable symptoms by age 7 years.

PATHOPHYSIOLOGY/ETIOLOGY

- Spectrum ranges from simple motor or vocal disorders to a combination of both (Tourette).
- Etiology unclear, but likely related to dopamine, serotonin, and norepinephrine neurotransmitter system abnormalities.
- Onset often between 4 and 6 years of age, peaking by 10 to 12 years, and then slowly resolving for most patients.
- More common in boys.
- Often associated with other conditions like obsessive-compulsive disorder (OCD) and attention deficit/hyperactivity disorder (ADHD).

SIGNS AND SYMPTOMS

- Rapid, involuntary, motor movements or vocalizations.
- Motor: range from single motor group (blink) to complex activity (tapping foot).
- Vocalization: range from throat clearing to complex vocalization (coprolalia).

DIAGNOSIS

- Multiple motor and vocal tics for more than 1 year.
- Waxing and waning pattern.
- Symptoms are enhanced by stress and anxiety.

TREATMENT

- Behavioral therapy
- Medications avoided unless symptoms interfere with child's development or cause undue social stress.

 EXAM TIP

Methylphenidate may unmask Tourette syndrome, but does not cause it.

 WARD TIP

When a child presents for evaluation of tics, it is imperative to look for comorbid symptoms of ADHD and OCD.

PROGNOSIS

- The majority have reduced symptoms into adulthood; a small number worsen.

PANS AND PANDAS

- PANS (Pediatric Acute-onset Neuropsychiatric Syndrome) and PANDAS (Pediatric Autoimmune Neuropsychiatric Disorder Associated with Streptococci) have nearly identical presentations.
- PANS is associated with a variety of infections, and PANDAS is always associated with streptococci.
- Characterized by the development or exacerbation of tics and/or obsessive-compulsive disorder (OCD).
- Diagnosis is considered controversial by some authorities.

Ataxias

Inability to coordinate muscle activities to regulate posture and also strength and direction of extremity movements (see Table 18-7)

ACUTE CEREBELLAR ATAXIA

PATHOPHYSIOLOGY/ETIOLOGY

- Usually seen in children less than 6 years old.
- Often follows common viral infections, especially varicella, by 2–3 weeks; thought to be an autoimmune response affecting the cerebellum.

SIGNS AND SYMPTOMS

- Sudden onset of severe truncal ataxia; often, the child cannot stand or sit.
- Horizontal nystagmus in 50%.

DIAGNOSIS

Diagnosis of exclusion

TREATMENT

Self-limited disease

EXAM TIP

Titubations are a disturbance of body equilibrium in standing or walking, resulting in an uncertain gait or swaying of the trunk or head, typically resulting from diseases of the cerebellum.

TABLE 18-7. **Ataxias**

TYPE	COMMON FEATURES	EXAMPLES
Sensory	Gait: wide based and high stepping Falls in dark or eyes closed (Romberg +) Difficulty of fine finger movements	Posterior column involvement similar to B$_{12}$ deficiency
Cerebellar	Gait: wide based and crunchy so cannot perform Romberg test Intention tremors, nystagmus, dysmetria, titubations, hypotonia	Spinocerebellar ataxia Pontocerebellar hypoplasia Vermian agenesis or dysgenesis Cerebellar degeneration in trisomies, etc.
Mixed	Both sensory and cerebellar components	Friedreich ataxia Vincristine side affect

PROGNOSIS

Complete recovery typically occurs within 3 months.

FRIEDREICH ATAXIA

PATHOPHYSIOLOGY/ETIOLOGY

- Autosomal-recessive mutation in Frataxin gene on chromosome 9.
- Degeneration of the dorsal columns and rootlets, spinocerebellar tracts, and, to a lesser extent, the pyramidal tracts and cerebellar hemispheres.
- Onset before age 10 years.

SIGNS AND SYMPTOMS

- Slow ataxia progression involving the lower limbs more than the upper limbs.
- Diminished deep tendon reflexes.
- Positive Babinski sign.
- Positive Romberg test.
- Explosive, dysarthric speech.
- Associated abnormalities include degeneration of the posterior columns (loss of vibration and proprioception), high arched feet, skeletal abnormalities (scoliosis), cardiomyopathy, and optic atrophy.

DIAGNOSIS

Clinical features establish the diagnosis, which is confirmed with genetic testing.

TREATMENT

There is no curative treatment available, but symptomatic treatment will improve quality of life.

PROGNOSIS

Hypertrophic cardiomyopathy with heart failure is the cause of death for most.

WARD TIP

Myoclonic epilepsy with ragged-red fibers (MERRF) is often confused with Friedreich ataxia.

ATAXIA-TELANGIECTASIA

PATHOPHYSIOLOGY/ETIOLOGY

- Autosomal-recessive disorder of nervous and immune system due to chromosome 11 gene mutation.
- The most common degenerative ataxia.
- Decreased or absent IgA, IgE, and IgG$_2$ subclass; IgM may be increased.

SIGNS AND SYMPTOMS

- Ataxia begins about age 2, with ambulation loss by adolescence.
- Oculomotor apraxia is common.
- Telangiectasia becomes evident by mid-childhood on the bulbar conjunctiva, bridge of nose, and sun-exposed surfaces of the ears and extremities.
- Frequent sinopulmonary infections occur.

DIAGNOSIS

- Increased AFP along with clinical picture to confirm the diagnosis.
- Genetic testing is available.

TREATMENT

- No specific treatment available; supportive care.
- Increased sensitivity to ionizing radiation; avoid imaging studies.

PROGNOSIS

- Have a 50- to 100-fold greater chance of brain and lymphoid tumors.

Peripheral Neuropathies

BELL PALSY

DEFINITION

- Acute, unilateral, isolated facial palsy.

ETIOLOGY

- Cause unclear but typically develops about 2 weeks after a viral infection.

CLINICAL MANIFESTATIONS

- Drooping of the mouth and inability to close eye on the affected side.
- Taste lost on anterior 2/3 of tongue on affected side in half of cases.

DIAGNOSIS

- Clinical history and physical examination.
- High resolution MRI can eliminate other causes if needed.

TREATMENT

- Steroids started early can improve outcome.
- Some recommend addition of acyclovir as HSV is a causative agent.
- The vast majority with full recovery.

GUILLAIN-BARRÉ SYNDROME

 A previously healthy 6-year-old boy has had difficulty walking for past few days and is now unable to walk. He has some upper extremity weakness but no respiratory distress. He had upper respiratory infection symptoms a few weeks ago. On examination, he is weaker more in the lower than upper extremities. Deep tendon reflexes are absent at knee and ankle. *Think: Guillain-Barré syndrome (GBS).*

GBS is an ascending paralysis. History of prior upper respiratory tract or viral infection may be present. Initial symptoms are pain, numbness, paresthesia, or weakness in the lower extremities, which rapidly progresses to bilateral and relatively symmetric weakness. Decreased or absent deep-tendon reflexes are often present. Lumbar puncture typically shows increased protein with normal CSF white cell count.

PATHOPHYSIOLOGY/ETIOLOGY

- A postinfectious demyelinating neuropathy predominantly of motor neurons.
- Most commonly seen after upper respiratory infection, *Campylobacter jejuni, Mycoplasma pneumoniae,* Epstein-Barr virus, and influenza.

SIGNS AND SYMPTOMS

- Weakness begins in the legs and progresses symmetrically upward to the trunk, arms, then to bulbar and ocular muscles.
- Tendon reflexes are absent.
- Respiratory muscles affected in 50%; autonomic dysfunction, pain, and paresthesia can be present.

DIAGNOSIS

- CSF protein elevation without cellular response, and polyneuropathy is diagnostic.
- Spinal MRI shows enhancement of nerve roots.
- Nerve conduction will show reduced velocities.

TREATMENT

- Hospitalization and monitoring for respiratory weakness.
- IVIG for rapidly progressive disease.
- Plasmapheresis for failed IVIG therapy.

PROGNOSIS

Generally full recovery over several months

BOTULISM

PATHOPHYSIOLOGY/ETIOLOGY

- Three natural forms: infant (most common type in US), foodborne, and wound.
- Botulinum toxin blocks neuromuscular transmission causing death by affecting airway and respiratory muscles.

SIGNS AND SYMPTOMS

- Symmetric flaccid paralysis of the cranial nerves with diplopia, dysphagia, dysarthria, and decreased gag.
- Infant botulism: first sign is absence of defecation, then loss of head control and caudally progressive weakness.
- Respiratory paralysis occurs.

DIAGNOSIS

- Identification of botulinum toxin in serum or stool.
- Electromyogram may show potentiation of the evoked muscle at high-frequency stimulation.

TREATMENT

- Human botulism immune globulin.
- Antibiotics not helpful.

PROGNOSIS

Prognosis is good in uncomplicated cases.

JUVENILE MYASTHENIA GRAVIS

PATHOPHYSIOLOGY/ETIOLOGY

- Decrease in postsynaptic acetylcholine receptors due to autoimmune degradation, resulting in rapid fatigability of muscles.

SIGNS AND SYMPTOMS

- Ptosis, often asymmetrical, and extraocular muscle weakness are early signs.
- Dysphagia and facial weakness, especially in infants.
- Poor head control.
- Fatigability of muscles, more prominent later in the day.

EXAM TIP

It is not possible to have botulism without having multiple cranial nerve palsies.

EXAM TIP

Infantile botulism classically associated with ingestion of honey (honey contains botulism spores). Avoid honey in the first year of life. Most cases are due to ingestion of environmental dust or soil from home-canned foods or construction at or near the home.

DIAGNOSIS

- EMG with repetitive stimulation demonstrated decremental response.
- Reversal of muscle weakness with cholinesterase inhibitor administration (age specific protocols are available).
- Acetylcholine receptor-binding or receptor-blocking antibodies may be found.

TREATMENT

- Cholinesterase drugs (neostigmine or pyridostigmine).
- Oral steroids may be required.
- A thymectomy is considered for those with elevated anti-ACh receptor antibodies.

PROGNOSIS

- Prognosis varies, with some children undergoing spontaneous remission, while in others, the disease persists into adulthood.

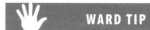

TRANSITORY NEONATAL MYASTHENIA

- Passive transfer of antibodies from myasthenic mothers.
- Generalized hypotonia developing a few hours after birth and lasting for weeks to months.
- Supportive care for poor suck and respiratory problems; neostigmine or exchange transfusion for more severe cases.

Electrolyte Imbalances

See Table 18-8 for common electrolyte imbalances affecting the nervous system.

WARD TIP

Children with myasthenic syndromes cannot tolerate neuromuscular blocking drugs, such as succinylcholine, and various other drugs. Most offenders are in the antibiotic, cardiovascular, and psychotropic categories.

WARD TIP

Rapid correction of hyponatremia can result in cerebellar pontine myelinolysis.

TABLE 18-8. Electrolyte Disturbances and the Nervous System

DISTURBANCE	MANIFESTATION	COMMON CAUSES
Hyponatremia	■ Rapid onset: brain swelling, lethargy, coma, and seizures ■ Slow onset: usually asymptomatic	■ Typically impaired renal water excretion in the presence of normal water intake
Hypernatremia	■ Intracranial bleeding is common in children (dehydrated brain shrinks and can tear bridging veins)	■ Most common cause is dehydration or inadequate intake of water
Hypokalemia	■ Neuromuscular: weakness, paralysis, rhabdomyolysis ■ Gastrointestinal: constipation, ileus ■ Nephrogenic diabetes insipidus ■ ECG changes: prominent U waves, T-wave flattening ■ Arrhythmias	■ Uptake into cells ■ Renal loss ■ Severe diarrhea, laxative abuse ■ Magnesium depletion is an important and often overlooked cause

Hyperkalemia	■ Severe cases are a medical emergency!
	■ Neuromuscular: weakness, ascending paralysis, respiratory failure
	■ Progressive ECG changes with increasing potassium:
	  ■ Peaked T and flattened P waves
	  ■ Long PR interval
	  ■ Idioventricular rhythm
	  ■ Wide QRS and deep S waves
	  ■ Sine-wave pattern and ventricular fibrillation
		■ Shift out of cells
		■ Aldosterone deficiency/unresponsiveness
		■ Renal failure

Headaches

MIGRAINE

This is the most common type of recurrent headache in pediatrics.

DEFINITION

A recurrent headache that can be associated with:
- Abdominal pain.
- Nausea and/or vomiting.
- Throbbing headache.
- Often bilateral (versus unilateral in adults).
- May be associated aura.
- Relieved by sleep.
- Family history of migraines.

Diagnosis of migraine is clinical. Neuroimaging (MRI) is indicated for unusual features, such as persistently occipital or with abnormal neurologic examination.

CLASSIFICATION

Migraines may be classified into the following subgroups:

Migraine Without Aura

- Most common form.
- Headache lasting 4–72 hours, perhaps a bit shorter in children.
- Two of the following: unilateral, pulsating, moderate/severe pain, aggravation of routine physical activity.
- Two of the following: nausea, vomiting, photophobia, phonophobia.

Migraine with Aura

- Headache with fully reversible aura symptoms: visual, sensory, speech, motor, brainstem, retinal.
- Aura is accompanied or followed by headache within 60 minutes, and it may last 5–60 minutes.
- Aura symptoms may spread gradually, or two or more symptoms May occur in succession.

Chronic Migraine

- Defined as headache on >15 days per month for more than 3 months.
- Daily headaches of less severity with less prominent migraine features.

Complicated Migraine

Transient neurologic signs develop during a headache and persist after the resolution of the headache for a few hours to days.

TREATMENT

- Avoid the possible triggers: psychological stress, strenuous exercise, sleep deprivation, cheese, chocolate, processed meat, or moving vehicles.
- Consider nonpharmacologic treatment, such as biofeedback.
- For acute attacks:
  - Dark, quiet environment and sleep.
  - Adequate fluid intake.
  - Pharmacologic therapy: acetaminophen and nonsteroidal anti-inflammatory drugs (NSAIDs) are first line.

WARD TIP

Episodic syndromes that may be associated with migraines include cyclic vomiting syndrome, abdominal migraine, benign paroxysmal vertigo, and benign paroxysmal torticollis.

WARD TIP

Prophylaxis should be offered to children with two or more migraines per month that interfere with activities such as school or recreation.

- Second-line drugs include triptans, caffeine, and ergot alkaloids (status migrainosus).
- Antiemetics are helpful at the start of headache.
- Treatment should be instituted as early as possible in an attack.

PROPHYLAXIS

- Antiepileptic drugs, such as topiramate, valproate, levetiracetam.
- Tricyclic antidepressants such as amitriptyline.
- β-blockers such as propranolol.

TENSION HEADACHE

Tension or stress headaches may be common but ignored since disability is uncommon. Sometimes it is described as "opposite of migraine."

PRESENTATION

- Described as constant hurting rather than throbbing.
- Present like a band around the head rather than focal.
- Is not worsened by activity.
- Less common than migraines to have nausea, vomiting, or photophobia.
- May be difficult to differentiate from migraine.

DIAGNOSIS

- Diagnosis of exclusion.
- EEG or CT is not necessary.

TREATMENT

Steps should be taken to minimize anxiety and stress:
- Mild analgesics often are sufficient.
- Other options include counseling and biofeedback.
- Sedatives or antidepressants are rarely necessary.

Coma

- Consciousness refers to the state of awareness of self and environment.
- Pediatric consciousness evaluation is dependent on age and developmental level.

DEFINITION

Pathologic cause of loss of normal consciousness

PATHOPHYSIOLOGY

- Consciousness is the result of communication between the cerebral cortex and the ascending reticular-activating system. Disruption results in altered consciousness.

ETIOLOGY

- Structural causes (trauma, vascular conditions, mass lesions).
- Metabolic and toxic causes (hypoxic-ischemic injury, toxins, infections, seizures).

EVALUATION

- ABCs; give O_2; obtain IV access, monitor vital signs, obtain bedside glucose; obtain additional labs and cultures, as indicated.
- Treat underlying cause (toxin antidote, reduce ICP, antibiotics, etc.).

WARD TIP

Headaches can occur in children secondary to refractive errors.

WARD TIP

Herniation is a result of increased intracranial pressure and often leads to coma or death.

Herniation syndromes that may result in coma:

- **Uncal herniation:** pressure on CN 6 with diplopia and inability to abduct eye
- **Central (trans-tentorial herniation):** blown (fixed and dilated) pupil, ptosis, CN 3 compression (down and out eye), ipsilateral hemiplegia

---

WARD TIP

Prognosis depends on the etiology of the insult and the rapid initiation of treatment!

PROGNOSIS

- Overall, children tend to do better than adults.
- Several general measurement scales have been published attempting to predict outcome. The most widely used is the Glasgow Coma Scale (see Emergency Medicine and Life Support chapter).

Increased Intracranial Pressure (ICP)

SYMPTOMS

- Headache, nausea, vomiting, diplopia, personality changes.
- Coughing or Valsalva maneuver increases ICP and worsens headache.

ETIOLOGY

Common causes include posterior fossa brain tumors (and other brain tumors), obstructive hydrocephalus, hemorrhage, meningitis, venous sinus thrombosis, pseudotumor cerebri, abscesses, and chronic lead poisoning.

DIAGNOSIS

- Thorough history and physical examination.
- Bulging fontanelle, impaired upward gaze in infants.
- Papilledema.
- Obtain CBC, erythrocyte sedimentation rate, and CT/MRI to narrow the differential.
- If CT/MRI is negative, consider lumbar puncture to measure pressure.

TREATMENT

- Varies with particular diagnosis, and should be directed at the underlying etiology.
- Techniques to lower ICP acutely include:
  - Intubation and hyperventilation, resulting in cerebral vasoconstriction.
  - Elevating the head 30 degrees to facilitate venous return.
  - Hyperosmolar agents such as mannitol or hypertonic 3% saline.
  - Extra-ventricular drain, providing relief and continuous monitoring of ICP.
  - Surgical decompression, if increased ICP persists.

WARD TIP

Any time you see papilledema, think increased ICP.

WARD TIP

Cushing triad: a sign of increased intracranial pressure and impending herniation of the brain
1. Irregular respirations
2. Decreased heart rate
3. Increased BP

WARD TIP

Never perform an LP if papilledema is present. Must obtain CT before LP if suspicious of increased ICP.

Aneurysms

- The pathogenesis is unclear.
- Most common in internal carotid artery, especially at the bifurcation.
- Early warning signs are related to the subarachnoid hemorrhage (SAH) onset, including headaches, vomiting, change in mental status, seizures, and cranial nerve palsy.
- More likely to rupture in patients <2 years of age or >8 years.

ETIOLOGY

- Most often are related to congenital diseases:
  - Ehlers-Danlos syndrome.
  - Marfan syndrome, tuberous sclerosis.
  - AVMs.
  - Coarctation of the aorta.
  - Polycystic kidney disease.

- Acquired aneurysms:
  - Bacterial embolization can result in cerebral vascular mycotic aneurysms.
  - Trauma, especially in the anterior cerebral artery or middle cerebral artery.

DIAGNOSIS

- CT- or MR-angiogram is the gold standard, especially for screening.
- Lumbar puncture and CT/MR imaging are appropriate for evaluation of a SAH.

TREATMENT

- Surgical clipping or endovascular coiling is definitive treatment.
- Administer antibiotics for mycotic aneurysms.

Arteriovenous Malformations (AVMs)

- Prenatal communication of arteries and veins occurs without intervening capillaries.
- Larger AVMs create a significant atrioventricular (AV) shunt (steal phenomenon) and considerable damage if they rupture.

PRESENTATION

- Small unruptured malformations present with headache or seizures.
- Larger malformations may present with progressive neurologic deficit.
- Hemorrhage is the most frequent presentation.

DIAGNOSIS

- Angiography is the test of choice and is required to direct the future therapy. MRA is also available.
- A CT is often performed at time of rupture to determine size and location.
- An MRI with angiography is often employed.

TREATMENT

- Treatment is evolving, but a surgical resection is the gold standard, if feasible.
- Other options, depending on size and risk of complications, include radiosurgery and embolization.

VEIN OF GALEN MALFORMATIONS

- May present as high-output congestive heart failure, failure to thrive, or hydrocephalus.
- Embolization is the preferred treatment; surgery has a higher mortality rate.
- A cranial bruit may be present.

CAVERNOUS HEMANGIOMAS

- Typically supratentorial lesions that present with bleeding or seizure.
- Observe; surgical resection if symptomatic.

Stroke

EPIDEMIOLOGY

- Biphasic incidence; peak incidence in neonates, then again in adolescence.
- Arterial ischemic events cause of strokes in neonates, followed by thrombosis.

SIGNS AND SYMPTOMS

- Sudden onset of neurologic deficit, especially hemiparesis, or seizures in neonates.

ETIOLOGY

- Pediatric causes of stroke differ from those in the adult population.
- Types of stroke include:
    - Ischemic: thrombosis (both arterial and venous) or embolic (arterial).
    - Hemorrhage.
- Risk factors that exist for stroke include:
    - AVMs.
    - Antiphospholipid antibodies/lupus anticoagulant.
    - Congenital coagulopathies (factor V Leiden, deficiencies of protein C, S, and antithrombin III).
    - Sickle cell anemia (sickling RBCs may cause thrombosis or endothelial injury).
    - Cardiac conditions: arrhythmias, myxoma, paradoxical emboli through a patent foramen ovale, and septic emboli from bacterial endocarditis.
    - Blunt trauma to the head and neck leading to arterial dissection.
    - Vasculitis (Kawasaki, hemolytic-uremic syndrome, meningitis).
    - Mitochondrial diseases.
    - Patients undergoing extracorporeal membrane oxygenation (ECMO) are at risk for intracranial hemorrhage and embolic ischemic stroke.

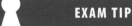

EXAM TIP

Cardiac abnormalities are the common causes of thromboembolic stroke in children.

ARTERIAL THROMBOSIS/EMBOLISM

- Intracerebral arterial dissection after head and neck trauma tears the vascular intima. Areas distally undergo infarction and produce focal symptoms.
- Cerebral symptoms such as a progressive hemiplegia, lethargy, or aphasia result from the shedding of small emboli into the carotid circulation.
- Seizures are common presenting symptom in neonates.

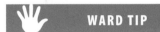

WARD TIP

A typical workup for a stroke syndrome will include head a CT or MRI scan, followed by an angiogram (if the CT/MRI is nondiagnostic), and an echocardiogram to exclude cardiac causes.

VENOUS THROMBOSIS

- May be subdivided into septic and nonseptic causes.
- Septic causes include bacterial meningitis, otitis media, and mastoiditis.
- Aseptic causes include severe dehydration, hypercoagulable states, congenital heart disease, and hemoglobinopathies.
- Neonates present with diffuse neurologic signs and seizures.
- In children, focal neurologic signs are more common.

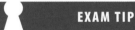

EXAM TIP

Low-molecular-weight heparin appears to be safe, effective, and well tolerated in children with strokes resulting from congenital heart disease, arterial dissection, and hypercoagulable states.

Closed Head Trauma

See Table 18-9 for a comparison of subdural and epidural hematomas. Clinically, it is not easy to differentiate the two, so head imaging helps differentiate.

SUBDURAL HEMATOMA (SDH)

EPIDEMIOLOGY

Intracranial brain injury seen in infants and as a sports-related injury.

ETIOLOGY

- Typically occurs when trauma ruptures the bridging vein between the dura and the brain.
- Occurs in neonates due to a tear in the tentorium cerebelli or the falx cerebelli.

TABLE 18-9. Features of Acute Epidural and Subdural Hematomas

SUBDURAL HEMATOMA	EPIDURAL HEMATOMA
Follows inner layer of dura	Follows outer layer of dura (periosteum)
"Rounds the bend" to follow to follow falx or tentorium	Crosses falx or tentorium
Not affected by sutures of skull	Limited by sutures of skull (typically)
Tendency for crescentic shapes	Tendency for lentiform shapes
More mass effect than expected for their size	Typical source of EDH: skull fracture with arterial or sinus laceration
Typical source of SDH: cortical vein	

WARD TIP

Subdural hematomas appear crescent shaped (concave) on CT and will not cross the midline, but they will cross ipsilateral suture lines.

- Skull fracture is not seen commonly.
- An SDH should be ruled out if changes in consciousness level develop after head injury.
- Typically frontoparietal location; can be acute, subacute, or chronic.

SIGNS AND SYMPTOMS

- These depend on age of the child and severity.
- Neonates: seizures, a bulging fontanelle, decreased activity.
- Increased ICP (irritability, lethargy, vomiting, papilledema, headache).
- Retinal hemorrhages are common in abused children.
- Brain damage is generally more severe than epidural hematoma.

DIAGNOSIS

Gold standard is CT scan showing crescent-shaped hyperdensity under the skull.

EPIDURAL HEMATOMA

EPIDEMIOLOGY

Seen most often in older children

ETIOLOGY

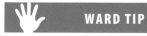
WARD TIP

Lucid interval. *Think: Epidural hematoma.*

- Commonly from a temporal-bone fracture lacerating the middle meningeal artery.
- A collection of blood between the skull inner table and the dura mater.
- Skull fracture seen commonly.
- Nearly always unilateral.

SIGNS AND SYMPTOMS

WARD TIP

Epidural hematomas appear lens shaped (convex) on CT and will not cross the midline or other cranial sutures.

- Classic progression involves an initial loss of consciousness, followed by a lucid interval (often missing in children), and then abrupt deterioration and death.
- Hemorrhage and acute brain swelling cause increased ICP, which can result in herniation with ipsilateral ptosis, dilated pupil, and hemiparesis.
- Retinal hemorrhages are not common.

DIAGNOSIS

Gold standard is CT scan with a lens-shaped (convex) area at the lesion.

TREATMENT

Epidural hematomas may progress rapidly, and immediate neurosurgical treatment is indicated.

COUP/CONTRECOUP INJURIES

Cerebral contusion injury associated with a sudden acceleration or deceleration of the head

Coup Injuries

- Located directly at the point of impact.
- More common in acceleration injuries such as being hit with a baseball bat.
- Multiple microhemorrhages as blood leaks into the brain tissue.

Contrecoup Injuries

- Located opposite (180 degrees) from the point of impact.
- More common in deceleration injuries, such as striking one's head after a fall.

DIFFUSE AXONAL INJURY

EPIDEMIOLOGY

- Tissues with differing elastic properties shear against each other, tearing axons.
- Caused by rapid deceleration/rotation of head.
- Locations:
  - Cerebral hemispheres near gray-white junction.
  - Basal ganglia.
  - Corpus callosum, especially splenium.
  - Dorsal brain stem.
- High morbidity and mortality—common cause of posttraumatic vegetative state.
- Initial CT often normal despite poor GCS.
- Lesions often nonhemorrhagic and seen only on MRI.
- Survivors often have substantial long-term cognitive and behavioral morbidity.

Concussion

A teenage girl experienced a head-to-head collision with another player during soccer 4 hours ago. She reports headache, dizziness, nausea, and difficulty concentrating and focusing since the injury. She has no focal neurologic findings on examination. *Think: Concussion.*

- Trauma-induced brain dysfunction without structural injury on standard neuroimaging.
- The signs and symptoms are nonspecific and may include:
  - Headache.
  - Fatigue.
  - Dizziness.

EXAM TIP

Old contusions develop an orange color secondary to hemosiderin deposition. Pathologists call these *plaques jaunes.*

EXAM TIP

Contrecoup injuries tend to be more severe than coup injuries.

WARD TIP

Diffuse axonal injury is best visualized on a T2-weighted MRI.

- Nausea/vomiting.
- Unsteadiness.
- Mental fogginess.
- Anterograde or retrograde amnesia.
- Difficulties with concentration.
- Sleep disturbances.
- Emotional lability.
- Neuroimaging typically is normal; it is rarely indicated to rule out other pathology.
- Management is physical and neurocognitive rest with strict adherence to "return to play" guidelines that limit sports until full recovery is evident.
- Most patients recover fully but caution is advised with repeat concussions.

Plagiocephaly

PHYSIOLOGY/ETIOLOGY

- Developmental flattening of the cranium usually due to consistently sleeping on the same area of the head.

CLINICAL MANIFESTATIONS

- Normal round head at birth that then develops a parallelogram shape.
- Ipsilateral ear anteriorly displaced (in contrast to craniosynostosis, which is posteriorly displaced.
- Absence of bony ridges (in contrast to craniosynostosis).

DIAGNOSIS

- History of sleep positioning and classic physical examination findings.

TREATMENT

- Repositioning.
- Occasionally helmet therapy.

Hydrocephalus

- Head circumference >2 SD above the mean is macrocephaly.
- If due to increased CSF in the CSF spaces, called hydrocephalus.

PHYSIOLOGY

- CSF is made by the choroid plexus in the walls of the lateral, third, and fourth ventricles.
- CSF flows from: lateral ventricles → foramen of Monro → third ventricle → cerebral aqueduct → fourth ventricle → foramina of Magendie and Luschka → subarachnoid space of spinal cord and brain → arachnoid villi.
- CSF is absorbed primarily by the arachnoid villi through tight junctions.

ETIOLOGY

- Obstructive (noncommunicating) hydrocephalus:
  - Stenosis of the aqueduct of Sylvius is most common.
  - Other causes include posterior fossa brain tumors, Arnold-Chiari malformations (type II), and Dandy-Walker syndrome.
  - Also seen in brain abscess, hematoma, infectious, vein of Galen malformation.

- Nonobstructive (communicating) hydrocephalus:
  - Due to either increased production or reduced CSF absorption.
  - Common causes include subarachnoid hemorrhage or meningitis, which obliterate the cisterns or arachnoid villi and obstruct CSF flow.
  - Venous sinus thrombosis, meningeal malignancy, and intrauterine infections are other causes.
- Ex vacuo: hydrocephalus resulting from decreased brain parenchyma.

CLINICAL MANIFESTATIONS

- Infants:
  - Enlargement of the head is the most prominent sign.
  - Bulging anterior fontanelle, cranial suture widening, sun-setting sign, and Parinaud syndrome can be seen.
- Children and adolescents:
  - Signs are more subtle because the cranial sutures are partially closed.
  - Elevated ICP signs (lethargy, vomiting, headache, etc.), as well as visual field disturbance, are seen. Papilledema can be present.
  - A gradual change in school performance due to a slowly obstructing lesion.

DIAGNOSIS

- A detailed history and physical exam is key to discovering the underlying etiology.
- Ultrasound and head CT/MRI can identify the cause of hydrocephalus.
- Familial (often X-linked) cases of aqueductal stenosis have been reported.

TREATMENT

- Medical management with acetazolamide (decrease CSF production) and furosemide may provide temporary relief.
- An extraventricular drain or ventriculoperitoneal shunt may be required.

EXAM TIP

Pneumococcal and tuberculous meningitis produce a thick exudate that can obstruct the basal cisterns leading to communicating hydrocephalus.

EXAM TIP

Parinaud syndrome is a group of gaze and pupil abnormalities associated with pressure on the vertical gaze center in the brainstem.

EXAM TIP

Premature infants with intraventricular hemorrhage are at higher risk to develop hydrocephalus.

Congenital Malformations

SPINA BIFIDA (INCLUDING ANENCEPHALY)

DEFINITION

- Congenital neural tube defect resulting in spine and spinal cord malformations.
- Manifestations range from spina bifida occulta to anencephaly.

ETIOLOGY

- The cause is unknown, but it is associated with a variety of syndromes and teratogens.
- Reduced incidence occurs with maternal folate supplementation.

CLINICAL MANIFESTATIONS

- Bulging sac at is observed the site of the neural tube defect.
- Most common site is the lumbar region.
- Hydrocephalus and Chiari II malformations are commonly seen.
- Spina bifida occulta may present with a subtle finding of a tuft of hair or mass over the spine that may result in symptoms, including back pain, incontinence, delay in walking, or lower extremity orthopedic deformities.

Diagnosis

- Prenatal USG often reveals defect.
- Elevated maternal serum α-fetoprotein.

Treatment

- Early surgical closure upon delivery.
- Treatment of hydrocephalus, if present.
- Prenatal diagnosis may allow in utero surgery in specialized centers.
- Long-term care includes a multidisciplinary team to manage the associated neurologic, orthopedic, urologic, and developmental complications.

AGENESIS OF THE CORPUS CALLOSUM

- Associated with many syndromes and inborn errors of metabolism, including lissencephaly, Dandy-Walker syndrome, Arnold-Chiari type 2 malformations, and Aicardi syndrome.
- MRI demonstrates absent parenchymal tissue.
- Consequences range from normal intelligence to marked developmental delay and seizures depending on associated syndromes.

SYRINGOMYELIA

A teenage girl has a headache and a cape-like distribution of pain and temperature sensory loss that developed after a minor motor vehicle accident. *Think: Cervical syringomyelia with undiagnosed Chiari I.*

The Chiari type I malformation is characterized by herniation of the cerebellar tonsils through the foramen magnum and may cause syringomyelia. Common presentations include headache, neck pain, vertigo, sensory changes, and ataxia. Typical scenario is occipital pain precipitated by cough or Valsalva maneuver. MRI is the modality of choice.

- A slowly progressive paracentral cavity formation within the brain or spinal cord, most often in the cervical or lumbar regions.
- MRI is the test of choice for diagnosis.
- Often develops post-traumatically in the setting of an undiagnosed Chiari I malformation or tethered cord.
- Symptoms include bilateral impaired pain and temperature sensation due to decussation of these fibers near the central canal. Weakness of the hand muscles and progressive symptoms develop as the cavity enlarges.

DANDY-WALKER MALFORMATION

- Results from failure of the fourth ventricle roof to form, causing cystic expansion into the posterior fossa.
- Most patients have hydrocephalus.
- Agenesis of the cerebellar vermis and corpus callosum is also common.
- Infants present with a rapidly increasing in head size.
- Management is via shunting of the cystic cavity to prevent hydrocephalus.
- Neurologic impairment is common.

ARNOLD-CHIARI MALFORMATIONS

- Four variations exist (see Figure 18-6). Type 2 is the most common, in which the cerebellum and medulla are shifted caudally, resulting in crowding of the upper spinal column.
- Type 2 is also associated with meningomyelocele.

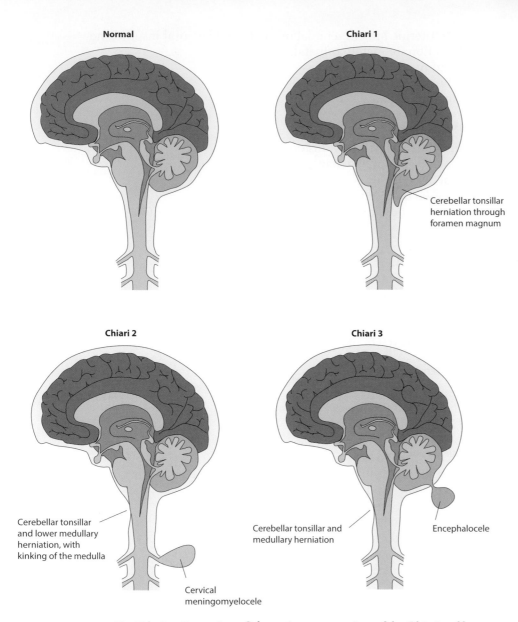

FIGURE 18-6. The Chiari malformations. Schematic representations of the Chiari malformations. Commonly associated hydrocephalus and syringomyelia not depicted.

- Infants with type 2 may present with stridor, weak cry, and apnea.
- Syringomyelia is common, especially with type 1.
- Management includes close observation with serial MRIs and surgery as required.

Cerebral Palsy (CP)

DEFINITION

- A **non-progressive** disorder of movement and posture resulting from damage to the developing brain prior to or surrounding birth.
- Most cases occur in the absence of identifiable causes.

ETIOLOGY/RISK FACTORS

- Prematurity with intraventricular hemorrhage.
- Birth or other asphyxia.

EXAM TIP

CP is a static disorder, meaning that it does not result in the loss of previously acquired milestones. If progressive symptoms or loss of previously attained milestones are seen, consider an alternative diagnosis.

- Intrauterine growth retardation (IUGR), placental insufficiency.
- Infection: prenatal/postnatal.
- Twin pregnancy.
- Chromosomal and genetic disorders.
- Head trauma.

SIGNS AND SYMPTOMS

- Prenatal and perinatal history.
- Delayed motor, language, or social skills.
- Not losing skills previously acquired.
- Feeding difficulties.
- Late-onset dystonia (ages 7–10 years).

EXAMINATION

- Hypertonia.
- Hyperreflexia.
- Posture and movement: may be spastic, ataxic, choreoathetoid, and dystonic.
- Abnormal primitive reflexes.
- Abnormal gait.
- Impaired growth of affected extremity.

ASSOCIATED PROBLEMS

- Seizure disorder.
- Intellectual disability.
- Developmental disorders.

CLASSIFICATION

- Hemiplegic cerebral palsy: upper limb involvement is greater than lower limb; many walk before 2 years.
- Diplegic cerebral palsy.
- Quadriplegic cerebral palsy: majority do not walk.
- Dystonic/athetoid cerebral palsy.
- Ataxic cerebral palsy.
- Monoplegic cerebral palsy: usually lower limb and appears late.

TREATMENT

- Multidisciplinary approach to maximizing function and minimizing impairment.
- Team includes general pediatrician, physiotherapist, occupational therapist, language therapist, neurologist, and social and educational support services.
- Orthopedic interventions are sometimes helpful.

Intellectual Disability (ID)

DEFINITION

- Below average intellectual functioning and deficits in adaptive behavior before 18 years of age.
- Significant impairment: intelligence quotient (IQ) or developmental quotient (DQ) <70 or <2 standard deviations (SDs).

EPIDEMIOLOGY

- Affects 1–3% of the population.
- Approximately 75% are mild cases.
- Males more commonly affected.

WARD TIP

For patients for whom the diagnosis of CP is considered, a lack of risk factors, a family history of neurologic disease, presentation in late infancy or early childhood, ataxic CP, or atypical features suggest the need for consideration of other diagnosis.

WARD TIP

Extensor plantar response (presence of Babinski sign) can be present up to 1 year of age, but should be present symmetrically.

EXAM TIP

DQ is often used as a rough estimator of IQ in infants and younger children. It is simply the mental age (estimated from historical milestones and exam) divided by the chronologic age, × 100.

SIGNS AND SYMPTOMS

- Significant delay in reaching developmental milestones.
- Delayed speech and language skills in toddlers with less severe ID.
- The child will continue to learn new skills depending on severity of ID.

DIAGNOSIS

- Thorough past medical, family and social history preclude intensive testing in many cases.
- Selective chromosomal, metabolic and neuroimaging as needed.

TREATMENT

- Identify and treat associated impairments such as behavioral and emotional disorder.
- Supportive medical home with interdisciplinary management.

EXAM TIP

The IQ is scaled such that the mean is 100 and the standard deviation (SD) is 15. So ID is simply defined as an IQ two SDs below the mean.

Learning Disability (LD)

- Significant discrepancy between a person's intellectual ability and academic achievement.
- Often learn best in unconventional ways.
- Often restricted to a particular realm such as reading or mathematics with correspondingly discrepant scores on standardized measures of intelligence or academic achievement.
- Significant improvement with appropriate interventions.

NOTES

HIGH-YIELD FACTS IN

Special Organs—Eye, Ear, Nose

Eye

AMBLYOPIA

DEFINITION

Amblyopia is a decrease in visual acuity in one or both eyes caused by blurred retinal images leading to failure of proper visual cortex development.

ETIOLOGY

- Strabismus.
- Refractive errors.
- Opacity in the visual path (e.g., cataract, ptosis, eyelid hemangioma).

DIAGNOSIS

Diagnosis is made by visual acuity testing.

TREATMENT

- Treatment of the pathology, such as removal of a cataract.
- Prescription glasses to correct refractive errors.
- Patching or application of atropine (blurs vision) in the good eye until the amblyopic eye has improved its vision.

STRABISMUS

DEFINITION

- Deviation or misalignment of the eye (see Figure 19-1).
- Strabismus can lead to vision loss, which can be permanent.

DIAGNOSIS

- Corneal light reflex: while the child looks into a light source, the clinician observes where the reflex lies in each eye; strabismus exists if the light reflex is asymmetric.
- Alternative cover test: while a child stares at a distant object, the clinician covers one of the child's eyes; movement of the uncovered eye when one eye is covered confirms strabismus.

TREATMENT

- Prescription glasses are the treatment for strabismus due to refraction error.
- Extraocular muscle surgery may be necessary.

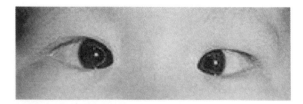

FIGURE 19-1. **Child with strabismus.**

OPTIC NEURITIS

DEFINITION

- Inflammation of the optic nerve.
- Retrobulbar optic neuritis: without ophthalmoscopically visible signs of disc inflammation.
- Papillitis or intraocular optic neuritis: ophthalmoscopically visible evidence of inflammation of the nerve head.
- Neuroretinitis: inflammation of both the retina and papilla.

ETIOLOGY

- Idiopathic in many cases.
- Secondary to underlying disease, such as multiple sclerosis or lupus.
- Recent viral infection, such as measles, mumps, varicella, polio, mononucleosis and influenza, and rarely following immunization for viral disease.
- Extension from an infection involving the teeth, sinuses, or meninges.
- Side effect of treatment with ethambutol.

SIGNS AND SYMPTOMS

- Loss of vision or central scotoma.
- Depressed color vision.
- Pain with extraocular motion.
- Pain to palpation of the globe.
- Afferent papillary defect (Marcus Gunn pupil).
- Bilateral in children (unilateral in adults).

TREATMENT

Data from adult studies adapted to pediatrics suggest that initial intravenous steroids followed by a short course of oral steroids may reduce symptom duration.

CONJUNCTIVITIS

DEFINITION

Inflammation of the conjunctiva

TYPES

Allergic

- Immunoglobulin E–mediated reaction to triggers such as pollen or dust.

SIGNS AND SYMPTOMS

- Watery, itchy, red eyes.
- Conjunctiva and lid edema.
- Typically bilateral.
- Pruritus and chemosis are common.

TREATMENT

- Removal of the trigger.
- Cold compresses.
- Antihistamines.

Viral

- Adenovirus is the typical cause.
- The pharyngoconjunctival fever triad is pharyngitis, fever, and conjunctivitis.
- Prolonged adenovirus type 8 infection can cause epidemic keratoconjunctivitis: fulminant vision-threatening condition with corneal involvement.

EXAM TIP

A deviated eye is described as being turned "eso" (inward), "exo" (outward), "hypo" (downward), or "hyper" (upward) -tropic.

EXAM TIP

In children, optic neuritis is less commonly associated with multiple sclerosis.

WARD TIP

Adenovirus is the most common viral cause of conjunctivitis.

SIGNS AND SYMPTOMS

- Watery, red eyes.
- Often has preauricular lymph nodes.

TREATMENT

- supportive.
- handwashing to prevent transmission.

Bacterial

- Typical causes are nontypeable *Haemophilus influenzae*, *Streptococcus pneumoniae*, and *Staphylococcus aureus*.
- Contagious outbreaks can occur.

SIGNS AND SYMPTOMS

- Mucopurulent discharge.
- Red eyes.
- Conjunctiva edema.
- Often unilateral, but can be bilateral.

TREATMENT

- Topical antibiotics (drops or ointment).
- Warm compresses.

BLEPHARITIS

DEFINITION

Inflammation of the eyelid margins

ETIOLOGY

- *Staphylococcus aureus* or *epidermidis*.
- Seborrheic.
- A combination of the above.

SIGNS AND SYMPTOMS

- Burning.
- Itching.
- Erythema.
- Scaling.
- Ulceration of the lid margin, especially with staphylococcal infection.

TREATMENT

- Daily eyelid cleansing to remove scales.
- Topical antibiotics.

DACRYOSTENOSIS

 A 4-month-old child presents with an exudative eye discharge and a painful, red lacrimal sac. *Think: Dacryocystitis.*

Dacryocystitis is the most common infection of the lacrimal system, often a complication of dacryocystocele. Excessive tearing, purulent eye discharge, and fever are common symptoms. S. *aureus* and streptococci are the common organisms. Patients may require admission for intravenous antibiotics. An incision and drainage may be needed for a lacrimal sac abscess.

DEFINITION

A congenital nasolacrimal duct obstruction

EPIDEMIOLOGY

Occurs in 20% of infants; appears a few weeks after birth

ETIOLOGY

Failure of the epithelial cells of tear duct to separate

SIGNS AND SYMPTOMS

- Chronic tearing.
- Crusty discharge, especially upon awakening, typically without conjunctival injection.

COMPLICATIONS

Dacryocystitis: nasolacrimal sac inflammation treated with topical or systemic antibiotic and warm compresses

TREATMENT

- Digital lacrimal sac massage and warm compresses.
- Eyelid cleansing.
- Vast majority resolve before 1 year of age.
- Probing/instrumentation >1 year of age to rupture the epithelial membrane.

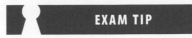

EXAM TIP

Dacryostenosis is the most common disorder of the lacrimal system.

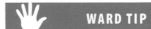

WARD TIP

Most dacryostenosis will resolve by 8 months of age.

CHALAZION

DEFINITION

Granulomatous inflammation of a meibomian (tarsal) gland

SIGNS AND SYMPTOMS

- Firm nodule on the eyelid.
- Nontender.

TREATMENT

- Warm compresses.
- Excision if necessary.
- Most subside spontaneously over months.

HORDEOLUM (STYE)

TYPES

- External hordeolum is an infection of the glands of Zeis or Moll.
- Internal hordeolum is infection of the meibomian gland.

ETIOLOGY

S. aureus

SIGNS AND SYMPTOMS

- Localized swelling.
- Tenderness.
- Erythema.

TREATMENT

- Warm compresses.
- Topical antibiotics often used but generally ineffective.
- Incision and drainage for no spontaneous rupture.

Periorbital cellulitis is pre-septal.

Periorbital cellulitis is much more common than orbital cellulitis.

The most common organisms causing both preorbital and orbital cellulitis—
SHIP

S. *aureus*

H. i*nfluenza* (now rare due to vaccine)

S. p*neumoniae* (reduced incidence due to vaccine)

Orbital cellulitis is post septal.

PERIORBITAL CELLULITIS

DEFINITION

Inflammation of the eyelids and periorbital tissue anterior to the septum

ETIOLOGY

Extension of local infections (trauma, such as an insect bite or scratch) or bacteremia

SIGNS AND SYMPTOMS

- Erythema.
- Edema.
- Induration and tenderness.
- Normal extraocular movements and without pain.

TREATMENT

Oral or IV antibiotics

ORBITAL CELLULITIS

DEFINITION

Inflammation/infection of the orbital tissues behind the septum

ETIOLOGY

- Extension of a local infection (paranasal sinusitis, dental abscess).
- Trauma.
- Most common site: medial orbital wall.
- The most common organisms are S. *aureus and streptococcal species.*, but some infections are polymicrobial.
- Orbital cellulitis is commonly caused by ethmoid sinusitis.

SIGNS AND SYMPTOMS

- Proptosis, ophthalmoplegia, and decreased vision in contrast to pre-septal cellulitis.
- Painful extraocular motion is often the first sign.
- Proptosis is a classic, but late, sign.
- Erythema in conjunctiva.
- Edema.

DIAGNOSIS

Orbital computed tomography (CT) scan with IV contrast

TREATMENT

- Ophthalmology consultation.
- Intravenous antibiotics, possible surgical drainage.

COMPLICATIONS

- Loss of vision.
- Meningitis.
- Central nervous system (epidural) abscess.

CORNEAL ULCER

ETIOLOGY

- Trauma (sand, contact lens, etc.) with secondary infection often after corneal abrasion.
- Bacterial: *Pseudomonas aeruginosa, Neisseria gonorrhoeae.*
- Fungal: especially in contact lens users.

SIGNS AND SYMPTOMS

- Corneal haze.
- Painful.
- Photophobia.
- Tearing.

COMPLICATIONS

- Perforation.
- Scarring.
- Blindness.

DIAGNOSIS

- Slit-lamp exam: fluorescein staining reveals an epithelial defect.
- Scraping of the cornea to identify infectious etiology.

TREATMENT

- Local antibiotics.
- In some cases, systemic treatment may be required.

RETINOBLASTOMA

- The most common primary ocular malignancy in children.
- Average age: 15 months in bilateral disease; 27 months for unilateral cases.

SIGNS AND SYMPTOMS

- Leukocoria: white pupillary reflex is the most common presentation.
- Strabismus is the second-most common presentation.
- Orbital inflammation occurs.
- Hyphema (blood) or pseudohypopyon (tumor cells) layering is visible anterior to the iris.

DIAGNOSIS

- Direct visualization during eye exam.
- Computed tomography (CT) or ultrasound (US) can help confirm and evaluate spread.
- Retinoblastoma gene is located on chromosome 13 at the 13q14 region.

TREATMENT

- Chemotherapy.
- Laser photocoagulation.
- Cryotherapy.
- Enucleation for unresponsive tumors.
- Genetic counseling for families with a history of retinoblastoma.

Ear

OTITIS MEDIA

DEFINITION

Inflammation of the middle ear

EPIDEMIOLOGY

- The incidence of otitis media is higher in:
  - Boys.
  - Children in day care.

EXAM TIP

Retinoblastoma gene is a mutation in the long arm of chromosome 13.

WARD TIP

Must evaluate for the presence of retinoblastoma in a child presenting with strabismus

EXAM TIP

Retinoblastoma is the most common primary malignant intraocular tumor in children.

WARD TIP

Family members of a patient with retinoblastoma should be evaluated; the tumor can be hereditary.

- Children exposed to secondhand smoke.
- Non-breast-fed infants.
- Immunocompromised children.
- Children with craniofacial defects such as cleft palate.
- Children with a strong family history for otitis media.
- Infection incidence is higher in children due to their eustachian tube anatomy, which is more horizontal, shorter in length, and more flaccid.

ETIOLOGY

- Bacteria: *S. pneumonia*, non-typeable *H. influenza*, and *Moraxella catarrhalis*.
- Viral: rhinovirus and respiratory syncytial virus.

COMPLICATIONS

- Hearing loss due to persistent middle-ear effusion.
- Perforation.
- Mastoiditis.
- Cholesteatoma: saclike epithelial structures.
- Facial-nerve paralysis.
- Labyrinthitis.
- Abscess formation.
- Tympanosclerosis: scarring of the tympanic membrane.
- Meningitis.

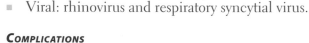

ACUTE OTITIS MEDIA

Eustachian tube dysfunction is the most important factor.

SIGNS AND SYMPTOMS

- Ear tugging.
- Ear pain.
- Fever.
- Malaise.
- Irritability.
- Hearing loss.
- Nausea and vomiting.

DIAGNOSIS

- Pneumatic otoscopy showing a hyperemic, bulging tympanic membrane with decreased mobility and loss of landmarks.
- Tympanocentesis is considered to obtain culture for patients who are <8 weeks old, are immunocompromised, have a complication, or fail multiple antibiotic courses.

TREATMENT

- First-line antibiotic: high-dose amoxicillin.
- Antipyretics: ibuprofen and/or acetaminophen.
- Topical anesthetic eardrops (e.g., benzocaine).
- For healthy children >2 years old with milder case, watchful waiting for 24–48 hours is an option.
- Pneumococcal vaccine has reduced the incidence of acute otitis media.

RECURRENT ACUTE OTITIS MEDIA

DEFINITION

Three to four episodes of acute otitis media in 6 months or 6 episodes in a year.

TREATMENT

- Prophylactic antibiotics.
- Myringotomy and pressure equalization (PE) tubes should be considered.

OTITIS MEDIA WITH EFFUSION

SIGNS AND SYMPTOMS

- Hearing loss.
- Dizziness.
- No fever.
- No ear pain.

DIAGNOSIS

Pneumatic otoscopy reveals a retracted tympanic membrane, loss of landmarks, and air-fluid levels or bubbles

TREATMENT

- If asymptomatic, observe child for 3 months to see if effusion resolves.
- If symptomatic or asymptomatic with effusions for >3 months of observation, treatment includes antibiotics and possibly myringotomy and insertion of PE tubes.

OTITIS EXTERNA

DEFINITION

- Inflammation of the external auditory canal.
- Occurs when trauma introduces bacteria into an excessively wet or dry canal.

ETIOLOGY

- Bacterial: *P. aeruginosa, S. aureus, Proteus mirabilis, Klebsiella pneumoniae*.
- Viral: HSV/Zoster.
- Fungal: *Candida*.

SIGNS AND SYMPTOMS

- Ear pain with movement of the tragus or pinna.
- Pruritus of the ear canal.
- Edema of the ear canal.
- Otorrhea: usually white.
- Palpable lymph nodes: peri- and preauricular.
- Normal tympanic membrane (may be difficult to see).

COMPLICATIONS

- Malignant otitis externa leads to hearing loss, vertigo, and facial-nerve paralysis.
- Temporary hearing loss is secondary to swelling.
- Necrotizing otitis externa:
  - *Pseudomonas* osteomyelitis in the temporal bone.
  - Risk factors: diabetes, immunocompromised (*Aspergillus fumigatus*).

DIAGNOSIS

Otoscopic examination

TREATMENT

Topical antibiotics and steroids are used to treat infection and reduce edema (e.g., Cortisporin suspension [hydrocortisone-polymyxin-neomycin])

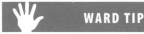

WARD TIP

Otitis externa is known as "swimmer's ear."

EXAM TIP

Malignant otitis externa is caused by *P. aeruginosa* and must be treated systemically (i.e., oral or IV antibiotics; NOT drops alone).

ACUTE MASTOIDITIS

DEFINITION

- Inflammation of the mastoid air cells in the temporal bone.

ETIOLOGY

- Most common pathogens: *S. pneumonia, group A streptococcus, and* non-typeable *H. influenza.*

PATHOPHYSIOLOGY

- Infection and destruction of the mastoid air space.
- Extension may include the petrous portion of the temporal bone.

EPIDEMIOLOGY

Mostly seen in children after/with an acute otitis media

SIGNS AND SYMPTOMS

- Fever.
- Pain and induration behind the ear overlying mastoid air cells and temporal bone.
- Erythema and tenderness over the mastoid area.
- Protruding ear on the affected side.
- Eye pain.

DIAGNOSIS

- Clinically. CT scan can help determine extent of spread.

TREATMENT

- Myringotomy with ventilation tube placement.
- IV antibiotics.
- Mastoidectomy may be necessary.

COMPLICATIONS

- Hearing loss.
- Facial nerve palsy.
- Subperiosteal abscess.
- Cranial osteomyelitis.
- Labyrinthitis.
- Intracranial spread (meningitis, epidural or cerebellar abscess, subdural empyema).
- Dural sinus thrombosis.

TINNITUS

DEFINITION

- Ringing in the ear.
- Seen in children with middle-ear disease, hearing loss, or with salicylate use.

VERTIGO

DEFINITION

Dizziness with the feeling that one's body is in motion

SIGNS AND SYMPTOMS

- Difficulty walking straight, or stumbling.
- Spinning sensation.
- Vomiting.

ETIOLOGY

May occur secondary to the following conditions:
- Otitis media.
- Labyrinthitis.
- Trauma.
- Cholesteatoma.
- BPV.
- Ménière disease.
- CNS disease.

TREATMENT

Address the underlying cause.

Nose

SINUSITIS

DEFINITION

Symptoms of sinus membrane inflammation lasting >10 days, with symptoms that are worsening or lasting a shorter period with severe symptoms, such as high fever

SINUS DEVELOPMENT

- Ethmoid and maxillary sinus at birth.
- Sphenoid sinus 5 years.
- Frontal sinus 7 years.

ETIOLOGY

- A child may be at risk for sinusitis if there is an obstruction or cilia impairment.
- *S. pneumonia*, non-typeable *H. influenza, M. catarrhalis.*
- Rhinovirus is the most common viral pathogen.
- Bacterial sinusitis is usually preceded by a viral upper respiratory infection.

PREDISPOSITIONS

- Occlusion of the sinus ostium.
- Cystic fibrosis.
- Allergy/asthma.
- Dental infections.

SIGNS AND SYMPTOMS

- Headache that worsens when bending forward.
- Sinus tenderness to palpation.
- Persistent nasal discharge (purulent) >10 days duration.
- Halitosis.
- Cough secondary to postnasal drip.
- Early AM nausea or emesis.

WARD TIP

Benign positional vertigo (BPV) will present with ataxia and horizontal nystagmus.

EXAM TIP

Ménière triad includes vertigo, tinnitus, and hearing loss.

EXAM TIP

At birth, only the maxillary and ethmoid sinuses are present.

The most common location for epistaxis in children is from the anterior nasal septum because Kiesselbach's plexus is located there.

Blood in vomit may be present if a child has swallowed blood from epistaxis; always ask about epistaxis if a patient presents with hematemesis.

Isolated nosebleeds are rarely a sign of a bleeding disorder.

Allergic rhinitis is the most common atopic disease.

The "allergic crease" seen in allergic rhinitis—horizontal crease on the nose that occurs from constant rubbing.

Children with allergic rhinitis may exhibit rabbit-like nose wrinkling because of pruritus.

COMPLICATIONS

- Cellulitis.
- Abscess formation.
- Osteomyelitis.
- Meningitis (spread of the ethmoid, sphenoid, or frontal sinuses).

DIAGNOSIS

- Diagnosis is made clinically.
- Rarely need CT scan (plain films are not as sensitive).

TREATMENT

- First line is amoxicillin for 10 days or for 7 days after symptom resolution.
- If no improvement occurs, a macrolide or amoxicillin-clavulanate may be used.
- Decongestants, nasal saline drops/mist, nasal irrigation are often tried, but few data support their use.

EPISTAXIS

DEFINITION

- Nosebleed.

ETIOLOGY/PATHOPHYSIOLOGY

- The most common location is the anterior septum (Kiesselbach plexus).
- The most common cause is trauma secondary to a fingernail.
- Other causes may include foreign bodies, inflammation, or dry air.
- If a child has recurrent, severe epistaxis, consider thrombocytopenia, clotting deficiencies, and angiofibromas.

EPIDEMIOLOGY

- Unusual during infancy; must consider coagulopathy or nasal organic causes (e.g., choanal atresia).

SIGNS AND SYMPTOMS

Bleeding may occur from one or both nostrils.

TREATMENT

- Compression for 10 minutes with head tilted forward.
- Cold compresses to the nose.
- Topical vasoconstrictors to visualize and identify of the bleeding site.
- Cauterization using silver nitrite.
- Packing the nose.

ALLERGIC RHINITIS

DEFINITION

An IgE-mediated nasal mucous membrane response to an allergen

SIGNS AND SYMPTOMS

- Sneezing.
- Watery nasal discharge.
- Red, watery eyes.

- Itchy ears, eyes, nose, and throat.
- Nasal obstruction secondary to edema.

DIAGNOSIS

Characteristic findings on physical examination include:
- Boggy, bluish mucous membranes of the nose.
- Dark circles under the lower eyelids ("allergic shiners").
- Allergic crease (transverse nasal crease from rubbing) and allergic salute (pushing the nose up with the hand).
- A smear of nasal secretions will show a high number of eosinophils.

TREATMENT

- Avoid triggers.
- Antihistamines.
- Decongestants.
- Cromolyn nasal solution.
- Topical steroids.

CHOANAL ATRESIA

DEFINITION

- A uni- or bilateral septum occurs between the nose and the pharynx. A bony septum is found in about 90% of cases.
- It is the most common congenital anomaly of the nose.

SIGNS AND SYMPTOMS

- The presentation depends on the child's ability to mouth breathe.
- Respiratory distress usually improves with crying (mouth is open).
- Cyanosis with feeding or sucking and relief of cyanosis with crying.

DIAGNOSIS

- Inability to pass a catheter through one or both nostrils.
- CT will show the extent of the atresia.

TREATMENT

- Placement of an oral airway, maintaining the mouth in an open position or intubation.
- Tracheostomy or intubation may be required, depending on the severity.
- The ultimate treatment is surgical correction.

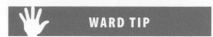

Allergic rhinitis in children may be a precursor for the development of asthma.

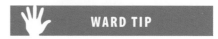

Fifty to seventy percent of children with choanal atresia have other associated congenital anomalies, including CHARGE, Treacher-Collins, Kallmann, VATER (vertebral defects, anal atresia, tracheoesophageal fistula, and renal defects), or Pfeiffer syndromes.

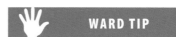

CHARGE syndrome:
Coloboma
Heart disease
Atresia choanae
Retarded growth
Genital anomalies
Ear involvement

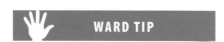

Restenosis of corrected choanal atresia is common.

NOTES

Musculoskeletal Disease

Pediatric Skeleton

- As compared to adults, a child's skeletal anatomy, biomechanics, and physiology result in differences in fracture pattern, diagnostic challenges, and treatment.
- Bone is more porous and elastic than in adults or older adolescents.
- In contrast to adults, pediatric bones have growth plates (physes) and a thick periosteum.
- The physis (growth plate) is a weak site in a child's bone.
- A thick periosteal sleeve helps stabilize fractures.
- Pediatric fractures along the physes are common as compared to adults where sprains are more common.

The Limping Child

- Thorough history and physical.
- Assess gait with patient barefoot.
- Plain-film radiographs typically initial study.
- Consider lab work based on differential diagnosis (i.e., CBC, ESR).
- Differential diagnosis of the limping child listed in Table 20-1.

Growing Pains

DEFINITION

- A diagnosis of exclusion in which children have bilateral, deep leg pain in the evenings or late afternoon

TABLE 20-1. **Differential Diagnosis of the Limping Child**

AGE RANGE	DIFFERENTIAL DIAGNOSIS
1–4	Developmental dysplasia of the hip
	Toxic synovitis
	Toddler's fracture
4–10 years old	Toxic synovitis
	Juvenile idiopathic arthritis
	Legg-Calvé-Perthes
10–18 years old	SCFE
	Osgood-Schlatter
	Gonococcal arthritis
	Fracture
All ages	Sprain
	Contusion
	Osteomyelitis
	Septic arthritis
	Neoplasm

EPIDEMIOLOGY

- Most commonly seen in 4- to 12-year-olds.

ETIOLOGY

- Unknown; is thought to be "overuse" and not "growth" related pain.

SIGNS AND SYMPTOMS

- Pain in late afternoon or evening, including awakening child from sleep.

MANAGEMENT

- Reassurance.
- NSAIDs.
- Exclusion of other diagnostic possibilities such as leukemia.

Newborn Conditions

DEVELOPMENTAL DYSPLASIA OF THE HIP (DDH)

 A 3-month-old female is noted on exam to have her left knee appear lower when her hips are flexed. The infant was born to a G1 now P1 mother via a breech vaginal delivery. *Think: DDH.*

Galeazzi sign, the apparent femur shortening on the side of the dislocated hip, is noted by placing the hips in 90 degrees of flexion and comparing the height of the knees. Screening examination should include the Ortolani test and the Barlow maneuver. DDH risk factors include female gender, breech presentation, and positive family history. Ultrasound can be obtained in infants younger than 6 months. DDH is a treatable condition with good outcomes with early intervention. Pavlik harness is the treatment of choice in the first 6 months of life.

DEFINITION

Abnormal hip growth and development result in an abnormal relationship between the proximal femur and the acetabulum.

EPIDEMIOLOGY

- One in 1000 live births.
- Increased risk with positive family history.
- Girls more common affected, especially if breech delivery.

PATHOPHYSIOLOGY

- At birth, there is a lack of development of both acetabulum and femur.
- Progressive with growth.

SIGNS AND SYMPTOMS

- Newborn:
  - **Ortolani:** maneuver reduces a displaced hip.
  - **Barlow:** provocative test attempting to dislocate an unstable nondisplaced hip.
  - Asymmetric skin folds.
- 3–6 months:
  - Limited abduction.
  - Galeazzi's sign: knee is lower on affected side when hips are flexed.

WARD TIP

A third of leukemias present with bone pain; the diagnosis of growing pains must be made after considering other possibilities.

EXAM TIP

Associated findings with DDH:
- Oligohydramnios
- Twin gestation
- Breech delivery
- Torticollis
- Metatarsus adductus

WARD TIP

Positive **Ortolani test:** Slowly abduct the flexed hip while pressing anteriorly on the greater trochanter. The femoral head will shift into the acetabulum producing a clunk.

WARD TIP

Positive **Barlow test:** The examiner dislocates the hip by flexing and adducting the hip while gently pushing posteriorly, demonstrating instability in the joint.

WARD TIP

X-ray is not helpful in the newborn. After 6–8 weeks, x-rays begin to show signs of dislocation (lateral displacement of the femoral head).

WARD TIP

Signs of instability are more reliable than x-ray in DDH.

EXAM TIP

In DDH, after 3–6 months, muscle development results in the Barlow and Ortolani tests becoming less reliable.

WARD TIP

Triple diapers have no place in the treatment of DDH.

- 12 months:
  - Painless limp and lurch to the affected side.
  - Galeazzi's sign.
  - Lumbar lordosis.

IMAGING

- <6 months: ultrasound.
- >6 months: radiographs (proximal femoral epiphysis ossifies by 4–6 months).
- Ultrasound of the hips recommended at 4 to 6 weeks for all breech newborns.

TREATMENT

- Newborn to 6 months: Pavlik harness (hip flexion and abduction for several months.
- 6 months to 2 years: closed reduction (high failure rate with Pavlik harness).
- >2 years: open reduction to correct acetabulum and femur abnormalities.

METATARSUS ADDUCTUS

DEFINITION

- Medial curvature of the mid-foot.

EPIDEMIOLOGY

- Identified in the first year of life, often at birth.

ETIOLOGY

- Often related to in utero constraint.

SIGNS AND SYMPTOMS

- A "c-shaped" foot.

TREATMENT

- If the foot easily overcorrects with passive motion: observation.
- A foot that corrects easily but does not overcorrect with passive motion: stretching exercises.
- For a foot that cannot be straightened: orthopedic referral, likely needs casting.

TALIPES EQUINOVARUS (CLUBFOOT)

DEFINITION

- Fixed inversion and plantar flexion of the foot.

EPIDEMIOLOGY

- Typically isolated.
- May be familial or associated with syndrome such as trisomy 18 and myelomeningocele.

SIGNS AND SYMPTOMS

- Reduced ankle range of motion.
- Ankle maintained in plantar flexion and inversion.
- Metatarsus adductus.

TREATMENT

- Serial casting.
- Achilles tendon release required if severe or poor outcome with casting.

TORTICOLLIS

DEFINITION

Twisted or wry neck

ETIOLOGY

- Congenital: injury during delivery to the sternocleidomastoid muscle.
- Acquired: rotatory subluxation of the upper cervical spine.

MANAGEMENT

- Congenital: physical therapy for stretching.
- Acquired:
  - Warm soaks.
  - Analgesics.
  - Mild anti-inflammatory agents.
  - Soft cervical collar.
  - Passive stretching.

EXAM TIP

Torticollis is a common cause of neck muscle strain.

The Lower Extremity

- Genu varum (bow legs): legs curve outward at the knees while the feet and ankles touch.
- Genu valgum (knock knees) in which legs are curved inward with knees touching.

INTERNAL TIBIAL TORSION

DEFINITION

- Medial rotation of the tibia.

EPIDEMIOLOGY/ETIOLOGY

- Common cause of intoeing in the child less than 3 years old.
- In utero constraint.

SIGNS AND SYMPTOMS

- Medially pointed foot with patella that faces forward.
- Typically bilateral.

TREATMENT

Observation; self-limited

BLOUNT DISEASE

DEFINITION

- Progressive proximal tibia angulation.

EPIDEMIOLOGY

- More common in obese children and those that walk early.
- Increased incidence in African Americans.

ETIOLOGY

- Inhibition of growth on the medial tibial growth plates resulting in relative lateral tibial overgrowth.

SIGNS AND SYMPTOMS

- Increased angulation at the proximal tibia.
- Lateral thrust with gait.

DIAGNOSIS

- Plain radiographs demonstrate angulation (beaking) of medial metaphysis.

MANAGEMENT

- Splints for mild disease.
- Surgery for severe disease for failed splinting.

RICKETS (SEE ENDOCRINE CHAPTER)

The Spine

IDIOPATHIC SCOLIOSIS

DEFINITION

A curvature of spine in the lateral plane due to an axial rotation of the involved vertebrae (see Figure 20-1)

ETIOLOGY

- Eighty percent of cases are idiopathic.
- Non-idiopathic scoliosis is associated with:
    - Neurofibromatosis.
    - Marfan syndrome.
    - Cerebral palsy.
    - Muscular dystrophy.
    - Poliomyelitis.
    - Myelodysplasia.
    - Congenital vertebral anomalies.

EPIDEMIOLOGY

- Four to five times more common in girls.
- Early adolescence.

SIGNS AND SYMPTOMS

- Usually asymptomatic.
- Severe curvature may lead to restrictive lung disease.

DIAGNOSIS

- On a patient bending forward at the waist, abnormal findings include unilateral asymmetry of the height of the ribs or paravertebral muscles.
- X-ray of entire spine in both the AP and lateral planes.

EXAM TIP

Thirty percent of family members of patients with scoliosis are also affected. Siblings of affected children should be carefully examined.

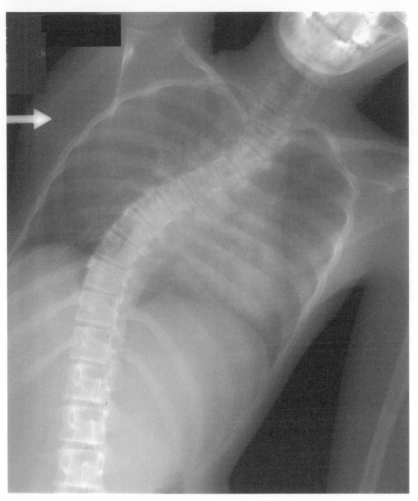

FIGURE 20-1.   **Radiograph of spine demonstrating marked scoliosis.**

MANAGEMENT

Treatment depends on the curve magnitude, skeletal maturity, and risk of progression:

- Curve <25°: physical therapy and back exercises (strengthening back muscles).
- Curve 25–45° in a skeletally immature child: orthopedic back brace, which prevents further curve progression.
- Curve >45°: spinal fusion to correct deformity.

PROGNOSIS

- Curve >60°: associated with poor pulmonary function and shortened life span.
- Curve <40°: usually do not progress; small curves are well tolerated.
- Risk of progression higher in younger childhood.

WARD TIP

Screening for scoliosis should begin at age 6–7 years.

KYPHOSIS

DEFINITION

Posterior curvature of the spine

ETIOLOGY

Scheuermann thoracic kyphosis is a structural deformity of the thoracic spine.

SIGNS AND SYMPTOMS

- Pain.
- Progressive deformity.
- Neurologic compromise.
- Cardiovascular complaints.
- Cosmetic issues.

RADIOLOGY

- Diagnosis is confirmed on lateral radiographs.
- X-ray shows anterior wedging of at least 5° of three or more adjacent thoracic vertebral bodies.

MANAGEMENT

- Bracing/casting for smaller curves and surgery for patients with significant pain.

SPONDYLOLYSIS

DEFINITION

Fracture of the pars interarticularis due to repetitive stress to this area

ETIOLOGY

New bone formation in areas where the annular ligament is stressed.

TYPES

- Congenital: cervical.
- Acquired: lumbar, most often at L5 (85% of cases).

SIGNS AND SYMPTOMS

- Cervical pain.
- Low back pain, worse during the adolescent growth spurt and with spine extension.
- Radicular symptoms are not common.

DIAGNOSIS

Oblique x-ray view of the spine will show the characteristic "Scottie dog sign."

TREATMENT

- NSAIDs.
- Strength and stretching exercises.
- Lumbosacral back brace.

SPONDYLOLISTHESIS

DEFINITION

Anterior or posterior displacement of one vertebral body on the next

SIGNS AND SYMPTOMS

- A palpable "step-off" at the lumbosacral area.
- Limited lumbar flexibility.
- Radicular symptoms more common than spondylolysis.

DIAGNOSIS

Lateral x-ray views show displacement of one vertebral body from another.

WARD TIP

Spondylolysis is the most common cause of low back pain in adolescent athletes. This injury is most commonly seen in gymnasts, dancers, and football players.

EXAM TIP

Degree of displacement in spondylolisthesis is described using the Meyerding classification:

Grade 1: 0–25% displacement
Grade 2: 25–50%
Grade 3: 50–75%
Grade 4: 75–100%
Grade 5: over 100% (spondyloptosis)

MANAGEMENT

Treatment depends on grade of lesion:

- <50% displacement: similar to spondylolysis with close follow-up.
- >50% displacement: surgical stabilization of the unstable segment.

COMPLICATIONS

- Deformity.
- Disability.

DISKITIS

DEFINITION

- Pyogenic infection of the intervertebral disk space.

ETIOLOGY

- Most present prior to 5 years of age.
- Hematogenous seeding of disk space, most commonly S. *aureus*.

SIGNS AND SYMPTOMS

- Moderate to severe pain.
- Fever.
- Pain is localized to the level of involvement and exacerbated by movement.
- Radicular symptoms (pain, weakness, numbness and tingling).

DIAGNOSIS

- MRI is the radiographic study of choice.
- Blood culture (30% positive); biopsy (50%–85% positive).
- Elevated ESR.

MANAGEMENT

- Intravenous antibiotics.
- Surgery is often not necessary unless abscess is identified.

KLIPPEL-FEIL SYNDROME

DEFINITION

Congenital fusion of a variable number of cervical vertebrae

ETIOLOGY

Failure of normal segmentation in the cervical spine

SIGNS AND SYMPTOMS

- Classic clinical triad:
  - Short neck.
  - Low hairline.
  - Limitation of neck motion.
- Associated with:
  - Renal anomalies.
  - Scoliosis.
  - Spina bifida.
  - Deafness.

EXAM TIP

Children at highest risk for diskitis:

- Immunocompromised
- Systemic infections
- Post surgery

WARD TIP

The lumbar spine is the most common site of involvement for diskitis.

WARD TIP

S. aureus is the most common organism causing diskitis.

WARD TIP

Plain radiographs are usually not helpful for early diagnosis of diskitis.

EXAM TIP

Children with Klippel-Feil syndrome are at risk for:

- Atlantoaxial instability
- Neurologic impairment

DIAGNOSIS

Children with Klippel-Feil syndrome should have the following tests performed:
- Renal ultrasound.
- Hearing test.
- Lateral flexion-extension radiographs of cervical spine under fluoroscopy.

TREATMENT

- Annual evaluation.
- Avoid high contact sports.
- Closely evaluate immediate family members.

Infection

OSTEOMYELITIS

 An 18-month-old girl refuses to walk. She has marked tenderness over the distal left femur. She has a temperature of 101.6°F (38.7°C), erythrocyte sedimentation rate (ESR) of 72 mm/hr, and white blood cell (WBC) count of 18,500/mL. Radiographs reveal no bony abnormalities. *Think: Osteomyelitis.*

The initial signs and symptoms are often nonspecific. Refusal to walk, limping, or reluctance to move the affected extremity are common. Fever is usually present. Focal tenderness over a long bone may be an important clue. The WBC count and ESR usually are elevated. Initial plain radiograph may be normal or show only soft tissue swelling. Radionuclide bone scans usually are positive within 48–72 hours of onset of illness. MRI is often used to diagnose focal areas. Bone aspiration may reveal an etiologic agent.

DEFINITION

- Infection of the bone, most commonly bacterial.
- Can be acute or chronic.

EPIDEMIOLOGY

- Median age about 6 years (school-age children).
- Male preponderance.
- Other than with patients with sickle cell disease, no racial differences noted.

ETIOLOGY

- Most often bacterial.
- See Table 20-2 for causes of osteomyelitis by age group.
- Overall, *Staphylococcus aureus* is the most common organism.

PATHOPHYSIOLOGY

- Primarily hematogenous.
- Sluggish blood flow in the capillary bed of the physis allows bacterial invasion. Subsequent inflammation results in infection.
- In smaller children, these blood vessels connect the metaphysis and epiphysis; presentation of osteomyelitis may be a septic joint.
- Other, less common routes:
  - Spread from contiguous infected structures.
  - Direct inoculation (i.e., steeping on nail).
  - Occult injury without breaking skin; disrupted blood flow making bacterial adherence more likely.

TABLE 20-2. Common Causes of Osteomyelitis by Age

AGE GROUP	ORGANISMS
Infants <1 year, especially under age 3 months	*Staphylococcus aureus* *Streptococcus agalactiae* *Escherichia coli* *Neisseria gonorrhoeae*
<5 years	*Staphylococcus aureus* *Streptococcus pyogenes* *Streptococcus pneumoniae* *Kingella kingae*
>5 years	*Staphylococcus aureus* *Streptococcus pyogenes*
Adolescent	*Staphylococcus aureus* *Streptococcus pyogenes* *Neisseria gonorrhoeae*

SIGNS AND SYMPTOMS

- Infants and young children:
  - Fever, irritability, and lethargy.
  - Refusal to walk or bear weight (pseudoparalysis).
- Older children:
  - Fever.
  - May localize pain.
  - Limping.
- Physical examination:
  - Painful local swelling.
  - Point tenderness.
  - Local warmth.
  - Erythema.

DIAGNOSIS

- Positive blood culture.
- Culture of infection site aspiration or bone biopsy.
- Leukocytosis.
- Elevated ESR and C-reactive protein are commonly elevated but not specific; they are commonly used to track response to and duration of therapy.
- Radiographic findings (see Figure 20-2):
  - Lucent areas in bone represent boney matrix destruction.
  - Periosteal and lytic bone changes are seen after substantial bone destruction.
  - Plain films may be normal for up to 14 days after infection.
- Magnetic resonance imaging (MRI):
  - Imaging modality of choice; high sensitivity and specificity.
  - Provides anatomic detail not seen with bone or CT scan.
  - Visualizes soft tissue abscess, bone marrow edema, and bone destruction.
  - Contrast enhancement with gadolinium.
- Radionuclide scintigraphy (bone scan):
  - Common isotopes used include technetium, gallium, and indium.
  - Can detect osteomyelitis onset within 48 hours with about 90% sensitivity.
  - Especially useful in multifocal lesions.

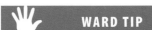

Consider osteomyelitis in any child with decreased use of a limb and fever.

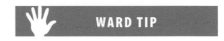

Every attempt should be made to establish a microbiologic diagnosis.

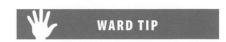

The ESR and CRP can be followed to assess response of osteomyelitis to therapy. They should decrease if treatment is working.

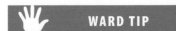

Osteomyelitis without radiographic change should not be treated with antibiotics until an osseous specimen is obtained.

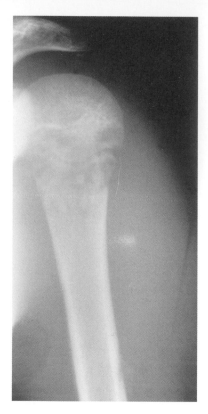

FIGURE 20-2. **Acute hematogenous osteomyelitis of the proximal humerus.** Mottling and patchy radiolucencies are present in the metaphyseal region. (Reproduced, with permission, from Wilson FC, Lin PP. *General Orthopedics.* New York: McGraw-Hill, 1997.)

WARD TIP

Most common cause of polyarticular septic arthritis is *Neisseria gonorrhoeae*.

WARD TIP

Septic arthritis may coexist with osteomyelitis at sites where the metaphysis lies *within* the joint capsule:

- Proximal femur–hip joint
- Proximal humerus–shoulder joint
- Distal lateral tibia–ankle joint
- Proximal radius–elbow joint

WARD TIP

Adolescent intravenous (IV) drug abusers are at risk for gram-negative septic arthritis.

DIFFERENTIAL DIAGNOSIS

- Septic arthritis (can coexist).
- Fracture.
- Cellulitis.
- Transient synovitis.
- Acute leukemia or neuroblastoma.
- Slipped capital femoral epiphysis (SCFE).
- Soft tissue injury or infection.

TREATMENT

- Hospital admission for parenteral antibiotics after obtaining blood, bone, and joint aspirate cultures.
- Infants and children: penicillinase-resistant penicillin (nafcillin or oxacillin) and cephalosporin (cefotaxime).
- Older children (>5 years): nafcillin or, if high rate of MRSA, use vancomycin.
- Consider surgical drainage if:
  - Clear abscess is noted on imaging.
  - Pus is obtained from aspirate.
  - No response occurs after 24–48 hours of antibiotics.
  - After penetrating injury, retained foreign body is suspected.

COMPLICATIONS

- Pathologic fractures.
- Chronic osteomyelitis.
- Leg length discrepancy.

SEPTIC ARTHRITIS

A 14-year-old boy has 2 days of right knee pain. Three days prior, he hit his knee on a pool table. Vitals: Temperature 100.6°F (38.1°C), pulse rate 100, respirations 24. On physical exam, the knee is swollen and tender and is held in flexion. This patient likely has septic arthritis. *Aspiration of the knee for smear and culture is the next step.*

Although more common in children, it occurs in all ages. Trauma can be the precipitant. *S. aureus* is the most common cause. Physical examination may show local erythema, warmth, and swelling. The diagnosis is made by detection of bacteria (culture and/or Gram stain) in synovial fluid aspiration.

DEFINITION

A microbial invasion of joint space

ETIOLOGY

- Neonates:
  - *S. aureus* (most common cause in all ages).
  - *S. agalactiae*.
  - Gram-negative enteric bacilli (*K. kingae*; *Haemophilus influenzae* type b is now rare).
- Older children (similar to osteomyelitis):
  - *S. aureus*
  - *S. pyogenes*
  - *S. pneumoniae*
  - Gonococcus (polyarticular in small joints or monoarticular in a large joint)

EPIDEMIOLOGY

Relatively common in infancy and childhood; can occur in all ages

PATHOPHYSIOLOGY

Organisms may invade the joint by:
- Hematogenous (most common route).
- Direct inoculation.
- Contiguous spread.

SIGNS AND SYMPTOMS

- Pain with passive range of motion.
- Joint stiffness.
- Erythema.
- Edema.
- Limp and unable to bear weight.

LABORATORY

- Complete blood count (CBC)—a normal WBC does not rule out diagnosis.
- ESR and CRP are elevated, although neither specific nor sensitive. They are commonly used to track response to therapy.
- Blood culture.
- Joint aspiration with fluid analysis is the definitive test.

MANAGEMENT

- Hospital admission for parenteral antibiotics after obtaining blood and joint aspirate cultures.
- Septic joints are orthopedic emergencies; intraoperative joint washout may be required.
- Antibiotic therapy is similar to osteomyelitis above.

COMPLICATIONS

- Potential for severe complications:
  - Hematogenous or local spread – can result in osteomyelitis.
  - Avascular necrosis.
  - Angular deformities.
  - Leg length discrepancy.

TRANSIENT SYNOVITIS (AKA TOXIC SYNOVITIS)

An 18-month-old infant has a limp that progressed to refusal to bear weight on her left leg. When lying in bed, she is not in distress but has left hip pain with range of motion. No swelling, redness, or warmth is noted. Patient had a febrile URI 4 days prior.

DEFINITION

- Reactive arthritis.
- Common cause of hip pain in children.
- Occurs in children between 3 and 10 years of age, more commonly in boys.

ETIOLOGY

- Cause remains uncertain.
- Often follows an upper respiratory infection (URI).

SIGNS AND SYMPTOMS

- Unilateral hip or groin pain is the most common complaint.
- Painful limp.
- Usually afebrile and nontoxic appearance.

EXAM TIP

The major consequence of bacterial invasion of a joint is permanent damage to joint cartilage.

WARD TIP

Candida albicans must be considered in neonates and premature infants with septic arthritis or osteomyelitis, especially if a central line is in place.

WARD TIP

Hip pathology may present as knee or anterior thigh pain secondary to referred pain. Remember to always evaluate the hip with complaints of knee pain.

EXAM TIP

Most cases of septic arthritis occur in weight-bearing (hip or knee) joints and involve a single joint (monoarticular).

EXAM TIP

The knee is the most frequently infected pediatric joint, but infection of the hip may also have severe consequences.

WARD TIP

Fever is not necessary for diagnosis of septic arthritis.

WARD TIP

The most common mimic of septic arthritis is transient synovitis. Examining the joint aspirate can differentiate.

DIAGNOSIS

- Transient synovitis and septic arthritis have similar presentations. Where doubt exists, ultrasound-guided or fluoroscopically guided diagnostic aspiration should be performed.
- Radiographs usually are normal.
- Most patients will have fluid in the joint visible on ultrasound, which does not distinguish septic arthritis from transient synovitis.
- ESR, CRP and WBC usually are normal.

MANAGEMENT

- First, rule out septic arthritis.
- Supportive therapy.
- Nonsteroidal anti-inflammatory drugs (NSAIDs).
- Complete recovery occurs within about a week.

Trauma

BUCKLE (TORUS) FRACTURE

- Definition: impaction injury in which the bone cortex is buckled but not disrupted (Figure 20-3).
- Occurs with axial loading onto long bone under compression (e.g. fall on outstretched hand).
- Treatment: 3 to 4 weeks of cast or splint for this stable fracture.

GREENSTICK FRACTURE

- Definition: a break in the convex cortex under tension caused by the bending of malleable bone (Figure 20-3).
- Incomplete fracture in which cortex is disrupted on one side only.
- Represents bone failure on the tension side and a plastic or bend deformity on the compression side.
- Treatment: Manipulative reduction is required for this unstable fracture.

TODDLER FRACTURE

- Definition: nondisplaced spiral fracture of the tibia (Figure 20-4).
- Typically seen in the 2- to 3-year-old.
- Symptoms include pain, refusal to walk, and minor swelling.
- No or minimal history of a twisting motion of the leg with a planted foot is present.
- Treatment: immobilization for a few weeks to protect the limb and to relieve pain.

SALTER-HARRIS FRACTURE CLASSIFICATION

See Figure 20-5.

INJURIES & OVERUSE

Sprains

DEFINITION

- **Sprain:** injury to ligament.
- **Strain:** injury to muscle-tendon unit.

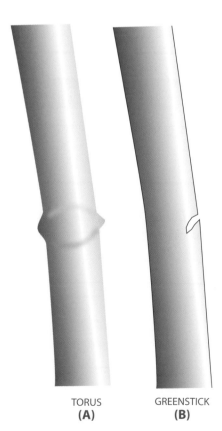

TORUS **(A)**   GREENSTICK **(B)**

FIGURE 20-3. Torus fracture (A) and Greenstick fracture (B).

ANKLE SPRAIN

- Inversion: injury to lateral ligament (85%)
  - Anterior talofibular injures first.
  - Posterior talofibular—severe pain.
- Eversion: injury to medial ligament (5%)
  - Deltoid ligament injury most common.
  - May be more severe than inversion.

SIGNS AND SYMPTOMS

- Grade I: minimal pain/tenderness without loss of motion; weakened.
- Grade II: pain/tenderness; some swelling; difficulty walking; ecchymosis.
- Grade III: significant swelling and ecchymosis; inability to bear weight; unstable joint; disruption of ligament; articular cartilage may be torn.

MANAGEMENT

- The treatment goal is to reduce local edema and residual stiffness.
- PRICE therapy: protection, rest, ice, compression, elevation.
- Protection includes joint immobilization, elastic bandage wrap, and Jones's dressing (a padded, bulky gauze bandage dressing and elastic wrap) for more severe injuries. Splinting protects against injury and relieves swelling and pain.
- Crutches and crutch gait training.
- NSAIDs as needed for analgesia.
- For milder injury, early joint use and rehabilitation are key to healing.

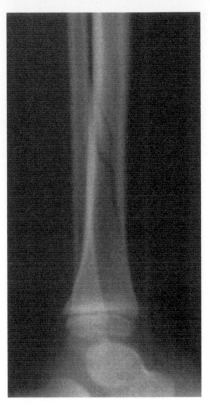

FIGURE 20-4. Toddler fracture. (Reproduced, with permission, from Schwartz DT, Reisdorff BJ. *Emergency Radiology.* New York: McGraw-Hill, 2000: 602.)

 WARD TIP

Sprain is a diagnosis of exclusion in children. Pain greater over the ligaments than bone suggests sprain. Pain greater over the bone than ligament suggests fracture.

Salter-Harris Type I:
- Fracture through the physis (growth plate only)
- Often seen in children < 5 years
- Only visible radiographically if the physis is widened, distorted or the epiphysis is distorted

Salter-Harris Type II:
- Through the metaphysis and the physis
- Most common sites are distal radius & tibia

Salter-Harris Type III:
- Through the epiphysis and physis
- Most common sites are knee ankle

Salter-Harris Type IV:
- Through the epiphysis, physis, and metaphysis
- Most common site is lateral condyle of humerus
- Can produce joint deformity and chronic disability

Salter-Harris Type V:
- Crush injury of the physis
- May appear as a narrowing of the growth plate lucency
- Often not radiographically visible
- May lead to premature fusion
- The proximal tibia is the most common site for growth disturbance
- Mechanism is axial compression

FIGURE 20-5. Salter-Harris fracture classification.

KNEE SPRAINS AND INJURIES

DEFINITION

- May be external (medial and lateral collateral ligaments), internal (anterior and posterior cruciate ligaments), or injuries to the menisci.
- The most common injuries are medial collateral and anterior cruciate ligaments.
- Valgus forces result in medial collateral, anterior cruciate, and, with external rotation, results in medial meniscus injury.
- Varus force results in lateral collateral and/or anterior cruciate ligament injury.
- Anterior and posterior forces with hyperextension result in anterior and posterior cruciate ligament injuries.

SIGNS AND SYMPTOMS

- Popping sound often heard with anterior cruciate ligament tear.
- Pain over damaged ligament or over the joint plane for meniscal injuries.
- Swelling.

DIAGNOSIS

- Clinical in most cases.
- Radiographs to exclude fractures.

TREATMENT

- PRICE therapy: protection, rest, ice, compression, elevation.
- Orthopedic referral for severe injuries.

SEVER DISEASE (APOPHYSITIS OF THE CALCANEUS)

DEFINITION

- Inflammation of the growth plate in the heel.

EPIDEMIOLOGY

- More common in late childhood and early adolescence.

ETIOLOGY

- Overuse of the tendons of the foot.

SIGNS AND SYMPTOMS

- Posterior and plantar heel pain, especially with physical activity.
- Outward signs are rare; pain with squeezing of the area.

THERAPY

- PRICE therapy: protection, rest, ice, compression, elevation.
- Pre-exercise stretching.
- NSAIDs as needed for analgesia.

PATELLOFEMORAL SYNDROME

DEFINITION

- Knee pain caused by increased contact pressure between the patella and femur.

EPIDEMIOLOGY

- Most common in adolescent girls.
- Worsened with walking on stairs.

ETIOLOGY

- Unknown.

SIGNS AND SYMPTOMS

Pain anteriorly around and under the patella

TREATMENT

- Rest.
- Quadriceps stretching exercises.

SUBLUXATION OF RADIAL HEAD (NURSEMAID'S ELBOW)

A 2-year-old boy has left arm pain. He holds his arm in a flexed, pronated position and refuses to supinate his forearm. His mother remembers pulling him by the arm yesterday after he tried to run into the street. *Think: Subluxation of the radial head (nursemaid's elbow).*

Subluxation of the radial head is a common elbow injury in the 2- to 4-year-old child. It is due to a sudden longitudinal forearm pull while the child's arm is in pronation. Child keeps his arm in passive pronation, with slight flexion at the elbow. Imaging is not required if the history is consistent.

DEFINITION

Subluxation of the radial head

ETIOLOGY

- Slippage of the radius head under a stretched annular ligament.
- The most common cause is axial traction (e.g., holding child's hand while falling).

EPIDEMIOLOGY

- Common age: 1–4 years.
- Rare after the age of 6 years (annular ligament becomes thick and strong by age 5 years).

SIGNS AND SYMPTOMS

- Child suddenly refuses to use an arm.
- Elbow fully pronated/inability of the child to supinate the arm.
- No swelling or bony tenderness on exam.

DIAGNOSIS

- Diagnosis is made primarily by history.
- Imaging studies are unnecessary.

MANAGEMENT

- Elbow is placed in full supination and slowly moved to full flexion.
- Alternatively, overpronation with full extension of the forearm.
- A click at the radial head signifies reduction (see Figure 20-6).
- Relief of pain is remarkable and rapid.

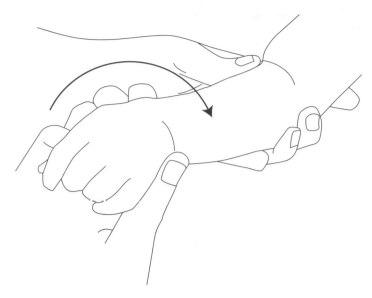

FIGURE 20-6. Reduction of nursemaid's elbow.

OSGOOD-SCHLATTER DISEASE

A 16-year-old boy has right knee pain. He is active in multiple sports. On examination, he has significant tenderness and swelling over the tibial tuberosity. He is otherwise healthy. *Think: Osgood-Schlatter disease;* treat with activity restriction.

Osgood-Schlatter disease is a common, chronic overuse injury of the knee. It occurs due to forceful contraction of the extensor mechanism in sports such as jumping. Tenderness over the proximal tibial tuberosity at the site of patellar insertion is often present. While clinically diagnosed, plain radiographs are helpful to rule out other causes of knee pain.

DEFINITION

- Proximal tibial physis inflammation where the patellar tendon inserts on the tibia.
- Benign, self-limited extra-articular disease.

ETIOLOGY

- Traction apophysitis/repetitive trauma.
- Chronic microtrauma to the tibial tuberosity due to quadriceps muscle overuse.

RISK FACTORS

- Boys between ages 10 and 15 years.
- Rapid skeletal growth.
- Involvement in repetitive jumping sports.

SIGNS AND SYMPTOMS

- Knee pain (tibial tuberosity pain).
- Reproduced by extending the knee against resistance.
- Normal knee joint examination.
- Tibial tuberosity swelling.
- Absence of effusion or condylar tenderness.

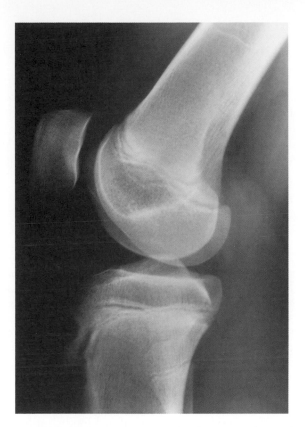

FIGURE 20-7. **Osgood-Schlatter disease.** Note the elevation and irregularity of the tibial tubercle. (Reproduced, with permission, from Wilson FC, Lin PP. *General Orthopedics.* New York: McGraw-Hill, 1997.)

DIAGNOSIS

- Diagnosis is clinical.
- Knee X-ray may show tibial tubercle fragmentation (see Figure 20-7) or patellar tendon calcification. Compare with opposite side.

TREATMENT

- Relative rest with graded return to activity.
- Knee immobilizer only for severe cases.

OSTEOCHONDRITIS DISSECANS

DEFINITION

Avascular necrosis of subchondral bone, often an overuse injury

SIGNS AND SYMPTOMS

- Vague pain (typically in the knee or ankle).
- With joint flexed, may be able to palpate defect below articular cartilage.
- May present as a loose body in the joint with a feeling of "catching" or locking."
- Most common in the lateral portion of medial femoral condyle.

DIAGNOSIS

- X-rays show characteristic appearance of subcondylar osteonecrosis.
- MRI may be useful to confirm diagnosis.

TREATMENT

- Children <11 years—typically observed with serial radiographs to assess healing.
- Adolescents—excision of loose fragments if small; replacement with fixation if large. Sometimes the area can be drilled to promote revascularization and healing.

PROGNOSIS

Typically good with appropriate intervention.

Legg-Calvé-Perthes Disease

 A 6-year-old boy has hip and knee pain, and he has been limping. He cannot abduct or internally rotate his hip. *Think: Legg-Calvé-Perthes disease.*
Legg-Calvé-Perthes disease is avascular necrosis of the femoral head. It is due to vascular changes within the proximal femur. Limping is the most common symptom. Pain may be poorly localized in the groin or referred to the thigh or knee joint. **Thigh or knee pain in the child may be due to hip pathology**. Plain x-rays of the hip are helpful in making the diagnosis. It occurs at an earlier age than slipped capital femoral epiphysis (SCFE).

DEFINITION

Avascular necrosis of femoral head occurs after blood supply disruption to the proximal femoral epiphysis.

ETIOLOGY

- Idiopathic; may be a combination of genetic and environmental factors.

EPIDEMIOLOGY

- Four times more common boys.
- Highest incidence between 4 to 8 years of age.

SIGNS AND SYMPTOMS

- Most common presentation is "painless limp."
- Pain (activity related and relieved by rest) can be a presenting sign.
  - Pain may be in groin, anteriorly in the hip region, around the greater trochanter, or **referred to the knee**.
- Hip motion is limited, particularly abduction and internal rotation.

WARD TIP

Classic presentation of Legg-Calvé-Perthes disease is a "painless limp."

RADIOLOGY

- Anteroposterior and frog-leg lateral position radiographic findings correlate with the progression and extent of necrosis (see Figure 20-8).
- Early: decreased size of ossification center, widening of the medial joint space.
- Middle: fragmentation of the epiphysis, collapse of the femoral head.
- Late: new bone (reossification) replaces necrotic femoral head.

MANAGEMENT

- Pediatric orthopedic consultation.
- Abduction orthoses to "contain" the femoral head on the acetabulum.
- Rest and NSAIDs.
- Surgery may be required, especially for children over 8 years of age.

COMPLICATIONS

Limb length discrepancy

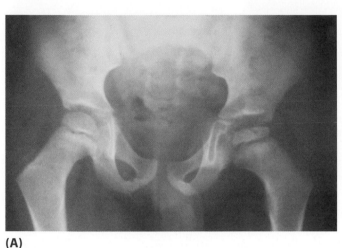
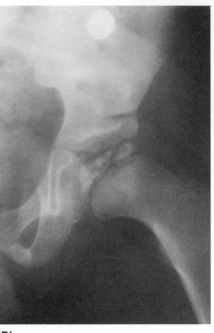

(A)   **(B)**

FIGURE 20-8. **Radiograph of pelvis demonstrating changes of Legg-Calvé-Perthes disease.** Note the sclerotic, flattened, and fragmented right femoral head. (Reproduced, with permission, from McMahon PJ, Skinner HB, eds. *Current Diagnosis & Treatment in Orthopedics.* 6th ed. New York: McGraw-Hill, 2021.)

Slipped Capital Femoral Epiphysis (SCFE)

 An obese 14-year-old boy has left anterior thigh pain for 2 months. He has limited passive flexion and internal rotation of his hip. *Think: SCFE.*
SCFE is a common adolescent hip disorder occurring with a pubertal growth spurt. Referred pain (groin, thigh, or knee pain) is common. AP and frog-leg lateral pelvic views should be obtained.

DEFINITION

- Type of Salter I fracture of the proximal femoral growth plate.
- Disruption of the proximal femoral epiphysis through the physial plate.
- Epiphysis usually displaced medially and posteriorly.

ETIOLOGY

- Most cases are idiopathic.
- The growth plate is weak (physis is weak prior to closure).

EPIDEMIOLOGY

- Occurs with a growth spurt: boys 13 to 15; girls 11 to 13.
- More common in African Americans.
- Between 20% and 40% present with or develop bilateral disease.

RISK FACTORS

- Obesity.
- Hypothyroidism.
- Hypopituitarism.
- Growth hormone (GH) administration.
- Renal osteodystrophy.

 WARD TIP

Knee pain in a child warrants a complete hip examination.

 EXAM TIP

SCFE is a commonly missed time-sensitive pediatric orthopedic problem.

 WARD TIP

Remember, slips can occur in children of normal weight.

 WARD TIP

MRI can reveal avascular necrosis, whereas conventional radiographs may appear normal.

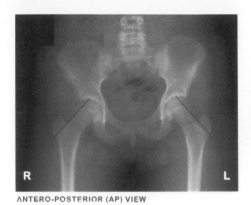

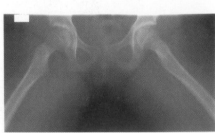

FROG LEG VIEW

ANTERO-POSTERIOR (AP) VIEW

FIGURE 20-9. Hip radiographs in a 13-year-old girl with mildly slipped capital femoral epiphysis (SCFE) on the right. Note on the AP view that a line drawn along the superior border of the femoral neck (Klein line) shows less femoral head superior to the line on the right than it does in the normal hip on the left.

SIGNS AND SYMPTOMS

- Limping, often painful.
- Pain can be located anywhere between the groin and medial knee.
- Obligate abduction and external hip rotation occurs with passive or active hip flexion.
- Leg tends to roll into external rotation at rest.

DIAGNOSIS

- Bilateral AP and frog-leg lateral radiographs (Figure 20-9)
  - Ice cream scoop (epiphysis) falling off its cone.
  - The frog-leg lateral film most helpful.
- Earliest sign is widening of epiphysis.
- Consider endocrinology evaluation for presentations less than 10 or greater than 16 years of age.

COMPLICATIONS

- Avascular necrosis of capital femoral epiphysis.
- Chondrolysis.
- Nonunion.
- Premature closure of the epiphyseal plate.

TREATMENT

- Orthopedic consultation.
- Immediate bedrest.
- *In situ* pinning with a single large screw (Figure 20-10).

Juvenile Idiopathic Arthritis (JIA)

DEFINITION

Chronic disease characterized by inflammation of the joints

ETIOLOGY

Unknown; autoimmune disorder, likely caused by a combination of immune mechanisms, genetics, and environmental exposure

DIAGNOSTIC CRITERIA

- Age of onset under 16 years.
- Arthritis in one or more joints.

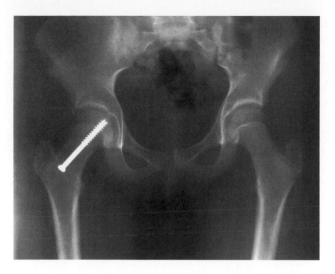

FIGURE 20-10. **SCFE after screw fixation (same patient as Figure 20-9).**

- Duration ≥6 weeks.
- Exclusion of other causes.
- See Table 20-3 for diagnosis based on joint fluid analysis.

SIGNS AND SYMPTOMS

- Polyarticular (about 25% of cases):
  - Five or more joints.
  - Female predominance; onset typically 1 to 3 years of age and early adolescence.
  - Symmetric, chronic pain and swelling of joints.
  - Both large and small joints.
  - Less prominent systemic features.
  - Two categories: rheumatoid factor (RF) positive and RF negative.
  - Long-term arthritis; symptoms wax and wane.
- Pauciarticular (about 40% of cases):
  - Fewer than five joints.
  - Female predominance; onset typically 1 to 3 years of age.
  - Asymmetric chronic arthritis of a few large joints.
  - Systemic features are uncommon.
  - Iridocyclitis (20%), 80% of which will be ANA positive.

TABLE 20-3. **Joint Fluid Analysis**

DISORDER	CELLS/ML	GLUCOSE
Trauma	RBC > WBC < 2000 WBC	Normal
Reactive arthritis	2000–10,000 mononuclear WBC	Normal
Juvenile idiopathic arthritis	5000–50,000 WBC, mostly neutrophils	Low to normal
Septic arthritis	>50,000 WBC, usually >90% neutrophils	Low to normal

(Reproduced, with permission, from Hay WW, et al. *Current Pediatric Diagnosis and Treatment,* 14th ed. New York: McGraw-Hill. 2002.)

- RF rarely positive; if positive, portends progression to polyarticular disease.
- ANA positive eventually positive in majority.
- Systemic (about 10% of cases):
  - No gender predominance; onset peaks at 5 to 10 years of age.
  - Salmon-pink macular rash.
  - Systemic symptoms: arthritis, fever, hepatosplenomegaly, leukocytosis, and polyserositis.
  - In contrast to oligo- or pauciarticular disease, leukocytosis, thrombocytosis, and elevated ESR and CRP are common.
  - RF is usually negative.
  - It may require bone marrow or lymph node biopsy to exclude malignant diseases.

TREATMENT

The goal of treatment is to restore function, relieve pain, and maintain joint motion.

- NSAIDs.
- Range-of-motion and muscle-strengthening exercises.
- Steroids, methotrexate, anti-tumor necrosis factor (TNF) antibodies, or antipyrimidine medication for patients who do not respond to NSAIDs.

Spondyloarthritides

DEFINITION

- A collection of diseases including juvenile ankylosing spondylitis, reactive arthritis following gastrointestinal or genitourinary infections, and arthritis related to inflammatory bowel disease or psoriasis.

ETIOLOGY

Unknown. RF, ANA, and other disease-specific markers are typically absent.

SIGNS AND SYMPTOMS/DIAGNOSIS

- Juvenile ankylosing spondylitis
  - Male predominance.
  - Associated with human lymphocyte antigen (HLA)-B27.
  - Sacroiliac joint or lumbosacral pain.
- Reactive arthritis
  - Reiter syndrome: triad of asymmetric arthritis, urethritis, and uveitis caused by *Chlamydia trachomatis*.
  - Enteric pathogen infection: *Salmonella*, *Shigella*, *Yersinia*, *Campylobacter*, *Mycoplasma*, and *Ureaplasma*.
  - Asymmetric, especially of the lower extremities.
- Arthritis related to inflammatory bowel disease
  - Waxing/waning pattern of disease in large joints of lower extremities.
  - If HLA B27 positive, pattern similar to ankylosing spondylitis.
- Arthritis related to psoriasis
  - Small or large joints.
  - Dactylitis, nail pitting, and onycholysis typically seen.
  - May not have psoriasis but rather history in first-degree relative.
  - About 50% are ANA positive.

TREATMENT

- The goal of treatment is to restore function, relieve pain, and maintain joint motion.
- NSAIDs.

Dermatomyositis/Polymyositis

DEFINITION

- Represent a group of autoimmune disorders of unknown etiology involving skeletal muscle and cutaneous inflammation.
- Polymyositis primarily affects skeletal muscle.
- Dermatomyositis: skin eruption and myopathy.

EPIDEMIOLOGY

- Girls are affected more commonly than boys.
- Age 5–14 years.

SIGNS AND SYMPTOMS

- Progressive symmetric proximal muscle weakness.
- Violaceous rash: symmetric, erythematous rash on extensor surfaces (Gottron papules), upper eyelids (heliotrope rash), and knuckles.
- Worrisome triad (not common):
  - Dysphagia.
  - Dysphonia.
  - Dyspnea.

DIAGNOSIS

- Classic presentation as described.
- ESR, serum CK, and aldolase reflect disease activity.
- Electromyography distinguishes myopathic from neuropathic muscle weakness.

TREATMENT

- Prednisone.
- Intravenous immune globulin, cyclosporine, or methotrexate in refractory cases.

PROGNOSIS

Prognosis has improved significantly with the use of steroids; however, some may have prolonged symptoms including impaired muscle function.

EXAM TIP

In adults, dermatomyositis and polymyositis are associated with malignancy and rheumatic disease. Myositis is not associated with cancer in children.

WARD TIP

Dermatomyositis affects proximal muscles more than distal muscles, and weakness usually starts in the legs. An inability to climb stairs may be the first warning sign.

Muscular Dystrophies

DUCHENNE MUSCULAR DYSTROPHY (DMD)

 A 3-year-old boy must use his hands to push himself up when rising from a seated position. *Think: Gower's sign.*
The Gower sign indicates proximal muscle weakness (decreased ability to rise from the floor without upper extremity assistance). DMD is an X-linked recessive trait. Children with DMD usually reach early motor milestones; the diagnosis may be delayed until 3 and 6 years of age. Creatine kinase (CK) is 50–100 times normal. DNA analysis confirms the diagnosis.

DEFINITION

Degenerative disease of muscles: DMD is characterized by early childhood onset, typically before 5 years of age.

EXAM TIP

DMD is the most common muscular dystrophy.

INHERITANCE

- X-linked recessive.
- One in 3,300 males.

SIGNS AND SYMPTOMS

- Clumsiness.
- Easy fatigability.
- Symmetric involvement.
- Proximal limb involvement before distal.
- Pelvic girdle, with shoulder girdle usually later.
- Rapid progression.
- Loss of ambulation by 13 years.
- Pseudohypertrophy of calves.
- Cardiomyopathy in all patients by about 18 years of age.

DIAGNOSIS

- Serum CK is markedly elevated.
- Muscle biopsy: degeneration, regeneration, variation in fiber size and proliferation of connective tissue; no dystrophin present.
- Genetic testing.

MANAGEMENT/PROGNOSIS

- Encourage ambulation.
- Prevent contractures with passive stretching.
- Death common by late teens/early 20s due to respiratory insufficiency or cardiomyopathy.

EXAM TIP

DMD is associated with:
- Intellectual disability
- Cardiomyopathy

EXAM TIP

Death in patients with DMD occurs through cardiac or respiratory failure.

BECKER MUSCULAR DYSTROPHY (BMD)

DEFINITION

Milder form of muscular dystrophy compared to DMD

INHERITANCE

X-linked recessive

SIGNS AND SYMPTOMS

- Late childhood onset, typically between 5 and 15 years.
- Slow progression.
- Proximal muscle weakness.
- Prominence of calf muscles.
- Inability to walk occurs after 16 years.
- Intellectual disability less common than DMD.
- About one third will have some form of intellectual disability.

DIAGNOSIS

- Serum CK is markedly elevated.
- It is similar to DMD, but dystrophin is present, although reduced or abnormal.
- Genetic testing.

MANAGEMENT/PROGNOSIS

Similar to DMD although death delayed until the 30s or beyond

MYOTONIC MUSCULAR DYSTROPHY (MMD)

INHERITANCE

Autosomal dominant

SIGNS AND SYMPTOMS

- Congenital MMD affects infants and can be severe.
- Adult-onset MMD has a variable onset, typically in the teens to adulthood.
- Voluntary muscle weakness in the face, distal limbs, and diaphragm.
- Involuntary clenching of hands and jaw, ptosis, and respiratory difficulty.
- Endocrinopathies commonly found.

DIAGNOSIS

- Genetic testing.

MANAGEMENT/PROGNOSIS

- Similar to DMD.
- Neonatal form has poor prognosis, often requiring ventilation and feeding tube.

LIMB GIRDLE MUSCULAR DYSTROPHY

DEFINITION

A muscular dystrophy that affects predominately proximal muscles early and sparing distal and facial muscles

INHERITANCE

Most cases autosomal recessive, with high sporadic incidence

SIGNS AND SYMPTOMS

- Variable age of onset; childhood (not congenital) to early adult.
- Pelvic girdle usually involved first and to greater extent.
- Shoulder girdle often asymmetric.

DIAGNOSIS

- Muscle biopsy shows dystrophic muscle changes.
- Genetic testing.

MANAGEMENT

- Promote ambulation.
- Physiotherapy.
- Mildly progressive, life expectancy mid to late adulthood.

FACIOSCAPULOHUMERAL MUSCULAR DYSTROPHY

INHERITANCE

Autosomal dominant

SIGNS AND SYMPTOMS

- Variable.
- Typically, slow progression with presentation in the second or third decade.
- Infantile form, rare, but rapidly progressive with early loss of ambulation.
- Diminished facial movements: inability to close eyes, smile, or whistle.

- Weakness of the shoulder girdle: difficulty raising arms over head.
- Normal life span for adult onset.

Connective Tissue Diseases

MARFAN SYNDROME

DEFINITION

Genetic defect of genes coding for the connective tissue protein fibrillin

INHERITANCE

Classically autosomal dominant

SIGNS AND SYMPTOMS

- Musculoskeletal:
    - Tall stature.
    - Long, thin digits (arachnodactyly).
    - Hyperextensible joints.
    - High arched palate.
- Cardiac: dilation of the aortic root.
- Pulmonary: propensity to develop spontaneous pneumothorax.
- Ocular: ectopia lentis—lens dislocation (which progresses over time).

DIAGNOSIS

- Clinical findings as described above.
- Genetic testing (mutation of FBN1 gene).

TREATMENT

- Early recognition and treatment of complications.
- Beta blockers to reduce myocardial contractility and aortic root dilation.

PROGNOSIS

Generally good with attention to cardiac complications

EHLERS-DANLOS SYNDROME (EDS)

DEFINITION

Group of genetically heterogenous connective tissue disorders

ETIOLOGY

- Quantitative deficiency of collagen causing poor cross-linking of collagen.
- Autosomal dominant.

SIGNS AND SYMPTOMS

- Children with EDS are normal at birth.
- Skin hyperelasticity.
- Fragility of the skin and blood vessels.
- Joint hypermobility.
- Propensity for tissue rupture.

EXAM TIP

The most worrisome complications of Marfan syndrome are aortic dilation, aortic regurgitation, and aortic aneurysms.

WARD TIP

Type IV EDS is associated with a weakened uterus, blood vessels, or intestines. It is important to identify patients with EDS type IV because of the grave consequences of the disease. Women with EDS type IV should be counseled to avoid pregnancy.

MANAGEMENT

DIAGNOSIS

- Clinical findings as described above.
- Genetic testing.

TREATMENT

- Symptomatic.
- Preventative including echocardiograms depending on diagnosed type.
- Prolonged wound fixation.
- Genetic counseling.

PROGNOSIS

Generally good but reduced life span with type IV

Benign Bone Lesions

OSTEOID OSTEOMA

DEFINITION

Reactive lesion of bone of unknown etiology

SIGNS AND SYMPTOMS

- Pain (evening or at night), relieved with NSAIDs.
- Point tenderness.

RADIOLOGY

Osteosclerosis surrounds a small radiolucent nidus.

MANAGEMENT

- NSAIDs relieve pain.
- Surgical resection of the nidus is curative.

PROGNOSIS

Prognosis is excellent. Malignant transformation does not occur; the lesion may recur.

ENCHONDROMA

DEFINITION

Cartilaginous lesions

SIGNS AND SYMPTOMS

- Swelling occurs in the tubular bones, most commonly, the hands.
- Pathologic fractures may be a presenting sign.
- Ollier disease (if multiple lesions are present).

RADIOLOGY

Radiolucent diaphyseal or metaphyseal lesion

MANAGEMENT

Surgical curettage

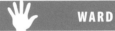

WARD TIP

Osteoid osteomas are most common in the femur and tibia.

EXAM TIP

Enchondromas have a predilection for the phalanges.

PROGNOSIS

Prognosis is good. Malignant transformation is very rare in childhood.

OSTEOCHONDROMA (EXOSTOSIS)

DEFINITION

- A common, benign cartilage-capped protrusion of osseous tissue arising from the bone surface.

SIGNS AND SYMPTOMS

- Painless, hard, nontender mass.
- Distal metaphysis of distal femur, proximal humerus, and proximal tibia.
- Grows with child until skeletal maturity.

RADIOLOGY

Pedunculated or sessile mass in the metaphyseal region of the bone

MANAGEMENT

Excision if symptomatic

PROGNOSIS

Prognosis is excellent. Malignant transformation is very rare in children.

BAKER (POPLITEAL) CYSTS

DEFINITION

- Isolated fluid filled bursa or a herniation of the knee joint synovium into the popliteal region.

SIGNS AND SYMPTOMS

- Popliteal mass, sometimes presents with discomfort.
- Commonly transilluminates.

DIAGNOSIS

- Plain radiographs to rule out other conditions.
- Ultrasound, MRI, or aspiration of mucinous fluid are rarely required.

MANAGEMENT

- This benign lesion typically resolves over time; surgery is rarely needed.
- Corticosteroid injection can reduce inflammation.

WARD TIP

It is important to exclude deep vein thrombosis (DVT) in patients with a popliteal cyst and leg swelling.

EXAM TIP

Baker cysts are the most common mass in the popliteal fossa.

Osteogenesis Imperfecta (OI)

A 2-year-old child has a right radial fracture after bumping his arm. An x-ray shows multiple healing fractures. He has blue sclera, thin skin, and hypoplastic teeth. *Think: OI.* Triad: fragile bones, blue sclerae, and early deafness. The teeth frequently have dentinogenesis imperfecta: normal enamel, but dysplastic dentin. Radiographic appearance may vary according to the disease type and its severity, and it may include osteopenia and fractures. In infancy, these features may result in evaluation for nonaccidental injury.

DEFINITION

- Inherited connective tissue disorder, characterized by poor bone mineralization leading to multiple and recurrent fractures.
- "Classic" OI is an autosomal-dominant disorder that occurs in all racial and ethnic groups.

ETIOLOGY

- More than 150 mutations in the genes that encode for type 1 collagen.
- Four commonly discussed types of OI:
  - Types I and IV are milder, presenting with increased fracture risk.
  - Type II is lethal in the newborn period.
  - Type III is severe, causing significant bony deformity secondary to multiple fractures.

SIGNS AND SYMPTOMS

- Bone fragility with repeated fracture after mild trauma.
- Easy bruising.
- Deafness.
- Blue sclera.
- Hyperextensibility of ligaments.
- Normal intelligence.

EXAM TIP

Type I collagen fibers are found in bones, organ capsules, fascia, cornea, sclera, tendons, meninges, and the dermis.

DIAGNOSIS

Radiographic findings:
- Osteopenia.
- Wormian bones ("floating" intrasutural bones of the skull seen in OI).
- Thin cortices.
- Bowing.
- Normal callus formation.
- Collagen synthesis analysis.

TREATMENT

- Bisphosphonates.
- Surgical correction of long-bone deformities.
- Trauma prevention.

PROGNOSIS

Prognosis is poor, and most patients are confined to wheelchairs by adulthood.

Charcot-Marie-Tooth

DEFINITION

- Hereditary motor and sensory neuropathy

EPIDEMIOLOGY/ETIOLOGY

- Most common form is autosomal dominant demyelinating polyneuropathy (CMT1).

SIGNS AND SYMPTOMS

- Slowly progressive gait difficulty, usually in late childhood or adolescence.
- Pes cavum.
- Hypo- or areflexia.
- Distal leg weakness with footdrop.

TREATMENT

- Orthotic devices as needed.

Renal Osteodystrophy

DEFINITION

Bone diseases resulting from defective mineralization due to renal failure

SIGNS AND SYMPTOMS

- Growth retardation.
- Muscle weakness.
- Bone pain.
- Skeletal deformities.
- Slipped epiphyses.

DIAGNOSIS

- Normal to decreased serum calcium.
- Normal to increased phosphorus.
- Increased alkaline phosphatase.
- Normal or increased parathyroid hormone (PTH) levels.
- Hand, wrist, and knee x-rays show subperiosteal bone resorption and metaphysis widening.

TREATMENT

- Normalization of serum calcium, phosphorus and PTH levels.
- Low-phosphate diet.
- Enhance fecal phosphate excretion with oral calcium carbonate.
- Vitamin D administration.

WARD TIP

In children, renal osteodystrophy resembles rickets.

Dermatologic Disease

Classification of Skin Lesions

PRIMARY SKIN LESIONS

- Macule: flat, nonpalpable, <1 cm skin discoloration.
- Patch: flat, nonpalpable >1 cm skin discoloration.
- Plaque: elevated, flat-topped, >1 cm diameter.
- Wheal: elevated, area of dermal edema, disappears within hours.
- Vesicle: circumscribed, elevated, fluid-filled, <1 cm diameter.
- Bullae: circumscribed, elevated, fluid-filled, >1 cm, diameter.
- Pustule: circumscribed, elevated, pus-filled.
- Papule: elevated, palpable, solid, <1 cm diameter.
- Nodule: elevated, palpable, solid, >1 cm.
- Petechiae: red-purple, nonblanching macule, usually pinpoint, caused by extravasated red blood cells.
- Purpura: red-purple, nonblanching macule, caused by extravasated red blood cells.
- Telangiectasia: blanchable, dilated blood vessels.

SECONDARY SKIN LESIONS

- Scale: accumulation of stratum corneum.
- Crust (scab): dried serum, blood, or purulent exudate on skin surface.
- Erosion: loss of epidermis, leaving a denuded, moist surface; heals without scar.
- Ulcer: loss of epidermis extending into dermis; heals with scar.
- Scar: replacement of normal skin with fibrous tissue during healing.
- Excoriation: linear erosion produced by scratching.
- Atrophy: thinning of skin.
- Lichenification: thickening of epidermis with accentuation of normal skin markings.

Diagnostic Procedures Used in Dermatology

- Diascopy: glass slide pressed firmly against red lesion—blanchable (capillary dilatation) or nonblanchable (extravasation of blood).
- Gram stain: stains bacterial cell wall dividing them into two main categories: gram-positive and Gram-negative; can be performed on body fluid and biopsies.
- KOH prep: identifies fungi and yeast under microscope.
- Tzanck smear: helps to microscopically identify virally infected cells (typically herpes) from the base of a vesicle or ulcer.
- Scabies prep: skin scraping to identify mites, eggs, or feces under microscope.
- Wood's lamp: tinea capitis will fluoresce green/yellow on hair shaft.
- Patch testing: detects type IV hypersensitivity reactions (allergic contact dermatitis).

Papulosquamous Reactions

PSORIASIS (FIGURE 21-1)

DEFINITION

- Chronic, noninfectious, hyperproliferative inflammatory disorder.
- Polygenic, chronic, relapsing, T cell–mediated inflammatory skin disease.

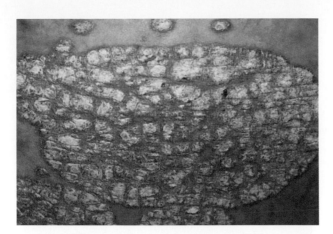

FIGURE 21-1. **Silvery scale plaque of psoriasis.** (Reproduced, with permission, from Fauci K.S., Kasper D.L., Braunwald E., et al. *Harrison's Principles of Internal Medicine*, 17th ed. New York: McGraw-Hill, 2008:311.)

ETIOLOGY

- Unknown, but with genetic predisposition.
- Triggering factors: trauma, infection, and medications.

PATHOPHYSIOLOGY

Increased epidermal cell proliferation and abnormal epidermal keratinocyte differentiation

EPIDEMIOLOGY

- Rarely presents at birth.
- One-third of cases of psoriasis present in patients under 20 years of age.

SIGNS AND SYMPTOMS

- Classic: thick, silvery-scaled, sharply defined, pink plaques.
- Common locations: scalp, elbows, knees, umbilicus, and diaper area.
- Nails commonly involved: pitting, onycholysis, subungual hyperkeratosis.
- Koebner phenomenon (lesions at site of trauma) and Auspitz sign (pinpoint bleeding at scale removal site) are common.
- May be associated with arthritis (psoriatic arthritis).
- Guttate variant: small, "droplike" papules with scale, group A streptococcus frequently a trigger.

DIAGNOSIS

- Clinical diagnosis.
- Potassium hydroxide (KOH) test and/or fungal culture to rule out fungal infection.

TREATMENT

- First line: emollients and topical corticosteroids.
- Additional topicals: coal tar, anthralin, synthetic vitamin D analogues (calcipotriene, calcitriol).
- If extensive or resistant: narrow band-ultraviolet B (NB-UVB) phototherapy, PUVA (psoralen and ultraviolet A [UVA]), retinoids, methotrexate, cyclosporine, TNF-alpha inhibitors.

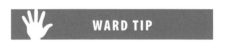

WARD TIP

For salmon-pink plaques with silvery scale, *think: Psoriasis.*

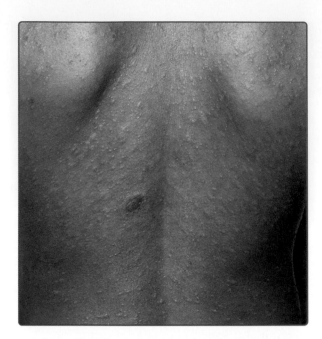

FIGURE 21-2. Vesicular pityriasis rosea, showing typical primary plaque and secondary papulovesicles. Note Christmas tree distribution. (Reproduced, with permission, from Kang S., Amagai M., Bruckner A.L., et al., eds. *Fitzpatrick's Dermatology*, 9th ed. New York, McGraw Hill, 2019.)

PITYRIASIS ROSEA (FIGURE 21-2)

DEFINITION

Common, self-limited eruption of single herald patch followed by a generalized secondary eruption

ETIOLOGY

Although a definitive cause has not been identified, suspected infectious agents include HHV-6, 7, and 8, as well as H1N1 influenza.

EPIDEMIOLOGY

Affects children and young adults

SIGNS AND SYMPTOMS

- Herald plaque: 1- to 10-cm solitary, oval, with fine scales.
- Typically, 5 to 10 days later, a generalized eruption of multiple smaller, pink, oval, scaly patches appear over trunk and upper extremities, following skin tension lines in a "Christmas tree" distribution.
- Symptoms can occur in an inverse form (extremities affected and trunk spared).
- Pruritus can be seen.

DIAGNOSIS

- Clinical.
- Rapid plasma reagin (RPR) to differentiate from syphilis.
- KOH to differentiate from fungal infection.

TREATMENT

- Self-limited, resolves in 2–12 weeks.
- Symptomatic: control pruritus (baths, calamine, topical corticosteroids, oral antihistamines).

Eczematous Reactions

ATOPIC DERMATITIS (AD, ECZEMA)

DEFINITION

Inflammatory skin disorder starting in early childhood.

ETIOLOGY

Complex interaction between impaired skin barrier, dysregulation of cutaneous inflammation, and environmental triggers.

EPIDEMIOLOGY

- Affects 10 to 30% of all children worldwide.
- Affects all ages, but onset usually in first year of life.
- Often outgrow by adolescence.
- Familial tendency and risk for other atopic disorders (allergic rhinitis, asthma, and food allergy).
- AD may be the initial manifestation of the "atopic march."

SIGNS AND SYMPTOMS

- Pruritic.
- Distribution varies with the patient's age.
- Infantile: red, exudative, **crusty,** and **oozing** lesions primarily affecting face (especially cheeks), trunk, and extensor surfaces.
- Nose, paranasal and diaper areas often spared.
- Juvenile/adult: dry, lichenified, pruritic plaques over flexural areas (antecubital, popliteal, neck).
- Susceptible to secondary bacterial (S. *aureus*) and viral (Molluscum contagiosum, herpes simplex virus) infections.

DIAGNOSIS

Clinical (pruritus, dermatitis, relapsing course); often personal or family history of atopy

TREATMENT

- Skin hydration with moisturizers.
- Topical corticosteroids for anti-inflammatory therapy.
- Sensitive skin care (non-perfumed lotions, soaps detergents) and irritant avoidance (wool).
- Oral antihistamines to manage itch.
- Bleach baths to decrease bacterial colonization.
- Oral antibiotics only if clinical signs of secondary infection.
- Oral corticosteroids avoided (steroid dependence or rebound flares possible).
- Resistant cases may require topical calcineurin (pimecrolimus or tacrolimus).

CONTACT DERMATITIS

DEFINITION

Inflammatory skin reaction resulting from contact with an external agent

ETIOLOGY

- Irritant: nonimmune-based, direct-cell injury from applied agent (saliva, feces, urine, detergents).
- Allergic: caused by a T-cell mediated reaction.

WARD TIP

Atopic dermatitis is part of the atopic triad: allergic rhinitis, asthma, and eczema.

WARD TIP

Skin colonization is common, especially with *Staphylococcus aureus*.

EXAM TIP

Rhus dermatitis is an allergic dermatitis caused by contact with poison ivy or oak.

SIGNS AND SYMPTOMS

- Sharply demarcated, erythematous vesicles and plaques at site of contact with agent.
- Chronic lesions may be lichenified.

DIAGNOSIS

- Clinical: consider location, relationship to external factors, particular configurations.
- History alone can identify the sensitizing agent in some cases, including:
  - Nickel.
  - Plant-associated (poison ivy).
- Patch testing is used to identify allergen.

TREATMENT

- Removal of offending agent.
- Topical corticosteroids.

SEBORRHEIC DERMATITIS

DEFINITION

Chronic skin inflammation occurring at sites with sebaceous gland activity, characterized by erythema and scaling

ETIOLOGY

Unknown; however, *Malassezia furfur* has been implicated.

PATHOPHYSIOLOGY

Unknown

EPIDEMIOLOGY

- Affects children and adults.
- Prevalence markedly increased in HIV+/AIDS patients.

SIGNS AND SYMPTOMS

- Children age 1–3 months: greasy scales on scalp (cradle cap), forehead, shoulders, and neck, axilla, or inguinal folds).
- Adults: flaking, greasy scales on erythematous background over scalp (dandruff), ears, eyelids (blepharitis), nasolabial fold, and central chest.

DIAGNOSIS

- Clinical.
- KOH or fungal culture to differentiate from fungal infection.

TREATMENT

- Symptomatic: antiseborrheic shampoo (selenium sulfide), short course of topical corticosteroids.
- Topical immunomodulatory agents (tacrolimus, pimecrolimus).
- Consider Langerhans cell histiocytosis and HIV for chronic seborrhea.

Bullous Diseases

EPIDERMOLYSIS BULLOSA

DEFINITION

A group of inherited disorders of cell-adhesion mechanisms characterized by trauma- or friction-induced skin blistering

ETIOLOGY

Mutation of cell-adhesion proteins at the basement membrane zone

EPIDEMIOLOGY

Various forms can present from infancy to young adulthood.

SIGNS AND SYMPTOMS

Blistering and erosions occur at sites of trauma; distribution can be both local or generalized.

DIAGNOSIS

- Skin biopsy for typical microscopic findings.
- Genetic testing to confirm mutation.

TREATMENT

- Wound dressing with nonstick or nonadherent dressings.
- Infection prevention.
- Pain management.

ERYTHEMA MULTIFORME (FIGURE 21-3)

DEFINITION

Targetoid lesions presenting in an acral distribution

> **EXAM TIP**
>
> Herpes simplex viruses are the most common cause of erythema multiforme.

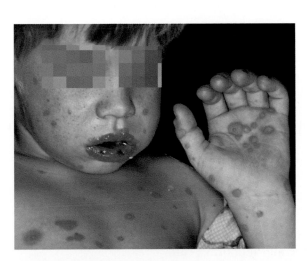

FIGURE 21-3. **Erythema multiforme.** Note the many different-sized lesions. (Reproduced, with permission, from Soutor C., Hordinsky M.K. *Clinical Dermatology.* New York, McGraw Hill, 2013.)

ETIOLOGY

- Herpes simplex virus 1, less often herpes simplex virus 2.
- Less common causes: Epstein-Barr virus, varicella, *Mycoplasma pneumoniae*, drugs.

EPIDEMIOLOGY

Older children and adults

SIGNS AND SYMPTOMS

- Pruritus or pain.
- Target lesion with three zones: peripheral red ring, pale zone, and dusky, violaceous center that may blister.
- Most commonly seen on upper extremity extensor surfaces. Mucosal lesions can be seen.

DIAGNOSIS

Clinical; skin biopsy for typical microscopic findings.

TREATMENT

- Supportive; topical emollients, antihistamines, and nonsteroidal anti-inflammatory agents assist with symptoms but not disease course.
- Heals in about 2 weeks.

STEVENS-JOHNSON SYNDROME

DEFINITION

Widespread erythematous macules, vesicles, bullae, and areas of denudation of <10% of total body surface area (BSA)

ETIOLOGY

- Often drug-induced: penicillin, sulfonamides, barbiturates, nonsteroidal anti-inflammatory drugs (NSAIDs), thiazides, phenytoin.
- Mycoplasma infection can lead to an SJS-like presentation.

SIGNS AND SYMPTOMS

- Mucosal surface burning, edema, and erythema may be presenting signs.
- Erythematous macules rapidly develop central necrosis, forming vesicles, bullae, and denuded areas on the face, trunk, and extremities.
- Symptoms affect two or more mucosal areas.
- Purulent uveitis/conjunctivitis may result in scarring or corneal ulcers.

DIAGNOSIS

Clinical.

TREATMENT

- Discontinue offending agent (if identified).
- Symptomatic and supportive care.
- Systemic steroids and IVIG are often used; efficacy is controversial.
- Observe closely for strictures developing upon mucous membrane healing.
- Ophthalmologic evaluation.
- Mouthwashes, topical anesthetics, pain control.

TOXIC EPIDERMAL NECROLYSIS (TEN)

DEFINITION

Sudden onset over 24 to 48 hours of widespread blistering (>30% body surface area) associated with skin tenderness, target lesions absence, and histologic findings of full-thickness epidermal necrosis without microscopic dermal infiltration.

ETIOLOGY

Hypersensitivity, triggered by medications listed above

PATHOPHYSIOLOGY

Damage to basal cell layer of epidermis

SIGNS AND SYMPTOMS

- Sudden onset of fever, malaise, and flu-like symptoms.
- Widespread morbilliform rash or erythema with tenderness that quickly blisters.
- Absence of targetoid lesions.
- May evince Nikolsky sign (separation of epidermis with gentle shear force).
- Complications: secondary skin infections, fluid and electrolyte abnormalities, prerenal azotemia.

DIAGNOSIS

- Clinical.
- Microscopic finding of full-thickness epidermal necrosis and a minimal to absent dermal infiltrate.

TREATMENT

- Removal of causative agent.
- Consider transfer to a burn unit.
- Fluid and electrolyte replacement.
- Role of IVIG or systemic steroids is controversial.
- Antibiotics for secondary bacterial infection.

EXAM TIP

Nikolsky's sign is present when direct pressure applied to surface of bullae causes them to extend laterally and sheer off the top layer of epidermis.

Cutaneous Bacterial Infections

IMPETIGO (FIGURE 21-4)

A 3-year-old girl had an upper respiratory infection for the past week. Two days ago, her parents noted a rash under her nose. She is afebrile with multiple round and oval areas of erythema with golden-colored crusts. *Think: Impetigo.*

Impetigo is a contagious superficial skin infection limited to the epidermis. It is transmitted by direct contact. The more common, nonbullous form begins as a single papule that quickly becomes a vesicle. When this vesicle ruptures and the contents dry, a characteristic honey or golden-colored crusts develops.

DEFINITION

- Contagious, superficial, bacterial infection transmitted by direct contact.
- Nonbullous in 70% of cases.
- Bullous impetigo most commonly affects neonates and young children.

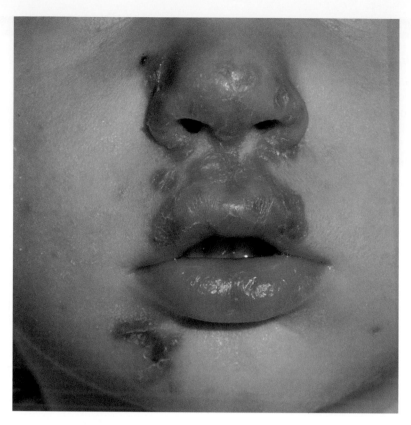

FIGURE 21-4. **Impetigo.** Note characteristic honey-colored crusted lesion, typically seen at corners of mouth and over face. (Reproduced, with permission, from Wolff K., Johnson R.A., Suurmond D. *Fitzpatrick's Color Atlas & Synopsis of Clinical Dermatology*, 6th ed. New York: McGraw-Hill, 2009:599.)

ETIOLOGY

- Non-bullous impetigo: *Staphylococcus aureus* and group A β-hemolytic *Streptococcus pyogenes* (GAS).
- Bullous impetigo: exfoliative strains of *Staphylococcus aureus*.

PATHOPHYSIOLOGY

Trauma to infections site; only involves the epidermis

EPIDEMIOLOGY

- Common in children.
- Warm and humid climates.
- Crowded conditions.

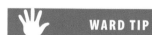

WARD TIP

"Honey-colored crust" is classic for impetigo.

SIGNS AND SYMPTOMS

- Mild burning or pruritus.
- Initial lesion is a transient erythematous papule or thin-roofed vesicle that ruptures easily and forms a honey-colored crust.

DIAGNOSIS

Clinical; can confirm with Gram stain and culture showing gram-positive cocci in clusters (*S. aureus*) or chains (GAS)

TREATMENT

- Remove crusts by soaking in warm water.
- Antibacterial washes.
- Topical antibiotic (mupirocin) for limited infection; oral antibiotics if extensive.

CELLULITIS

DEFINITION

Acute, deep infection of dermis and subcutaneous tissue

ETIOLOGY

- *S. aureus*, often MRSA, and group A β-hemolytic *S. pyogenes*.

PATHOPHYSIOLOGY

- Precipitating factors include trauma, mucosal infections, underlying dermatosis, and preexisting lymphatic stress.
- Risk factors include cancer, chemotherapy, immunodeficiency, diabetes, cirrhosis, neutropenia, and malnutrition.

EPIDEMIOLOGY

Any age

SIGNS AND SYMPTOMS

- Erythematous, edematous, shiny area of warm and tender skin with poorly demarcated, non-elevated borders.
- Fever, chills, and malaise can develop rapidly.

DIAGNOSIS

- Clinical; confirmed by Gram stain demonstrating gram-positive cocci in clusters or chains.
- Lesional and blood cultures are only positive in 15% and 2% of cases, respectively.

TREATMENT

- In communities with high rates of MRSA, consider clindamycin or trimethoprim-sulfamethoxazole (TMP/SMX).
- TMP/SMX does not cover for GAS, so a first-generation cephalosporin can be added to TMP/SMX or, if MRSA is unlikely, may be used as monotherapy.

Toxin-Mediated Diseases

STAPHYLOCOCCAL SCALDED SKIN SYNDROME

DEFINITION

Toxin-mediated blistering disease

ETIOLOGY

S. aureus.

PATHOPHYSIOLOGY

- Colonization/infection of the nose, umbilicus, perioral region, perineum, or conjunctivae.
- Produces exfoliatin and epidermolytic toxins that spread hematogenously to skin, resulting in sloughing of the epidermis and superficial blistering.

EPIDEMIOLOGY

Infants and children less than 5 years of age

SIGNS AND SYMPTOMS

- Skin is initially red and tender with flaccid bullae.
- Epidermis sloughs appearing wrinkled, often around the mouth, neck, axillae, and groin.
- Becomes widespread within 24–48 hours, resembling scalding.
- Nikolsky's sign.
- Self-limited, although death can occur in neonates with extensive disease.

DIAGNOSIS

Clinical; skin biopsy in challenging cases; infection confirmed by culture of colonized site (nose, eyes, throat) revealing gram-positive cocci

TREATMENT

- Hospitalize for extensive skin sloughing.
- Systemic antibiotics.
- Pain control.
- Intravenous (IV) fluids in severe cases.

SCARLET FEVER

DEFINITION

Toxin-mediated disease of sore throat, fever, and mucous membrane erythema

ETIOLOGY

Group A *Streptococcus*

PATHOPHYSIOLOGY

Toxin-mediated

EPIDEMIOLOGY

- Children.
- Untreated streptococcal throat infection.

SIGNS AND SYMPTOMS

- Pharynx is beefy red, and tongue is initially white, but within 4–5 days, the white coating sloughs and the tongue becomes bright red.
- Fine pink-scarlet papules first appear on the neck and upper chest, and become a sandpaper-like diffuse rash, including the extremities.
- Fades in 4–5 days, followed by desquamation.
- Circumoral pallor.
- Linear petechiae evident in body folds (Pastia's sign).

DIAGNOSIS

- Clinical; confirmed by culture from throat or wound.
- Rapid direct antigen tests detect GAS antigens.

TREATMENT

- Acetaminophen for fever and pain.
- Antibiotics for the pharyngitis (penicillin, macrolide, or cephalosporin).
- Follow-up is recommended if a history of rheumatic fever is present.

Cutaneous Viral Infections

HAND, FOOT, AND MOUTH DISEASE

DEFINITION

Oral ulcers and a macular or maculopapular eruption of the hands and feet

ETIOLOGY

Most commonly caused by coxsackievirus A16.

EPIDEMIOLOGY

More common in infants and children.

SIGNS AND SYMPTOMS

- Mild oropharyngeal pain, difficulty feeding, fever.
- Oral lesions: inflamed oropharynx with vesicles that leave 4-8 mm ulcers.
- Skin lesions: oval 3 to 7 mm maculopapular, vesicular, or pustular lesions on the hands, feet, and buttocks; usually resolve within 1 week.

DIAGNOSIS

Clinical: identification of the causative agent is typically unnecessary.

TREATMENT

Supportive care; ensure adequate hydration

VERRUCAE (WARTS)

DEFINITION

Viral infection of skin and mucous membranes spread by direct contact

ETIOLOGY

Human papillomavirus (HPV)

EPIDEMIOLOGY

Increased incidence in atopic and immunocompromised patients

SIGNS AND SYMPTOMS

- Tender if irritated.
- Types:
    - Verrucae vulgaris: hands, fingers, knees; skin-colored papule.
    - Verrucae plantaris: rough; on plantar aspect of foot.
    - Verrucae planar: flat; on face and dorsum of hands and fingers.
    - Condyloma acuminata: anogenital warts.

DIAGNOSIS

Clinical

TREATMENT

Cryotherapy, topical keratolytic agents (e.g., salicylic acid), destructive agents (podophyllin), curettage and desiccation, topical imiquimod

EXAM TIP

HPV genotypes 6 and 11 cause 90% of condyloma acuminate cases, while genotypes 16 and 18 are most strongly associated with cervical dysplasia (precancerous).

HERPES GINGIVOSTOMATITIS (FEVER BLISTERS, COLD SORES)

DEFINITION

Painful oral mucosa vesicles, typically due to herpes simplex virus type I infection

ETIOLOGY

Herpes simplex virus (HSV) type 1

PATHOPHYSIOLOGY

- Transmitted by direct contact with skin and mucous membranes.
- After primary infection, the virus remains latent in a neural ganglion.
- Latent virus reactivation results in recurrent disease (lip blisters).
- Recurrences become less frequent over time.

EPIDEMIOLOGY

- Primary infection affects children and young adults.
- Increased incidence in immunocompromised patients.

SIGNS AND SYMPTOMS

- Erythema and edema of gingiva and oral mucosa, followed by vesicles on an erythematous base.
- Perioral lesions may develop.
- Erosions and crusted lesions form after a couple of days.
- Fever, malaise, headache, dehydration, and adenopathy may occur with primary infection.
- Prodrome of burning, tingling, or itching occurs with recurrent infection.
- Complications include dehydration, herpetic whitlow, or cutaneous HSV infection (eczema herpeticum) in atopic dermatitis patients.

DIAGNOSIS

- Clinical; rarely Tzanck preparation (multinucleated giant cells), culture, or PCR.

TREATMENT

- Oral acyclovir, valacyclovir, or famciclovir decrease viral shedding time and accelerate healing time. Consider treatment if herpetic whitlow is present or there is risk for severe disease.
- Suppressive therapy with acyclovir for more than six recurrences per year.

MOLLUSCUM CONTAGIOSUM

DEFINITION

Self-limited, contagious, viral infection transmitted by direct contact

ETIOLOGY

Molluscum contagiosum virus (poxvirus)

EPIDEMIOLOGY

- Affects children and sexually active adults.
- Increased incidence in atopic and immunocompromised patients.

SIGNS AND SYMPTOMS

- Single or multiple, 1- to 5-mm, umbilicated, skin-colored or pearly papules (Figure 21-5).
- Commonly found on face, eyelids, axillae, and anogenital region.
- Multiple facial lesions seen with HIV infection.

WARD TIP

Herpetic whitlow (herpes-infected finger)—can occur in children with herpes gingivostomatitis secondary to sucking of fingers.

WARD TIP

Do not try to excise herpetic whitlow—opening the lesion will only serve to spill more virus onto surrounding skin and spread the infection.

WARD TIP

For umbilicated, pearly papules, *think: Molluscum contagiosum.*

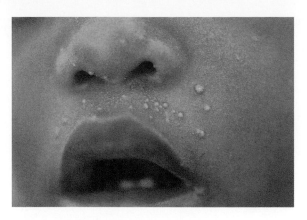

FIGURE 21-5.   Molluscum contagiosum. (Reproduced, with permission, from Soutor C., Hordinsky M.K. *Clinical Dermatology*. New York, McGraw Hill, 2013.)

DIAGNOSIS

Clinical

TREATMENT

Observation (self-resolves); curettage, cantharidin, or cryosurgery, if needed

Cutaneous Fungal Infections

TINEA (DERMATOPHYTOSES)

DEFINITION

- Noninvasive fungi that infect keratinized tissue of epidermis, nails, and hair.

ETIOLOGY

Trichophyton, Microsporum, Epidermophyton

EPIDEMIOLOGY

Exacerbated by warm, humid climates

SIGNS AND SYMPTOMS

- Tinea pedis ("athlete's foot").
- Tinea cruris ("jock itch") – groin.
- Tinea corporis ("ringworm"): – body (see Figure 21-6).
- Tinea capitis – scalp.
- Tinea barbae – beard/mustache area.
- Onychomycosis – nails.

DIAGNOSIS

- Clinical presentation and history.
- KOH preparation reveals multiple, septated hyphae.
- Occasionally, Wood's lamp shows bright green hair-shaft fluorescence in tinea capitis.
- Fungal culture of the affected area may demonstrate dermatophyte.

TREATMENT

- Topical antifungal agents (imidazoles and terbinafine) for skin infection.
- Systemic antifungal agents for tinea capitis and onychomycosis (griseofulvin, terbinafine).

 WARD TIP

Tinea corporis lesions are annular with peripheral scale and central clearing.

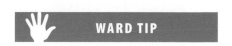 **WARD TIP**

Griseofulvin can cause elevation of liver enzymes.

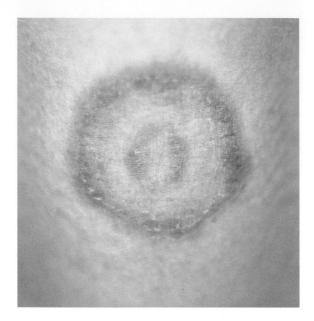

FIGURE 21-6. **Tinea corporis (ringworm).** (Reproduced, with permission, from Soutor C., Hordinsky M.K. *Clinical Dermatology.* New York, McGraw Hill, 2013.)

CANDIDAL SKIN INFECTIONS (CANDIDA)

DEFINITION

Superficial infection occurring in moist cutaneous sites

ETIOLOGY

Candida albicans

PATHOPHYSIOLOGY

Predisposing factors: diabetes mellitus, obesity, immunosuppression, recent antibiotic use

SIGNS AND SYMPTOMS

- Pruritus and soreness.
- Confluent, bright-red papules and pustules forming a sharply demarcated eroded plaque with pustular lesions at the periphery (satellite lesions).
- Most commonly found in the diaper area in children.
- Can occur in other intertriginous areas: axilla, inframammary creases.
- Vaginal infection in adolescents leads to a vulvovaginitis.
- The oral form is thrush: thick white plaque not easily removed on tongue and cheeks.

DIAGNOSIS

Clinical; KOH preparation reveals pseudohyphae and budding spores with positive cultures of lesion.

TREATMENT

- Keep intertriginous areas dry.
- Topical antifungals (nystatin and azoles).
- Topical corticosteroids for symptomatic relief.

WARD TIP

Thrush is a candidal infection of oral mucosal surfaces, presenting as creamy white (sometimes described as cottage cheese-like) plaques on an erythematous surface.

WARD TIP

Diaper rash is often superinfected with *Candida*, which manifests as erythematous satellite lesions.

Infestations

LICE (PEDICULOSIS)

DEFINITION

- Pediculosis corporis—body.
- Pediculosis capitis—scalp hair.
- Pediculosis pubis—pubic hair.

ETIOLOGY

- *Pediculus humanus corporis.*
- *Pediculus humanus capitis* (Figure 21-7).
- *Pthirus pubis.*

PATHOPHYSIOLOGY

Lice are obligate parasites, feeding on human blood.

EPIDEMIOLOGY

- Poor hygiene in some cases.
- Head-to-head contact, sharing hair items.
- Sexual contact.

SIGNS AND SYMPTOMS

- Pruritus.
- Superficial bacterial infections may develop from scratching.
- Corporis: primary lesion is an intensely pruritic, small, red macule or papule with central hemorrhagic punctum on shoulders, trunk, or buttocks; secondary lesions include excoriations, wheals, and eczematous, secondarily infected plaques.

DIAGNOSIS

Nits are detectable on hair/fibers.

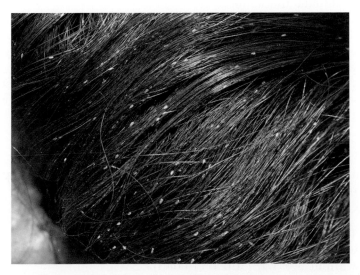

FIGURE 21-7. **Lice.** (Reproduced, with permission, from Richard P. Usatine, MD.)

TREATMENT

- Hot water laundering.
- Boil or dispose of implements such as combs.
- Comb hair and mechanically remove lice.
- Some areas with high resistance patterns: pyrethroids, malathion, lindane, spinosad, and ivermectin are choices.

SCABIES

👤 A 4-year-old boy has a pruritic, papular rash on his arms and legs. On examination, he is afebrile with diffusely distributed papules on the trunk and extremities, concentrated in the intertriginous areas. Burrows are noted. *Think: Scabies.*

Scabies is a contagious condition caused by the mite *Sarcoptes scabiei* spreading in households via contact or sharing of inanimate object. Schoolchildren are at higher risk. Typical presentation is generalized, intense nocturnal itching, classically described in interdigital web spaces of fingers and toes, popliteal fossae, flexor surfaces of the wrists, and gluteal region. The presence of skin burrows is a supportive finding. A definitive diagnosis is established by finding the scabies mites. Treatment is topical 5% permethrin, usually with a second treatment one week after the first.

ETIOLOGY

Female mite *Sarcoptes scabiei hominis*

PATHOPHYSIOLOGY

- Female mite burrows into the stratum corneum, depositing eggs and feces.
- Eggs hatch, the mites mature in 2–3 weeks, and repeat the cycle.

EPIDEMIOLOGY

- Physical contact with infected individual.
- Rarely transmitted by fomites, as isolated mites die within 2–3 days.

SIGNS AND SYMPTOMS

- Pruritus at initial infestation.
- First sign: 1- to 2-mm red papules, some excoriated, crusted, or scaling.
- Threadlike burrows.
- Common locations: interdigital web space, axilla, wrists, ankles, buttock, belt area, and penis; typically avoids scalp or face.
- Infants have nodules and papules on palms, soles, scalp, and occasionally face, or in axilla from mites transferred from parent's hands when holding the child.

DIAGNOSIS

Clinical; microscopic lesion scrapping with mites, ova, and feces is confirmation

TREATMENT

- Permethrin, neck down, in children >2 years for 8–12 hours; repeat in 1 week.
- Permethrin to face and scalp in children <2 years old.
- Alternatives include sulfur ointment and oral ivermectin.

WARD TIP

Threadlike burrows are classic for scabies but may not be seen in infants.

WARD TIP

Transmission of scabies mites is unlikely 24 hours after treatment.

Growths

INFANTILE HEMANGIOMA

DEFINITION

Benign vascular proliferation, not fully formed at birth, that grows over first months

ETIOLOGY/PATHOPHYSIOLOGY

Abnormal vascular angiogenesis

EPIDEMIOLOGY

Approximately 4% of infants

SIGNS AND SYMPTOMS

- Red papules or nodules that develop soon after birth, increases in size over the first 5–6 months of life and then slowly involute over years (see Figure 21-8).
- If >5 infantile hemangiomas are present, hepatic hemangiomas and an acute platelet-consumption phenomenon called Kasabach-Merritt are possible.

TREATMENT

- Most resolve without treatment, but topical timolol may be used.
- Oral propranolol is required for hemangiomas that are disfiguring or functionally impactful (feeding, breathing, vision).

MELANOCYTIC NEVUS (MOLE)

DEFINITION

Benign proliferation of melanocytes, which can be classified according to location of clustering on histopathology: dermal-epidermal junction (junctional), dermis (dermal), or both (compound) (Figure 21-9).

EPIDEMIOLOGY

Nevi usually arise in childhood and peak during adolescence. A decreased development of new nevi is seen in adulthood.

TREATMENT

- Serial observation for early recognition of premalignancy.
- Early excision of suspicious lesions.

MALIGNANT MELANOMA

DEFINITION

Malignant proliferation of melanocytes

ETIOLOGY

May arise from normal-appearing skin or from preexisting mole or skin lesion

PATHOPHYSIOLOGY

- Horizontal growth phase: lateral extension within the epidermis and dermis.
- Vertical phase: penetrates into dermis, increasing risk of metastasis.

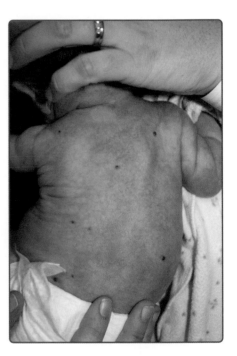

FIGURE 21-8. Capillary hemangioma. (Reproduced, with permission, from Kang S., Amagai M., Bruckner A.L., et al., eds. *Fitzpatrick's Dermatology*, 9th ed. New York, McGraw Hill, 2019.)

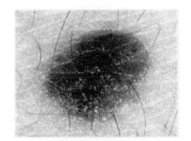

FIGURE 21-9. Melanocytic nevus. (Reproduced with permission from Wang S.Q., Katz B., Rabinovitz H., et al.: Lessons on dermoscopy. Compound congenital melanocytic nevus, *Dermatol Surg.* 2000;26(4):397–398.)

EPIDEMIOLOGY

- Increased incidence in fair-skinned people and with sun exposure.
- Adolescents.
- Increased risk in patients with large congenital melanocytic nevi.

SIGNS AND SYMPTOMS

Characteristics of a mole suspicious for melanoma include:
- Asymmetric.
- Border (irregular).
- Color (variegated and mottled).
- Diameter (>0.6 cm).
- Elevated.
- Enlarging.

DIAGNOSIS

Microscopic evaluation: prognosis based on thickness of the primary tumor

TREATMENT

- Surgical excision.
- Close follow-up.

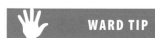

WARD TIP

Characteristics of mole suspicious for melanoma:
- Asymmetric
- Borders irregular
- Color uneven
- Diameter >0.6 cm
- Elevated
- Enlarging

Other Skin Conditions

HENOCH-SCHÖNLEIN PURPURA

DEFINITION

The most common vasculitis of childhood (Figure 21-10).

ETIOLOGY/PATHOPHYSIOLOGY

- Immunoglobulin A (IgA) deposition in small vessel walls.
- May occur following an upper respiratory infection.

EPIDEMIOLOGY

Pediatric age group

WARD TIP

Palpable purpura is the classic sign of small-vessel damage.

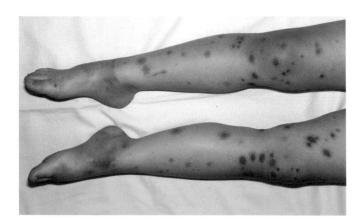

FIGURE 21-10. Henoch-Schönlein purpura. (Reproduced, with permission, from Lawrence B. Stack, MD.)

SIGNS AND SYMPTOMS

- Palpable purpura.
- Arthritis.
- Abdominal pain or GI bleeding.

DIAGNOSIS

Clinical; may biopsy

TREATMENT

- Usually benign, self-limited.
- Non-steroidal anti-inflammatory drugs for pain.
- Steroid often used to treat GI involvement/pain.
- Monitor for renal dysfunction for months after diagnosis (see also Renal chapter).

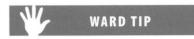

WARD TIP

Intestinal wall purpura can serve as a lead point for intussusception.

ACNE VULGARIS

DEFINITION

Disorder of pilosebaceous glands.

ETIOLOGY/PATHOPHYSIOLOGY

- Results from a combination of hormonal (androgens), bacterial (*Propionibacterium acnes*), and genetic factors.
- The initial pathology is microscopic microcomedones.

EPIDEMIOLOGY

Adolescents

SIGNS AND SYMPTOMS

- Comedone: plug of sebaceous and dead skin, lipid, and bacteria; open comedone (blackhead) or closed (whitehead).
- Pustules, papules.
- Painful nodules and cysts if severe.
- Seborrhea of face and scalp (greasy skin).
- Depressed or hypertrophic scars may develop with healing.

DIAGNOSIS

Clinical; confirmed by presence of comedones

TREATMENT

- Benzoyl peroxide wash.
- Topical antibiotics (clindamycin or erythromycin):
  - Oral tetracyclines (exert antibacterial and anti-inflammatory effects).
- Topical retinoid: increases cell turnover and prevents comedones.
- Oral isotretinoin (Accutane) for severe, recalcitrant, nodular acne.
- Dermabrasion or laser for treatment of scars.

WARD TIP

Accutane is teratogenic; therefore, **monthly pregnancy monitoring is required for females.**

DIAPER RASH

DEFINITION

Rash occurring in the diaper area

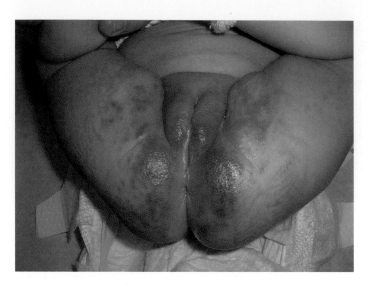

FIGURE 21-11. **Candida Diaper Rash.** (Reproduced with permission from Richard P. Usatine, MD.)

ETIOLOGY

- Irritant contact dermatitis: prolonged dampness, interaction of urine (ammonia) and feces with the skin.
- Candidal or bacterial secondary infection can occur (Figure 21-11).
- May be any other dermatologic condition in diaper distribution such as psoriasis, Langerhans cell histiocytosis, or a nutritional deficiency.

PATHOPHYSIOLOGY

Overhydration, friction, maceration, allergy, etc.

EPIDEMIOLOGY

Most children who wear diapers, to some degree

SIGNS AND SYMPTOMS

- Red, scaly, fissured, eroded skin.
- Patchy or confluent.
- Symptoms involve the convex portion of the buttock (the part touching the diaper); candida involves the inguinal creases and has satellite lesions.

TREATMENT

- Keep infant dry, and change diapers often.
- Ointments and thick barrier creams (zinc oxide) can protect skin irritation.
- Avoid powders (infant lung injury if inhaled accidentally).
- Use nystatin or other antifungal cream for yeast infection.

VITILIGO

DEFINITION

Disorder of skin depigmentation

ETIOLOGY/PATHOPHYSIOLOGY

- Unknown, possibly autoimmune.
- Trauma may be associated with initiation of the lesions.
- Associated with Addison disease, Hashimoto thyroiditis, and hypoparathyroidism.

EPIDEMIOLOGY

Half of all cases present before 20 years of age.

SIGNS AND SYMPTOMS

Depigmented macules and patches.

DIAGNOSIS

Clinical, although skin biopsy can confirm diagnosis

TREATMENT

- Phototherapy, e.g., narrow-band UVB therapy.
- Potent topical steroids, or topical tacrolimus or pimecrolimus.

URTICARIA-ANGIOEDEMA

A 12-year-old boy with a history of multiple food allergies ate a candy bar at school. He complained of throat discomfort and a rash. On examination, he is afebrile but is wheezing. Multiple discrete erythematous papules are noted on trunk and extremities. *Think: Urticaria.*

Urticaria with or without angioedema is common. Angioedema is due to an urticarial process that involves deeper layers of the skin. Acute urticaria is more common in children. History is often able to identify an inciting factor, especially if the hives occur shortly after ingestion of a food or drug such as milk, eggs, peanuts, and shellfish. The mast cell is the mediator in urticarial development. These lesions are typically pruritic and erythematous, often showing central clearing. Systemic symptoms develop if it is associated with anaphylaxis.

DEFINITION

Allergic response causing edema of the tissues

ETIOLOGY/PATHOPHYSIOLOGY

Type 1 hypersensitivity reaction of immunoglobulin E (IgE) with mast cells causes the release of histamine, vasodilation, increased vascular permeability, and axonal response

EPIDEMIOLOGY

Can occur in response to a large number of entities: ingestion, contact, infectious agents, environmental factors, or genetic conditions

SIGNS AND SYMPTOMS

- Urticaria: Symptoms are well circumscribed and often migratory, but can be coalescent, erythematous, raised lesions (wheals or welts) (see Figure 21-12). Individual lesions last <24 hours.
- Angioedema involves the deeper layers of skin, submucosa, and subcutaneous tissues.

TREATMENT

- Usually self-limited.
- Antihistamines.
- Watch for signs of airway compromise (especially with angioedema).
- Epinephrine for signs of anaphylaxis.

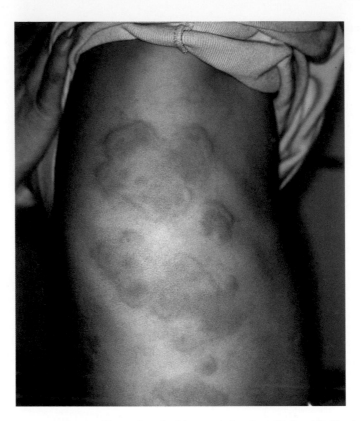

FIGURE 21-12. **Urticaria.** (Reproduced with permission from Richard P. Usatine, MD.)

Erythema Nodosum

DEFINITION

A panniculitis that affects subcutaneous fat in the skin

ETIOLOGY

Unknown in about half of the cases, but it can be associated with group A streptococcal infection, tuberculosis, *Yersinia enterocolitica* gastroenteritis, medications (antibiotics, birth control), and inflammatory bowel disease.

PATHOPHYSIOLOGY

Panniculitis infiltrate of neutrophils acutely and monocytes or histiocytes in chronic inflammation

EPIDEMIOLOGY

Adolescents or older

SIGNS AND SYMPTOMS

- 1 to 6 cm painful, red or violet oval lesions that extend in a parallel fashion on the extremities.
- The non-ulcerative lesions are found mostly commonly over shins, but also on the arms and other areas.
- Prodrome of fever, malaise, and arthralgia may be seen.
- Lesions resolve in 1–2 weeks, but they may recur for 2 to 6 weeks.

DIAGNOSIS

Clinical; occasionally biopsy required

TREATMENT

- Supportive (pain control).
- Treatment of underlying condition.

 Neonatal Dermatologic Conditions

See Table 21-1.

 Hair Loss

TRICHOTILLOMANIA (HAIR PULLING)

DEFINITION

- Traumatic hair pulling resulting in breaking of hair shafts at different lengths.
- Can also involve eyebrows or eyelashes.

ETIOLOGY

- Habitual.
- Sign of psychiatric disorder.
- Reaction to stress.

SIGNS AND SYMPTOMS

- Patchy hair loss of scalp (often on side of dominant hand).
- Loss of eyebrows, eyelashes.
- Close examination of hair demonstrates hair shafts broken at different lengths.

TREATMENT

- Behavioral modification.
- Consider psychiatry/psychology referral.

TABLE 21-1. **Neonatal Dermatology**

CONDITION	ETIOLOGY	APPEARANCE	RESOLUTION
Sebaceous hyperplasia	Maternal and infant hormones	Shiny yellow papules	A few weeks
Acne neonatorum	Transferred maternal androgens	Similar to minor acne vulgaris	Peaks at 2 months
Milia	Retention of dead skin and oily material in hair follicles	White papules on face	Within first month
Erythema toxicum neonatorum	Unknown, possible hypersensitivity	Blotchy red spots with overlying white or yellow papules or pustules	A few days
Congenital dermal melanocytosis (previously known as "Mongolian spots")	Melanocytes arrested in migration from neural crest to epidermis	Congenital, blue-gray macules, especially in nonwhite infants	First few years of life, although some never disappear
Pustular melanosis	Unknown; common in dark-skinned newborns	1-2 mm pustule that breaks leaving a collarette of scale and an underlying hyperpigmented lesions	Resolves in about 10 to 14 days

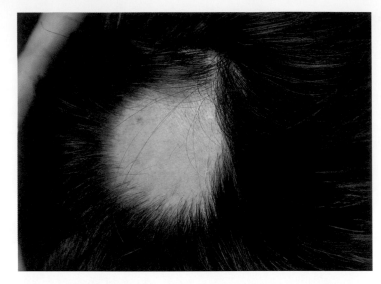

FIGURE 21-13. **Alopecia areata of scalp: Solitary lesion.** This is a sharply outlined portion of the scalp with complete alopecia without scaling, erythema, atrophy, or scarring. Empty follicles can still be seen on the involved scalp. The short, broken-off hair shafts (so-called exclamation-point hair) appear as very short stubs emerging from the bald scalp. (Reproduced, with permission, from Wolff K., Johnson R.A., Suurmond D. *Fitzpatrick's Color Atlas & Synopsis of Clinical Dermatology*, 5th ed. New York: McGraw-Hill, 2005:956.)

ALOPECIA AREATA (FIGURE 21-13)

DEFINITION

Non-scarring hair loss

ETIOLOGY

Immune-mediated loss of hair; course can be relapsing/remitting in some children

SIGNS AND SYMPTOMS

- Smooth circular areas of hair loss.
- Exclamation-point hairs.

TREATMENT

- High rates of spontaneous resolution/regrowth occur within 12 months.
- In some cases, steroids (systemic, topical, or local injection) occur.

Dermatologic Manifestations of Infectious Diseases

See Table 21-2.

TABLE 21-2. **Dermatologic Manifestations of Infectious Diseases**

Rubella (German measles)	▪ Pink macules and papules, initially on face and spread inferiorly within 24 hours ▪ Rash lasts 3 days, i.e., the "3-day measles"
Rubeola (measles)	▪ Erythematous macules and papules initially along hairline, spreading inferiorly within 2–3 days, fade within 4–6 days ▪ Koplik's spots: Bluish-white papules on erythematous base appear on day 2 of fever, over buccal mucosa, adjacent to second molars
Rocky mountain spotted fever (*Rickettsia rickettsii*)	▪ 2–6 mm erythematous macules that appear peripherally on wrists, forearms, ankles, palms, and soles ▪ Spreads to trunk, proximal extremities, and face within 6–18 hours ▪ Evolves to deep-red papules and petechiae over 1–3 days ▪ Within 2–4 days, exanthema is no longer blanchable
Erythema infectiosum (fifth disease; Parvovirus B19)	▪ "Slapped cheeks"—red papules coalesce on face ▪ Lacey rash on buttocks and upper arms that spreads ▪ Palms and soles may be involved
Meningococcemia (*Neisseria meningitidis*)	▪ Discrete, petechiae, and pink or purpuric macules, and papules over trunk, extremities, and palate
Gonococcemia (*Neisseria gonorrhoeae*)	▪ Erythematous macules over arms and legs evolve into hemorrhagic, painful pustules within 2–3 days
Syphilis (*Treponema pallidum*)	▪ Primary: painless ulcer (chancre) with indurated borders ▪ Secondary: Multiple, "ham-colored" papules scattered symmetrically over trunk, palm, soles, and genitals; condyloma lata—soft, flat-topped, pink papules in anogenital region ▪ Tertiary: Gummas—brown, firm plaques on body
Lyme disease (*Borrelia burgdorferi*)	▪ Erythema chronicum migrans—expanding, erythematous, annular plaque with central clearing
Bacterial endocarditis	▪ Osler's nodes: Tender, violaceous subcutaneous nodules on palms and soles ▪ Janeway lesions: Multiple, hemorrhagic, nontender macules on fingers and toes ▪ Subungual splinter hemorrhages ▪ Multiple petechiae on upper chest and mucous membranes

Dermatologic Manifestations of Systemic Disease

See Table 21-3.

TABLE 21-3. **Dermatologic Manifestations of Systemic Disease**

Sturge-Weber syndrome	■ Port-wine stain: Capillary malformation in a segmental distribution on the face ■ Port wine stains are fully formed at birth, persist into adulthood, and can thicken over time ■ Appear as a well-demarcated red to purple patch
Dermatomyositis	■ Heliotrope sign: Lilac color and edema of upper eyelids ■ Gottron papules: Pink to violaceous, flat-topped papules on the knuckles ■ Shawl sign: Violaceous erythema of the neck, shoulders, and upper back ■ Calcinosis cutis: Calcification in the skin common in juvenile dermatomyositis ■ Samitz sign: Ragged and frayed cuticles
Systemic lupus erythematosus	■ Malar rash: Erythematous plaques on the cheeks ■ Photosensitivity ■ Oral ulcers ■ Discoid lupus: Annular erythema, atrophy, scale, and hypo- or hyperpigmentation; common locations: hard palate, conchal bowl, head and neck
Obesity, metabolic syndrome	■ Acanthosis nigricans: Velvety, hyperpigmented plaques; occur on the neck, axilla, groin
Peutz-Jeghers syndrome	■ Lentigines: Hyperpigmented macules on nose, mouth, oral cavity, hands, and feet
Kawasaki disease (etiology unknown)	■ Erythematous macules and plaques appear in a stocking-and-glove distribution 1–3 days after onset of fever ■ Spreads to involve trunk and extremities within 2 days, lasts an average of 12 days

The Adolescent

Puberty

DEFINITION

Process of sexual maturation and secondary sexual characteristic development

EPIDEMIOLOGY

- For boys, onset of puberty is about 11.4 years (range 9.5 to 13.5 years).
- For girls, African Americans generally begin puberty earlier than Caucasians.
  - African American, 8.1 years (range 6.1 to 10.1 years).
  - Caucasian, 9.7 years (range 7.8 to 11.6 years).
- Strong genetic component is noted.
- A trend toward earlier start of puberty in recent generations has been noted.

SIGNS AND SYMPTOMS

- In boys, first signs include testicular enlargement and thinning of the scrotum, followed by growth of the penis and pubic hair (pubarche). Facial and axillary hair occur next, and accelerated growth occurs towards the end of puberty (about 2 years later than in girls). (see Figure 22-1).

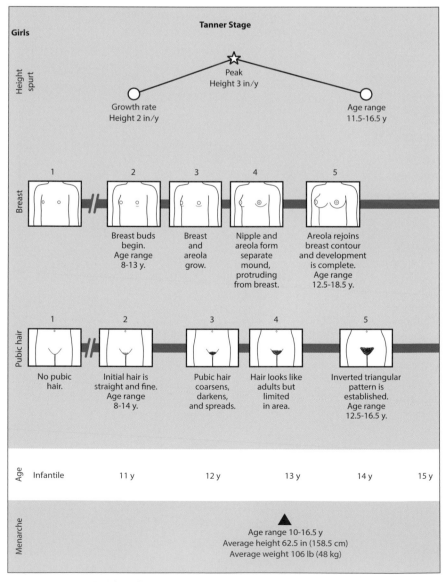

A

FIGURE 22-1. *(Continued)*

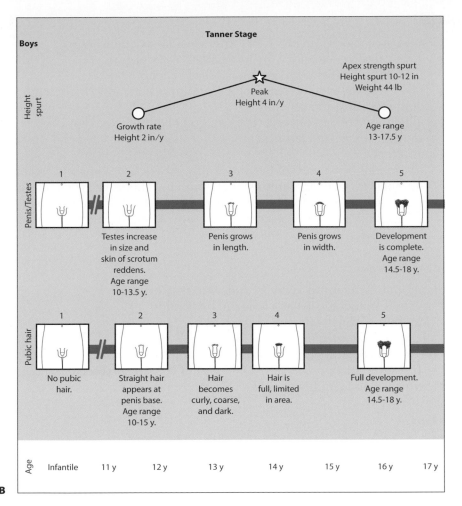

FIGURE 22-1. **A.** Female Tanner staging. **B.** Male Tanner staging. (Reproduced, with permission, from Toy E.C., Hormann M.D., Yetman R.J., et al. *Case Files: Pediatrics*, 6th ed. New York, McGraw Hill, 2022, Figs. 45-1 and 45-2.)

- In girls, first sign includes breast buds (thelarche) followed by growth of pubic hair; menarche occurs about 2–2.5 years after breast buds. Peak growth velocity occurs earlier in puberty than in boys. (see Figure 22-1).

DELAYED PUBERTY

DEFINITION

- In girls, no puberty signs are evident by 13 years or no menarche by 16 years.
- In boys, no puberty signs are evident by 14 years or more than 5 years have passed since initiation.

ETIOLOGY

Causes include gonadal failure, chromosomal abnormalities (e.g., Turner syndrome, Klinefelter syndrome), hypopituitarism, chronic disease, and malnutrition.

PRECOCIOUS PUBERTY

DEFINITION

Pubertal developmental in boys less than 9 years of age, African American girls less than 7 years of age, and Caucasian girls less than 8 years of age.

ETIOLOGY

- Central precocious puberty (CPP; early gonadal axis activation)
  - The cause is idiopathic in more than 90% of girls, but a structural CNS abnormality is present in 25% to 75% of boys.
  - CNS lesions without neurologic symptoms are rarely malignant, seldom requiring neurosurgery.
- Peripheral precocious puberty (PPP; no gonadal axis activation).
- Secondary sex characteristics are either iso- or contra-sexual (gender inconsistent).
  - Exogenous hormones (birth control pills, estrogen, testosterone cream).
  - Adrenal or gonadal tumors, beta-human chorionic gonadotropin–secreting tumors in males (e.g., hepatoblastoma, choriocarcinoma).
  - Congenital adrenal hyperplasia, McCune-Albright syndrome, neurofibromatosis, tuberous sclerosis.

SIGNS AND SYMPTOMS

- Syndromic skin lesions, oiliness, and acne may be seen.
- Findings can include axillary hair and body odor.
- Assess Tanner (SMR) staging (Figure 22-1).
- Palpate the abdomen for masses.
- GU exam to determine if testes are different in size or consistency
  - Transillumination may differentiate solid vs cystic (hydrocele) mass.
- Neuro exam to identify signs of CNS abnormality.

DIAGNOSIS

- Elevated serum levels of estradiol in girls and testosterone in boys.
- LH assay is undetectable in prepubertal children but is detectable in most cases of CPP.
- A gonadotropin-releasing hormone (GnRH) stimulation test may be required if LH and FSH levels are inconclusive.
- Bone-age radiographs are advanced beyond chronologic age.
- Organic CNS causes of CPP may require CT or MRI.
- A pelvic ultrasonography may be indicated if PPP is suspected on examination.

TREATMENT

- For CPP, GnRH analogues (leuprolide or histrelin) are used.
- For PPP, treat the underlying cause.

Adolescent Psychosocial Development

EARLY ADOLESCENCE (10 TO 13 YEARS)

- Concern about the developing body.
- Expands friendships from family to concentrate with peers.
- Transitioning from concrete to abstract thinking.

MIDDLE ADOLESCENCE (14 TO 16 YEARS)

- Emergence of sex drive.
- Peer values begin to impact behavior although family value predominate.
- Conflict over independence begin to emerge.
- Abstract thinking begins to predominate, but questionable decision making.

LATE ADOLESCENCE

- Body maturation and gender role clearer.
- Idealistic features emerge, potentially resulting in family/authority conflict.
- Exploration of life roles.
- Completion of cognitive development.

Adolescent Health Screening

- Complete a HEEADDSSS evaluation (see also Chapter 6)
- Testicular and breast self-examination taught at initiation of puberty.

SUBSTANCE ABUSE

- Screen for tobacco, alcohol, and other drug use at all visits.
- CRAFFT screening tool often employed (see Figure 22-2).

EPIDEMIOLOGY

- Alcohol and cigarettes are the most prevalent drugs.
- Marijuana is the most commonly reported illicit drug.
- Substance abuse varies according to age, gender, geographic region, race, and other demographic factors.

SIGNS AND SYMPTOMS

See Table 22-1 for signs and symptoms of intoxication and withdrawal due to substances of abuse.

WARD TIP

Adolescent HEEADDSSS assessment

Home
Education
Eating
Activities
Drugs and Alcohol
Depression
Safety
Sex
Suicide

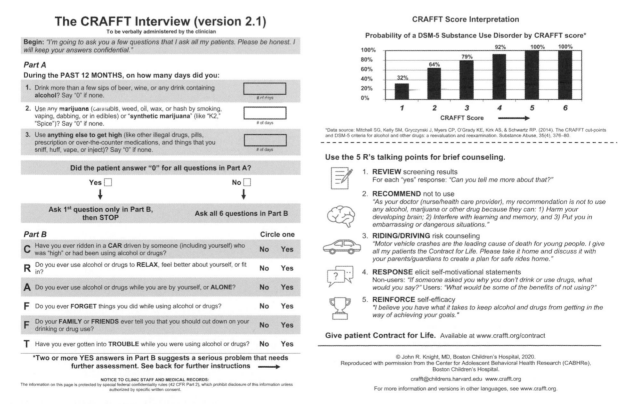

FIGURE 22-2. CRAFFT screening tool. Reproduced with permission from the Center for Adolescent Behavioral Health Research (CABHRe), Boston Children's Hospital. crafft@childrens.harvard.edu www.crafft.org For more information and versions in other languages, see www.crafft.org.)

TABLE 22-1. **Substances of Abuse—Intoxication and Withdrawal**

SUBSTANCE	INTOXICATION/OVERDOSE	WITHDRAWAL

Alcohol	Decreased fine motor control
	Impaired judgment and coordination
	Ataxic gait and poor balance
	Lethargy, difficulty sitting upright
	Respiratory depression
	Rx: Benzodiazepines, folate, thiamine, vitamin B12
		Irritability, insomnia, disorientation,
		    tremor, diaphoresis (6–24 hours)
		Alcoholic hallucination (1–2 days)
		Delirium tremens (2–5 days)—
		    generalized tonic-clonic seizures

Sedative-hypnotics
    (benzodiazepines,
    barbiturates)
	Drowsiness, slurred speech
	Incoordination, ataxia
	Mood lability, impaired judgment
	Nystagmus
	Respiratory depression, coma, death
	Rx: Benzodiazepines—flumazenil (careful, may precipitate seizures);
	    barbiturates—alkalinize urine; both—activated charcoal
		Autonomic hyperactivity
		Insomnia, anxiety, tremor
		Nausea, vomiting
		Delirium, hallucinations
		Seizures—may be life-threatening

Stimulants (cocaine, amphetamines)	Euphoria, sweating, chills, nausea Autonomic instability, cardiac arrhythmias Psychomotor agitation, dilated pupils Vasoconstriction—MI, CVA **Rx:** Benzodiazepines (haloperidol if severe)	Not life-threatening Dysphoric "crash," depression, anxiety Hunger, craving Constricted pupils

Opioids (heroin, codeine,
    morphine, methadone,
    meperidine)
	Drowsiness, slurred speech
	Nausea, vomiting, constipation
	Constricted ("pinpoint") pupils
	Seizures
	Respiratory depression
	Rx: Naloxone/naltrexone, methadone taper
		Not life-threatening
		Dysphoria, insomnia
		Lacrimation, rhinorrhea
		Yawning, weakness, muscle aches
		Sweating, piloerection, dilated pupils
		Nausea, vomiting
		Rx: Clonidine, methadone taper

Hallucinogens (mushrooms,
    mescaline, LSD)
	Perceptual changes, papillary dilation
	Tachycardia, palpitations
	Tremors, incoordination
	Rx: "Talk down," benzodiazepines for agitation
		May have flashbacks later due to
		    reabsorption of lipid stores

PCP (hallucinogen)	Violence, recklessness, impulsivity Impaired judgment, nystagmus, ataxia Hypertension, tachycardia Muscle rigidity, high pain tolerance Seizures, coma **Rx:** Benzodiazepines, acidify urine	As with other hallucinogens, flashbacks may occur

Marijuana (THC)	Euphoria, impaired concentration
	Mild tachycardia
	Conjunctival injection
	Dry mouth, ↑ appetite
		No withdrawal syndrome, but mild
		    irritability, insomnia, nausea, and ↓
		    appetite may occur in heavy users

(continued)

TABLE 22-1. *(Continued)*

SUBSTANCE	INTOXICATION/OVERDOSE	WITHDRAWAL
Inhalants	Impaired judgment, belligerence, impulsivity	Irritability, nausea, vomiting, tachycardia
	Perceptual disturbances, slurred speech	Occasional hallucinations
	Ataxia, dizziness	
	Nystagmus, tremor, hyporeflexia	
	Lethargy, euphoria, stupor, coma	
	Respiratory depression, cardiac arrhythmias	
Caffeine	Anxiety, insomnia, twitching	Headache, nausea, vomiting, drowsiness
	Flushed face, rambling speech	Anxiety, depression
	GI disturbance, diuresis	
Nicotine	Restlessness, insomnia, anxiety	Dysphoria, anxiety, irritability, insomnia ↑
	Increased GI motility	appetite, craving

CVA, cerebrovascular accident; GI, gastrointestinal; LSD, lysergic acid diethylamide; MI, myocardial infarction; PCP, phencyclidine; Rx, treatment; THC, tetrahydrocannabinol.

TREATMENT

- Non-pharmacologic: group therapy, narcotics anonymous.
- Hospitalizations may be necessary for acute withdrawal.
- Alcohol abuse: rule out medical complications, start benzodiazepine for withdrawal symptoms, and give thiamine before glucose to prevent Wernicke encephalopathy.

DEPRESSION AND SUICIDE (SEE PSYCHIATRY CHAPTER)

- Screening at all visits beginning at 12 years of age.
- Several tools available; most common include Patient Health Questionnaire for Adolescents (PHQ-A) and the Beck Depression Inventory.

LABORATORY

- Pap: the U.S. Preventative Services Task Force (USPSTF) recommends all females should receive Pap smear cytologic testing every 3 years to screen for cervical dysplasia starting at the age of 21. Women under 21 need not be screened, regardless of sexual history.
- Lipids: universal lipid screening is recommended between 9 and 11 and again at 17 and 21 years of age.
- A fasting lipid profile is done beginning at age 2 years for children with positive history of lipid and cholesterol disorders and/or positive family history continues.
- Anemia: selective testing is done for poor iron intake, food insecurity, and for girls with extensive menstrual blood loss.
- HIV: universally at 15 and 18 years.
- Selective HIV testing: sexually active, IV drug users, infection with other STIs
- Screening for sexually transmitted infections (chlamydia, gonorrhea, syphilis) performed annually for sexually active patients.
- Tuberculosis screening annually for adolescents with HIV or at high risk (group homes, incarceration, former residents of countries with TB high rate).
- Vision and hearing: screening is performed once at each of the early, middle, and late adolescent visits.

IMMUNIZATIONS

At 11 to 12 years, initiate the following:

- Tetanus, diphtheria, and acellular pertussis booster (Tdap).
- Human papillomavirus (HPV) and can be given as early as 9 years of age.
- Meningococcal (with booster at 16 years).
- Continue annual flu.

Confirm series are likely already completed:

- Measles, mumps, and rubella (MMR).
- Hepatitis A and B.
- Varicella.
- SARS-CoV-2.

Eating Disorders

DEFINITION

Two subtypes:

- Restricting—limiting any oral intake.
- Binge eating/purging—binge eating or purging for 3 months.

ANOREXIA NERVOSA

> A 16-year-old girl has a 6-month history of amenorrhea and a 25-lb weight loss. She is thin, with Tanner stage 4 breast and pubic hair development. She complains of constipation and bloating. When asked about her weight loss, she states that she is "overweight." *Think: Anorexia nervosa.*
>
> Anorexia nervosa is an eating disorder characterized by weight loss, and psychiatric disturbance reflected as distorted body image. Common symptoms include constipation, cold intolerance, dry skin, and hair loss. It predominantly affects females. The associated hormonal abnormalities result in amenorrhea. Electrolyte abnormalities (hyponatremia, hypokalemia, hypophosphatemia, hypoglycemia) may be present.

DIAGNOSIS

- Restriction of energy intake, leading to low body weight (BMI < 18.5) in context of age, sex, developmental trajectory, and physical health.
- Even though underweight, an intense fear of gaining weight.
- Disturbance in self-perception of body weight or lack of insight into the seriousness of physical condition.

ETIOLOGY

- Genetic predisposition.
- Psychological need to control, perfectionism.
- Desire to conform to society's ideal of beauty.
- Can occur with life events such as leaving for college or family death.

PATHOPHYSIOLOGY

- Altered levels of leptin and serotonin have been found in some patients.
- Endocrine abnormalities include increased growth hormone levels, loss of cortisol diurnal variation, reduced luteinizing hormone, follicle-stimulating hormone, impaired response to luteinizing hormone–releasing hormone, abnormal glucose tolerance test.

EXAM TIP

The most common cause of death in anorexia nervosa is cardiac arrhythmias due to electrolyte disturbances, particularly hypokalemia.

EPIDEMIOLOGY

- Ten to 1 female predominance.
- Bimodal onset at 13–14 and 17–18 years.
- More common in industrialized countries.
- Common in individuals participating in ballet, gymnastics, and modeling
- Comorbid conditions include major depression, bulimia, somatic symptom disorders, or schizophrenia.

SIGNS AND SYMPTOMS

- Extreme dieting, special diets such as vegetarianism.
- Refusal to eat meals with family members or in public.
- Preoccupation with food and its preparation.
- Denial of hunger.
- Obsessive interest in physical exercise.
- Abuse of laxatives, diuretics, or stimulants to enhance weight loss.
- Multiorgan involvement: amenorrhea, hypothermia, constipation, low blood pressure, bradycardia, lanugo, hair loss, petechiae, pedal edema, dry skin, osteopenia.
- Electrolyte abnormalities: hyponatremia, hypochloremic hypokalemic alkalosis if vomiting.
- Lab abnormalities: anemia, leukopenia, transaminitis, elevated triglycerides.

TREATMENT

- Anorexic patients deny health risks of the behavior and are resistant to treatment.
- Individual and family psychotherapy.
- Behavior modification to restore normal eating behavior, set specific weight goals.
- Nutritional rehabilitation: restore nutritional state and weight.
- SSRIs for comorbid anxiety or depression.

BULIMIA NERVOSA

 A 15-year-old girl has bilateral parotid gland swelling and dental enamel erosion of her posterior upper incisors. She reports frequent vomiting after meals. *Think: Bulimia nervosa.*

Bulimia nervosa is characterized by recurrent episodes of binge eating defined as the rapid consumption of a large amount of food in a reasonably short time. The hallmark of bulimia is a fear of not being able to stop eating when the binge is in progress. Self-induced vomiting and excessive exercise are the compensatory behaviors. Parotid enlargement, dental problems, and abrasions of knuckles are due to biting down on them during self-induced vomiting. The typical age of presentation is during the teenage years.

DIAGNOSIS

- Recurrent episodes of binge eating.
- Episodes occur at least once a week for 3 months.
- Recurrent compensatory behavior to compensate for eating and to prevent weight gain includes vomiting, laxatives, diuretics, enemas, excessive exercise.
- Body shape and weight is the basis of self-evaluation.
- Does not occur exclusively during episodes of anorexia nervosa.

ETIOLOGY

Genetics, environment (stress), psychological, and cultural influences

WARD TIP

Electrocardiography (ECG) in anorexia nervosa may show low-voltage T-wave inversion and flattening, ST depression, supraventricular or ventricular arrhythmias, and/or prolonged QT intervals.

EXAM TIP

The long-term mortality of anorexia nervosa is about 5% per decade due to starvation, suicide, or cardiac failure.

WARD TIP

Beware of complications occurring during rehabilitation for anorexia nervosa, including congestive heart failure (CHF), cardiac arrhythmias, and overcorrection of electrolyte abnormalities (refeeding syndrome).

WARD TIP

Refeeding syndrome can lead to fatal electrolyte abnormalities. Look especially for hypokalemia and hypophosphatemia that can result in fatal arrhythmias.

PATHOPHYSIOLOGY

- Early puberty and childhood obesity are risk factors.
- The psychodynamic theory proposes displaced anger over one's body and masochistic displays of control.

EPIDEMIOLOGY

- Ten to 1 female predominance.
- Onset typically late adolescence or early adulthood.
- More common in industrialized countries.
- Comorbid conditions include mood, anxiety, and impulse disorders; a history of drug abuse or physical/sexual abuse is common.

SIGNS AND SYMPTOMS

- Secretive binge-eating and purging behaviors.
- Laxatives, diuretics, or stimulants abuse to enhance weight loss.
- Obsessive interest in physical activity.
- Physical manifestations include parotid gland enlargement, dental caries, scars on dorsum of fingers (teeth scraping during self-induced vomiting), petechiae.
- Laboratory abnormalities include: hypochloremic hypokalemia alkalosis (vomiting); metabolic acidosis (laxative effect); elevated bicarbonate (compensation); hypernatremia; elevated BUN and amylase; and altered thyroid hormone levels.

TREATMENT

- Behavioral, group, and family therapy and medication.
- SSRIs first line medication.
- Chronic and relapsing; half fully recover.
- Increased risk of suicide compared to general population.

Female Health Issues

BREAST MASS

DEFINITION

A palpably discrete area of any size on the breast, ideally found on self-examination (Table 22-2).

EPIDEMIOLOGY

- The common adolescent breast mass is fibroadenoma.
- Primary breast cancer in teens is rare.

ETIOLOGY

Possibly due to local response to estrogen stimulation

SIGNS AND SYMPTOMS

- Fibroadenomas are 2–3 cm solid masses in the upper-outer breast quadrant.
- Lesions are rubbery, nontender, and mobile.

TABLE 22-2. **Breast Masses in Adolescent Females**

Common	Rare (malignant or malignant potential)
Fibroadenoma	Juvenile secretory carcinoma
Fibrocystic changes	Intraductal carcinoma
Breast cysts (including subareolar cysts)	Cystosarcoma phyllodes
Breast abscess or mastitis	Sarcomas (fibrosarcoma, malignant fibrous
Fat necrosis (after trauma)	histiocytoma, rhabdomyosarcoma)
Less common (benign)	Metastatic cancer (hepatocellular
Lymphangioma	carcinoma, lymphoma, neuroblastoma,
Hemangioma	rhabdomyosarcoma)
Intraductal papilloma	
Juvenile papillomatosis	
Giant fibroadenoma	
Neurofibromatosis	
Nipple adenoma or keratoma	
Mammary duct ectasia	
Intramammary lymph node	
Lipoma	
Hematoma	
Hamartoma	
Galactocele	

(Reproduced, with permission, from Hay W.W. Jr, Levin M.J., Abzug M.J., et al, eds. *Current Diagnosis & Treatment: Pediatrics*. 25th ed. New York: McGraw Hill, 2020.)

DIAGNOSIS

Clinical examination typically is sufficient; USG may be required.

TREATMENT

- Close observation with serial USG if spontaneous regression does not occur.
- Fine needle aspiration for mass that is growing.

AMENORRHEA

DEFINITION

- Primary amenorrhea is defined as no menstrual period or secondary sex changes by age 13 years, or no menses by age 15 years in the girl with secondary sex changes.
- Secondary amenorrhea is absence of menses for 3 consecutive months or 6 months of irregular cycles in the girl with prior menses.

ETIOLOGY

The causes of primary and secondary amenorrhea are myriad (Table 22-3).

SIGNS AND SYMPTOMS

May be normal exam, signs of androgen excess, or evidence of syndromes

TABLE 22-3. Differential Diagnosis of Amenorrhea by Anatomic Site of Cause

Hypothalamic-pituitary axis	**Uterovaginal outflow tract**
Hypothalamic suppression	Müllerian dysgenesis[a]
Chronic disease	Congenital deformity or absence of uterus, uterine tubes, or vagina
Stress	Imperforate hymen, transverse vaginal septum, vaginal agenesis, agenesis of the cervix[a]
Malnutrition	Androgen insensitivity syndrome (absent uterus)[a]
Strenuous athletics	Uterine lining defect
Drugs (haloperidol, phenothiazines, atypical antipsychotics)	Asherman syndrome (intrauterine synechiae post-curettage or endometritis)
Central nervous system lesion	Tuberculosis, brucellosis
Pituitary lesion: adenoma, prolactinoma	**Defect in hormone synthesis or action (virilization may be present)**
Craniopharyngioma, brainstem, or parasellar tumors	Adrenal hyperplasia[a]
Head injury with hypothalamic contusion	Cushing disease
Infiltrative process (sarcoidosis)	Adrenal tumor
Vascular disease (hypothalamic vasculitis)	Ovarian tumor (rare)
Congenital conditions[a]	Drugs (steroids, ACTH)
Kallmann syndrome (anosmia)	
Ovaries	
Gonadal dysgenesis[a]	
Turner syndrome (XO)	
Mosaic (XX/XO)	
Injury to ovary	
Autoimmune disease (oophoritis)	
Infection (mumps)	
Toxins (alkylating chemotherapeutic agents)	
Irradiation	
Trauma, torsion (rare)	
Polycystic ovary syndrome	
Ovarian failure	

ACTH, adrenocorticotropic hormone.

[a]Indicates condition that usually presents as primary amenorrhea.

(Reproduced, with permission, from Hay W.W. Jr, Levin M.J., Abzug M.J., et al, eds. *Current Diagnosis & Treatment: Pediatrics.* 25th ed. New York: McGraw Hill, 2020.)

DIAGNOSIS

- A suggested algorithm for diagnosis is shown (Figure 22-3).
- A thorough history and physical examination is the first step.
- Further testing is dependent on the presence or absence of normal female anatomy.
    - For normal anatomy, LH, FSH, TSH, prolactin levels are commonly required.
    - For abnormal anatomy, karyotype may be indicated.

TREATMENT

Dependent upon the cause identified in the evaluation

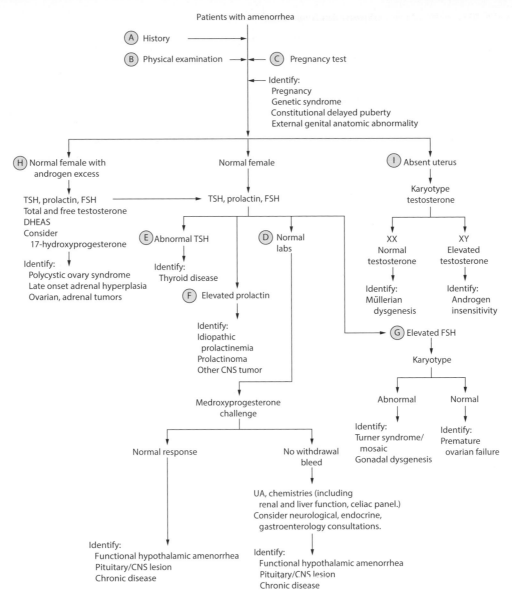

FIGURE 22-3. **Evaluation of Primary Amenorrhea and Secondary Amenorrhea.** CNS, central nervous system; DHEAS, dehydroepian-drosterone sulfate; FSH, follicle-stimulating hormone; TSH, thyroid-stimulating hormone; UA, urine analysis. (Reproduced, with permission, from Hay W.W. Jr, Levin M.J., Abzug M.J., et al, eds. *Current Diagnosis & Treatment: Pediatrics*, 25th ed. New York, McGraw Hill, 2020.)

DYSMENORRHEA

DEFINITION

Pain with menstrual flow

EPIDEMIOLOGY

About 60% of girls have pain by middle to late adolescence.

ETIOLOGY

- Primary: prostaglandin- and leukotriene-stimulated uterine and myometrial contractions lead to pain.
- Secondary: a variety of physiologic and pathologic conditions occur, such as ectopic pregnancy, pelvic infections, and endometriosis.

SIGNS AND SYMPTOMS

- For primary dysmenorrhea, painful cramping occurs in the first 36 to 48 hours of menses.
- Headache, fatigue, nausea, and vomiting may occur.

DIAGNOSIS

Thorough history and physical examination to eliminate secondary causes

TREATMENT

- For primary dysmenorrhea, NSAIDs or oral contraceptives.
- For secondary dysmenorrhea, treatment of the specific condition.

ABNORMAL UTERINE BLEEDING (AUB)

DEFINITION

- Change to the expected menstrual regularity, volume, frequency, or duration in the absence of pregnancy.
- May be further categorized as heavy menstrual bleeding (AUB/HMB) or intermenstrual bleeding (AUB/IMB).
- Terminology has evolved, and older terms such as menorrhagia and menometrorrhagia have been abandoned. AUB encompasses:
  - Amenorrhea (absence of menses).
  - Irregular intervals of menses.
  - Intervals <21 days or >45 days.
  - More than 7 days of bleeding.
  - Heavy bleeding soaking through one or more pads or tampons every hour.
  - Breakthrough (intermenstrual) bleeding.

ETIOLOGY

- Anovulatory cycle is most common in adolescents with endometrium exposed to unopposed estrogen levels and lack of progesterone production
  - Common in the first 2 to 3 years after menarche.
  - Consider polycystic ovary syndrome (PCOS), hyper- or hypothyroidism.

OVULATORY CYCLE

- Prolonged progesterone secretion with relatively low estrogen production
  - Consider also PCOS, endometriosis, medications such as hormonal contraceptives.

SIGNS AND SYMPTOMS

- History of bleeding, as outlined above.
- Pallor if significant blood loss.
- Physical evidence of polycystic ovary syndrome or thyroid disease.

DIAGNOSIS

- Pallor if significant blood loss.
- Urine pregnancy test.
- CBC.
- Thyroid studies.
- Sexually transmitted disease testing.
- Consider progesterone levels during luteal phase to determine ovulatory vs. anovulatory bleeding.
- Coagulation studies, especially for family history of bleeding.
- For PCOS: serum glucose, lipid, testosterone and dehydroepiandrosterone sulfate levels.

TREATMENT

- Hormone therapy with oral contraceptives is first line in non-smoking patients with no underlying etiology.
- NSAIDs reduce bleeding and relive dysmenorrhea (contraindicated in bleeding disorders).
- Tranexamic acid.

Male Health Issues

 A 16-year-old boy presents with lower-left abdominal pain and left testicular pain for 2 weeks. Palpation of the testes is normal except for isolated tenderness of the epididymis. Cremasteric reflex is normal. *Think: Epididymitis.*

   Patients with epididymitis experience gradual scrotal pain and tenderness is localized to the epididymis +/− pyuria. Congenital genitourinary anomalies may predispose to recurrent infection. It can be difficult to differentiate from torsion.

EPIDIDYMITIS

DEFINITION

Inflammation of the epididymis due to infection or trauma

EPIDEMIOLOGY AND ETIOLOGY

About two-thirds of cases occur in sexually-active boys due to *C. trachomatis* or *N. gonorrhoeae.*

SIGNS AND SYMPTOMS

- Acute onset of unilateral testicular and/or scrotal pain and swelling.
- Urethral discharge.
- Swollen and tender epididymis.
- Cremasteric reflex may be absent.

DIAGNOSIS

- STI evaluation.
- Ultrasound, if unable to differentiate from torsion.

TREATMENT

- Antibiotics for likely chlamydial or gonococcal infection.
- Scrotal elevation and analgesics.

TESTICULAR TORSION (SEE RENAL CHAPTER)

VARICOCELE

DEFINITION

Dilation of the pampiniform venous plexus in the scrotum

EPIDEMIOLOGY

Found in about 15% of healthy men and about 35% of men with infertility

ETIOLOGY

Unknown, but theories include incompetent values in the spermatic cord or increased pressure on the pampiniform venous plexus due to left renal vein compression

WARD TIP

Testicular torsion would cause decreased flow on ultrasound, while epididymitis causes increased flow with ultrasound. Epididymitis also presents with fever and presents with more gradual pain localized to the epididymis.

SIGNS AND SYMPTOMS

- Typically asymptomatic, but can cause dull, achy scrotal pain.
- "Bag of worms" palpable and visible through the scrotal skin.

DIAGNOSIS

Classic history and physical examination

TREATMENT

Generally reassurance although repair if infertility is an issue

PUBERTAL GYNECOMASTIA

DEFINITION

Glandular swelling of breast tissues in boys

EPIDEMIOLOGY

Occurs in 40 to 60% of boys between 10 and 16 years of age, peaking at about age 14 (SMR 2 to 4)

ETIOLOGY

- In most cases, reduced ratio of serum levels of androgens to estrogens.
- May be associated with drugs, especially marijuana.
- Rarely associated with estrogen excess states such as with tumors, thyroid abnormalities, Klinefelter syndrome.

SIGNS AND SYMPTOMS

Firm, sometimes tender, asymmetric breast swelling

DIAGNOSIS

Usually clinical evaluation

TREATMENT

- Usually none (90% spontaneous resolution).
- Surgical if especially large or psychologically impactful.

Sexually Transmitted Infections (Table 22-4)

BACTERIAL VAGINOSIS

ETIOLOGY

Replacement of normal vaginal *Lactobacillus sp.* with *Bacteroides sp.*, *Mobiluncus sp.*, *Gardnerella vaginalis*, and *Mycoplasma hominis*.

SIGNS AND SYMPTOMS

- Thin, white vaginal discharge.
- "Fishy" odor classically described.

DIAGNOSIS

KOH preparation (whiff test) and findings of "clue cells" on microscopic evaluation of discharge.

TREATMENT

- Oral metronidazole.
- Alternatives intravaginal clindamycin or metronidazole gel.

WARD TIP

Due to the high rate of concurrent gonorrhea and chlamydia infection, treatment for gonorrhea (ceftriaxone) should always be included with that for chlamydia (azithromycin or doxycycline) and vice versa.

WARD TIP

Positive "whiff test": KOH mixed with vaginal discharge on a slide produces a fishy smell. This is characteristic of bacterial vaginosis.

TABLE 22-4. **Summary of Infectious Agents Associated with STI**

DISEASE	PATHOGEN	SYMPTOMS	DIAGNOSIS	TREATMENT
Chlamydia	*Chlamydia trachomatis*	Asymptomatic, mucopurulent cervicitis, PID, urethritis, most common cause of epididymitis if sexually active. Can cause conjunctivitis in newborns born to infected mothers	Nucleic acid amplification test (NAAT) of urine or discharge	Ceftriaxone and azithromycin
Gonorrhea	*Neisseria gonorrhoeae*	Asymptomatic, urethritis, cervicitis, PID, epididymitis, greenish mucoid discharge. Can cause conjunctivitis in newborns born to infected mothers	NAAT. If unavailable, do microscopy (for men only, shows gram-intracellular diplococci) or culture endocervical or urethral specimens	Ceftriaxone and azithromycin
HPV	Human papillomavirus	Condyloma acuminata are large flesh-colored, pink, or brown papules that can coalesce into "cauliflower" plaques. In children, more HPV strains cause genital warts. Can progress to cervical cancer in adults	Typically clinical. 5% acetic acid can turn HPV infected warts white. Biopsy can be done if uncertain. Do not do cervical screenings until age 21	Watch and wait. Many regress on own. Multiple therapies available for condyloma acuminata, but recurrence is common
Herpes*	Herpes simplex virus	Multiple painful vesicles on an erythematous base (HSV1 and HSV2) +/− urethritis	PCR testing, direct fluorescence antibody, or serologic tests of lesion	Antiviral (e.g., acyclovir) and supportive care (sitz bath, topical creams)
Syphilis	*Treponema pallidum*	Primary syphilis: painless chancre. If not treated, can present with systemic symptoms	Non-treponemal RPR or VDRL followed by treponemal FTA-ABS	Penicillin
Trichomoniasis	*Trichomonas vaginalis*	Urethritis, vulvovaginitis, yellow-green discharge	Microscopy with flagellated organisms is the first test for women. If negative or in men, do culture or NAAT	Metronidazole
Bacterial vaginosis**	Anaerobic bacteria (e.g., *Gardnerella vaginalis*)	White-gray vaginal discharge with fishy odor, vulvovaginitis	Clinical diagnosis +/− microscopy with +KOH "whiff test," visualization of clue cells (epithelial cells coated with bacteria), and pH >4.5	Metronidazole, male partners do not need treatment
Yeast infection**	*Candida albicans*	Itchy curd-like discharge with vulvovaginitis	Clinical diagnosis +/− visualization of budding yeast with a KOH stain	Topical azoles
HIV	Human immunodeficiency virus	Many systemic presentations	Immunoassay	Antiretroviral therapy

* May be caused by sexual contact OR auto-inoculation (herpetic whitlow, herpetic stomatitis).

** Non-STI causes of vaginal complaints.

WARTS

ETIOLOGY

Human papillomavirus

SIGNS AND SYMPTOMS

Small, cauliflower-like lesions that can occur throughout the anogenital regions of both genders.

DIAGNOSIS

Visual inspection for typical lesions

TREATMENT

- Cryotherapy.
- Topical antiviral agents such as imiquimod or podofilox.
- Prevention for many types with adolescent HPV vaccination.

CERVICITIS

ETIOLOGY

Infection of the endocervix, typically with C. *trachomatis* or N. *gonorrhoeae*.

SIGNS AND SYMPTOMS

- Mucopurulent discharge from cervical os.
- Friable cervix.
- Pelvic pain with manipulation of cervix with N. *gonorrhoeae*.
- Asymptomatic infection common.

DIAGNOSIS

Nucleic acid amplification tests (NAATs) on urine, vaginal, or endocervical fluid.

TREATMENT

- Oral azithromycin for isolated chlamydia
  - Alternatives include doxycycline, erythromycin, levofloxacin, or ofloxacin.
- Ceftriaxone for isolated N. *gonorrhoeae*.
- Simultaneous treatment for both chlamydia and gonorrhea is typical.

URETHRITIS

ETIOLOGY

- Infection of the urethra, typically with C. *trachomatis* or N. *gonorrhoeae*.
- Far more common in men.

SIGNS AND SYMPTOMS

- Purulent urethral discharge.
- Dysuria, frequency, and meatal erythema.

DIAGNOSIS

Nucleic acid amplification tests (NAATs) on urine or urethral fluid.

TREATMENT

- Oral azithromycin for isolated chlamydia
  - Alternatives include doxycycline, erythromycin, levofloxacin, or ofloxacin.

- Ceftriaxone for isolated N. *gonorrhoeae*.
- Simultaneous treatment for both chlamydia and gonorrhea is typical.

ULCERS

ETIOLOGY

- Most commonly due to herpes simplex virus 1, 2 or 3; primary syphilis; chancroid (*Haemophilus ducreyi*).
- In children, also think of systemic causes (e.g., Crohn's) and other syndromes.
- Lipschütz ulcers ("virginal" or "aphthous" ulcers): large, painful necrotic ulcers with purulent base, raised edges, systemic symptoms (ages 10–15 years); etiology may be viral.
- With oral ulcers, arthritis, uveitis, think: Behçet syndrome.
- With ulcers in oropharynx and conjunctivitis, think: Stevens-Johnson syndrome and toxic epidermal necrolysis.

SIGNS AND SYMPTOMS

- HSV
    - Painful, shallow ulcers.
    - Systemic signs and symptoms similar to flu may be seen.
    - Tender regional adenopathy.
- Primary syphilis
    - Painless, single ulcer with sharp edge.
    - Painless regional adenopathy.
- Chancroid
    - Multiple, painful ulcers with irregular borders.
    - Fluctuant, painful, regional adenopathy.

DIAGNOSIS

- HSV
    - PCR, direct fluorescent antibody, or culture (Tzanck smear rarely used now).
- Primary syphilis
    - Serum testing including RPR, FTA-ABS, VDRL.
- Chancroid
    - Culture of lesion fluid.

TREATMENT

- HSV
    - Antiviral agents including acyclovir, valacyclovir, and famciclovir.
- Primary syphilis
    - Intramuscular penicillin.
- Chancroid
    - Oral macrolide (azithromycin or erythromycin) or parenteral ceftriaxone.

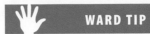

WARD TIP

PainFUL ulcers:
Chancroid (*Hemophilus ducreyi*)
Herpes
PainLESS ulcers:
Lymphogranuloma venereum (LGV)
Chancre in primary syphilis

A 15-year-old female presents to the ED with a fever and lower abdominal pain for 1 day, dyspareunia (pain with sex), and vaginal discharge. She had unprotected sexual intercourse with a new male partner recently. Physical exam reveals adnexal tenderness, cervical motion tenderness, and a friable cervix. *Think: Pelvic inflammatory disease (PID).*

Acute PID should be suspected in young females with pelvic pain. Empiric antibiotic treatment is recommended in **all** sexually active women with lower abdominal pain and cervical motion, adnexal, or uterine tenderness. Elevated temperature, leukocytosis, and purulent discharge may help with diagnosis, but treatment should be initiated even without these findings.

PELVIC INFLAMMATORY DISEASE

DEFINITION

An inflammatory process of the uterus, ovaries, peritoneal tissues and fallopian tubes

EPIDEMIOLOGY

- About 1.25 million cases yearly in the United States.
- The leading cause of reproductive morbidity (sterility, ectopic pregnancy).

ETIOLOGY

STIs, including *C. trachomatis*, *N. gonorrhoeae*, and a variety of other vaginal organisms.

SIGNS AND SYMPTOMS

- Lower abdominal pain.
- Vaginal discharge.
- "Chandelier sign" – patient jumps towards the ceiling from pain with cervical motion.
- Uterine and adnexal tenderness.
- Can progress to tubo-ovarian abscesses, peritonitis, and perihepatitis (Fitz-Hugh-Curtis syndrome).

DIAGNOSIS

See Table 22-5.

TREATMENT

- Outpatient therapy with a combination of third-generation cephalosporins and doxycycline, with or without metronidazole.

TABLE 22-5. Diagnostic Criteria for Pelvic Inflammatory Disease

Minimum criteria

Empiric treatment of PID should be initiated in sexually active young women and others at risk for sexually transmitted infections if one or more of the following minimum criteria are present:

- They are experiencing pelvic or lower abdominal pain and no other cause(s) for the illness can be identified
- Cervical motion tenderness or uterine tenderness or adnexal tenderness

Additional supportive criteria

Oral temperature > 38.3°C (101°F)

Abnormal cervical or vaginal mucopurulent discharge or cervical friability

Presence of abundant white blood cells on microscopic evaluation of vaginal secretions diluted in saline

Elevated erythrocyte sedimentation rate or elevated C-reactive protein

Laboratory documentation of infection with *Neisseria gonorrhoeae* or *Chlamydia trachomatis*

Definitive criteria (selected cases)

Histopathologic evidence of endometritis on endometrial biopsy

Tubo-ovarian abscess on sonography or other radiologic tests

Laparoscopic abnormalities consistent with PID

(Adapted, with permission, from the Centers for Disease Control and Prevention: Sexually transmitted diseases treatment guidelines 2015.)

- Initial inpatient antibiotic treatment and transition to oral therapy for uncertain diagnosis, concern for surgical abdomen, pelvic or tubo-ovarian abscess, pregnancy, inability to take oral medications, failed outpatient therapy, or severe disease.

Contraception

BARRIER

- Includes male and female condoms
  - Latex brands reduce the risk of transmitting STIs to a partner.
  - Pregnancy prevention improved when combined with spermicide.
- Diaphragms and cervical caps are generally not effectively used in adolescents.

INTRAUTERINE DEVICE (IUD)

- Copper and hormonal IUDs available.
- Misperception that these cause infection or not safe for teens.
- More expensive and less readily available than condoms.

IMPLANT

- Single progestin-only rod inserted in upper arm provides 3 years of pregnancy protection.
- Irregular bleeding and occasionally prolonged bleeding noted.

VAGINAL RING

- About a 2-inch, flexible ring inserted into the vagina by the patient.
- Backup contraception needed if out of place for more than 48 hours.

TRANSDERMAL PATCH

- Applied to lower abdomen, upper body, or buttocks for 7 days and then replaced twice, with no patch the 4th week allows for bleeding to occur.

ORAL CONTRACEPTIVES

- Variety of estrogen and progesterone combination pills.
- Can assist in regulation of menstrual cycles, especially for teens with dysmenorrhea or bleeding challenges.
- Nausea and weight gain often cited as reasons for failure.
- Remembering to take a pill daily can be challenging for some teens.

CONTRACEPTIVE INJECTIONS

- Injectable medroxyprogesterone acetate
  - Administered every 3 months.
  - Irregular bleeding problematic for some, but amenorrhea a benefit for those with heavy cycles.
  - Reversible osteoporosis later in life potential risk.

NOTES

Psychiatric Disease

Psychiatric Examination of Children

- Consult multiple sources:
  - Child: young children usually report information in concrete terms but give accurate details about their emotional states.
  - Parents, teachers, child welfare, and social services workers.
- Methods of gathering information from children:
  - Play, stories, drawing.
  - Kaufman Assessment Battery for Children: cognitive test for ages 3 to 18.
  - Wechsler Intelligence Scale for Children–Revised: intelligence quotient (IQ) for ages 6–16.
  - Peabody Individual Achievement Test: tests scholastic achievement.

Intellectual Disability

See Neurologic Disease chapter.

Learning Disability

See Neurologic Disease chapter.

Behavioral Disorders

DEFINITION

Behavioral disorders include oppositional defiant disorder and conduct disorder.

OPPOSITIONAL DEFIANT DISORDER

 A 9-year-old boy is defiant toward his teacher, refusing requests to follow the rules. His parents report similar scenarios at home, and he often becomes argumentative with them. *Think: Oppositional defiant disorder (ODD).*

Some oppositional behavior may be normal. However, normal defiance should not **impair significant social relationship or academic performance**. Children with ODD have substantially impaired relationships with parents, teachers, and peers, but they might not show oppositional behavior in the pediatrician office. The diagnosis is based on parent and teacher reports. Attention deficit hyperactivity disorder (ADHD) and other mood disorders may coexist.

DIAGNOSIS

- *Diagnostic and Statistical Manual of Mental Disorders*, 5th ed. (DSM-V) definition: recurrent pattern of argumentative, defiant, vindictive, and hostile behavior for more than 6 months.
- Consistent pattern of disobedience toward authority figures.
- Four or more of the following criteria are usually present:
  - Loses temper.
  - Argues with adults.

- ▪ Refuses to follow rules.
- ▪ Deliberately annoys others.
- ▪ Does not take responsibility for mistakes or behavior.
- ▪ Sensitive, touchy, easily annoyed.
- ▪ Angry, resentful.
- ▪ Spiteful, vindictive.
- ▪ Behavior causes impairment in social and academic functioning.
- ▪ Rule out other causes of clinical presentation.

PATHOPHYSIOLOGY

Low self-esteem, low frustration tolerance, often with comorbid substance abuse

EPIDEMIOLOGY

- ▪ Prevalence: 2–16%.
- ▪ May be a precursor of a conduct disorder.
- ▪ Increased incidence of substance abuse, mood disorders, ADHD.

TREATMENT

- ▪ Behavioral therapy, problem-solving skills.
- ▪ Early intervention is more effective than waiting for a child to grow out of it.
- ▪ Parental management training.

CONDUCT DISORDER

 The school reports a 9-year-old boy has been hitting other children and stealing pens. The mother reports that he often pokes their family cat with sharp objects. *Think: Conduct disorder (CD).*

This disorder involves a variety of problematic behaviors, including oppositional and defiant behaviors and antisocial activities, such as lying, stealing, running away, and physical violence. This pattern of behavior violates the basic rights of others. CD is more common in boys, is difficult to treat, and is more likely to persist into adulthood.

DIAGNOSIS

- ▪ Chronic conflict with parents, teachers, or peers.
- ▪ A repetitive and persistent behavior pattern that involves violation of the basic rights of others or of social norms and rules, with at least three of the following in 1 year:
    - ▪ Aggression toward people and animals.
    - ▪ Destruction of property.
    - ▪ Deceitfulness or theft.
    - ▪ Serious violation of rules.
- ▪ The behavior causes significant impairment in social, academic, or occupational functioning.

ETIOLOGY

- ▪ Lack of empathy is an important risk factor.
- ▪ Involves genetic and psychosocial factors.

EPIDEMIOLOGY

- ▪ High risk of developing antisocial personality disorder in adulthood.
- ▪ Increased incidence of ADHD, learning disorders, mood disorders, substance abuse, and criminal behavior in adulthood.

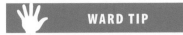

WARD TIP

Temper tantrums and breath holding are manipulative behaviors.

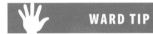

WARD TIP

ODD can be a developmental antecedent to conduct disorder. The former does not involve any violation of the basic rights of others.

EXAM TIP

Conduct disorder is one of the most difficult mental health problems during adolescence. There is a high correlation with antisocial personality disorder in adulthood.

TREATMENT

- Multimodal:
    - Structured environment, firm rules, consistent enforcement.
    - Psychotherapy: behavior modification, problem-solving skills.
    - Optimize comorbid treatment of ADHD.

Attention Deficit/Hyperactivity Disorder (ADHD)

 An 11-year-old does not complete his homework. He claims that he did not know about the assignments. He interrupts other kids, is often restless, and gets up during class. His parents report that he cannot sit still at the dinner table. *Think: ADHD— inattentive, and hyperactive **in at least two settings.***

DEFINITION

- Three types predominantly:
    - Inattentive.
    - Hyperactive-impulsive.
    - Combined: most children have the combined type.

DIAGNOSIS

- Six or more of the following present for more than 6 months:
    - **Inattention:** problems listening, concentrating, paying attention to details, organizing tasks, easily distracted, forgetful.
    - **Hyperactivity-impulsivity:** unable to inhibit impulses, blurting out, interrupting, fidgeting, leaving seat, talking excessively.
    - **Combined subtype:** six or more symptoms of inattention and hyperactivity-impulsivity.
    - Behavior inconsistent with age and development.
    - Impairment interferes in at least two settings (social, academic, occupational).
- The above may lead to:
    - Difficulty getting along with peers and family.
    - School underachievement secondary to poor organizational skills.
    - Poor sequential memory, deficits in fine motor skills.
- Medical conditions and sleep conditions must be ruled out.
- Eliminate other causes: death in the family, divorce, hearing deficits, anxiety or depression, learning disability, child abuse.

ETIOLOGY

- Genetic predisposition and environmental factors (including family dysfunction).
- Perinatal complications, maternal nutrition and substance abuse, obstetric complications, viral infections.
- Neurochemical/neurophysiologic factors (e.g., lead poisoning).
- Psychosocial factors, including emotional deprivation and parental anxiety and inexperience.

PATHOPHYSIOLOGY

- Catecholamine hypothesis: a decrease in norepinephrine metabolites.
- Hypodopaminergic function, low levels of homovanillic acid.

EPIDEMIOLOGY

- Prevalence: 4–12% among young and school-age children.
- Male to female ratio 2 to 3:1.
- Seen with mood, personality, conduct, and oppositional defiant disorders.
- ADHD may continue into adulthood resulting in work and personal challenges.

TREATMENT

- Pharmacotherapy:
  - **First line**: psychostimulants such as methylphenidate (Ritalin), dextroamphetamine.
- **Second line**:
  - Atomoxetine (Strattera).
  - Tricyclic antidepressants (work by blocking dopamine).
  - Clonidine and guanfacine (affect norepinephrine discharge rates).
- Non-pharmacotherapy:
  - Behavior modification, cognitive behavioral therapy, group therapy.
  - Parental counseling: positive reinforcement, firm nonpunitive limit setting, reduced external stimulation.

Autism Spectrum Disorders (ASD)

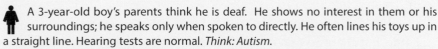

A 3-year-old boy's parents think he is deaf. He shows no interest in them or his surroundings; he speaks only when spoken to directly. He often lines his toys up in a straight line. Hearing tests are normal. *Think: Autism.*

Autism is a spectrum of behaviors that include abnormalities in social interactions, aberrant communication, and restricted repetitive and stereotyped behaviors. The onset is before age 3 years. Speech is typically delayed or may regress. It is often associated with intellectual disability.

DEFINITION

- Group of conditions that involve problems with social skills, language, and behaviors.
- Apparent early in life with multiple areas of developmental delay.
- Asperger syndrome, pervasive developmental disorder, and childhood disintegrative disorders are included in ASD with the DSM-5 revision.

ETIOLOGY

- Unknown. Possibilities include:
  - Genetic predisposition: higher incidence in siblings, especially twins.
  - Prenatal neurologic insult.
  - Immunologic and biochemical factors.

PATHOPHYSIOLOGY

- Neuroanatomic structural abnormalities
  - Initial rapid brain growth is followed by slow growth in areas responsible for higher functions of cognition, language, emotion, and social function.

EPIDEMIOLOGY

- Prevalence: about 1:68
  - Increased incidence may be due to improved screening, understanding, and diagnostic accuracy.

WARD TIP

Stimulants used appropriately for ADHD do not cause addiction.

EXAM TIP

ADHD in teens and adults can be linked to increased risk-taking behavior and depression.

EXAM TIP

There is a high degree of comorbidity in children with ADHD to also have conduct disorder or ODD.

EXAM TIP

Many children with autism spectrum disorder have intellectual disability, although a few have narrow remarkable abilities (savants).

EXAM TIP

Autism spectrum disorders are not caused by thimerosal-containing vaccines.

EXAM TIP

Characteristic triad in autism:
Impairments in social interaction, impairments in communication, and restricted interests and repetitive behaviors

WARD TIP

Standard developmental screening tests have poor sensitivity for autism spectrum disorders.

- 4:1 male to female (except in Rett syndrome, which is more common in girls).
- Significant comorbidity occurs with fragile X syndrome, Rett syndrome, tuberous sclerosis, intellectual disability, and seizures.

DIAGNOSIS

- Persistent deficits in all three forms of social communication and interaction:
  - Social-emotional reciprocity (back and forth conversation).
  - Nonverbal communication (abnormal eye contact, cannot understand gestures).
  - Maintaining and understanding relationships (difficulty or disinterest in making friends).
- Repetitive, restrictive behavioral patterns or activities:
  - Echolalia or repetitive movements, unwavering adherence to routine/sameness.
  - Increased or decreased response to sensory input (a sound, excessive touching objects).
- Symptoms must be present in early development and must impair life either in early or later development.

TREATMENT

- No curative treatment exists.
- Supportive modalities are used to manage symptoms and improve social skills.
  - Early childhood intervention (ECI): free or low cost services for children less than 3 years of age focusing on strengthening and achieving developmental milestones.
  - Applied behavioral analysis: encourages positive behaviors and discourages negative behaviors.
- Medication to decrease harmful or negative sequelae (self-injury, irritability, etc.): Risperidone is FDA approved, and other non-FDA-approved medications include SSRI, TCA, stimulant, anti-convulsants.

WARD TIP

Computed tomography (CT) and magnetic resonance imaging (MRI) in autistic disorder may be normal or may show ventricular enlargement; polymicrogyria; histologically may show small, densely packed, immature cells in the limbic system and cerebellum.

WARD TIP

Those with autistic disorder and who do speak often exhibit echolalia, pronoun reversal, inappropriate cadence or intonation, impaired semantics, and failure to use language for social interaction.

WARD TIP

Fifty to sixty percent of individuals with a single depressive episode can be expected to have a second episode.

Mood Disorders

MAJOR DEPRESSIVE DISORDER (MDD)

DEFINITION

- Pathologic sadness or despondency, not explained as a normal response to stress, that causes impairment in function.
- Recurrent condition, often continues into adulthood.

ETIOLOGY/PATHOPHYSIOLOGY

- Genetic predisposition; 2 to 4 times more common if first degree relatives with MDD.
- Unknown. Heterogeneous disease with biological, genetic, environmental, and psychosocial factors contributing
  - Catecholamine hypothesis: a norepinephrine deficit at brain-nerve terminals.
  - Cortisol hypothesis: larger quantities of blood and urine cortisol metabolites, abnormal diurnal variation.

EPIDEMIOLOGY

- The prevalence is 0.5% to 1.4% in children and 11.4% in adolescents.
- Incidence rises post pubertal, especially in girls.
- Comorbidities include anxiety/panic disorders, OCD, eating disorders, substance abuse, borderline personality disorder, ADHD, and ODD.
- Up to 15% of patients with depression attempt or contemplate suicide.
- Can persist into adulthood.

DIAGNOSIS

- Five of the following signs for ≥2 weeks:
  - Depressed mood most of the day.
  - Loss of interest in activities.
  - Sleep disturbance (insomnia or hypersomnia) nearly every day.
  - Weight change or appetite disturbance.
  - Decreased concentration.
  - Suicidal ideation or thoughts of death.
  - Psychomotor agitation or retardation.
  - Fatigue or loss of energy.
  - Feelings of worthlessness or inappropriate guilt.
- Eliminate other causes, such as hypothyroidism, nutritional deficiency, chronic infection/systemic disease, and substance abuse.

TREATMENT

- If the patient is suicidal or homicidal, admit them to the hospital.
- If there is no harm or risk to the patient or others, use:
  - Biopsychosocial approach, cognitive behavior therapy (CBT), individual and/or group therapy, family intervention.
- If failed non-pharmacological treatment start SSRI, often fluoxetine or escitalopram.

PERSISTENT DEPRESSIVE DISORDER (DYSTHYMIA)/CHRONIC DEPRESSION

- Depressed mood, more days than not, for at least 1 year
  - Two of the following symptoms: appetite disturbance, sleep disturbance, fatigue, low self-esteem, poor concentration, difficulty making decisions, or feelings of hopelessness.
  - No manic, hypomanic, or disturbance better explained by schizophrenic behavior.

UNSPECIFIED DEPRESSIVE DISORDER

Clinically significant depressive symptoms that cause distress or impairment in functioning, but do not meet full criteria for depressive disorder. These can be used where the physician does not have sufficient information to make diagnosis of depression (e.g., emergency room setting).

Suicide

RELEVANT DEFINITIONS

- **Suicidal ideation:** with or without a plan.
- **Suicide gesture:** for attention, without intent for death.
- **Suicide attempt:** intention for death.

WARD TIP

In suspected cases of depression, be sure to look for other signs or risk factors such as school failure or family history of mental health disorders.

WARD TIP

A combination of treatments for depression may be necessary. Childhood depression often can be treated with behavior modification. More severe mood disorders are managed by a child psychiatrist and often require medications. A combination may be optimal.

WARD TIP

Use of antidepressant medications, particularly SSRIs, in adolescents reportedly may increase risk of suicidal thoughts and behaviors during initial weeks due to disinhibition. These data are controversial.

EXAM TIP

One percent of suicide gestures are lethal.

EXAM TIP

Thirty to seventy percent of suicides occur with significant alcohol or drug abuse. Substance abuse disinhibits the individual to complete the act.

ETIOLOGY

- Suicide is a complex human behavior with biologic, sociologic, and psychological roots.
- Psychiatric disorders: correlations of suicidal behavior and mood or disruptive disorders, substance abuse, and personality disorders (borderline personality disorder).
- Environmental factors: stressful life events; family disruption due to death or separation, illness, birth, or siblings; peer pressure; physical or sexual abuse.
- Parental influence: psychiatric illness, substance abuse, violence, physical or sexual abuse.

EPIDEMIOLOGY

- Second leading cause of death for young adults age 10–19.
- Boys attempt suicide less often but are more successful than girls; girls tend to choose less-lethal methods like overdose or cutting; boys choose firearms or hanging.
- The rate of suicide is higher in Alaskan, Asian-American, and Native-American youth.
- Risk factors include history of psychiatric disorders, prior attempts, family clustering of suicides, substance use/abuse, history of sexual abuse, or major depression.

ASSESSMENT

- Assess signs and symptoms, correlate with other clinical variables, such as psychiatric and substance abuse history, gender, age, race, prior history of suicide attempts, and recent traumatic life events.
- Key questions: Are you having any thoughts about harming yourself or taking your life? Have you developed a plan? What is your plan?

TREATMENT

- Immediate hospitalization; remove all potentially lethal items.
- Psychotherapeutic intervention, trustful atmosphere, coping strategies; remove motivation for suicide; involve parents and relatives, guidance counselor.
- Pharmacotherapy depends on the accompanying diagnosis.

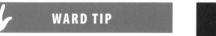

Violent Behavior

EPIDEMIOLOGY

- Homicide is the third leading cause of death among 15- to 19-year-olds and the leading cause of death in African-American adolescents.
- Rates of homicide are higher in males than in females.
- Death by firearm homicide is highest in the 15- to 24-year-old age group.

RISK FACTORS

- Intellectual disability, moderate to severe language disorder, learning disorder, ADHD, mood disorders, anxiety disorders, personality disorders, conduct disorders, and ODD.
- Other risk factors include substance abuse, gang involvement, history/exposure to domestic/child abuse, and access to firearms.

SCREENING

Ask about recent involvement in physical fights, carrying a weapon, firearms in household, gang involvement, concerns about the person's safety, past trauma episodes, and school or home social problems.

Anxiety Disorders

SEPARATION ANXIETY DISORDER

DEFINITION

- Excessive anxiety beyond that expected for the child's developmental level related to separation or impending separation from the attachment figure.
- Separation anxiety is normal until age 3–4 years.

EPIDEMIOLOGY

- Prevalence: 4% of school-age children.
- Males and females are affected equally.

ETIOLOGY

Possibly genetic; higher incidence when first-degree relative is affected. Contribution by anxiety when excessive parental concern is expressed.

SIGNS AND SYMPTOMS

- May refuse to sleep alone or go to school.
- May complain of physical symptoms to avoid anxiety-provoking activities (somatization).
- Becomes extremely distressed when forced to separate, and may worry excessively about losing their parents forever.

TREATMENT

- Family therapy.
- Supportive psychotherapy.
- Low-dose SSRIs.

OBSESSIVE-COMPULSIVE (OCD) AND RELATED DISORDERS

DEFINITION

- **Obsessions:** persistent, intrusive thoughts, images, impulses involuntarily intruding into consciousness. Common themes are contamination and fear of harm to self or others.
- **Compulsions:** actions are due to an internal obligation to follow certain rituals and rules.

ETIOLOGY

Genetic predisposition, higher concordance among monozygotic versus dizygotic twins

EPIDEMIOLOGY

One-fourth of cases begin by 14 years of age.
High comorbidity occurs with anxiety disorders, depression, and tic disorders.

DIAGNOSIS

Obsession and/or compulsions causing impairment in social, academic, or work functioning

WARD TIP

Separation anxiety may lead to complaints of somatic symptoms to avoid school/work.

SIGNS AND SYMPTOMS

- Preoccupied with details, rules, lists, order, organization, or schedules, resulting in loss of the goal of activity.
- Perfectionism that prohibits task completion.
- Social impairment due to preoccupation with work and level of productivity.
- Overconscientious, scrupulous, and inflexible about matters of morality, ethics, or values.
- Unable to discard objects of no worth or sentimental value.
- Preference to work as an individual and not in a group.
- Miserly spending to save for future catastrophes.
- Inflexible, rigid, stubborn.
- Characteristics must be ego-dystonic and functionally disruptive versus ego-syntonic and functionally adaptive in OCD.

TREATMENT

- Long-term therapy is required.
- Behavioral therapy, such as self-observation, extinction, operant conditioning, and modeling.
- Pharmacotherapy:
  - First-line agents are SSRIs.
  - Clomipramine is a second-line agent.

EXAM TIP

Habit reversal: substituting another, more benign behavior for the previous habit

Body Dysmorphic Disorder

- Preoccupation with an imagined defect in appearance or excessive concern about a slight physical anomaly (e.g., large nose, small muscles) occurs.
- Multiple visits to plastic surgeons or dermatologists are common.
- Mean age of onset is 15 years.
- Risk factors include child maltreatment such as abuse.
- Comorbidities include depression, substance abuse, social anxiety disorder, and OCD.
- Treatment: CBT, SSRI, or combination has been effective.

Selective Mutism

DEFINITION

Not speaking in certain situations (e.g., school)

EPIDEMIOLOGY

- Onset usually around age 3 or 4.
- May be preceded by a stressful life event.

TREATMENT

Supportive psychotherapy, behavior therapy, family therapy
Fluoxetine when school performance severely affected

Gender Dysphoria

DIAGNOSIS

- A difference between the gender assigned and inner gender identity.
- The discrepancy causes stress and functional impairment in social, academic, and personal settings.

EPIDEMIOLOGY

- Coexisting anxiety or depression disorders are common.
- Increased risk of suicide exists.

SIGNS AND SYMPTOMS

- Persistent discomfort with assigned sex
  - Desire to be rid of assigned sex characteristics.
  - Strong desire for sex characteristics of the opposite gender.
  - Desire to be the opposite gender.
  - Preference to be treated like the opposite gender.
  - Conviction that their feelings and reactions are those of the other gender.

TREATMENT

General support in accepting patient's desired gender through psychotherapy or hormone therapy to slow progression of puberty (considered reversible). Gender affirming surgery is typically deferred until 18 years of age, as it is not reversible.

Eating Disorders

ANOREXIA NERVOSA (SEE ADOLESCENT CHAPTER)

BULIMIA NERVOSA (SEE ADOLESCENT CHAPTER)

RUMINATION

DIAGNOSIS

- Repeated regurgitation and rechewing of food for a period of at least 1 month following a period of normal functioning.
- Other medical, psychiatric conditions (including other eating disorders) have been ruled out.

ETIOLOGY

- Adverse psychosocial environment.
- Individuals with intellectual disability.

PATHOPHYSIOLOGY

- Unsatisfactory mother–infant relationship.
- Positive reinforcement when attention follows rumination.
- Negative reinforcement when rumination reduces anxiety.

EPIDEMIOLOGY

Highest prevalence occurs in normal infants and intellectually disabled adults.

SIGNS AND SYMPTOMS

- Presents with "spitting up" or frequent vomiting.
- Effortless regurgitation, does not involve retching.
- Malnutrition, weight loss, failure to thrive.

TREATMENT

- Counseling to improve parent–child dynamics.
- Behavioral intervention.
- Aversive techniques—withdrawal of positive attention.
- In infants, the disorder frequently remits spontaneously.

PICA

DIAGNOSIS

- Persistent eating of nonnutritive substances for ≥1 month (e.g., clay, dirt, etc.)
- The activity is inappropriate to the level of development.
- Behavior is not culturally sanctioned.
- Other psychiatric disorders have been ruled out.

ETIOLOGY

- Intellectual disability.
- Vitamin or mineral deficiencies (e.g., iron deficiency anemia, particularly in pregnancy).
- Poverty, neglect, lack of parental supervision, developmental delays.
- Cultural belief.

EPIDEMIOLOGY

- In children aged 18 months to 2 years, the ingestion and mouthing of nonnutritive substances is normal behavior.
- Most common during 2 and 3 years of age.
- The prevalence increases with the severity of intellectual disability.

SIGNS AND SYMPTOMS

- Presenting complaint is— "puts everything in his or her mouth."
- Complications include:
  - Ingestion of paint chips is associated with lead poisoning.
  - Hair or large objects can cause bezoar with bowel obstruction.
  - Sharp objects such as pins or nails can cause intestinal perforation.
  - Ingestion of feces or dirt can result in parasitic infections.

TREATMENT

- Often remits spontaneously.
- Treat underlying vitamin deficiency, if present.
- Psychotherapy—assess why pica is occurring.
- Behavior modification.
- Direct observation and removal of potential pica.

WARD TIP

Pica is found more commonly in patients with autism spectrum disorders, intellectual disability, OCD, and schizophrenia.

Somatic Symptom and Related Disorders

See Table 23-1 comparing somatoform disorders, factitious disorders, and malingering.

TABLE 23-1. Somatic Symptoms versus Factitious Disorders versus Malingering

DISORDER	DEVELOPMENT OF SYMPTOMS	REASON FOR SYMPTOMS
Somatic symptoms	Unconscious	Unconscious
Factitious disorder	Conscious	Unconscious (primary gain)
Malingering	Conscious	Conscious (secondary gain)

DEFINITION

- Somatic symptoms occur with significant distress or impairment in social, occupational, or other areas of functioning.
- These include somatic symptom disorder, conversion disorder, pain disorder (functional neurological symptom disorder), illness anxiety disorder, factitious disorder, psychological factors affecting other medical conditions.

TREATMENT

- Psychodynamic therapy: gain insight into unconscious conflicts and understand how psychological factors have influenced symptom maintenance.
- Identify and eliminate sources of secondary gain to avoid symptom reinforcing.
- Improve self-esteem, promoting assertiveness, and teach non-somatic ways to express distress.
- Group therapy: learn better coping strategies and improved social skills.

SOMATIC SYMPTOM DISORDER

- One or more somatic symptoms that results in disruption of daily life.
- It must meet two of the following criteria:
  - High health-related anxiety.
  - Disproportionate and persistent concerns about the medical seriousness of one's symptoms.
  - Excessive time and energy devoted to these concerns.
- Symptoms do not necessarily have to be medically explained, but they must be accompanied by excessive thoughts, feelings, and behavior.
- Comorbidities include depression, IBS, fibromyalgia, chronic pain, PTSD, and history of sexual or physical abuse.

CONVERSION DISORDER

DIAGNOSIS

- Sensory symptoms or motor deficits that are not intentionally produced.
- Symptoms cannot be explained by an organic etiology.
- Initiation of the symptom or deficit is preceded by a psychological stressor.
- Symptoms can cause impairment in social functioning.
- Other etiologies for the clinical presentation are ruled out.

EPIDEMIOLOGY

- Onset may occur at any age, but it is more common in adolescence or adulthood.
- More common in women than men.
- Increased incidence occurs in children who have experienced physical or sexual abuse and in those whose parents are seriously ill or have chronic pain.

SIGNS AND SYMPTOMS

- Paralysis, abnormal movements, inability to speak, see, hear; pseudoseizures.
- Associated with comorbid neurologic, depressive, or anxiety disorders.
- *La belle indifference*, the lack of interest in potentially life-altering symptoms, is common in adults, but rarely occurs in children.

WARD TIP

Favorable prognosis for conversion disorder is associated with acute onset, definite precipitation by a stressful event, good premorbid health, and the absence of previous psychiatric illness.

EXAM TIP

Conversion disorder may be associated in some cases with history of a traumatic brain injury.

EXAM TIP

A proportion of patients diagnosed with conversion disorder go on to develop demonstrable organic pathology (e.g., multiple sclerosis or seizure nidus).

A 17-year-old girl is concerned that a small left breast lump is malignant cancer despite a benign histopathology report. You are the fourth doctor she consults for an opinion. *Think: Illness anxiety disorder.*

She has hypochondriasis, defined as a preoccupation with fears of having, or the belief that one has, a serious disease despite evidence to the contrary. The key feature in this condition is an abnormal concern that one is developing or has a serious illness. Psychotherapy that includes exploration of current life problems often result in symptom resolution.

DIAGNOSIS

- Preoccupation with having or fear of having a disease for >6 months.
- Somatic symptoms are mild or nonexistent.
- Persistent preoccupation occurs despite adequate medical evaluation and assurance.
- Causes impairment in social functioning.
- Illness preoccupation cannot be explained by other mental disorders.

ETIOLOGY

- Associated with anxiety, depression, and narcissistic traits.
- Past experience with serious illness as a child or of a family member.

SIGNS AND SYMPTOMS

- Many visits to different doctors and deterioration of doctor–patient relationships.
- Complain they are not receiving proper care so they pursue more opinions.
- Receive many evaluations and unnecessary surgeries.
- Drug addiction may result due to their chronic ongoing physical complaints.

TREATMENT

- Help the patient identify and manage the fear of serious illness.
    - Include behavior-modification techniques.
    - Treat comorbid anxiety and depressive disorders, as needed.

EXAM TIP

Anxiety disorder can lead to strained social relationships because of preoccupation with perceived condition and the patient's expectation of receiving special treatment.

Factitious Disorders

DEFINITION

- Intentional fabrication or actual symptom production in a child by a caregiver (usually the mother) to gain attention for themselves.
- Also known as "Factitious Disorder by Proxy" and "Medical Child Abuse."

EPIDEMIOLOGY

- Adults who commit MBP may have a personal history of factitious disorders.
- Most offenders are women and the parent of the child.

SIGNS AND SYMPTOMS

- Conditions unresponsive to treatment or unusual disease course often include:
    - Vomiting/diarrhea (ingestion, syrup of ipecac).
    - Rashes (due to scrubbing with solvents).
    - Failure to thrive (food withholding).
    - Seizures (exogenous insulin administration).
    - Infections (injecting feces into IV line).
    - Adding blood or other substances to urine specimens.
- Physical or laboratory findings that are unusual, discrepant, or clinically impossible or occur only in the parent's presence.
- Medically knowledgeable mother who appears connected to the hospital setting, who is reluctant to leave the child, and may be dramatic and desires attention.
- Family history of similar problems or unexplained sibling death.
- Signs or history of factitious disorder in mother.

DIAGNOSIS

Appropriate physician suspicion, good medical records, and reporting of abuse (often multiple doctors have been visited, with little continuity)

TREATMENT

The caregiver requires psychiatric therapy, such as for other factitious disorders.

MALINGERING

DEFINITION

Intentional symptom creation of secondary gain (e.g., getting out school or doing chores)

WARD TIP

Malingering	Munchausen
Secondary gain (avoiding chores/school)	Primary gain (gain attention for self)

Personality Disorders

- These patterns of behavior deviate from cultural standards and can begin in adolescence or early adulthood. See Table 23-2.
- Cluster A: "Weird"
    - Paranoid Personality: distrustful and suspicious.
    - Schizoid Personality: wants to be isolated, a loner type with limited emotional expression.

TABLE 23-2.   Personality Disorder Distinctions

DISORDER	IDENTIFYING FEATURE
OCPD	Find pleasure after completing actions
OCD	Feel distressed after actions
Avoidant	Wants relationships
Schizoid	Wants to be alone

- **Cluster B: "Wild"**
  - Borderline Personality: unstable mood, impulsive, splitting (a relationship is either awful or perfect).
  - Histrionic Personality: attention seeking (including seductive behavior), excessive emotionality (think soap operas).
  - Narcissistic Personality: demands the best, needs admiration, entitled, lacks empathy.
  - Antisocial Personality: lacks remorse, violates laws of society, breaks the law (if <18 years = Conduct Disorder).
- **Cluster C: "Worried"**
  - Obsessive-compulsive Personality: find pleasure in completing ritualistic actions.
  - Avoidant Personality: wants relationships with others but intense fear of ridicule and being disliked.
  - Dependent Personality: needs to be taken care of, cannot be on their own, submissive.

Pediatric Emergencies

General Approach to the Acutely Ill Child

- The approach to a child with a potentially life-threatening condition should be focused and systematic. Trauma provides a good model that can be adapted for any medical problem.
- **ABCDE** for a primary survey:
  - **Airway**: Is the airway patent, or obstructed/compromised? Does the patient require intubation? Are airway maneuvers, such as chin-lift/jaw-thrust, required?
  - **Breathing**: Is the patient's respiratory effort normal, excessive, or insufficient? Provide supplemental oxygen, bag-mask ventilation, or other airway support, as necessary.
  - **Circulation**: Does the patient have a life-threatening hemorrhage? (If an obvious, life-threatening hemorrhage is present, apply manual pressure during the primary survey to gain control.) Is the patient warm and well perfused, with strong pulses? Or are they cold and poorly perfusing? Establish IV access and provide fluids or blood products, as appropriate.
  - **Disability/Dextrose**: What is the patient's level of consciousness? (AVPU: <u>a</u>lert, responsive to <u>v</u>oice, responsive to <u>p</u>ain, or <u>u</u>nresponsive or check 15-point Glasgow Coma Score [GCS, Table 24-1]). Check glucose level for altered mental status (AMS).
  - **Exposure**: Does the patient require treatment for environmental exposure? Is the patient hyper- or hypothermic? Do they require decontamination of clothes, skin, hair, or mucus membranes?
- Once all life-threatening problems are being addressed, a more formal history and physical examination can be obtained, while still focusing on acute problems. The **SAMPLE** history may be useful:
  - **S**igns and **s**ymptoms: may help decide treatment plan.
  - **A**llergies: to medications or other.
  - **M**edications: current medications may alter treatment decisions.
  - **P**ast medical history: may give clues to underlying cause or provide information to guide treatment.
  - **L**ast meal: if control of the airway is needed, patient's NPO status may alter intubation plans. If NPO status cannot be confirmed, rapid-sequence intubation is preferred to decrease aspiration risk.
  - **E**vents: what was happening immediately prior to illness?

Acute Respiratory Failure

- History and physical with special attention to:
  - Acute increase in work of breathing, with or without fever, cough, tachypnea.
  - Examine for tachypnea, work of breathing, retractions, abnormal lung sounds, alterations to chest percussion.
  - Must include cardiac and abdominal examinations.

COMPARTMENT MODEL OF RESPIRATORY FAILURE (TABLE 24-2):

- Upper airway: obstruction from the upper aerodigestive tract to the large conducting airways:
  - Stridor is a common finding.

TABLE 24-1. Glasgow Coma Scale (GCS)

EYE OPENING (TOTAL POINTS: 4)

Spontaneous	4
To Voice	3
To Pain	2
None	1

VERBAL RESPONSE (TOTAL POINTS: 5)

INFANTS AND YOUNG CHILDREN		OLDER CHILDREN	
Appropriate words; smiles, fixes, and follows	5	Oriented	5
Consolable crying	4	Confused	4
Persistently irritable	3	Inappropriate	3
Restless, agitated	2	Incomprehensible	2
None	1	None	1

MOTOR RESPONSE (TOTAL POINTS: 6)

Obeys	6
Localizes pain	5
Withdraws	4
Flexion	3
Extension	2
None	1

Note minimum score is 3, not 0.

- Lower airways:
  - Wheezing is characteristic, crackles may be present.
  - Causes include asthma, bronchiolitis.
- Lung parenchymal disease:
  - Disorders of the alveoli (pulmonary edema, pneumonia, ARDS) disrupting gas exchange; results in shunt physiology (blood flow with no ventilation to affected lung region).
  - Disorders of the pulmonary vasculature: will cause dead space physiology (ventilation with no blood flow to affected lung region).
  - CNS system disorders: responsible for control of respiration, airway protection, clearance of secretions.
  - Disorders of the respiration muscles and peripheral nervous system: responsible for ability to expand lungs for adequate ventilatory effort and ability to maintain normal lung volumes (with sighing for example).

TABLE 24-2. **Compartment Model of Respiratory Failure**

COMMON CAUSES OF RESPIRATORY FAILURE	COMPARTMENT AFFECTED	HISTORY AND PHYSICAL EXAM	TREATMENT (IN ADDITION TO SUPPORTIVE CARE)
Croup (viral laryngotracheobronchitis)	Upper airway	Acute onset of fever, respiratory distress, and stridor. Often viral etiology	O_2 Racemic epinephrine Steroids (dexamethasone)
Retropharyngeal or peritonsillar abscess	Upper airway	Acute onset of fever, drooling, neck pain, trismus (inability to open jaw), respiratory distress Can diagnose with physical exam, or neck imaging if needed	Antibiotics Incision and drainage
Foreign body (FB) aspiration	Upper airway	Acute onset of respiratory distress, cough, inability to clear secretions, especially in a toddler (exploring environment). May have focal crackles or wheezing in affected area Radio-opaque FB may be visible on CXR. Otherwise, inspiratory/expiratory films may show hyperinflation in affected side (90% right side due to angle of airway)	Removal with bronchoscopy
Anaphylaxis	Upper airway Lower airway	Exposure to allergen, followed by respiratory distress, fever, vomiting, hypotension, hives.	IM epinephrine, steroids Intubation if upper airway
Asthma exacerbation (status asthmaticus)	Lower airway	PMH may include asthma or history of ectopy (allergies, eczema). Family history of asthma Acute onset of wheezing and respiratory distress	Glucocorticoids (methylprednisolone, dexamethasone) Bronchodilators albuterol ± ipratropium Magnesium CPAP or BiPAP may be needed
Bronchiolitis	Lower airway, lung parenchyma	Acute onset of fever and respiratory distress, with wheezing or crackles CXR shows peribronchial cuffing, perihilar fullness, ± patchy atelectasis or infiltrates Viral etiology, especially RSV	Supportive management including supplemental humidified oxygen, escalating to invasive or non-invasive ventilation as needed
Pneumonia	Lung parenchyma	Acute onset of fever, respiratory distress. Often with focal crackles or dullness to percussion. Tachypnea is a sensitive sign. CXR will often show focal consolidation, but may be normal early Etiology of pneumonia may be viral, bacterial, fungal, mycobacterial, or non-infectious	Empirical antibiotics (for community acquired pneumonia in otherwise healthy and fully vaccinated child, amoxicillin or ampicillin) Supportive therapy

DISORDERS OF CONTROL OF BREATHING AND APNEA

- Respiratory effort is controlled in brain stem, increasing respiratory effort (rate and depth) in response to increasing $PaCO_2$ or decreasing PaO_2.
- Apnea is defined as an absence of respiratory effort for more than 20 seconds, or for a shorter time if cyanosis, bradycardia, pallor, or marked hypotonia occurs.
  - May cause hypoxemia, hypercarbia, or hemodynamic instability. Typically improves with bag-mask ventilation (BMV).
  - Neonatal apnea is often due to an immature respiratory drive; an apneic event will be followed by bradycardia and desaturation.
- Causes of disorders of breathing:
  - **BRUE** (**B**rief **R**esolved **U**nexplained **E**vent)
    - Previously known as apparent life-threatening event (ALTE).
    - Observer notes apnea or breathing irregularity, limpness or marked change in tone, unresponsiveness, pallor, or cyanosis.
    - Lasts less than one minute and resolves.
    - History, examination, and vital signs are reassuring.
    - No known explanation can be identified.
    - No association between BRUE and sudden infant death syndrome. Safe sleep and environmental practices, including smoke exposure, should be reviewed.
    - Maintain a high index of suspicion for child abuse.
    - For low-risk patients (more than 32 weeks' gestation, older than 60 days of age, no CPR by trained clinician required during event, first event, no family or social history concerns):
      - Educate about BRUEs, provide CPR training to caregiver.
      - Consider: 12 lead ECG, pertussis testing, brief period of observation and pulse oximetry monitoring.
  - Seizures
    - Hypoventilation due to alterations in respiratory control or diaphragm activity may occur.
    - Treat seizure with abortive medications, although some medications may exacerbate respiratory depression.
  - Respiratory infections: especially RSV and pertussis
    - Can cause apnea, especially in former premature neonates.
    - Provide supportive care and treat underlying condition.
  - Sepsis
    - CNS and non-CNS infections can cause respiratory-drive alternation.
    - Provide supportive care and treat underlying condition.
  - GERD
    - The low tone of the gastroesophageal sphincter may result in regurgitation, triggering laryngospasm (airway protective reflex).
    - Treat with histamine receptor antagonist or proton pump inhibitors.
  - Cardiac dysrhythmia
    - Usually will have other signs or symptoms.
    - Screen with EKG.
  - Breath-holding spells
    - Paroxysmal episodes with pallor or cyanosis and unresponsiveness.
    - Often begin at 6 to 18 months of age.
    - Cyanotic type: precipitated by anger or frustration, followed by loud cry then involuntary breath holding in expiration.
    - Pallid type: precipitated by pain or fear, with minimal or silent cry, then breath holding.
    - Apneic period followed by loss of consciousness, then inspiration, and then resolution of breath-holding spell.

Shock

DEFINITION

Inadequate tissue and organ oxygenation due to either inadequate oxygen delivery, increased oxygen consumption, decreased oxygen utilization by cells, or some combination of these

SIGNS AND SYMPTOMS

- Hypotension is often a late finding in shock due to a child's ability to increase systemic vascular resistance.
- Tachycardia, abnormal capillary refill, and organ dysfunction (poor urine output, elevated creatinine, encephalopathy) may occur.
- Decreased urine output and altered mental status are clinical signs of acute organ dysfunction.

PATHOPHYSIOLOGY

States of shock often alter oxygen delivery via one or more of the following mechanisms:
- Low oxygen content of blood: severe anemia or hypoxemia
  - Low cardiac output (CO; the amount of blood pumped from the heart to the systemic circulation in liters per minute).
  - CO = Heart rate × Stroke volume.
  - Causes of low heart rate include heart block, sinus node dysfunction, drug toxicity.
  - Stroke volume is a function of filling (preload), resistance against which the ventricle is pumping (afterload), and contractility.
  - Blood pressure can be calculated by the product of cardiac output and systemic vascular resistance (SVR), i.e., BP = CO × SVR.
- Shock can be classified as warm (warm skin and flash capillary refill due to low SVR) and cold (poor perfusion and prolonged capillary refill, high SVR but poor cardiac output).
  - Infants and young children are more likely to present with cold shock.
- Categorization of shock based on etiology (Table 24-3).

TREATMENT

- Consider the type of shock to determine the appropriate treatment
- Hypovolemia is treated with rapid crystalloid or colloid volume expansion AND maintenance fluids.
  - Estimate fluid loss and replace half the deficit in the first 8 hours and the rest of the deficit over the next 16 hours.
  - Note that patients with hypo- or hyper-natremic dehydration should be corrected more slowly, over 48 hours, to avoid rapid osmotic fluid shifts in the brain.
  - Maintenance fluids follow 4:2:1 rule: 4 mL/kg/hr for first 10 kg, 2 mL/kg/hr for second 10 kg, then 1mL/kg/hr for any additional weight.
    - Example: 13 kg toddler requires 46 mL/hr of maintenance IV fluids.
  - Adult rates reached at about 60 kg (100 mL/hr).
- Catecholamine-resistant shock (shock despite fluid resuscitation and use of epinephrine or norepinephrine) may be due to adrenal insufficiency.
  - Absolute: due to a known mineralocorticoid enzyme deficiency. See endocrine chapter (17) for specific enzyme deficiencies.

WARD TIP

Hyponatremia can cause an osmotic fluid shift into the brain within a few hours. Patients with hyponatremic dehydration should be rehydrated slowly, as aggressive rehydration can lead to **osmotic demyelination syndrome.**

TABLE 24-3. Etiologies of Shock

Type of Shock	Examples	Pathophysiology	Treatments to Consider
Obstructive	Tension pneumothorax Cardiac tamponade	Increased intrathoracic pressure or obstruction to venous return to the heart, lowering cardiac preload	IV fluid bolus Relieve obstruction with needle decompression or pericardiocentesis
Hemorrhagic shock (subtype of hypovolemic)	Hemorrhage	Low preload from depletion of blood volume Depletion of clotting factors often leads to more bleeding	Blood products preferred over crystalloids Provide balanced resuscitation with PRBC, platelets, and FFP
Hypovolemic	Severe gastroenteritis Burns: loss of skin protective barrier, increased insensible losses	Low preload from depletion of extracellular fluid Decreased CO Increased SVR	IV fluid bolus Diagnose problem
Cardiogenic	Decompensated congestive heart failure Prolonged SVT with poor CO Critical congenital heart disease (e.g. severe aortic stenosis), ductal dependent lesions	Decreased CO Increased SVR	Inotropes (epinephrine, milrinone), vasodilators In neonates, consider prostaglandin E to maintain ductal patency Arrhythmia management Monitor for fluid overload: if decompensated, fluid overload will make contractility worse
Distributive	Anaphylaxis Septic shock may present with distributive shock Some ingestions Neurogenic – due to interrupted sympathetic outflow from spinal cord injury, resulting in shock and bradycardia	Low SVR leading to low BP and maldistribution of blood flow CO often high	IV fluid bolus Vasopressor to increase SVR (norepinephrine, vasopressin) IM epinephrine (anaphylaxis)
Septic shock	Bacterial, viral, parasitic infection associated with severe inflammatory response Diffuse vasodilation	Low SVR leading to low BP and maldistribution of blood flow Cardiac output often high Elements of hypovolemia, decreased SVR, septic cardiomyopathy (low cardiac output), and mitochondrial toxicity may all lead to shock	IV fluid bolus Vasopressor to increase SVR (norepinephrine, vasopressin, others) Early, appropriate antibiotic therapy decreases mortality Monitor for fluid overload (want adequate preload but overload may lead to pulmonary edema, AKI, or organ failure)

- Relative: inability of catecholamine synthesis to meet needs of overwhelming shock
  - Includes suppression of adrenal gland due to chronic steroid use.
- Both forms improve with use of mineralocorticoid steroids.
  - Patients with chronic adrenal suppression may require higher than normal doses.

Neurological Emergencies (see also Neurology Chapter)

- Initial approach:
  - Perform brief neurological exam as part of the initial **ABCDE** assessment described above.
  - Assign GCS or evaluate AVPU (described above).
  - Evaluate cranial nerve, motor, or sensory deficits if patient is stable.
- Diagnostic testing:
  - Glucose level, point of care.
  - Electrolytes.
  - CT if suspect intracranial hemorrhage or hydrocephalus.
  - Lumbar puncture if meningitis/encephalitis are in the differential and noncommunicating hydrocephalus has been ruled out.
  - EEG can show seizures or encephalopathy.
  - Ammonia level.
- Syndromes associated with altered mental status - See Table 24-4.

Pediatric Injuries

WARD TIP

Be on the lookout for intentionally inflicted injuries in children (nonaccidental trauma). Look for patterns of injuries, injuries not consistent with the child's development, and for histories that don't make logical sense.

EXAM TIP

Motor vehicle collisions are the leading cause of pediatric injuries.

- Trauma is the most common fatal disease in toddlers and young children.
  - Motor vehicle collision
    - Most common cause of death after infancy.
    - Risk factors include improper securement (car seats, seat belts), improper use of airbags, adolescent drivers, intoxicated drivers.
    - Car safety: rear-facing car seats for infants and children up to 2 years old (or as long as the child does not exceed the car seat's weight limit), front-facing until outgrows car seat, then booster seat for children less than 4'9" tall.
  - Pedestrian injuries: common cause of injury and death.
  - Bicycle injuries: helmets reduce the head and brain injuries by 85–90%.
  - Submersion injuries/drownings
    - Children less than 4 years of age are at high risk.
    - Adolescent submersion injury is often associated with intoxication.
  - Burns
    - 80% of fatalities occur from house fires and are associated with smoke inhalation.
    - Contact burns, electrical burns, and scaldings affect children below the age of 4 years.
  - Firearms
    - Second leading cause of death in adolescent males.
    - Two-thirds of American households have firearms; one-third have a handgun.
    - Gun safety should be included in anticipatory guidance.

TRAUMATIC BRAIN INJURY (TBI)

- In patients with low-risk mechanism of injury, prediction rules can help distinguish patients who do not require neuro-imaging and those who can be discharged after observation. PECARN prediction rule is one such rule (see also Chapter 18; Concussion). Indicators to perform CT scan include:
  - GCS less than 15.
  - Palpable skull fracture.

TABLE 24-4. Syndromes Associated with Altered Mental Status or Encephalopathy

SYNDROME	CLINICAL PRESENTATION	DIAGNOSTIC TESTING	TREATMENT
Traumatic brain injury	Recent head injury, followed by altered mental status and sometimes focal findings	CT brain can reveal epidural, subdural, or subarachnoid hemorrhage	Neurosurgical drainage or removal of bone flap ICP lowering therapy
Increased ICP	Focal findings of CN alterations, altered mental status, seizures	CT brain for hydrocephalus, herniation, loss of grey-white differentiation, effacement of sulci	ICP lowering therapy: hypertonic saline, mannitol, controlled hyperventilation
Substance induced	Often toddler or adolescent, history of ingestion, presenting with altered mentation and other toxidrome signs	Electrolytes, blood gas, osmolality, liver panel CT brain Salicylate and acetaminophen levels	Supportive care Ingestion-directed therapy
Infection – encephalitis or meningitis	Altered mental status associated with fever, neck stiffness, or signs and symptoms of inflammation	CSF chemistry, cell count, and culture after excluding non-communicating hydrocephalus MRI may show inflammatory changes of brain or meninges	Empirical antibiotics
Diabetic Ketoacidosis (DKA)	DKA can be associated with cerebral edema and AMS Risk factors for cerebral edema: younger age, new onset DKA, severe acidosis, administration of sodium bicarbonate	ABG/VBG, electrolytes, calculated osmolality	Slow correction of acidosis, extracellular volume deficits and glucose levels
Abuse	A common cause of morbidity and mortality. Mechanism of injury may not match severity of disease or inappropriate activity for child's level of development. May have signs of elevated ICP or intracranial hemorrhage	CT brain Skeletal survey at index visit and in follow up identify acute, healing, or chronic fracture Ophthalmology for retinal hemorrhages Careful social history	Medical professionals are mandatory reporters of child abuse in many states of the USA
Shock and Hypoxemia	Poor oxygen delivery results in end-organ dysfunction. In the brain, this causes encephalopathy and delirium. Patients in shock are often confused and interfere with care	Workup for sepsis	Measures to restore oxygen delivery
Intussusception	Intermittent agitation due to abdominal pain Possibly hematochezia	Abdominal ultrasound	Barium enema
Subclinical status epilepticus	Persistent failure to return to baseline may indicated ongoing seizure activity, even without visible seizures	EEG	Anti-epileptic drugs (benzodiazepines are first line, but can also use levetiracetam, barbiturates, fosphenytoin or valproate,)

- Altered mentation or abnormal behavior per parent.
- Loss of consciousness >5 seconds.
- Parietal, occipital, or temporal scalp hematoma.
- Severe mechanism of injury (including fall >3 feet).

SUICIDE ATTEMPTS (SEE ALSO CHAPTER 23 [PSYCHIATRY CHAPTER])

- May include ingestion, but also penetrating traumatic injury, hanging or falls.
- Stabilize patient and attend to **ABCDE**s.
- Evaluate for co-ingestions or other injuries that might not be apparent.
- Evaluate for all likely injuries (for example, in a hanging, evaluate for bony or ligamentous injury to the cervical spine, vascular injury to structures of the neck, and hypoxic-ischemic injury to brain).
- When stabilized, evaluate for depression using the HEADDSSS exam.
- High-risk situations for recurrent suicide attempts may include poor social support, prior suicide attempts, and a high-lethality attempt. These patients often require hospitalization in an inpatient psychiatric unit.

SUBMERSION INJURIES

- Prevention and anticipatory guidance are key:
    - Pool safety—locks to prevent children from accessing the pool, pool covers.
    - Swimming lessons/water-safety lessons.
    - Constant vigilance around water for at risk children (especially toddlers).
- Patterns of injury include pulmonary injury from aspiration of water or negative-pressure pulmonary edema due to inspiration against closed glottis when water triggers airway protective reflexes.
    - If aspirating clean pool water, chemical pneumonitis is common, and antibiotics are not indicated.
    - If water is not clean, treatment must be directed at likely organisms (anaerobes, *Aeromonas*, *Pseudomonas*, amoeba).

BURNS

- Epidemiology
    - Is a leading cause of pediatric accidental death.
    - Common in toddlers.
    - Nonaccidental burns account for up to 20% of admissions.
- Pathophysiology
    - Disruption of function of skin leading to abnormalities in:
        - Thermal regulation.
        - Increased insensible fluid losses.
        - Barrier to infection.
- Classification of burn injury is based on depth, percent body surface area (BSA), and location.
    - Depth:
        - Superficial: 1st degree. Only epidermis is involved. Erythema, pain, absence of blisters occur. It generally heals within one week without scarring. Example: sunburn.
        - Partial thickness: 2nd degree. Involves epidermis and portions of dermis.
            - Superficial partial thickness: blisters, painful, red, and weeping, skin blanches with pressure occur; usually heals one to three weeks without scarring.

- Deep partial thickness: extends more deeply into dermis. Blisters, damaged hair follicles, loss of soft touch sensation; does not blanch with pressure. Takes longer to heal (more than 3 weeks) and may have hypertrophic scarring.
- Full thickness: 3rd degree. Destroys epidermis and dermis. Leftover eschar (dead dermal layer). Painless and anesthetic. Dry, will not blanch. No blisters.
  - Circumferential full thickness burn with eschar may lead to compromised blood supply as edema occurs (eschar will not swell).
  - Healing may involve wound contractures.
- Extension to deep tissues: fourth degree may involve muscle and bone. Can be life threatening.
- Percentage of BSA
  - Burn size determines resuscitation and level of care; superficial (1st degree) burns are not included in calculations.
    - Rule of nines: fastest, may use for adolescents. Infants and young children have relatively larger heads, limiting accuracy.
      - Each leg 18%.
      - Each arm 9%.
      - Front and back of trunk 18% each.
      - Head 9%.
    - Palm method: for small or patchy burns. The palmar surface of hand without fingers is 0.5% BSA, and with fingers is 1%.
  - Location:
    - Assess risk for disability.
    - Worse outcomes for burns on face, eyes, ears, feet, perineum, or hands. Risk for poor cosmesis with healing or contractures.
    - Burns traversing joints may cause decreased functional mobility. Requires physical therapy.
  - Treatment:
    - Support airway, breathing, circulation first! (**ABCs**).
    - Airway: evaluate for facial or neck burns, singed nose hair; soot around mouth or nares, or hoarseness, may indicate inhalation injury and high risk of airway compromise and significantly increased risk of mortality.
    - Breathing: oxygenation, ventilation, and carbon-monoxide levels.
    - Circulation: IVF resuscitation
      - For infants with more than 10% BSA and children with more than 15% BSA establish IV or IO access and resuscitate with balanced crystalloid solution.
      - Parkland formula:
        - Total fluid requirement over first 24h = maintenance fluid requirement + (wt [kg] × %BSA × 4 mL).
        - Administer ½ over first eight hours and ½ over next 16 hours.
    - Wound care for superficial and partial thickness:
      - Analgesia.
      - Cold compresses.
      - Antiseptic cleaning.
      - Debride open blisters (intact blisters need not to be unroofed).
      - Topical antibiotics (silver sulfadiazine, bacitracin).
      - Protect skin with bulky dressings.
      - Reassess after 24 hours and serially for healing and to detect wound infection.

- Care for full thickness or more extensive superficial:
    - Attend **ABC**s.
    - Fluid and electrolyte replacement.
    - Sedation and analgesia often required with extensive wound debridement.
    - Clean and care for wounds as above.
- Criteria for admission to hospital or burn unit:
    - Admit:
        - 2–5% full thickness burn.
        - 5–10% full or partial thickness burn.
- Other indications for admission:
    - Suspicion of abuse, unsafe home environment.
    - Burns of face, hands, genitalia, perineum, major joints.
    - Circumferential burns of extremity.
    - High voltage electrical burns.
    - Significant chemical burns.
    - Signs of inhalational injury.
- Indications for transfer to burn unit:
    - Involvement of more than 10% BSA.
    - More than 5% full thickness.
    - Requiring advanced therapy.

Pediatric Poisonings and Toxic Ingestions

- Epidemiology
    - Developmentally stratified:
        - Children under about 4 years often engage in exploratory ingestion or confusing brightly colored pills with candy.
        - Adolescents often intentional as a suicide attempt.
    - A frequent reason for pediatric emergency visits
- Prevention and anticipatory guidance:
    - Childproof home, including cabinets/containers.
    - Store toxic substances in original childproof container, out of children's reach.
    - Childproof caps or locked containers.
    - Supervise children appropriately.
- Initial evaluation
    - History of ingestion:
        - Timing, total number of pills and dose (to calculate dose per kg), formulation (extended formulations will have prolonged absorption phase).
        - Route of exposure.
        - Progression of symptoms.
    - General medical history.
- Decontamination
    - Skin decontamination: many toxins rapidly absorbed through skin
        - Remove potentially contaminated clothes.
        - Use gloves.
        - Rinse patient with water.
        - Use mild soap or shampoo for substances that will not rinse with water alone.
        - Some agents require specialized topical treatments: hydrofluoric acid (calcium soaks), oxalic acid (calcium soaks), phenol (mineral or other oil, isopropyl alcohol), white phosphorous (copper sulfate).

- Ocular decontamination: cornea is especially sensitive to corrosive agents can lead to permanent scarring.
  - Remove contacts.
  - Rinse eyes copiously for 15 minutes.
  - Emergent ophthalmologic exam.
- Respiratory decontamination:
  - Protect healthcare and emergency workers from toxic gases or fumes.
  - Remove victim from exposure.
  - Provide supplemental oxygen and ventilatory support as needed.
- Gastrointestinal exposure:
  - Inducing emesis not recommended: not effective, potential for a second esophageal exposure if a caustic substance.
  - Nasogastric lavage generally not recommended: only removes fraction of pills.
    - Contraindicated in patients who cannot protect their airway (airway not secured with cuffed endotracheal tube, or patient not awake and protecting own airway).
  - Activated charcoal recommended in select poisonings only.
    - Lack of prospective data regarding its use.
    - Indications:
      - Risk of poisoning justifies use of charcoal.
      - Can be administered within 60 minutes of the ingestion.
    - Not effective for heavy metals, iron, lithium, alcohols, hydrocarbons, cyanide.
  - Whole-bowel irrigation:
    - Thought to decrease absorption via enterohepatic recirculation.
    - Only recommended in a small number of indications; consult with poison control center.
- Diagnosis and Treatment:
  - Severe poisonings cause myriad signs and symptoms.
  - Agitation from substance ingestion often treated with benzodiazepines.
  - See Tables 24-5, 24-6, and 24-7 for various poisonings.
  - Provide emotional support for family, who may experience emotions of guilt and anxiety.

WARD TIP

Typically activated charcoal is only administered if within one hour of the ingestion.

WARD TIP

In the United States, Poison Control (1-800-222-1222) can provide expert consultation in the care of the poisoned patient, including access to toxicologists. They also provide epidemiological data about calls to track poisonings. It is a good idea to call for all ingestions.

Pediatric Life Support

PEDIATRIC CARDIAC ARREST

- Epidemiology
  - More than 5,000 pediatric out-of-hospital cardiac arrests annually in the United States.
  - Majority of these occurs with parents or caretakers nearby; basic life support (BLS) courses should be targeted toward these.
  - Pediatric arrest generally results from respiratory failure or progression of shock (in contrast to cardiac arrest in adults).
  - Leading causes of arrest in children less than one year of age: SIDS (most common in USA), respiratory disease, airway obstruction, sepsis, drowning, injuries (unintentional and intentional), congenital heart disease, other congenital abnormalities.
  - For children older than 1 year, the leading cause of death is injury (accidental or intentional).

EXAM TIP

Leading causes of pediatric death:
Under 1 year – Congenital malformations, SIDS, and conditions related to prematurity
Over 1 year – Unintentional injury

TABLE 24-5. "Toxidromes:" Symptoms and Representative Causes

TOXIDROME	EXAMPLE POISONINGS	SYMPTOMS
Anticholinergic	Diphenhydramine Tricyclic antidepressants	Hyposecretion, dry mucus membranes, urinary retention. Flushed skin Dilated pupils Delirium, seizures
Cholinergic	Organophosphate insecticides, black widow spider bite, tobacco, chemical warfare (many agents inhibit acetylcholinesterase)	Hypersecretion, muscle fasciculation, weakness Bronchorrhea Bronchospasm Seizures, coma
Opiates	Morphine, oxycodone, codeine	CNS depression, dilated pupils, hypothermia, hypotension, constipation Respiratory depression and respiratory acidosis
Sympathomimetic	Amphetamines, cocaine, theophylline, caffeine	Hyperthermia, hypertension, tachypnea Dilated pupils Psychosis and convulsions
Extrapyramidal toxicity	Haloperidol Metoclopramide	Tremor and rigidity
Hypermetabolic	Salicylate	Fever, tachycardia Metabolic acidosis Hyperpnea, restlessness, seizures Metabolic acidosis
Hydrocarbon aspiration	Aspiration or ingestion of a volatile hydrocarbon substance	GI symptoms Respiratory symptoms, including development of ARDS

- Administration of Pediatric BLS:
  - Determine unresponsiveness: stimulate and check for response.
  - If no response, shout for help (send a particular person to call 911) and get automated external defibrillator (AED). If lone provider: phone 911 and get AED. Feel for pulse. If no pulse, start chest compressions.
    - Check pulse every 2 minutes. If no pulse, continue with cycles of compressions/rescue breaths.
    - Unwitnessed arrest: can perform 2 minutes compression before AED application.
  - Airway: head-tilt chin lift (no suspected cervical spinal injury) or jaw thrust (if C-spine injury suspected).
  - Breathing:
    - Rescue breaths, as recommended, with compressions.
    - Infants less than 1 year: mouth over mouth and nose to create seal.
    - Children older than 1 year: pinch nose, create mouth-to-mouth seal.
  - Compressions:
    - Rate of 100–120 beats per minute.
    - Minimize interruptions to compressions.

TABLE 24-6.   Selected Drug Toxicities

Drug	Toxicity	Treatment
Sulfonamides	Kernicterus in infants	
Chloramphenicol	Gray baby syndrome: vomiting, ashen color, cardiovascular collapse	
Quinolones	Cartilaginous defects in children Achilles tendon rupture in animal studies	
Tetracycline	Gray enamel of permanent teeth, affects bone growth	Avoid in children < 9y Toxicity unlikely unless massive ingestion
Salicylate	Reye syndrome: hepatic injury, hypoglycemia, vomiting. Associated with viral illness Hypermetabolic toxicity with metabolic acidosis and simultaneous primary respiratory acidosis	Dialysis
Acetaminophen	Generalized malaise, nausea, vomiting Latent period Jaundice, hepatocellular necrosis, coagulopathy Metabolic acidosis, renal and myocardial damage, coma	N-acetylcysteine regenerates glutathione and is given as a prolonged infusion Check acetaminophen level at 4h, use Rumack-Matthew Nomogram for single ingestion in absence of chronic use
Tricyclic antidepressants	Anticholinergic symptoms EKG changes with widened QRS, flattened T waves	Sodium bicarbonate IV Intubation and activated charcoal if altered mental status
Organophosphates	Cholinergic toxicity	Atropine and pralidoxime
Heavy metals	Lead: chronic exposure related to neurodevelopmental and behavioral problems. Screen at well child check	Dimercaprol Dimercaptosuccinic acid (succimer, DMSA), EDTA
Iron	Abdominal pain Vomiting Shock Late: GI strictures	Deferoxamine
Methanol, ethylene glycol	Intoxication Blindness (methanol) Metabolic acidosis which may have osmolar gap Oxalate crystals in urine (ethylene glycol)	Fomepizole Ethanol (rarely used as will cause intoxication)
Benzodiazepines	Sedation Respiratory depression Negative inotropy	Flumazenil generally NOT recommended especially with chronic use, as will precipitate seizures
Opiates/narcotics	Respiratory depression Pinpoint pupils	Naloxone Supportive management for hypoventilation or hypotension
Anticholinergics	"Mad as a hater, dry as a bone, blind as a bat, red as a beet, and hot as hell"	Supportive management for ABCs and benzodiazepines for agitation Acetylcholinesterase inhibitors in rare cases when co-ingestion (esp TCAs) can be excluded and symptoms are severe

TABLE 24-7. Emergent Alterations of Hemoglobin or the Electron Transport Chain

SYNDROME	PATHOPHYSIOLOGY	SYMPTOMS	NOTES
Carboxyhemoglobinemia	Exposure to carbon monoxide (formed by hydrocarbon combustion, including fires) CO binds Hb with extremely high affinity, diminishing its ability to offload O_2 in peripheral tissue COHb reads on pulse oximeter as 100%, so will have high SPO_2 but low oxyhemoglobin when co-oximetry is checked.	Headache, nausea/vomiting, alteration of consciousness, symptoms of inadequate oxygen delivery (shock) Diagnosis by co-oximetry will directly measure COHb level	Supportive management plus supplemental FIO_2 @ 100%, consider hyperbaric oxygen for severe illness or COHb level >25% Evaluate for cyanide toxicity
Cyanide toxicity	Mitochondrial toxin Commonly due to domestic fires, occupation exposure may occur Inhibits mitochondrial electron transport chain, stopping oxidative phosphorylation	HA, confusion, AMS Tachycardia, hypertension followed by bradycardia, dysrhythmia, hypotension Vomiting, abdominal pain Cherry-red skin flushing Shock and multi-organ failure Bitter almond scent Rapidly lethal if untreated	Decontamination, supportive management Evaluate for carbon monoxide toxicity Cyanide antidotes: hydroxocobalamin and sodium thiosulfate; sodium nitrite and sodium thiosulfate (contraindicated if methemoglobinemia)
Methemoglobinemia	Occurs when the iron in hemoglobin is oxidized from ferrous (Fe^{+2}) to ferric (Fe^{+3}), which does not bind O_2 and can shift oxy-hemoglobin dissociation curve to the left, impairing oxygen delivery	Abrupt development of symptoms of hypoxia after exposure to an oxidizing substance (possibly in setting of G6PD deficiency) Dyspnea, headache, fatigue, lethargy progressing to shock, respiratory depression, seizure, or coma	Levels from 3%-10% usually asymptomatic, >30-40% may be life-threatening Discontinue offending substance Supportive care Methylene blue is first line treatment for severe disease (avoid in G6PD deficiency or patients on serotoninergic meds, use ascorbic acid (vitamin C) instead)

- Infant less than 1 year of age:
  - Two fingers (index and middle) on the sternum about a finger-width below the nipple line or encircle infant with both hands placing thumbs together over the sternum (preferred for two provider).
  - Compress at least one-third of the chest anterior-posterior diameter.
  - One provider: 30 compressions to 2 breaths.
  - Two providers: 15 compressions to 2 breaths.
  - Advanced airway in place: continuous compressions, RR 10/min.
- Child older than 1 year of age
  - Chest compressions indicated if:
    - Patient pulseless or HR less than 60 beats/min with impaired respirations.

- Heel of one hand on the lower half of sternum (avoid xiphoid); chest compression at 2 inches of depth.
  - Single rescuer: 30:2 compressions: breaths.
  - Two rescuer, child: 15:2 compression: breaths.
- AED application:
  - Pads come with instructions indicating where to apply.
  - Turn AED on, follow AED instructions; AED will identify shockable rhythms.
  - AED will prompt to continue compressions (no shockable rhythm) or prompt to clear and deliver shock (shockable rhythm).

PEDIATRIC ADVANCED LIFE SUPPORT

- Initiate BLS.
- Shockable rhythms:
  - 10% of pediatric cardiac arrests are initially a shockable rhythm.
  - Early defibrillation is key.
  - Initial shockable rhythm = better outcomes than PEA/asystole arrest.
  - Later shockable rhythms are not associated with good prognosis.
- Medications
  - Epinephrine
    - Given every 3–5 minutes.
    - Increases systemic vascular resistance, increasing "diastolic" blood pressure and improving coronary artery perfusion.
    - Delay in first administration of epinephrine is associated with poor outcomes in pediatric cardiac arrest.
  - Anti-arrhythmics
    - If ventricular fibrillation or pulseless VT is refractory to shocks, can consider amiodarone or lidocaine.
  - Calcium and sodium bicarbonate:
    - Frequently used, not associated with better outcomes.
    - Can consider for specific indications.
- Evaluate reversible causes – the H's and the T's.
  - H's: hypoxemia, hypovolemia, H+ (acidosis), hyperkalemia, hypocalcemia.
  - T's: thrombosis (PE, MI), tension pneumothorax, cardiac tamponade.

NOTES

Index

NOTES

NOTES